OXFORD MEDICAL PUBLICATIONS

Genetics of Mitochondrial Disease

OXFORD MONOGRAPHS ON MEDICAL GENETICS

General Editors

ARNO G. MOTULSKY

MARTIN BOBROW

PETER S. HARPER

CHARLES SCRIVER

CHARLES J. EPSTEIN

JUDITH G. HALL

Genetics of Mitochondrial Disease

Edited by

IAN JAMES HOLT

*Dunn Human Nutrition Unit, Wellcome Trust/MRC Building,
Hills Road, Cambridge, UK*

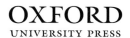

OXFORD

UNIVERSITY PRESS

OXFORD
UNIVERSITY PRESS

Great Clarendon Street, Oxford OX2 6DP

Oxford University Press is a department of the University of Oxford.
It furthers the University's objective of excellence in research, scholarship,
and education by publishing worldwide in

Oxford New York

Auckland Bangkok Buenos Aires Cape Town Chennai
Dar es Salaam Delhi Hong Kong Istanbul Karachi Kolkata
Kuala Lumpur Madrid Melbourne Mexico City Mumbai Nairobi
São Paulo Shanghai Taipei Tokyo Toronto

Oxford is a registered trade mark of Oxford University Press
in the UK and in certain other countries

Published in the United States
by Oxford University Press Inc., New York

A catalogue record for this title is available from the British Library.

Library of Congress Cataloging in Publication Data
(Data available)
ISBN 0 19 850865 4 (Hbk)

10 9 8 7 6 5 4 3 2 1

Typeset by Newgen Imaging Systems (P) Ltd., Chennai, India
Printed in Great Britain
on acid-free paper by
Biddles Ltd, Guildford and King's Lynn

Foreword

The diseases caused by mitochondrial dysfunctions, the first of which was described ~40 years ago in the classic paper by Roft Luft and co-workers, have become an important area of human pathology. This area has seen striking developments in the past fifteen years as a result of the elucidation of the structure and function of the human mitochondrial genome and of the discovery of the first pathogenic mitochondrial DNA (mtDNA) deletions and point mutations in the late 1980s. Almost 100 mtDNA point mutations, a large number of mtDNA rearrangements (including large deletions and duplications) and more recently, numerous nuclear gene mutations have been shown to be associated with a variety of disorders affecting the skeletal muscles, the brain, the heart, the liver, the cochlea and other organs. These extraordinary developments have had the effect of stimulating basic research aimed at understanding in depth the origin, transmission and segregation of mtDNA mutations, as well as the fundamental processes of mtDNA replication and transcription, mtDNA repair, mitochondrial translation, protein and RNA import from the cytosolic-nuclear compartment into mitochondria, mitochondrial division, fission and movement, and, in general, the processes whereby the nuclear and mitochondrial genomes communicate with each other. The advances in our knowledge of the basic processes, in turn, have provided new insights into the way in which alterations in the processes caused by mtDNA mutations listed above, result in pathological or ageing-related phenotypes.

Another factor that has played an important role in expanding our basic knowledge of the mitochondrial processes, as well as our understanding of the pathogenetic mechanisms of mtDNA mutations, has been the introduction of powerful methodological tools. Such was the development of an approach for the construction of cellular models of mtDNA-linked disease by mitochondria-mediated transformation of mtDNA-less cells. This approach provided a rapid and effective method for differentiating an mtDNA from a nuclear gene alteration as being the cause of any pathological mitochondrial dysfunction. The recent successful construction of the first mito-mouse to carry a natural pathogenic mouse mtDNA mutation has opened the possibility of creating animal models of mtDNA-linked diseases for the analysis of their pathogenesis and the possible development of therapeutic approaches. Another set of powerful techniques, which have extended the analysis of mitochondrial dysfunctions to the single cell level, have been refined histochemical and immunohistochemical methods, *in situ* hybridization assays, utilizing standard oligodeoxynucleotide or peptide-nucleic acid probes, and the laser capture microdissection approach combined with PCR. Finally, one should mention that a variety of imaginative approaches have started being applied for correcting mtDNA-linked defects, by cellular or genetic manipulation, with a potential therapeutic application as a goal.

It is clear that success in the development of genetic approaches for the therapy of mtDNA-linked diseases will depend on our understanding of fundamental aspects of human mitochondrial genetics. Significant progress has indeed been made in the past 15 years in this area.

Due to the large number of genomes contained in each cell, mammalian mitochondrial genetics is substantially an intracellular population genetics, with the associated phenomena of selection and segregation. The recognition that the fundamental units of inheritance of mtDNA, in mammalian cells as in yeast, are not the individual mtDNA molecules, but polyploid complexes of mtDNA molecules and proteins (nucleoids), which are restricted in their capability to mix and have, furthermore, a limited sphere of influence, tending to remain associated with their transcription and translation products, has been an important conceptual advance. The validity of this new concept has been confirmed by the observations of a restricted mitotic segregation of mutations by mitochondrial division and of a limited complementation capacity of recessive mutations in cellular model systems. On the other hand, the demonstration of the dynamic nature of the mitochondrial organization and the identification of several nuclear gene products which participate in mitochondrial fusion and division have called attention to the multiplicity of functional, developmental and environmental factors which can participate in the control of mitochondrial gene segregation.

Another area where significant advances have been made in recent years is that of the very complex genetic control of mtDNA maintenance. Particularly significant has been the recognition that alterations in nucleotide metabolism can have a profound effect on mtDNA integrity and balance, and the discovery of nuclear gene products like the transcription factor Tfam and the Twinkle primase/helicase, which play an important role in mtDNA maintenance.

This volume presents a highly comprehensive and critical overview of the area of mitochondrial diseases, with an emphasis on genetics. The topics discussed herein by specialists in each field cover a broad variety of aspects of such diseases and the relevant background information. In particular, these topics range from the structure, function and biogenesis of mitochondria to the multiplicity of mtDNA or nuclear gene mutations which affect them, from the effects of mtDNA mutations on cell function to the clinical aspects of mitochondrial encephalomyopathies, from the pathogenetic mechanisms of the various mutations to the prospects of gene therapy, and finally, from the cellular and animal models of mitochondrial diseases to prenatal diagnosis of such diseases and genetic counselling. Some chapters are appropriately devoted to the dynamics of mitochondrial DNA, to the role of mitochondrial dysfunctions in neurodegenerative diseases, and to the mechanisms operating in the age-related accumulation of mtDNA mutations. Because of the broad context in which the genetics of mitochondrial diseases is presented here and because of its timely appearance, one can be very confident that this volume will be invaluable not only to investigators involved in mitochondrial research but also to many outside the circle of mitochondria specialists.

Giuseppe Attardi

Preface

In order to understand the causes of mitochondrial diseases the reader is first presented with an overview of mitochondrial structure and function. Clinically orientated readers may wish to skip this section, at least initially; however, this is not recommended, for it is increasingly difficult to describe and hence understand any disease without reference to the underlying cell and molecular biology.

The emphasis of the book is on mitochondrial diseases involving the mitochondrial genome and so the first two chapters detail the means by which mitochondrial DNA is maintained, copied, and expressed. An outline of how the many nuclear protein components of mitochondria are imported, processed, and assembled is set out in Chapter 3. The central role of mitochondria in cellular ATP production (oxidative phosphorylation) is discussed in Chapter 4, as many mitochondrial diseases manifest themselves as deficiencies of ATP production; this fourth chapter concludes the summary of mitochondrial structure and function.

Section II opens with a review of neuromuscular diseases caused by mutations in human mitochondrial DNA. Mitochondrial DNA mutations can be divided into three classes, and a chapter is devoted to each; these are rearrangements, that is partial deletions and partial duplications (Chapter 6), point mutations affecting translation (Chapter 7), and mutations in structural elements of the oxidative phosphorylation system (Chapter 8).

Owing to the size of the nuclear genome, identifying defective nuclear genes associated with mitochondrial disease has proved more difficult than for mitochondrial DNA. Nevertheless, much progress has been made in recent years and this is reviewed in Section III. The first of two chapters deals exclusively with nuclear gene mutations that impact on mitochondrial DNA (Chapter 9). The second (Chapter 10) is more wide ranging, covering mutations in structural components of the oxidative phosphorylation system, assembly factors and other mutant proteins that perturb mitochondrial function.

Section IV takes the reader into deeper and sometimes contentious water: none more so than Chapter 13, which reviews the role of mitochondrial DNA in ageing. The section opens with a discussion of the possible myriad effects of mitochondrial DNA mutations on mitochondrial and cellular function, beyond the straightforward impairment of ATP production (Chapter 11). Chapter 12 deals with common neurodegenerative disorders and asks to what extent mitochondrial dysfunction features and whether it is a consequence, or cause of the disease. Issues such as the role of mitochondria in calcium homeostasis and apoptosis appear in both Chapters 11 and 12, emphasizing the need for a comprehensive understanding of mitochondrial function in order to explain, and ultimately develop rational therapies for mitochondrial diseases.

For a number of years no animal model of mitochondrial disease was available and so cell culture was the dominant model system. Studies on cultured cells strengthened the hypothesis that mitochondrial DNA mutations were a cause of human disease. They also unexpectedly threw up a mass of data on the behaviour of different mitochondrial genotypes when contained in the same cell, which is discussed in Chapter 14. Although animal models of mitochondrial disease caused by mutations in mtDNA lagged behind human cell culture models, considerable progress has been made by studying the disruption of mitochondrial genes encoded in the nucleus of mice, in particular via disruption of a gene that is essential for mitochondrial DNA maintenance. These studies have taught us much about the essential role of mitochondrial DNA and mitochondrial function in development of specific tissues and the whole organism, thereby providing insights into various aspects of mitochondrial disease. More recently, a breakthrough has been made with the creation of a mouse that carries and transmits rearranged mitochondrial DNA molecules to its offspring. These and other advances in the field of mouse models are reviewed in Chapter 15.

The penultimate chapter details the extent to which our current knowledge allows us to predict the likelihood of transmission of mitochondrial DNA disease to offspring, a prerequisite to offering prenatal diagnosis. The book ends with an assessment of the prospects for novel therapeutic strategies for a group of diseases that remains for now largely untreatable.

Cover plate

Transverse section of skeletal muscle from a patient with mitochondrial disease. Many of the muscle fibres stain reddish-purple particularly at the fibre periphery, whereas this phenomenon is rare or absent in muscle sections of normal healthy subjects. The heavy stain is indicative of mitochondrial proliferation, and is the hallmark of mitochondrial myopathy. Many such patients carry mutant mitochondrial DNA within their mitochondria.

Acknowledgements

First and foremost I would like to thank the authors for their contributions, and the patience and tolerance they showed in their dealings with me. On a personal note I would like to thank all those who have supported me in my scientific endeavours throughout my career, most notably Professors Anita Harding, Giuseppe Attardi and Howard Jacobs. Particular thanks are also owed to the current members of my laboratory, without their efforts I could not have afforded myself the indulgence of editing this volume. Finally, I offer heartfelt thanks to my daughter, Anna Holt, who helped collate the manuscript.

Contents

List of contributors

B Bigger, Department of Neurology, Medical School, The University of Newcastle upon Tyne, Newcastle upon Tyne NE2 4HH, UK

J Mark Cooper, Department of Clinical Neurosciences, Royal Free and University College Medical School, Rowland Hill Street, London NW3 2PF, UK

J Antonio Enriquez, Departamento de Bioquimica y Biologia Molecular y Celular, Universidad de Zaragoza, Espana, Zaragoza, Spain

Aubrey de Grey, University of Cambridge, Department of Genetics, Downing Street, Cambridge CB2 3EH, UK

Carolino Graff, Department of Medical Nutrition, Karolinska Institutet NOVUM, Huddinge Hospital, S-141 86 Huddinge, Sweden

Michael G Hanna, University Department of Clinical Neurology, National Hospital for Neurology and Institute of Neurology, Queen Square, London WC1N 3BG, UK

Neil Howell, Biology Division 0656, Department of Radiation Oncology and the Department of Human Biological Chemistry and Genetics, The University of Texas Medical Branch, Galveston, TX 77555-0656, USA

Howard Jacobs, Institute of Medical Technology and Tampere University Hospital, FIN-33014 Tampere, Finland

Andrew M James, Dunn Human Nutrition Unit, Wellcome Trust/MRC Building, Hills Road, Cambridge, CB2 2XY, UK

Carla Koehler, Department of Chemistry and Biochemistry, UCLA Box 951569, Los Angeles, CA 90095-1569, USA

Nils-Göran Larsson, Department of Medical Nutrition, Karolinska Institutet NOVUM, Huddinge Hospital, S-141 86 Huddinge, Sweden

Robert N Lightowlers, Department of Neurology, Medical School, The University of Newcastle upon Tyne, Newcastle upon Tyne NE2 4HH, UK

Vincent Macaulay, University of Oxford, Department of Paediatrics, John Radcliffe Hospital room 4406, Headington, Oxford, UK

David R Marchington, University of Oxford, Department of Paediatrics, John Radcliffe Hospital room 4406, Headington, Oxford, UK

Michael P Murphy, Dunn Human Nutrition Unit, Wellcome Trust/MRC Building, Hills Road, Cambridge CB2 2XY, UK

Massimo Pandolfo, Service de Neurologie Hospital Erasme, Université Libre de Bruxelles, Brussels, Belgium

Joanne Poulton, University of Oxford, Department of Paediatrics, John Radcliffe Hospital room 4406, Headington, Oxford, UK

T Pulkes, University Department of Clinical Neurology, National Hospital for Neurology and Institute of Neurology, Queen Square, London WC1N 3BG, UK

Eric A Schon, Departments of Neurology and of Genetics and Development, Columbia University New York, New York 10032, USA

Johannes Spelbrink, Institute of Medical Technology and Tampere University Hospital, 33101 Tampere, Finland

Anu Suomalainen-Wartiovaara, Biomedicum Helsinki, r. c522B, Programme of Neurosciences and Department of Neurology, Helsinki University, Haartmaninkatu 8, 00290 Helsinki, Finland

Jan-Willem Taanman, Department of Clinical Neurosciences, Royal Free and University College Medical School, University College, London, Rowland Hill Street, London NW3 2PF, UK

Robert W Taylor, Department of Neurology, Medical School, The University of Newcastle upon Tyne, Newcastle upon Tyne NE2 4HH, UK

Douglass M Turnbull, Department of Neurology, Medical School, The University of Newcastle upon Tyne, Newcastle upon Tyne NE2 4HH, UK

Marten Wikstrom, Helsinki Bioenergetics Group, Department of Medical Chemistry, Institute of Biomedical Sciences, POB 8, 00014 University of Helsinki, Finland

Massimo Zeviani, Division of Biochemistry and Genetics, National Neurological Institute "C. Besta", via Celoria, 11, 20133–Milano, Italy

Glossary

A, G, C, and T: Single letter code for the four bases of DNA, adenine, guanine, cytosine, and thymine. Thus A3243G denotes a (substitution) mutation: adenine to guanine at 3243 bp of human mitochondrial DNA.

AdPEO, autosomal dominant progressive external ophthalmoplegia: A mitochondrial disorder associated principally with multiple and varied partial deletions of mitochondrial DNA. Because the disease followed a Mendelian pattern of inheritance it was clear that the disease locus must be in nuclear rather than mitochondrial DNA.

ANT-1, adenine nucleotide translocator: It exchanges ADP and ATP between mitochondria and the cytosol. An ANT-1 *knockout* mouse displays features of mitochondrial myopathy. In humans, mutations in the gene are a cause of multiple deletions (see adPEO).

ATP, Adenosine triphosphate: The major energy currency of the cell.

ATP synthase, the enzyme which utilizes the proton gradient generated by the respiratory chain to produce ATP from ADP and inorganic phosphate.

Complex I, NADH–ubiquinone oxidoreductase: The first enzyme of the respiratory chain, mutations in the mitochondrially encoded subunits are associated with LHON, and more rarely MELAS-like phenotypes. Nuclear gene mutations are associated with infantile Leigh's syndrome.

COX, cytochrome *c* oxidase: The terminal respiratory chain enzyme; widely analysed in respiratory chain disorders as the assay is simple and reliable, and a histochemical assay can be performed on tissue sections and cultured monolayers of cells.

Cybrids: Cells containing mitochondrial DNA and nuclear DNA originating from different cells. Cybrids have proved a valuable tool in the study of mitochondrial diseases as the transfer of mitochondria/mtDNA from cells of patients with mitochondrial disease to a different cell enables one to assess mtDNA fitness. A critical step in developing this technology was the creation of human cell lines lacking mitochondrial DNA (see ρ^0 cells).

KSS, Kearn–Sayre syndrome: A neurological disorder commonly the result of rearranged mitochondrial DNA.

LHON, Leber's hereditary optic neuropathy: A mitochondrial disease associated with degeneration of the optic nerve. Recognized as a mitochondrial DNA disorder owing to its strict pattern of maternal transmission.

LS, Leigh's syndrome: A neurological disorder associated specifically with grey matter degeneration: associated with mutations in structural mitochondrial genes of both mitochondrial and nuclear DNA and of a respiratory chain assembly factor (SURF-1).

MELAS: Mitochondrial encepahlomyopathy, lactic acidosis, and stroke-like episodes: A specific form of mitochondrial myopathy most commonly associated with a point mutation in the mitochondrial transfer RNA gene specifying leucine (UUR) (see also MIDD and tRNA).

Membrane potential $\Delta\psi$: The electrochemical gradient across the inner mitochondrial membrane created primarily by the respiratory chain. Respiratory deficiency is predicted to result in a decrease in $\Delta\psi$. Cells with no respiratory capacity have a membrane potential around one-third of cells with a fully functional respiratory chain.

MERRF, myoclonic epilepsy and ragged red fibres: A specific form of mitochondrial myopathy most commonly associated with a tRNA^{Lys} point mutation in mitochondrial DNA (see tRNA).

MIDD, maternally inherited diabetes and deafness: Commonly caused by the same point mutation as that associated with MELAS (see above).

Mitochondrial DNA, mtDNA: In humans a small closed circular molecule of 16,569 bp that is exclusively transmitted through the maternal line. The protein products are all components of the oxidative phosphorylation system. Mutations in this molecule are a recognized cause of disease (see also much of the rest of the book).

Mitochondrial myopathy: Muscle disease presenting as weakness or fatigue associated with mitochondrial proliferation (see also ragged red fibres), functional tests of mitochondria often reveal respiratory deficiency.

MNGIE, mitochondrial neurogastrointestinal encephalomyopathy: Caused by mutations in the thymidine phosphorylase gene, which induce multiple deletions.

mTERF, mitochondrial transcription termination factor: The binding of this protein attenuates transcription downstream of the two ribosomal RNA genes, thereby increasing the ratio of ribosomal to messenger RNA (see Chapter 2 for details). Interest in the protein increased when it was discovered that the most common point mutation in human mitochondrial DNA is located within the mTERF binding site, which is itself wholly contained within a mitochondrial transfer RNA gene (see also MELAS and MIDD).

NARP/MILS, Neurogenic muscle weakness, retinitis pigmentosa/maternally inherited Leigh's syndrome: A neurological disease resulting from mutations in a mitochondrial gene encoding a subunit of ATP synthase. The disease is not associated with a classical mitochondrial myopathy. Unlike many other mitochondrial DNA mutations it does show a good correlation between proportion of mutant mtDNA and disease severity.

OXPHOS or OP(S), Oxidative phosphorylation system: The respiratory chain and ATP synthase; OP is the major energy producing system of the cell that is often compromised in mitochondrial diseases, almost invariably so where mitochondrial DNA is involved.

Pearson's syndrome: An often fatal infantile disorder due to rearranged mitochondrial DNA.

PEO, progressive external ophthalmoplegia: Inability to coordinate the muscles of the eye. A classical feature of mitochondrial myopathy and universal in, patients carrying partially deleted mitochondrial DNA.

POLG, polymerase γ: Currently the one well-characterized mitochondrial DNA polymerase.

ρ^0 **cells**: Cells that lack mtDNA and therefore have no respiratory activity whatsoever—can be re-populated with mitochondria/mtDNA from normal individuals or from patients with mitochondrial disease (see cybrids). These cells are useful as a reference (null) when determining the phenotypic severity of particular mitochondrial DNA mutations.

Respiratory chain: A series of multiprotein enzyme complexes that pump protons across the inner mitochondrial membrane to create an electrochemical gradient. The respiratory chain is now generally regarded by many as comprising Complexes I, III, and IV. Complex II, succinate dehydrogenase that is a component of the tricarboxylic acid cycle is no longer considered an integral part of the chain.

RRF, Ragged red fibres: Respiratory deficiency in muscle generally leads to mitochondrial proliferation, particularly at the fibre periphery (the subsarcolemmal region) this can be highlighted with a histochemical stain that appears red or purple, see Plate 1.

RP, Retinitis pigmentosa or pigmentory retinopathy: Clumping of pigment in the retina leading to impaired vision or even blindness.

ROS, AOS (re)active oxygen species: Highly reactive molecules with an unpaired electron which are formed as unwanted byproducts of many chemical reactions. The mitochondrial respiratory chain is a major source of ROS; ROS can stimulate cell proliferation.

SURF-1: An assembly factor for COX; mutations in the gene cause one particular form of mitochondrial disease—Leigh's syndrome.

TFAM or mtTFA or mtTF1: A mitochondrial transcription factor.

tRNA, transfer RNA: It is essential for protein synthesis. Human mitochondria contain a complete set of tRNAs distinct from those involved in synthesizing proteins coded in nuclear DNA. A three-letter code after the tRNA denotes the amino acid that the tRNA carries (e.g tRNA^{Lys} for Lysine). Where more than one tRNA carries the same amino acid the specific codon it recognizes is also indicated. Thus, there are two tRNAs in mitochondria that carry Leucine, one recognizes UUR codons, the other CUN. The commonest pathogenic mtDNA mutation is at 3243 bp in the tRNA^{LeuUUR} gene.

Twinkle: A mitochondrial protein that associates with mitochondrial DNA and is concentrated in distinct foci within the mitochondrial network; regarded as supporting the idea that animal mitochondrial DNA is arranged in multigenomic nucleoprotein complexes, or nucleoids. Shares homology with a viral DNA helicase/primase, although its function in mitochondria is still uncertain its importance is attested to by the fact that particular mutations in the Twinkle gene cause multiple mitochondrial DNA deletions.

Introduction

Mitochondria are currently enjoying something of a renaissance. A number of factors have contributed to the renewed interest in these organelles. Mitochondria generate most of the energy required by every cell in the body, via a process known as oxidative phosphorylation (OP or OXPHOS). OP is mediated by four multi-protein enzymes; the respiratory chain and ATP synthase. In the past decade, structures of several key enzymes in the energy generation process have been solved, providing profound insights into this complex process. Moreover, mitochondria are now known to play an important role in the orchestrated death of cells, apoptosis. Last but by no means least, the small piece of DNA located in mitochondria has become the focus of interest for many groups studying mitochondrial diseases in humans. It is the last area of study that forms the core of this volume.

Mitochondria are traditionally regarded as cylindrical structures of 0.5–1 μm diameter. Recently, it has become clear that mitochondria are dynamic entities that can fuse and branch and are capable of forming an extensive network. In yeast, specific genes have been shown to play critical roles in promoting mitochondrial fusion and fission. Mitochondria comprise an outer and inner membrane and a matrix. The outer membrane permits the free movement of ions and small molecules, whereas the inner membrane is ion-impermeable. The inner membrane is highly folded and protein rich. These proteins include three respiratory enzyme complexes, which pump protons from the matrix across the inner mitochondrial membrane. The controlled re-entry of protons to the matrix via ATP synthase drives ATP synthesis, from ADP and inorganic phosphate.

The OPS is constructed from the products of two genomes. The majority of proteins are nuclear coded but 13 polypeptides, in the case of humans, are products of mitochondrial DNA (mtDNA). Human mtDNA is a small gene-rich, circular molecule of 16,569 bp. Besides, the 13 components of OP it encodes transfer RNAs and ribosomal RNAs necessary for protein synthesis in mitochondria. Owing to its small size, human mtDNA was one of the earliest genomes to be sequenced in its entirety. mtDNA was inferred to exist well over 50 years ago, as studies in yeast indicated that some traits were transmitted via the cytoplasm rather than the nucleus. Yet, it was not until 1963 that mtDNA was first 'visualized' by electron microscopy, in rat liver cells. The early yeast geneticists recognized that traits transmitted via the cytoplasm did not follow classical Mendelian rules; rather mtDNA was uniparentally transmitted. In metazoans, including humans, mtDNA is transmitted exclusively through the maternal line. Therefore, any deleterious mutation located in mtDNA should be exclusively maternally transmitted.

Around the time that mitochondrial DNA was viewed for the first time, the concept of mitochondrial disease was advanced. Respiratory chain activity is ordinarily tightly linked, or coupled to ATP synthesis. Thus, when ADP is plentiful the respiratory chain is highly active. When mitochondria of a patient with hypermetabolism were analysed they were found to maintain a high respiratory chain flux even when ADP was scarce. Over the next 25 years, other patients were identified with dysfunctional mitochondria associated with muscle disease. These later cases almost invariably had a deficiency in one or more of the respiratory chain enzymes. The hallmark of these diseases was mitochondrial proliferation in muscle fibres (see cover plate); hence they were named mitochondrial myopathies, or more generally mitochondrial cytopathies. The idea that mitochondrial disease could be the result of aberrant mitochondrial DNA gained credence over a number of years. Families with maternally transmitted disease pointed the way, particularly where these were associated with mitochondrial abnormalities of muscle.

The fields of human mitochondrial genetics and disease converged in the late 1980s with the discovery of pathological mutations of mtDNA, giving fresh impetus to both areas of research. Currently, the number of pathological mutations stands somewhere between 50 and 100. There is uncertainty because strict criteria should be applied before designating a mutation as pathological, and these have not always been rigorously applied. The mutation should segregate with the disease and be absent from a large number of healthy controls from the same ethnic group. A deficiency in OP associated with the mutation strengthens the case for a causal link between mutation and disease.

Inducing the loss of mtDNA in yeast is relatively straightforward and was achieved over 30 years ago. The idea that cells derived from obligate aerobes could grow without oxidative phosphorylation was simply not countenanced by most mitochondrial researchers, yet this was shown to be the case, first for chicken cells in 1985 and 4 years later for human cells. Cells without mtDNA are called ρ^0 cells. ρ^0 cells are able to survive and proliferate without aerobic ATP production because the high glucose concentration in the growth medium allows the cell to generate its entire ATP requirement from glycolysis. In the case of human ρ^0 cells, a decrease in glucose concentration from 25 to 5 mM causes rapid cell death. Unfortunately complex multicellular organisms are inviable without mtDNA; a decrease in the number of copies of mtDNA is associated with a severe often-fatal neonatal syndrome, and mice engineered without the capacity to maintain their mtDNA die *in utero*.

Human ρ^0 cells have provided a useful tool for studying mitochondrial disease as they can be repopulated with mitochondria containing mtDNA of patients. The nuclei of the patient-derived cells is first detached to create a *cytoplast* and the cytoplasts then fused with ρ^0 cells. The products of such a fusion are called *cybrids* (as two cytoplasms have been combined in a cell with only one nucleus). Where a defect in OP is transferred to the cybrid along with the mitochondria, the underlying mutation must logically reside in mtDNA. A dozen or more putative pathological mutations have been analysed in this way and shown to produce a biochemical phenotype, that is, mitochondrial dysfunction.

That nuclear genes were also a cause of mitochondrial disease was long recognized, however, identifying specific mutations was a demanding task. Assays of mitochondrial function were often unhelpful, although occasionally deficiency of a particular respiratory complex has been found to result from a mutation in a structural component of the complex. Complex I of the respiratory chain is the best example of its type, however, isolated Complex I deficiency need not be the result of a mutation in a structural gene and with 46 polypeptides in the holoenzyme screening for all possible mutations is a daunting task. In other cases such as cytochrome *c* oxidase deficiency, genetic linkage analysis, micro-cell mediated chromosome transfer and intelligent guesswork each played a role in the process of identifying the causative mutation. An ever more detailed map combined with the complete sequence of the human nuclear genome will aid future attempts to identify nuclear mutations causing mitochondrial disease.

The past decade and a half have given rise to a whole host of new findings impinging on mitochondrial genetics and function, yet as even a superficial reading of the text will impart there much remains to be unravelled and the decade ahead may well prove to be the most exciting yet. Currently, the one sour note is that mitochondrial diseases are largely untreatable and this may well remain the case for some time to come. That said novel and elegant solutions to the problems of creating animal models of human mitochondrial disease have already been fashioned, and a similar level of ingenuity applied to disease treatment may well reap reward.

Section 1 Mitochondrial structure and function

1 Replication, repair, and recombination of mitochondrial DNA

Johannes N Spelbrink

Faithful copying and maintenance of the mitochondrial genome is fundamental to aerobic metabolism and therefore life. Many of the factors involved in mitochondrial DNA metabolism are unknown, or poorly characterized and even the basic mechanism of mitochondrial DNA replication is not well understood. Nevertheless, considerable progress has been made in recent years and this is undoubtedly a field that will benefit enormously from the characterization of the human genome sequence. Current knowledge of the machinery of mtDNA replication is discussed together with a review of the often-contentious areas of repair and recombination. Other topics covered here include the organization and segregation of mtDNA, and auxiliary requirements for mtDNA maintenance, notably nucleotide metabolism.

Introduction

Mitochondrial DNA (mtDNA) in mammals is a closed circular molecule of about 16 kb. The human and mouse mitochondrial genomes were the first to be completely sequenced 20 years ago[1-3] (Fig. 1.1). Like other animal mitochondrial genomes, they contain 22 transfer RNA and two ribosomal RNA genes; which are essential to implement translation in mitochondria (Chapter 2) of 13 genes encoding subunits of the oxidative phosphorylation system (Chapter 4).

Notwithstanding its small size, mtDNA plays an essential part in a cell's energy metabolism. Although ATP can be produced via glycolysis without the need for respiration, this is inefficient and cannot sustain complex multicellular organisms, such as humans, flies, or worms. The importance of mtDNA in humans is evidenced by both hereditary and sporadic disorders resulting from recessive mtDNA mutations. Defects include point mutations (Chapters 7 and 8) as well as large-scale partial deletions or duplications (Chapter 6), which can cause rare multisystem disorders or more common diseases such as diabetes. Collectively, mtDNA mutations are probably one of the commonest causes of genetic disease. They may be sporadic, maternally inherited or the indirect result of a nuclear gene mutation. Despite its importance in cellular metabolism and human disease, mtDNA maintenance has until recently been widely regarded as an evolutionary curiosity and been paid scant attention.

The machinery of mtDNA replication

Mammalian mitochondrial DNA is wholly reliant on nuclear-encoded proteins for its maintenance and faithful propagation. Many of the proteins involved in mtDNA maintenance

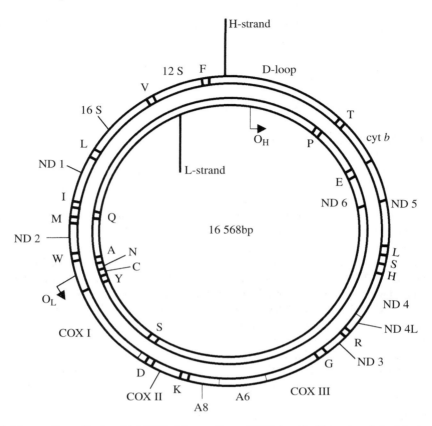

Fig. 1.1 Mammalian mitochondrial DNA. Mammalian mtDNA is a double—stranded, closed, circular molecule of 16.6 kb(1–3). Single letters indicate the positions of the corresponding tRNA genes. ND, NADH dehydrogenase genes; cyt *b*, cytochrome *b* gene; COX, cytochrome *c* oxidase genes; A6/8, ATP synthase genes 6 and 8; 12S/16S, ribosomal RNA genes.

remain to be identified or fully characterized. Purifying and identifying these proteins is problematic due to the difficulty of separating mitochondrial fractions from nuclear contaminants. The situation is complicated further by the fact that the nuclear and mitochondrial compartments of the cell share some gene products. For example, a single gene encodes mitochondrial and nuclear DNA ligase III, whereas mitochondrial RNA polymerase has a dedicated gene. Fortunately, cloning of the gene generally resolves the issue as most, if not all, mitochondrial proteins involved in mtDNA metabolism carry a characteristic canonical presequence that targets the protein to mitochondria. Another problem in delineating the mitochondrial replication machinery is that the repertoire of proteins involved in mtDNA replication varies between species.

So far only four protein components involved in mammalian mtDNA replication have been well characterized. These are transcription factor A of mitochondria (TFAM, formerly called mtTFA), DNA polymerase gamma (POLG), the accessory subunit of POLG (POLG2 by the HUGO nomenclature) and mitochondrial single-stranded DNA-binding protein (SSBP). Other proteins have been described, though these are not fully characterized, or else their role in mtDNA maintenance is still under debate.

TFAM

Two heavy (H) strand promoters and one light (L) strand promoter exist in human mtDNA. *In vitro* and *in organello* TFAM binding has been shown for one of the H-strand promoters and the L-strand promoter.[4,5] *In vitro* binding of TFAM is, however, not very sequence specific.[4,6,7] *In organello* and *in vitro* footprinting experiments suggest that TFAM binds at regular intervals throughout most of the D-loop region, implying a possible DNA-packaging function analogous to that of histones.[5,8] Nevertheless, the affinity of TFAM for the various binding sites is variable and the level of TFAM present in cells is supposed not always to be adequate to achieve complete occupancy.

In humans TFAM is a protein of ~25 kDa and belongs to a family of high-mobility (HMG)-box proteins.[9] HMG-box proteins are believed to activate DNA transactions by melting the two strands downstream of their binding site, a process induced by wrapping and bending duplex DNA.[8] Orthologues of TFAM have been identified in a variety of species, including yeast and frog.[10,11] The yeast TFAM homologue, Abf2p, does stimulate transcription somewhat but its primary role is in packaging the whole yeast mitochondrial genome.[8,12,13] A second transcription factor, Mtf1p, with similarity to bacterial σ factors, provides promoter specificity.[14,15] It is surprising to note that human TFAM can recognize the mouse L-strand promoter and vice versa, even though the promoter sequences are not all that similar.[12,16] This suggests that specificity of transcription initiation in humans does not depend on TFAM alone but requires an as yet unidentified factor or factors. Strong candidates for these factors are the recently identified TFB1M and TFB2M,[17,18] that show similarity to the yeast Mtf1p.

The above results point to at least two unrelated functions for TFAM: facilitating transcription initiation, and playing a structural role in DNA maintenance. Since high- and low-affinity binding-sites for TFAM exist, regulation of TFAM levels might determine the level of expression and replication of mtDNA.[19] For instance, high concentrations of TFAM might be necessary to ensure transcription from both the high-affinity L-strand promoter and the low-affinity H-strand promoter. Rather than promoting replication as previously proposed, TFAM might inhibit replication at high concentrations by analogy with the function of the bacterial histone like protein HU,[20,21] with which it shares many features. At low TFAM concentration, and in the absence of H-strand transcription, sites within the major non-coding region might become available for the binding of replication licensing factors, leading to initiation of DNA synthesis from O_H.

Either role of TFAM is compatible with an important function in mtDNA homeostasis, which was shown unequivocally by the embryonic lethal phenotype associated with complete loss of mtDNA in the mouse TFAM knockout.[22]

POLG and its accessory subunit

In most species the only well-characterized mitochondrial polymerase activity is that of DNA polymerase γ. In humans it is encoded by the nuclear POLG gene and has a molecular weight of ~140 kDa.[23,24] It bears similarity with prokaryotic A-type DNA polymerases, such as *E. coli* DNA polymerase I and T7 DNA polymerase. Conserved regions include a COOH-terminal domain responsible for polymerase activity and an NH_2-terminal 3'-5'-exonuclease domain involved in proofreading. These two activities were attributed to different subunits of the enzyme, however, cloning of polymerase γ from the yeast *S. cerevisiae* and subsequently that of *X. laevis, D. melanogaster* and humans has shown that they are combined in a single polypeptide of ~125–140 kDa.[23–26]

Null mutations in yeast POLG result in loss of mtDNA on a fermentable carbon source.[25,27] In *Drosophila* several mutations in the POLG gene, called *tamas*, result in larval lethality.[28] Last, POLG missense mutations have very recently been identified as a cause for adPEO and arPEO.[29,30] These data suggest an important role for POLG in mtDNA maintenance, but at least in mammals there is no formal proof that POLG is the replicative polymerase. The properties of POLG have been partly characterized in yeast and in human cultured cells.[27,31–33] In both cases, expression of a semi-dominant mutant form of the protein, deficient in 3'-5'-exonuclease activity results in the accumulation of mtDNA point mutations. The mutation patterns differ markedly, however, with transversions predominating in yeast and C–G to T–A transitions dominating in human cells. This could reflect differences in intrinsic properties of the enzymes, in their intracellular milieu, or in mtDNA repair. In any event, overexpression of variants deficient in 5'-3'-polymerase activity results in loss of mtDNA in yeast and human cells.

Another factor that might underpin the observed difference in mutation bias between yeast and human discussed above is the existence of a 40–55 kDa accessory subunit in the latter (and several other species) but not yeast. This subunit is also termed the POLG β-subunit and it consistently co-purifies with polymerase γ.[34,35] The recent crystal structure of the accessory subunit shows that it forms a homodimer, thus suggesting that the polymerase holoenzyme is an $\alpha\beta_2$ heterotrimer, at least in mammals.[36] One can speculate that this conformation would allow for transient interactions between one of the two β-subunits in the heterotrimer and a second POLG subunit to facilitate coupled leading and lagging-strand synthesis, as proposed by the synchronous replication model (see Section below). The β-subunit is thought to be important in maintaining catalytic efficiency or structural integrity of the holoenzyme. It has also been proposed that the accessory subunit is involved in recognition of the RNA primer in the D-loop region, guiding the catalytic subunit to the primer terminus.[35,37] *In vitro*, the accessory subunit has been shown to greatly increase processivity during strand elongation,[38,39] but the crystal data do not support the idea that the protein is a sliding clamp.[36] Thus, POLG and its accessory subunit form a stable, high fidelity, enzyme with high processivity suggesting that it is the replicative polymerase for mitochondrial DNA. A second putative mitochondrial DNA polymerase similar to nuclear β polymerase has been detected in trypanosomes and more recently in bovine heart mitochondria.[40] By analogy with the nuclear enzyme, such a β-like polymerase could function in gap-filling during mitochondrial DNA repair or lagging-strand synthesis in the synchronous replication model.

Unlike most nuclear DNA polymerases, POLG is relatively resistant to aphidicolin.[25] Recently, this fact has been exploited to develop a mitochondrial specific DNA-radiolabelling assay in cultured human cells.[41] Since it has reverse transcriptase activity, POLG can prime ribohomopolymer templates. A bizarre, yet medically important consequence of this property of the enzyme is that reverse transcriptase inhibitors such as AZT inhibit POLG and so can induce mitochondrial myopathy in AIDS patients treated with AZT.[42]

Single-stranded DNA-binding protein

The mitochondrial single-stranded DNA-binding protein (mtSSB) has been cloned from a variety of species including human and rat.[43] Multiple sequence alignments identify the proteins as similar to prokaryotic-type SSB proteins,[43] with the highest identity in the N-terminal region that functions in tetramerization or DNA binding.[44,45] The protein preferentially binds to single-stranded DNA, generally as a homotetramer.[44] By analogy with bacterial and phage SSB proteins,[46–48] the C-terminus may be involved in multiple protein interactions. In both *X. laevis* and *Drosophila*, SSB enhances POLG activity, but a direct physical interaction between the proteins has not been demonstrated.[49,50] Mitochondrial SSB is probably needed to stabilize single-stranded regions of mtDNA, both in the D-loop and in replicative intermediates.[51] SSB proteins are usually required to stabilize single-stranded regions at replication forks,[52] but could of course have a wider role in protecting extensive single-stranded regions that form during asynchronous mtDNA replication.

Other proteins

RNase MRP and Endonuclease G
Two enzymatic activities, RNase MRP and EndonucleaseG have been postulated to modify the D-loop RNA primer from the L-strand transcription unit near O_H and therefore play a role initiation of replication. The RNase MRP is a ribonucleoprotein complex consisting of a single RNA moiety and several proteins.[53–55] The enzyme was first isolated from mouse and human mitochondria, and shown to specifically cleave D-loop RNA templates near the origin of H-strand replication.[53,56,57] However, the protein was subsequently found to be much more abundant in the nucleus, where it is involved in ribosomal RNA processing and possibly tRNA processing.[58–61] The very low levels of the enzyme found in mitochondria sparked debate as to whether or not it was merely a nuclear contaminant of mitochondrial preparations.[58,62,63] Subsequently, the evidence in support of a specific intramitochondrial pool of RNase MRP has become more solid. (i) *In situ* hybridization experiments, show both mitochondrial and nuclear-specific labelling;[64] (ii) an RNase MRP fraction can be isolated that is resistant to nuclease following digitonin treatment, a detergent that disrupts the mitochondrial outer membrane,[63] suggesting that a proportion of RNase MRP is located within the mitochondrial matrix; (iii) survival of *S. pombe* with a mutation in the RNase MRP RNA gene requires an additional nuclear mutation, *ptp1*-1, which is implicated in mitochondrial function.[61] But, the *ptp*1 gene has not yet been identified making it difficult to assess the value of the last study.

Even assuming RNase MRP is present in mitochondria, its role in replication remains to be established. The experiments performed to date have been chiefly *in vitro* assays with purified enzyme and lacking other proteins believed to interact with the processing region. Moreover, the inherent properties of the unusual RNA–DNA hybrid structure near O_H may make it susceptible to processing by RNases generally; two other proteins believed to be present in mitochondria, RNase P and endonuclease G (EndoG), are also capable of processing L-strand transcripts near O_H.[65,66] RNase P is a ribonucleoprotein present in mammalian mitochondria involved in 5'-tRNA (transfer RNA) processing, and has many aspects in common with RNase MRP,[54] including some but not all of its protein components.[67,68] Given that a mutant RNase MRP allele in *S. pombe* has a nuclear tRNA processing phenotype,[69] a role in mitochondrial tRNA processing for RNase MRP should be considered. The Endo G was originally isolated as a nuclease with a preference for duplex DNA (dG).(dC) tracts and single stranded dC tracts, it too is found in nuclei and mitochondria. In addition, it was shown to possess RNase H-like activity, as do RNase MRP and RNase P.[65] One or more of these activities, may process L-strand-transcripts that form primers for DNA synthesis, but there is no *in vivo* evidence as yet. Moreover, detection of similar processed transcripts *in vivo* would not necessarily indicate that this was an essential prerequisite for mitochondrial DNA replication.

Mitochondrial RNA polymerase

Mitochondrial RNA polymerase has been identified in a variety of species, including *S. cerevisiae* and human[70,71] and shows similarity with T7 RNA polymerase. The protein has been extensively studied in yeast, but not yet so in human. The yeast, mammalian, and possibly the frog enzyme require one or more sigma-like factors for promoter-specific binding of the enzyme.[11,17,18,72,73]

Twinkle

Twinkle is a recently identified protein with similarity to the T7 primase/helicase gene 4 protein (gp4).[74] The similarity is restricted largely to the C-terminal helicase domain. Like T7 gp4 and many other 'ring' helicases, Twinkle is likely to adopt a hexamer conformation. The N-terminal domain, which in T7 gp4 has been identified as essential for primase activity, is of unknown function. Furthermore, sequence alignment of the few, eukaryotic Twinkle-like proteins known, shows homology to be weakest for the N-terminal regions. The plasmodium homologue POM1, lacks a region equivalent to the N-terminal portion of T7 gp4 or Twinkle, instead it possesses a long C-terminal extension of unknown function. Thus, it would be premature to concluded that Twinkle functions as a primase in human mitochondria.

Although the precise role of Twinkle has not yet been established, it is clear that it plays a role in mtDNA metabolism since mutations in the Twinkle gene lead to the formation of multiple partial deletions (Chapter 9). An interesting feature of Twinkle is the unusual mitochondrial localization pattern, examined using green fluorescent protein (GFP) tagged fusion proteins. In contrast to for example, POLG–GFP and TFAM–GFP, which show uniform mitochondrial fluorescence, Twinkle shows punctate mitochondrial fluorescence, a consequence of its localization in mtDNA nucleoids. A natural splice variant, that lacks the C-terminal 105 amino acids and terminates with four unique amino acids, appears unable to form hexamers and does not target to nucleoids.

Models for mammalian mtDNA replication

Although DNA is the standard repository of genetic information, a number of different mechanisms has evolved for the perpetuation and quality control of DNA synthesis.[52] Moreover, a diverse range of molecular machinery underpins these mechanisms.

Replication of mammalian mtDNA has long been recognized as unusual; many apparent mtDNA replication intermediates contain long stretches of partially single-stranded DNA and their characterization led to the proposal of a strand-asynchronous, asymmetrical model of mammalian mtDNA replication.[75] The strand-asynchronous model stipulates two sites of initiation of DNA synthesis, one for each strand, which lie far apart (hence asymmetrical).[75]

In this model, synthesis of the leading H-strand* starts at a point in the major non-coding region of mtDNA denoted as O_H; O_H is defined by the 5'-ends of the newly synthesized leading-strands, and is located on the L-strand upstream of three conserved sequence blocks (CSBs), as demonstrated mainly by 5'-end-mapping methods. Leading-strand synthesis proceeds two-thirds of the way around the molecule, displacing the original H-strand in the process (see Fig. 2(a–c)). At this point, the site of second (lagging) strand synthesis (O_L) is exposed allowing DNA synthesis of the light strand to begin (hence asynchronous). The critical nucleotides that support initiation of lagging-strand synthesis at O_L have been character-ized,[76,77] yet it is important to note that this does not establish O_L as the unique lagging-strand start point.

Recently a more conventional model of mammalian mtDNA replication has been proposed also to occur.[78] This second mechanism is coupled, that is, the leading and lagging-strands of mtDNA are synthesized simultaneously, or synchronously[78] (Fig. 1.2(a)/(b + d)). Coupled mtDNA replication starts from a single origin (also at or near O_H) and proceeds around the molecule in one direction, in contrast to many other systems including nuclear DNA where coupled replication is bidirectional. Since DNA synthesis *always* proceeds in the 5'–3'-direction the new model predicts formation of short segments of DNA, so-called Okazaki fragments,[79] on the lagging strand. The two models, or modes of mammalian mtDNA replication, could be unified into a single model if a variety of replication intermediates exist with different num-bers of lagging-strand start sites. That is, that the strand-synchronous and strand-asynchronous modes of replication may represent extremes of a spectrum where the frequency of lagging-strand initiation is the only variable. Support for this idea would require the identification of replication intermediates with two or more instances of lagging-strand initiation that were nevertheless demonstrably partially single-stranded.

Both mechanisms or modes of replication clearly operate in mammalian mitochondria, yet the abundance of the two types of replication intermediate is highly variable. Replication intermediates of both types are readily detectable in solid tissues examined to date (placenta, liver, and cardiac muscle). However, synchronous replication intermediates are of low abun-dance ordinarily in cell lines cultured in the laboratory examined to date, yet they greatly out-number strand-asynchronous replication intermediates in cell lines that require a net increase in mtDNA copy number, for example, during mtDNA amplification after drug-induced tran-sient mtDNA depletion.[78]

Another well-established peculiarity of mammalian mtDNA is the widespread and often abundant occurrence of molecules with a short triplex region. The third strand of approxi-mately 0.5 kb of DNA arises from O_H, and is termed the displacement-loop (D-loop) form of mtDNA.[75] The widespread assumption is that D-loops represent aborted replication interme-diates, most if not all are degraded, thus of the total number of leading strand initiation events that occur few extend beyond the end of the D-loop. Regulation of termination of leading-strand DNA synthesis is poorly understood, although it may involve the so-called Termination Associated Sequences (TAS) in the major non-coding region.[80] Extended leading-strand

---

* The nomenclature for the two strands of mitochondrial DNA is based on the apparent mobility of the two strands in a denaturing caesium chloride gradient. One strand has a relatively high guanine nucleotide content and is therefore called the Heavy- or H-strand, the other strand with its high cytosine content is termed Light- or L-strand.

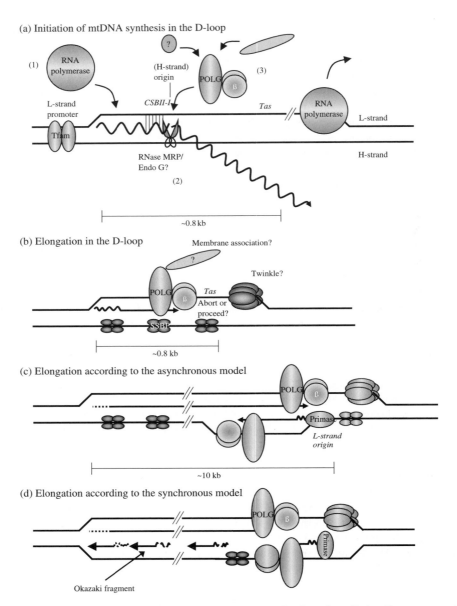

Fig. 1.2 Mechanisms and proteins in mammalian mtDNA replication. Compilation figure summarizing protein and mechanistic aspects of mtDNA replication in mammals. DNA is represented by a straight line, RNA by a wavy line. (a) MtDNA replication is initiated by transcription from the L-strand promoter involving at least TFAM and RNA polymerase (1). A transition to DNA synthesis is thought to occur following processing of the L-strand transcript by RNase MRP, endonuclease G or other processing activity (2) and assembly of the replication machinery (3). (b) Extension of D-loop replication beyond TAS sequences represents a dedicated replication event. Most nascent D-loop DNA, however, is terminated and turned over. (c) Continuation of H-strand replication and initiation of the L-strand replication according the asymmetrical, asynchronous mode of replication.[75] L-strand replication is initiated only after 10 kb of the H-strand has been synthesized, leaving most of the parental H-strand, single-stranded. (d) Unidirectional, coupled leading and lagging strand replication.[78] Lagging-strand synthesis initiates at the same time as leading strand synthesis, short (Okazaki) fragments are generated in the process of lagging-strand synthesis.

replicative intermediates and D-loop strands are indistinguishable at their 5′-ends, consistent with an attenuation model.

In humans and mouse, newly synthesized D-loop-containing mtDNA contains a 5′-RNA moiety fro example,[81,82] which forms a strong RNA–DNA hybrid particularly at CSB II.[82,83] Thus, D-loop DNA synthesis appears to be preceded by synthesis of an RNA primer originating at the L-strand promoter, implicating the mitochondrial transcription machinery in initiation of mtDNA replication. Indeed, a mouse knockout of the mitochondrial transcription factor, TFAM, results in embryonic lethality associated with complete loss of mtDNA.[22] However, TFAM may have multiple functions and therefore the loss of mtDNA need not necessarily stem from its role in transcription. If indeed the RNA primer for mtDNA replication is transcribed starting from the L-strand promoter, which also gives rise to complete L-strand polycistronic transcripts, then transition to DNA synthesis must occur, either by processing of the nascent RNA-strand near O_H, or by direct replacement of transcription machinery with DNA synthesis machinery at O_H. Although two specific enzyme activities have been proposed to generate the RNA primer by processing, there is no hard evidence that this is the favoured mechanism.

Continuation of nascent H-strand synthesis beyond the TAS-associated pause site is thought to mark a dedicated replication event. The two models for replication, from this point onwards, predict quite different events and replication intermediates. The asynchronous model predicts a large single stranded DNA-loop, representing the parental H-strand that is displaced by ongoing synthesis of the new H-strand. Intermediates of this nature have been observed by electron microscopy.[75] The synchronous model predicts a loop structure in which one strand of the loop is duplex, while the other strand is substantially duplex, yet has short gaps, owing to discontinuous synthesis of DNA on the lagging-strand. It is worth noting that lagging-strand synthesis is almost seamless, that is, the gaps must be closed efficiently and rapidly, otherwise the products of coupled replication would be cleaved by a single-strand-specific nuclease, which was demonstrably *not* the case in the neutral/neutral agarose gel electrophoresis study.[78] Coupled replication intermediates have also been observed by electron microscopy,[75] but have not been screened for under conditions that favour synchronous replication. A further experiment showing the validity of the synchronous model would be the demonstration of Okazaki fragments. Small RNA primers, often at specific sites usually initiate Okazaki-fragment synthesis. RNA primers should subsequently be removed, the small gaps filled with DNA, and the fragments end-joined by a DNA ligase. The process can however be very efficient making it difficult to isolate individual Okazaki fragments. The long-standing observation, of rare ribonucleotide (rNTP) sites in mtDNA,[84] could be explained by incomplete removal of RNA primers from Okazaki fragments. In a very recent study,[85] the observation of rNTPs in mtDNA has been extended by showing that they are widespread in replicating mtDNA, frequently consisting of patches of uninterrupted rNTPs. Interestingly, these patches appeared to be preferentially incorporated in the L-strand, especially in the region that is suggested to be extensively single-stranded in the asynchronous replication model. The authors suggest that the single-stranded replication intermediates of the asynchronous model could well be artefacts caused by endogenous RNase H-like activity acting on mtDNA during the isolation procedure. If correct, the above refutes the asynchronous model and will have far-reaching implications for our understanding of mtDNA maintenance.

The site of lagging-strand DNA synthesis initiation (O_L) in the asynchronous model, is also partly defined by retention of ribonucleotides at O_L in closed circular mtDNA.[84] Moreover, 5′-ends of replication intermediates map at a precise position near O_L.[82,86] Finally, in a variety of species, a strong stem–loop structure is predicted to form at O_L when the H-strand template is rendered single-stranded.[76] These observations suggest that O_L is a regulatory element with conserved features and accordingly argues that it has an important role in mtDNA replication. The widely accepted view is that its role is as the major or sole site of lagging-strand initiation. Nevertheless, O_L has proved dispensable in several animal groups including birds.[87] Priming at O_L (or elsewhere on the lagging-strand) is probably not mediated by the transcription machinery, yet a specific primase remains to be identified.

mtDNA repair and recombination

Over the years, a number of unsubstantiated dogmas arose in relation to repair and recombination of mammalian mitochondrial DNA, in fact repair of vertebrate mitochondrial DNA was long considered not to occur. However, there is now unequivocal evidence that mitochondria contain the complete machinery for base excision repair (for an overview see Bogenhagen).[88] Other repair pathways that are present in the nucleus, nucleotide excision repair, and mismatch repair, have not yet been identified. Recombination has been suggested to occur mainly as a gene conversion event,[89] possibly as a way to achieve mismatch repair. However, based on population genetics, more conventional homologous recombination has been proposed also to exist. Although in some minds the issue remains controversial, it is highly likely that a basic machinery for recombination is present in mammalian mitochondria if only to restart replication after stalling—via recombination-dependent replication.[90,91]

Mitochondrial DNA has often been described as 'naked' lacking as it does any obvious equivalent of nuclear histones and this was presumed to make it prone to damage in the highly oxidative environment within the mitochondrial matrix (Chapter 11). Now it appears that mtDNA is not in fact naked but exists in mitochondria as large nucleoprotein complexes, termed nucleoids. It has long been accepted that the mutation-fixation rate of mtDNA in mammalians is high compared to that of nuclear DNA, and the assumption has been that this reflects a high mutation rate, at least in female gametes. By the same line of reasoning, somatic mutation rates for mtDNA are believed to be high and moreover have been proposed as a significant contributing factor to ageing in humans and other animals (Chapter 13). Nevertheless, it is clear from recent studies that several types of mtDNA damage can be repaired effectively. These include 8-oxo-dG and deoxyuridine that result from oxidative damage to deoxyguanosine (dG) and deamination of deoxycytidine, respectively. These and other types of oxidative damage are dealt with by the base-excision repair (BER) machinery. Base excision repair comprises five steps. (i) Removal of the unconventional base by a damage-specific DNA glycosylase, which results in an apurinic/apyrimidinic (AP) site; (ii) nicking of the phosphate backbone by an AP endonuclease; (iii) removal of the deoxyribose moiety by an AP lyase; (iv) gap-filling by a DNA polymerase; and (v) re-ligation. Several DNA glycosylases have now been shown to reside in mitochondria as well as in the nucleus. The various genes are commonly single-copy nuclear genes that code for both the nuclear and mitochondrial versions of the protein.[92–99] Alternative-splicing, or alternative translational start sites, commonly provide the differentially targeted proteins. An AP endonuclease activity has been isolated from *X.laevis* mitochondria but the protein has not been positively identified. AP lyase activity has been demonstrated for POLG and also for *E.coli* polymerase I.[100] Nuclear polymerase β, however, contains a much more efficient lyase activity,[101] suggesting a possible role for a polymerase β-like protein in mitochondrial DNA repair (see Section on PoLG and its accessory subunit). Gap-filling of mtDNA could be mediated by POLG or a β-like polymerase, while DNA ligase III is presumed to be responsible for closure.[102] Antisense inhibition of DNA ligase III resulted in mtDNA depletion as well as accumulation of single-stranded nicks and possible gaps in mtDNA, suggesting an additional role in BER.[103]

Other types of DNA damage such as chemically induced crosslinks or simply the misincorporation of a base during replication are not usually repaired by the action of BER. Either nucleotide excision repair for the former or mismatch repair for the latter are required. Neither of these processes has been demonstrated in mitochondria.[88] The need for an efficient mismatch repair may be partially circumvented by the proofreading activity of POLG, as, compared to cells that express a proofreading deficient POLG, cells that express only endogenous POLG accumulate very few mtDNA mutations.[33] Because *S.cerevisiae* contains a partially functional mismatch repair pathway[32,104,105] and has a significantly lower mutation fixation rate than mammalian mtDNA, one could argue, nonetheless, that the relatively high mutation-fixation rate in mammalian mitochondria is attributable to the lack of mismatch repair activity. This would agree with the pattern of human polymorphisms and disease mutations; predominantly A → T to G → C transitions, which in yeast are effectively suppressed by mismatch repair. Proofreading and possibly BER by POLG seem to prevent mostly C → G to T → A transitions and A → T to T-A transversions.[32,33] One should consider, however, that high mutation-fixation rates are usually seen on an evolutionary timescale, and do not necessarily imply high rates of somatic mutation. Moreover, the discussion above focuses purely on mutation occurrence and ignores the fact that fixation of mtDNA variants need not occur simply by a random process of genetic drift (see nucleoids below and Chapter 14).

Evidence for possible homologous recombination events in mammals is scarce and mostly genetic. First, interconversion of rearranged mtDNA molecules has been observed in human cell lines, suggesting a recombination event. Cells homoplasmic for partially duplicated mtDNA were observed consistently to regain wild-type mtDNA (Wt-mtDNA), in one cell type.[106] Also on an occasion a deleted mtDNA species that would be predicted from an intramolecular recombination event in a partially duplicated molecule has been detected.[107] In addition, disease-associated mtDNA deletions as well as deletions and duplications of low abundance, 'sublimons', could be generated by recombination[108–110] as might the higher multiple rearrangement seen in one study.[106] Second, population genetic studies in human and chimpanzee have suggested a gradual loss of linkage between mtDNA loci with distance,[111] which was explained by a combination of paternal leakage of mtDNA and recombination. The interpretation of the population genetics data are, however, highly controversial,[112,113] and at least two additional studies that used larger data sets have directly questioned the original findings.[114,115] Combined these studies at least suggest the possibility of mtDNA recombination, albeit as a rare event.

Homologous recombination activity was demonstrated using ingenious *in vitro* assays with isolated mitochondria.[89] The activity could be inhibited using an antibody against *recA*, an essential component of eubacterial recombination machineries. The assays used could not, however, distinguish between reciprocal (crossover) recombination, and gene conversion, a process that copies the genetic information from one DNA molecule into a second molecule and involves extensive *de novo* DNA synthesis. The authors suggested, based partially on yeast studies, that mammalian mitochondria might only possess a gene-conversion type of recombination which could function for example, in mismatch and double-strand break repair. Surprisingly, double-strand break rejoining, especially on blunt-ended DNA, using similar mitochondrial extracts, resulted in low-frequency deletions of the template involving short, direct repeats,[116] possibly the result of a gene-conversion type of break repair. Based on these observations, it was suggested that deletions of mtDNA in pathological states could be the results of defective double-strand break repair. Of course, a certain degree of slippage during gene conversion or intermolecular template switching facilitated by gene-conversion machinery could bring about the same effect at a low frequency, in healthy individuals. Identification of the proteins involved in recombination and repair will clarify this issue and give insights into the mutability of mtDNA.

Organization and segregation of mtDNA

As alluded to above, mammalian mtDNA is now believed to occur as multiple copies organized in nucleo-protein complexes termed nucleoids. Nucleoids have been suggested to be the unit of mtDNA inheritance. Control of nucleoid size and organization will therefore be an important determinant of mitochondrial gene segregation with important implications for mutation fixation and disease transmission.

Evidence for nucleoid organization of mtDNA in mammalian cells is not only genetic and biochemical but also relies on modern fluorescence and electron microscopy techniques. A mammalian nucleoid model has been reviewed recently.[117] The genetic argument in favour of nucleoids is as follows. First, two different alleles of mtDNA, both harbouring a disease mutation, and introduced in mtDNA-less cells, only on very rare occasions complement each other.[118–120] Nevertheless, mitochondria in various species frequently undergo fusion and fission events.[121–125] This strongly suggests that, in mammalian cells as in yeast,[121] mitochondrial genetic units have a limited sphere of influence and are somehow restricted in their capability to mix, for example, by simple random diffusion. Second, cell lines harbouring heteroplasmic mtDNA mutations do not always show segregation of mtDNA genotypes, even after many cell generations.[117,121,126] This implies that the unit of segregation is in itself heteroplasmic and stable. Third, high levels of mtDNA point mutations are tolerated in the POLG mutator cell lines described above, without a severe adverse effect on mitochondrial function. Combined with the limited sphere of influence, each genetic unit must consist of several mtDNA molecules to enable high mtDNA mutation loads to be tolerated. Microscopy studies confirm two aspects of nucleoid organization of mtDNA. The first is the presence of various copies of mtDNA per nucleoid. Using DAPI staining of mtDNA it has been estimated that the number of mtDNA foci within a human cell is significantly less than the mtDNA copy number.[127] This was recently confirmed by estimating mtDNA nucleoids numbers using a GFP tagged version of Twinkle.[74] The second, electron-microscopic, observation is that complexes containing both DNA and protein exist in mitochondria of various species.[128,129] Biochemical evidence for mtDNA nucleoids as nucleo-protein complexes that constitute the unit of mtDNA inheritance comes mainly from yeast.[13,121,128,130] An important constituent of nucleoids in yeast is Abf2p, the yeast orthologue of mammalian TFAM. Disruption of the *Abf2* gene results in altered nucleoid appearance and mtDNA inheritance.[13,130] Various other proteins have been proposed as nucleoid constituents on the basis of stable DNA interaction, *in situ* fluorescent studies, or both.[131,132] Surprisingly these include, HSP60 and an α-ketoglutarate dehydrogenase subunit, both with established roles distinct from mtDNA maintenance. The association was based on *in organello* crosslinking experiments.[132] The caveat is that not all proteins that interact with mtDNA are necessarily nucleoid constituents. In human cells, various proteins known to interact with mtDNA do not show specific nucleoid localization when overexpressed as a GFP fusion protein. This could be due to a limitation in the occupancy of mtDNA by these proteins, while expression levels are artificially high, but could also mean that these proteins only interact transiently with mtDNA.

Physical association of nucleoids to the mitochondrial inner and possibly even outer membrane, would provide a handle by which mtDNA can be distributed (mitokinesis) during cell division.[117] Inner-membrane association of nucleoids can and has been inferred from direct observation, from co-purification of membrane patches with nucleoids or from copurification with membrane proteins.[132–136] Curiously, human mitochondrial sub-fractionation and subsequent lysis with laurylmaltoside showed partial purification of various mtDNA-maintenance proteins with the outer membrane fraction while the remainder co-purified with the inner-membrane fraction.[33] The same outer membrane fraction was completely free from cytochrome *c* oxidase subunit II, a *bona fide* integral inner membrane protein. These observations might indicate a physical (protein?) connection between nucleoids and the outer mitochondrial membrane. An obvious candidate is the mitochondrial fission apparatus, some components of which are cytosolic or outer-membrane-associated proteins.[125]

Understanding the dynamics of nucleoid organization during different stages of development and in dividing and post-mitotic cells will be helpful in understanding mitochondrial gene segregation, in health and especially human mitochondrial diseases. Studies in yeast will again be informative in this respect as shown in a study addressing nucleoid number and size in relation to amino acid metabolism,[137] although yeast and mammals may well have evolved different segregation strategies. In a second study using human cybrids, a gain of chromosome 9 was inferred to affect nucleoid organization at least transiently, since segregation was significantly altered,[126] but we have no clue yet as to what factors might affect nucleoid size and number.

Other requirements for mtDNA maintenance: nucleotide metabolism

Apart from the many proteins that directly participate in mtDNA maintenance, various metabolites play an essential role in mtDNA homeostasis. These include magnesium, and ribo- and deoxyribonucleotides that are the immediate building blocks for RNA and DNA synthesis, and the metabolism of the physiological anion, which in *E.coli* has been identified as glutamate.[52]

Nucleotide pools in mitochondria appear to rely mainly on intramitrochondrial nucleoside to nucleotide interconversion and direct import from the cytoplasm, rather than on *de novo* pathways. Since ribonucleotide reductase which can convert ribonucleotides to deoxyribonucleotides, has not been demonstrated yet as an intramitochondrial protein, both ribonucleotides and deoxyribonucleotides are probably imported in mitochondria from the cytosol. Indeed, a transporter-activity capable of importing one deoxyribonucleotide has recently been identified, but other nucleotides were not tested.[138] However, the recent identification of a human cDNA, encoding a member of the carrier family with NTP and dNTP transport capability has allowed for a more detailed study by reconstitution of the protein in lipid vesicles after overexpression in bacteria.[139] Thus, this carrier was shown to have broad substrate specificity and depend on dNDPs, ADP, or ATP to serve as exchange factors. Once inside mitochondria, (deoxy) ribonucleotides/nucleosides can undergo interconversion steps mediated by (deoxy)ribonucleotidases, which remove a phosphate residue from a (deoxy)ribonucleoside-monophosphate, and (deoxy)ribonucleotide kinases which adds a single phosphate from ATP to (deoxy)ribonucleosides. Some of these enzymes, including a uracil/thymine deoxyribonu-cleotidase, a thymidine kinase and a deoxyguanosine kinase, have now been positively iden-tified in mammalian mitochondria.[140–145] Both thymidine and deoxyguanosine kinase have broad substrate specificity, being able to metabolize not only natural substrates but also a vari-ety of nucleoside analogues, which can be a serious problem for patients undergoing chemotherapy or who are treated for viral infection, because of mitochondrial toxicity.[146]

So, how do cytoplasmic nucleoside/nucleotide pools affect mtDNA maintenance? Since it is unlikely that there exists a *de novo* nucleoside synthesis pathway in mammalian mitochondria, any imbalance in the cytoplasmic pools of nucleosides and nucleotides is likely to impact upon intramitochondrial pools as well. In yeast, overexpression of the *RNR1* gene, encoding the cyto-plasmic ribonucleotide reductase, in yeast POLG (*MIP1*) mutants alleviates the negative effects of the POLG mutants on mtDNA synthesis.[147] It was suggested that the overexpression of *RNR1* results in increased pools of dNTPs, suggesting that dNTP levels could be rate-determining for mtDNA synthesis. A second protein was identified, deletion of which, resulted in the suppres-sion of mutations in two (cell-cycle) checkpoint genes. A strong case was made that this second protein, Sml1, is in fact an inhibitor of the Rnr1 protein.[148,149] Indeed, deletion of the *Sml*1 gene had the same effect on the POLG mutants as overexpression of *Rnr*1. The best evidence that dNTP imbalance in humans can affect mtDNA integrity is MNGIE (see Section on 'Twinkle' above). The MNGIE is an autosomal recessive disorder caused by mutations in the thymidine phosphorylase (TP) gene.[150] The mutations invariably result in almost complete loss of TP activity.[150,151] Although TP catalyses a reversible reaction, thymidine + $P_i\Delta$thymine + deoxyribose-1-P, synthesis of thymidine does not appear to be the problem probably because of *de novo* synthesis. The problem is rather the breakdown of excess thymidine. Indeed, TP defi-ciency results in the accumulation of thymidine in the blood stream.[152] This is thought to affect cellular, and thus also mitochondrial thymidine levels.[151,152] How an excess of thymidine and its nucleotide derivatives induces mtDNA deletions is still a matter for speculation. It might result in enhanced misincorporation of dTTP followed by elevated recombination–repair or even turnover of mtDNA. The last idea is attractive, as it is known that TP deficiency can also lead to mtDNA depletion;[153] episodes of mtDNA depletion followed by repopulation could favour the amplification of deleted mtDNA molecules[154] constitutively present at low levels in various tissues.[110] Perturbed nucleotide homeostasis is also proposed as the cause for multiple mtDNA deletions in adPEO associated with ANT1 and Twinkle mutations (Chapter 9), and may well be the cause of other autosomal mtDNA-associated disorders. Indeed, very recently two of the above mentioned proteins involved in nucleotide metabolism have been implied in mtDNA-depletion syndromes. Mutations in the gene for mitochondrial deoxyguanosine kinase were found associated with mtDNA depletion in liver/brain.[155] In muscle-specific mtDNA depletion, the gene for the mitochondrial thymidine kinase was found to be mutated.[156]

Concluding remarks and future prospects

Current understanding of mtDNA maintenance stems from: (i) the identification of various nuclear disease genes that affect the process; (ii) the realization that specific types of mtDNA damage can be repaired; (iii) the identification of various proteins involved in mitochondrial fission and the distribution of mitochondria in the cell; and (iv) the creation of animal models that address the function of particular mtDNA maintenance proteins.

Notwithstanding these advances, a thorough understanding of the underlying processes is still lacking in many areas. Of particular interest will be how the various components of the maintenance machinery interact with one another and with the fission machinery; how mitochondrial nucleoid number and size are regulated, in particular during development, and how this may help us better understand mtDNA segregation. Further understanding of the mechanisms of mtDNA replication and repair will be closely linked to the identification of components involved in these processes. The importance of proper functioning of the mtDNA maintenance machinery in health is indisputable and understanding this process may provide a paradigm for related processes in the nucleus.

Acknowledgements

I would like to thank Ian Holt for critically reading the manuscript, Howy Jacobs for many stimulating discussions and Johanna Kurkela for help in making Fig. 1.1.

References

1. Anderson S, Bankier AT, De Bruijn MHL, Coulson AR, Drouin J, Eperon IC, *et al.* (1981). Sequence and organization of the human mitochondrial genome. *Nature* **290**: 457–465.
2. Bibb MJ, Van Etten RA, Wright CT, Walberg MW, and Clayton DA. (1981). Sequence and gene organization of mouse mitochondrial DNA. *Cell* **26**(2 Pt 2): 167–180.
3. Andrews RM, Kubacka I, Chinnery PF, Lightowlers RN, Turnbull DM, and Howell N (1999). Reanalysis and revision of the Cambridge reference sequence for human mitochondrial DNA. *Nat. Genet.* **23**(2): 147.
4. Fisher RP, Topper JN, and Clayton DA (1987). Promoter selection in human mitochondria involves binding of a transcription factor to orientation-independent upstream regulatory elements. *Cell* **50**(2): 247–258.
5. Ghivizzani SC, Madsen CS, Nelen MR, Ammini CV, and Hauswirth WW (1994). In organello footprint analysis of human mitochondrial DNA: human mitochondrial transcription factor A interactions at the origin of replication. *Mol. Cell. Biol.* **14**: 7717–7730.
6. Fisher RP and Clayton DA (1988). Purification and characterization of human mitochondrial transcription factor 1. *Mol. Cell. Biol.* **8**(8): 3496–3509.
7. Ikeda S, Sumiyoshi H, and Oda T (1994). DNA binding properties of recombinant human mitochondrial transcription factor 1. *Cell Mol. Biol. (Noisy-le-grand)* **40**(4): 489–493.
8. Fisher RP, Lisowsky T, Parisi MA, and Clayton DA (1992). DNA wrapping and bending by a mitochondrial high mobility group-like transcriptional activator protein. *J. Biol. Chem.* **267**(5): 3358–3367.
9. Parisi MA and Clayton DA (1991). Similarity of human mitochondrial transcription factor 1 to high mobility group proteins. *Science* **252**(5008): 965–969.
10. Fisher RP, Lisowsky T, Breen GA, and Clayton DA (1991). A rapid, efficient method for purifying DNA-binding proteins. Denaturation-renaturation chromatography of human and yeast mitochondrial extracts. *J. Biol. Chem.* **266**(14): 9153–9160.
11. Antoshechkin I and Bogenhagen DF (1995). Distinct roles for two purified factors in transcription of Xenopus mitochondrial DNA. *Mol. Cell. Biol.* **15**(12): 7032–7042.

12. Shadel GS and Clayton DA (1993). Mitochondrial transcription initiation. Variation and conservation. *J. Biol. Chem.* **268**(22): 16083–16086.

13. Newman SM, Zelenaya-Troitskaya O, Perlman PS, and Butow RA (1996). Analysis of mitochondrial DNA nucleoids in wild-type and a mutant strain of Saccharomyces cerevisiae that lacks the mitochondrial HMG box protein Abf2p. *Nucleic Acids Res.* **24**(2): 386–393.

14. Jang SH and Jaehning JA (1991). The yeast mitochondrial RNA polymerase specificity factor, MTF1, is similar to bacterial σ factors. *J. Biol. Chem.* **266**: 22671–22677.

15. Xu B and Clayton DA (1992). Assignment of a yeast protein necessary for mitochondrial transcription initiation. *Nucleic Acids Res.* **20**(5): 1053–1059.

16. Fisher RP, Parisi MA, and Clayton DA (1989). Flexible recognition of rapidly evolving promoter sequences by mitochondrial transcription factor 1. *Genes Dev.* **3**(12B): 2202–2217.

17. McCulloch V, Seidel-Rogol BL, and Shadel GS (2002). A human mitochondrial transcription factor is related to RNA adenine methyltransferases and binds S-adenosylmethionine. *Mol. Cell. Biol.* **22**(4): 1116–1125.

18. Falkenberg M, Gaspari M, Rantanen A, Trifunovic A, Larsson NG, and Gustafsson CM (2002). Mitochondrial transcription factors B1 and B2 activate transcription of human mtDNA. *Nat. Genet.* **31**(3): 289–294.

19. Dairaghi DJ, Shadel GS, and Clayton DA (1995). Human mitochondrial transcription factor A and promoter spacing integrity are required for transcription initiation. *Biochim. Biophys. Acta* **1271**(1): 127–134.

20. Mensa-Wilmot K, Carroll K, and McMacken R (1989). Transcriptional activation of bacteriophage lambda DNA replication in vitro: regulatory role of histone-like protein HU of Escherichia coli. *EMBO J.* **8**(8): 2393–2402.

21. Skarstad K, Baker TA, and Kornberg A (1990). Strand separation required for initiation of replication at the chromosomal origin of *E.coli* is facilitated by a distant RNA–DNA hybrid. *EMBO J.* **9**(7): 2341–2348.

22. Larsson NG, Wang J, Wilhelmsson H, Oldfors A, Rustin P, Lewandoski M, *et al.* (1998). Mitochondrial transcription factor A is necessary for mtDNA maintenance and embryogenesis in mice. *Nat. Genet.* **18**(3): 231–236.

23. Ropp PA and Copeland WC (1996). Cloning and characterization of the human mitochondrial DNA polymerase, DNA polymerase gamma. *Genomics* **36**(3): 449–458.

24. Lecrenier N, Van Der Bruggen P, and Foury F (1997). Mitochondrial DNA polymerases from yeast to man: a new family of polymerases. *Gene* **185**: 147–152.

25. Foury F (1989). Cloning and sequencing of the nuclear gene *MIP1* encoding the catalytic subunit of the yeast mitochondrial DNA polymerase. *J. Biol. Chem.* **264**(34): 20552–20560.

26. Ye F, Carrodeguas JA, and Bogenhagen DF (1996). The gamma subfamily of DNA polymerases: cloning of a developmentally regulated cDNA encoding Xenopus laevis mitochondrial DNA polymerase gamma. *Nucleic Acids Res.* **24**(8): 1481–1488.

27. Hu J, Vanderstraeten S, and Foury F (1995). Isolation and characterization of ten mutator alleles of the mitochondrial DNA polymerase- encoding MIP1 gene from *Saccharomyces cerevisiae. Gene* **160**: 105–110.

28. Iyengar B, Roote J, and Campos AR (1999). The tamas gene, identified as a mutation that disrupts larval behavior in Drosophila melanogaster, codes for the mitochondrial DNA polymerase catalytic subunit (DNApol-gamma125). *Genetics* **153**(4): 1809–1824.

29. Van Goethem G, Dermaut B, Lofgren A, Martin JJ, and Van Broeckhoven C (2001). Mutation of POLG is associated with progressive external ophthalmoplegia characterized by mtDNA deletions. *Nat. Genet.* **28**(3): 211–212.

30. Lamantea E, Tiranti V, Bordoni A, Toscano A, Bono F, Servidei S, *et al.* (2002). Mutations of mitochondrial DNA polymerase gammaA are a frequent cause of autosomal dominant or recessive progressive external ophthalmoplegia. *Ann. Neurol.* **52**(2): 211–219.

31. Foury F and Vanderstraeten S (1992). Yeast mitochondrial DNA mutators with deficient proofreading exonucleolytic activity. *EMBO J.* **11**(7): 2717–2726.
32. Vanderstraeten S, Van den Brule S, Hu J, and Foury F (1998). The role of 3'-5' exonucleolytic proofreading and mismatch repair in yeast mitochondrial DNA error avoidance. *J. Biol. Chem.* **273**(37): 23690–23697.
33. Spelbrink JN, Toivonen JM, Hakkaart GA, Kurkela JM, Cooper HM, Lehtinen SK, *et al.* (2000). *In vivo* functional analysis of the human mitochondrial DNA polymerase POLG expressed in cultured human cells. *J. Biol. Chem.* **275**(32): 24818–24828.
34. Wang Y, Farr CL, and Kaguni LS (1997). Accessory subunit of mitochondrial DNA polymerase from Drosophila embryos. Cloning, molecular analysis, and association in the native enzyme. *J. Biol. Chem.* **272**(21): 13640–13646.
35. Carrodeguas JA and Bogenhagen DF (2000). Protein sequences conserved in prokaryotic aminoacyl-tRNA synthetases are important for the activity of the processivity factor of human mitochondrial DNA polymerase. *Nucleic Acids Res.* **28**(5): 1237–1244.
36. Carrodeguas JA, Theis K, Bogenhagen DF, and Kisker C (2001). Crystal structure and deletion analysis show that the accessory subunit of mammalian DNA polymerase gamma, Pol gamma B, functions as a homodimer. *Mol. Cell* **7**(1): 43–54.
37. Fan L, Sanschagrin PC, Kaguni LS, and Kuhn LA (1999). The accessory subunit of mtDNA polymerase shares structural homology with aminoacyl-tRNA synthetases: implications for a dual role as a primer recognition factor and processivity clamp. *Proc. Natl Acad. Sci. USA* **96**(17): 9527–9532.
38. Lim SE, Longley MJ, and Copeland WC (1999). The mitochondrial p55 accessory subunit of human DNA polymerase gamma enhances DNA binding, promotes processive DNA synthesis, and confers *N*-ethylmaleimide resistance. *J. Biol. Chem.* **274**(53): 38197–38203.
39. Carrodeguas JA, Kobayashi R, Lim SE, Copeland WC, and Bogenhagen DF (1999). The accessory subunit of Xenopus laevis mitochondrial DNA polymerase gamma increases processivity of the catalytic subunit of human DNA polymerase gamma and is related to class II aminoacyl-tRNA synthetases. *Mol. Cell. Biol.* **19**(6): 4039–4046.
40. Nielsen-Preiss SM and Low RL (2000). Identification of a beta-like DNA polymerase activity in bovine heart mitochondria. *Arch. Biochem. Biophys.* **374**(2): 229–240.
41. Emmerson CF, Brown GK, and Poulton J (2001). Synthesis of mitochondrial DNA in permeabilised human cultured cells. *Nucleic Acids Res.* **29**(2): E1.
42. Dalakas MC, Illa I, Pezeshkpour GH, Laukaitis JP, Cohen B, and Griffin JL (1990). Mitochondrial myopathy caused by long-term zidovudine therapy. *N. Engl. J. Med.* **322**(16): 1098–1105.
43. Tiranti V, Rocchi M, DiDonato S, and Zeviani M (1993). Cloning of human and rat cDNAs encoding the mitochondrial single-stranded DNA-binding protein (SSB). *Gene* **126**(2): 219–225.
44. Curth U, Urbanke C, Greipel J, Gerberding H, Tiranti V, and Zeviani M (1994). Single-stranded-DNA-binding proteins from human mitochondria and Escherichia coli have analogous physico-chemical properties. *Eur. J. Biochem.* **221**(1): 435–443.
45. Li K and Williams RS (1997). Tetramerization and single-stranded DNA binding properties of native and mutated forms of murine mitochondrial single-stranded DNA-binding proteins. *J. Biol. Chem.* **272**(13): 8686–8694.
46. Kong D and Richardson CC (1998). Role of the acidic carboxyl-terminal domain of the single-stranded DNA-binding protein of bacteriophage T7 in specific protein–protein interactions. *J. Biol. Chem.* **273**(11): 6556–6564.
47. Yuzhakov A, Kelman Z, and O'Donnell M (1999). Trading places on DNA—a three-point switch underlies primer handoff from primase to the replicative DNA polymerase. *Cell* **96**(1): 153–163.
48. Genschel J, Curth U, and Urbanke C (2000). Interaction of E. coli single-stranded DNA binding protein (SSB) with exonuclease I. The carboxy-terminus of SSB is the recognition site for the nuclease. *J. Biol. Chem.* **381**(3): 183–192.

49. Mikhailov VS and Bogenhagen DF (1996). Effects of Xenopus laevis mitochondrial single-stranded DNA- binding protein on primer-template binding and 3′ → 5′ exonuclease activity of DNA polymerase gamma. *J. Biol. Chem.* **271**(31): 18939–18946.

50. Farr CL, Wang Y, and Kaguni LS (1999). Functional interactions of mitochondrial DNA polymerase and single-stranded DNA-binding protein. Template-primer DNA binding and initiation and elongation of DNA strand synthesis. *J. Biol. Chem.* **274**(21): 14779–14785.

51. Zeviani M, Amati P, Comi G, Fratta G, Mariotti C, and Tiranti V (1995). Searching for genes affecting the structural integrity of the mitochondrial genome. *Biochim. Biophys. Acta* **1271**: 153–158.

52. Kornberg A and Baker TA (1992). *DNA Replication.* Second edition New York: W.H. Freeman and Company.

53. Chang DD and Clayton DA (1989). Mouse RNAase MRP RNA is encoded by a nuclear gene and contains a decamer sequence complementary to a conserved region of mitochondrial RNA substrate. *Cell* **56**(1): 131–139.

54. Gold HA, Topper JN, Clayton DA, and Craft J (1989). The RNA processing enzyme RNase MRP is identical to the Th RNP and related to RNase P. *Science* **245**(4924): 1377–1380.

55. Topper JN and Clayton DA (1990). Characterization of human MRP/Th RNA and its nuclear gene: full length MRP/Th RNA is an active endoribonuclease when assembled as an RNP. *Nucleic Acids Res.* **18**(4): 793–799.

56. Chang DD and Clayton DA (1987). A mammalian mitochondrial RNA processing activity contains nucleus-encoded RNA. *Science* **235**(4793): 1178–1184.

57. Bennett JL and Clayton DA (1990). Efficient site-specific cleavage by RNase MRP requires interaction with two evolutionarily conserved mitochondrial RNA sequences. *Mol. Cell. Biol.* **10**(5): 2191–2201.

58. Kiss T and Filipowicz W (1992). Evidence against a mitochondrial location of the 7–2/MRP RNA in mammalian cells. *Cell* **70**: 11–16.

59. Kiss T, Marshallsay C, and Filipowicz W (1992). 7-2/MRP RNAs in plant and mammalian cells: association with higher order structures in the nucleolus. *EMBO J.* **11**: 3737–3746.

60. Chu S, Archer RH, Zengel JM, and Lindahl L (1994). The RNA of RNase MRP is required for normal processing of ribosomal RNA. *Proc. Natl Acad. Sci. USA* **91**(2): 659–663.

61. Paluh JL and Clayton DA (1996). Mutational analysis of the gene for Schizosaccharomyces pombe RNase MRP RNA, mrp1, using plasmid shuffle by counterselection on canavanine. *Yeast* **12**(14): 1393–1405.

62. Topper JN, Bennett JL, Clayton DA (1992). A role for RNAase MRP in mitochondrial RNA processing. *Cell* **70**: 16–20.

63. Puranam RS and Attardi G (2001). The RNase P associated with HeLa cell mitochondria contains an essential RNA component identical in sequence to that of the nuclear RNase P. *Mol. Cell. Biol.* **21**(2): 548–561.

64. Li K, Smagula CS, Parsons WJ, Richardson JA, Gonzalez M, Hagler HK, *et al.* (1994). Sucellular partitioning of MRP RNA assesed by ultrastructural and biochemical analysis. *J. Cell. Biol.* **124**: 871–882.

65. Côté J and Ruiz-Carillo A (1993). Primers for mitochondrial DNA replication generated by endonuclease G. *Science* **261**: 765–769.

66. Potuschak T, Rossmanith W, and Karwan R (1993). RNase MRP and RNase P share a common substrate. *Nucleic Acids Res.* **21**(14): 3239–3243.

67. Lygerou Z, Mitchell P, Petfalski E, Séraphin B, and Tollervey D (1994). The POP1 gene encodes a protein component common to the RNAase MRP and RNase P ribonucleoproteins. *Genes Dev.* **8**: 1423–1433.

68. Schmitt ME and Clayton DA (1994). Characterization of a unique protein component of yeast RNase MRP: an RNA-binding protein with a zinc-cluster domain. *Genes Dev.* **8**(21): 2617–2628.

69. Paluh JL and Clayton DA (1996). A functional dominant mutation in Schizosaccharomyces pombe RNase MRP RNA affects nuclear RNA processing and requires the mitochondrial–associated nuclear mutation ptp1-1 for viability. *EMBO J.* **15**(17): 4723–4733.

70. Masters BS, Stohl LL, and Clayton DA (1987). Yeast mitochondrial RNA polymerase is homologous to those encoded by bacteriophages T3 and T7. *Cell* **51**(1): 89–99.

71. Tiranti V, Savoia A, Forti F, D'Apolito MF, Centra M, Rocchi M, *et al.* (1997). Identification of the gene encoding the human mitochondrial RNA polymerase (h-mtRPOL) by cyberscreening of the Expressed Sequence Tags database. *Hum. Mol. Genet.* **6**(4): 615–625.

72. Shadel GS and Clayton DA (1995). A Saccharomyces cerevisiae mitochondrial transcription factor, sc-mtTFB, shares features with sigma factors but is functionally distinct. *Mol. Cell. Biol.* **15**(4): 2101–2108.

73. Bogenhagen DF (1996). Interaction of mtTFB and mtRNA polymerase at core promoters for transcription of Xenopus laevis mtDNA. *J. Biol. Chem.* **271**(20): 12036–12041.

74. Spelbrink JN, Li FY, Tiranti V, Nikali K, Yuan QP, Tariq M, *et al.* (2001). Human mitochondrial DNA deletions associated with mutations in the gene encoding Twinkle, a phage T7 gene 4-like protein localized in mitochondria. *Nat. Genet.* **28**(3): 223–231.

75. Clayton DA (1982). Replication of animal mitochondrial DNA. *Cell* **28**: 693–705.

76. Chang DD, Wong TW, Hixson JE, and Clayton DA (1985). Regulatory sequences for mammalian mitochondrial transcription and replication. In: E Quagliariello, EC Slater, F Palmieri, C Saccone, and AM Kroon (eds), Achievements and Perspectives of Mitochondrial Research. Volume II: Biogenesis. Amsterdam: Elsevier; pp. 135–144.

77. Wong TW and Clayton DA (1985). *In vitro* replication of human mitochondrial DNA: accurate initiation at the origin of light-strand synthesis. *Cell* **42**(3): 951–958.

78. Holt IJ, Lorimer HE, and Jacobs HT (2000). Coupled leading- and lagging-strand synthesis of mammalian mitochondrial DNA. *Cell* **100**(5): 515–524.

79. Kurosawa Y, Ogawa T, Hirose S, Okazaki T, and Okazaki R (1975). Mechanism of DNA chain growth. XV. RNA-linked nascent DNA pieces in Escherichia coli strains assayed with spleen exonuclease. *J. Mol. Biol.* **96**(4): 653–664.

80. Doda JN, Wright CT, and Clayton DA (1981). Elongation of displacement-loop strands in human and mouse mitochondrial DNA is arrested near specific template sequences. *Proc. Natl Acad. Sci. USA* **78**(10): 6116–6120.

81. Gillum AM and Clayton DA (1978). Displacement-loop replication initiation sequence in animal mitochondrial DNA exists as a family of discrete lengths. *Proc. Natl Acad. Sci. USA* **75**(2): 677–681.

82. Kang D, Miyako K, Kai Y, Irie T, and Takeshige K (1997). *In vivo* determination of replication origins of human mitochondrial DNA by ligation-mediated polymerase chain reaction. *J. Biol. Chem.* **272**(24): 15275–15279.

83. Xu B and Clayton DA (1996). RNA–DNA hybrid formation at the human mitochondrial heavy-strand origin ceases at replication start sites: an implication for RNA–DNA hybrids serving as primers. *EMBO J.* **15**(12): 3135–3143.

84. Brennicke A and Clayton DA (1981). Nucleotide assignment of alkali-sensitive sites in mouse mitochondrial DNA. *J. Biol. Chem.* **256**(20): 10613–10617.

85. Yang MY, Bowmaker M, Reyes A, Vergani L, Angeli P, Gringeri E, *et al.* (2002). Biased incorporation of ribonucleotides on the mitochondrial L-strand accounts for apparent strand-asymmetric DNA replication. *Cell* **111**: 495–505.

86. Tapper DP and Clayton DA (1982). Precise nucleotide location of the 5′ ends of RNA-primed nascent light strands of mouse mitochondrial DNA. *J. Mol. Biol.* **162**(1): 1–16.

87. Desjardins P and Morais R (1990). Sequence and gene organization of the chicken mitochondrial genome. A novel gene order in higher vertebrates. *J. Mol. Biol.* **212**(4): 599–634.

88. Bogenhagen DF (1999). Repair of mtDNA in vertebrates. *Am. J. Hum. Genet.* **64**(5): 1276–1281.

89. Thyagarajan B, Padua RA, and Campbell C (1996). Mammalian mitochondria possess homologous DNA recombination activity. *J. Biol. Chem.* **271**(44): 27536–27543.

90. Haber JE (1999). DNA recombination: the replication connection. *Trends Biochem. Sci.* **24**(7): 271–275.

91. Kowalczykowski SC (2000). Initiation of genetic recombination and recombination-dependent replication. *Trends Biochem. Sci.* **25**(4): 156–165.

92. Slupphaug G, Markussen FH, Olsen LC, Aasland R, Aarsaether N, and Bakke O, *et al.* (1993). Nuclear and mitochondrial forms of human uracil-DNA glycosylase are encoded by the same gene. *Nucleic Acids Res.* **21**(11): 2579–2584.

93. Kang D, Nishida J, Iyama A, Nakabeppu Y, Furuichi M, Fujiwara T, *et al.* (1995). Intracellular localization of 8-oxo-dGTPase in human cells, with special reference to the role of the enzyme in mitochondria. *J. Biol. Chem.* **270**(24): 14659–14665.

94. Takao M, Aburatani H, Kobayashi K, and Yasui A (1998). Mitochondrial targeting of human DNA glycosylases for repair of oxidative DNA damage. *Nucleic Acids Res.* **26**(12): 2917–2922.

95. Nishioka K, Ohtsubo T, Oda H, Fujiwara T, Kang D, Sugimachi K, *et al.* (1999). Expression and differential intracellular localization of two major forms of human 8-oxoguanine DNA glycosylase encoded by alternatively spliced OGG1 mRNAs. *Mol. Biol. Cell* **10**(5): 1637–1652.

96. Takao M, Zhang QM, Yonei S, and Yasui A (1999). Differential subcellular localization of human MutY homolog (hMYH) and the functional activity of adenine:8-oxoguanine DNA glycosylase. *Nucleic Acids Res.* **27**(18): 3638–3644.

97. Miyako K, Takamatsu C, Umeda S, Tajiri T, Furuichi M, Nakabeppu Y, *et al.* (2000). Accumulation of adenine DNA glycosylase-sensitive sites in human mitochondrial DNA. *J. Biol. Chem.* **275**(16): 12326–12330.

98. Parker A, Gu Y, and Lu AL (2000). Purification and characterization of a mammalian homolog of Escherichia coli MutY mismatch repair protein from calf liver mitochondria. *Nucleic Acids Res.* **28**(17): 3206–3215.

99. Ohtsubo T, Nishioka K, Imaiso Y, Iwai S, Shimokawa H, Oda H, *et al.* Identification of human MutY homolog (hMYH) as a repair enzyme for 2- hydroxyadenine in DNA and detection of multiple forms of hMYH located in nuclei and mitochondria. *Nucleic Acids Res.* **28**(6): 1355–1364.

100. Pinz KG and Bogenhagen DF (2000). Characterization of a catalytically slow AP lyase activity in DNA polymerase gamma and other family A DNA polymerases. *J. Biol. Chem.* **275**(17): 12509–12514.

101. Matsumoto Y and Kim K (1995). Excision of deoxyribose phosphate residues by DNA polymerase beta during DNA repair. *Science* **269**(5224): 699–702.

102. Lakshmipathy U and Campbell C (1999). The human DNA ligase III gene encodes nuclear and mitochondrial proteins. *Mol. Cell. Biol.* **19**(5): 3869–3876.

103. Lakshmipathy U, and Campbell C (2001). Antisense-mediated decrease in DNA ligase III expression results in reduced mitochondrial DNA integrity. *Nucleic Acids Res.* **29**(3): 668–676.

104. Chi NW and Kolodner RD (1994). The effect of DNA mismatches on the ATPase activity of MSH1, a protein in yeast mitochondria that recognizes DNA mismatches. *J. Biol. Chem.* **269**(47): 29993–29997.

105. Reenan RA and Kolodner RD (1992). Isolation and characterization of two Saccharomyces cerevisiae genes encoding homologs of the bacterial HexA and MutS mismatch repair proteins. *Genetics* **132**(4): 963–973.

106. Holt IJ, Dunbar DR, and Jacobs HT (1997). Behaviour of a population of partially duplicated mitochondrial DNA molecules in cell culture: segregation, maintenance and recombination dependent upon nuclear background. *Hum. Mol. Genet.* **6**(8): 1251–1260.

107. Tang Y, Manfredi G, Hirano M, and Schon EA (2000). Maintenance of human rearranged mitochondrial DNAs in long-term cultured transmitochondrial cell lines. *Mol. Biol. Cell* **11**(7): 2349–2358.

108. Schon EA, Spadari S, Moraes CT, Nakase H, Zeviani M, and DiMauro S (1989). A direct repeat is a hotspot for large-scale deletion of human mitochondrial DNA. *Science* **244**: 346–349.

109. Mita S, Spadari S, Moraes CT, Shanske S, Arnaudo E, Fabrizi GM, *et al.* (1990). Recombination via flanking direct repeats is a major cause of large scale deletions of human mitochondrial DNA. *Nucleic Acids Res.* **18**: 561–567.

110. Kajander OA, Rovio AT, Majamaa K, Poulton J, Spelbrink JN, Holt IJ, *et al.* (2000). Human mtDNA sublimons resemble rearranged mitochondrial genoms found in pathological states *Hum. Mol. Genet* **9**(19): 2821–2835.

111. Awadalla P, Eyre-Walker A, and Smith JM (1999). Linkage disequilibrium and recombination in hominid mitochondrial DNA. *Science* **286**(5449): 2524–2525.

112. Kivisild T and Villems R (2000). Questioning evidence for recombination in human mitochondrial DNA. *Science* **288**(5473): 1931.

113. Parsons TJ and Irwin JA (2000). Questioning evidence for recombination in human mitochondrial DNA. *Science* **288**(5473): 1931.

114. Ingman M, Kaessmann H, Paabo S, and Gyllensten U (2000). Mitochondrial genome variation and the origin of modern humans. *Nature* **408**(6813): 708–713.

115. Elson JL, Andrews RM, Chinnery PF, Lightowlers RN, Turnbull DM, and Howell N (2001). Analysis of European mtDNAs for recombination. *Am. J. Hum. Genet.* **68**(1): 145–153.

116. Lakshmipathy U and Campbell C (1999). Double strand break rejoining by mammalian mitochondrial extracts. *Nucleic Acids Res.* **27**(4): 1198–1204.

117. Jacobs HT, Lehtinen SK, and Spelbrink JN (2000). No sex please, we're mitochondria: a hypothesis on the somatic unit of inheritance of mammalian mtDNA. *Bioessays* **22**(6): 564–572.

118. Yoneda M, Miyatake T, and Attardi G (1994). Complementation of mutant and wild-type human mitochondrial DNAs coexisting since the mutation event and lack of complementation of DNAs introduced seperately into a cell within distinct organelles. *Mol. Cell. Biol.* **14**: 2699–2712.

119. Hayashi J-I, Takemitsu M, Goto Y-I, and Nonaka I (1994). Human mitochondria and mitochondrial genome function as a single dynamic cellular unit. *J. Cell. Biol.* **125**: 43–50.

120. Enriquez JA, Cabezas-Herrera J, Bayona-Bafaluy MP, and Attardi G (2000). Very rare complementation between mitochondria carrying different mitochondrial DNA mutations points to intrinsic genetic autonomy of the organelles in cultured human cells. *J. Biol. Chem.* **275**(15): 11207–11215.

121. Nunnari J, Marshall WF, Straight A, Murray A, Sedat JW, and Walter P (1997). Mitochondrial transmission during mating in Saccharomyces cerevisiae is determined by mitochondrial fusion and fission and the intramitochondrial segregation of mitochondrial DNA. *Mol. Biol. Cell* **8**(7): 1233–1242.

122. Yaffe MP (1997). Mitochondrial morphogenesis: fusion factor for fly fertility. *Curr. Biol.* **7**(12): R782–R783.

123. Yaffe MP (1999). The machinery of mitochondrial inheritance and behavior. *Science* **283**(5407): 1493–1497.

124. Labrousse AM, Zappaterra MD, Rube DA, and van der Bliek AM (1999). C. elegans dynamin-related protein DRP-1 controls severing of the mitochondrial outer membrane. *Mol. Cell. Biol.* **4**(5): 815–826.

125. van der Bliek AM (2000). A mitochondrial division apparatus takes shape. *J. Cell. Biol.* **151**(2): F1–F4.

126. Lehtinen SK, Hance N, El Meziane A, Juhola MK, Juhola KM, Karhu R, *et al.* Genotypic stability, segregation and selection in heteroplasmic human cell lines containing np 3243 mutant mtDNA. *Genetics* **154**(1): 363–380.

127. Satoh M and Kuroiwa T (1991). Organization of multiple nucleoids and DNA molecules in mitochondria of a human cell. *Exp. Cell. Res.* **196**(1): 137–140.

128. Miyakawa I, Sando N, Kawano S, Nakamura S, and Kuroiwa T (1987). Isolation of morphologically intact mitochondrial nucleoids from the yeast, Saccharomyces cerevisiae. *J. Cell. Sci.* **88**(Pt 4): 431–439.

129. Kuroiwa T, Kuroiwa H, Sakai A, Takahashi H, Toda K, and Itoh R (1998). The division apparatus of plastids and mitochondria. *Int. Rev. Cytol.* **181**: 1–41.
130. Zelenaya-Troitskaya O, Newman SM, Okamoto K, Perlman PS, and Butow RA (1998). Functions of the high mobility group protein, Abf 2p, in mitochondrial DNA segregation, recombination and copy number in Saccharomyces cerevisiae. *Genetics* **148**(4): 1763–1776.
131. Meeusen S, Tieu Q, Wong E, Weiss E, Schieltz D, Yates JR, *et al.* (1999). Mgm101p is a novel component of the mitochondrial nucleoid that binds DNA and is required for the repair of oxidatively damaged mitochondrial DNA. *J. Cell. Biol.* **145**(2): 291–304.
132. Kaufman BA, Newman SM, Hallberg RL, Slaughter CA, Perlman PS, and Butow RA (2000). In organello formaldehyde crosslinking of proteins to mtDNA: identification of bifunctional proteins. *Proc. Natl Acad. Sci. USA* **97**(14): 7772–7777.
133. Albring M, Griffith J, and Attardi G (1977). Association of a protein structure of probable membrane derivation with HeLa cell mitochondrial DNA near its origin of replication. *Proc. Natl. Acad. Sci. USA* **74**(4): 1348–1352.
134. Kuroiwa T, Kawano S, and Hizume M (1997). Studies on mitochondrial structure and function in Physarum polycephalum. V. Behaviour of mitochondrial nucleoids throughout mitochondrial division cycle. *J. Cell. Biol.* **72**(3): 687–694.
135. Hillar M, Rangayya V, Jafar BB, Chambers D, Vitzu M, and Wyborny LE (1979). Membrane-bound mitochondrial DNA: isolation, transcription and protein composition. *Arch. Int. Physiol. Biochim.* **87**(1): 29–49.
136. Barat M, Rickwood D, Dufresne C, and Mounolou JC (1985). Characterization of DNA-protein complexes from the mitochondria of Xenopus laevis oocytes. *Exp. Cell. Res.* **157**(1): 207–217.
137. MacAlpine DM, Perlman PS, and Butow RA (2000). The numbers of individual mitochondrial DNA molecules and mitochondrial DNA nucleoids in yeast are co-regulated by the general amino acid control pathway. *Embo J.* **19**(4): 767–775.
138. Bridges EG, Jiang Z, and Cheng YC (1999). Characterization of a dCTP transport activity reconstituted from human mitochondria. *J. Biol. Chem.* **274**(8): 4620–4625.
139. Dolce V, Fiermonte G, Runswick MJ, Palmieri F, and Walker JE (2001). The human mitochondrial deoxynucleotide carrier and its role in the toxicity of nucleoside antivirals. *Proc. Natl Acad. Sci. USA* **98**(5): 2284–2288.
140. Wang L, Hellman U, and Eriksson S (1996). Cloning and expression of human mitochondrial deoxyguanosine kinase cDNA. *FEBS Lett.* **390**(1): 39–43.
141. Johansson M and Karlsson A (1996). Cloning and expression of human deoxyguanosine kinase cDNA. *Proc. Natl Acad. Sci. USA* **93**(14): 7258–7262.
142. Wang L and Eriksson S (2000). Cloning and characterization of full-length mouse thymidine kinase 2: the N-terminal sequence directs import of the precursor protein into mitochondria. *Biochem J.* **351**(Pt 2): 469–476.
143. Jullig M and Eriksson S (2000). Mitochondrial and submitochondrial localization of human deoxyguanosine kinase. *Eur. J. Biochem.* **267**(17): 5466–5472.
144. Milon L, Meyer P, Chiadmi M, Munier A, Johansson M, Karlsson A, *et al.* (2000). The human nm23-H4 gene product is a mitochondrial nucleoside diphosphate kinase. *J. Biol. Chem.* **275**(19): 14264–14272.
145. Rampazzo C, Gallinaro L, Milanesi E, Frigimelica E, Reichard P, and Bianchi V (2000). A deoxyribonucleotidase in mitochondria: involvement in regulation of dNTP pools and possible link to genetic disease. *Proc. Natl Acad. Sci. USA* **97**(15): 8239–8244.
146. Wang L, Munch-Petersen B, Herrstrom Sjoberg A, Hellman U, Bergman T, Jornvall H, *et al.* (1999). Human thymidine kinase 2: molecular cloning and characterisation of the enzyme activity with antiviral and cytostatic nucleoside substrates. *FEBS Lett.* **443**(2): 170–174.
147. Lecrenier N and Foury F (1995). Overexpression of the RNR1 gene rescues Saccharomyces cerevisiae mutants in the mitochondrial DNA polymerase-encoding MIP1 gene. *Mol. Gen. Genet.* **249**: 1–7.

148. Zhao X, Muller EG, and Rothstein R (1998). A suppressor of two essential checkpoint genes identifies a novel protein that negatively affects dNTP pools. *Mol. Cell.* **2**(3): 329–340.
149. Chabes A, Domkin V, and Thelander L (1999). Yeast Sml1, a protein inhibitor of ribonucleotide reductase. *J. Biol. Chem.* **274**(51): 36679–36683.
150. Nishino I, Spinazzola A, and Hirano M (1999). Thymidine phosphorylase gene mutations in MNGIE, a human mitochondrial disorder. *Science* **283**(5402): 689–692.
151. Nishino I, Spinazzola A, and Hirano M (2001). MNGIE: from nuclear DNA to mitochondrial DNA. *Neuromuscul. Disord.* **11**(1): 7–10.
152. Spinazzola A, Marti R, Nishino I, Andreu AL, Naini A, Tadesse S, *et al.* (2002). Altered thymidine metabolism due to defects of thymidine phosphorylase. *J. Biol. Chem.* **277**(6): 4128–4133.
153. Nishino I, Spinazzola A, Papadimitriou A, Hammans S, Steiner I, Hahn CD, *et al.* Mitochondrial neurogastrointestinal encephalomyopathy: an autosomal recessive disorder due to thymidine phosphorylase mutations. *Ann. Neurol.* **47**(6): 792–800.
154. Spelbrink JN, Zwart R, Van Galen MJM, and Van den Bogert C (1997). Preferential amplification and phenotypic selection in a population of deleted and wild-type mitochondrial DNA in cultured cells. *Curr. Genet.* **32**: 115–124.
155. Mandel H, Szargel R, Labay V, Elpeleg O, Saada A, Shalata A, *et al.* (2001). The deoxyguanosine kinase gene is mutated in individuals with depleted hepatocerebral mitochondrial DNA. *Nat. Genet.* **29**(3): 337–341.
156. Saada A, Shaag A, Mandel H, Nevo Y, Eriksson S, and Elpeleg O (2001). Mutant mitochondrial thymidine kinase in mitochondrial DNA depletion myopathy. *Nat. Genet.* **29**(3): 342–344.

2 Mitochondrial DNA expression

Jan-Willem Taanman

Introduction

In vertebrates, the mitochondrial genome consists of double-stranded, covalently-closed DNA molecules that are present as multiple copies per mitochondrion. The two strands of DNA can be distinguished on the basis of G + T base composition, which results in different buoyant densities of each strand ('heavy' and 'light') in an isopycnic gradient. In metabolically active vertebrate cells, a ~1-kb non-coding region of a large fraction of the mitochondrial DNA (mtDNA) molecules contains a triplex structure, in which a short (7S) DNA strand complementary to the light (L) strand displaces the heavy (H) strand. This region, which is flanked by the genes for the transfer RNAs (tRNAs) tRNA^Phe and tRNA^Pro, is called the displacement loop or D-loop region and is the least conserved part of mitochondrial genomes. It has evolved as the major control site for both replication and transcription. Mammalian mtDNA shows exceptional economy of organization. A map of human mtDNA is shown in Fig. 2.1. The genes are closely packed and lack introns. Except for the D-loop region, intergenic sequences are absent or limited to a few bases and some genes even overlap. Furthermore, the tRNA and rRNA molecules are unusually small[1] and in most protein genes part of the termination codon is generated post-transcriptionally by polyadenylation of messenger RNA.[2]

Soon after the first mtDNA sequences became available, comparisons with mitochondrial protein sequences revealed deviations from the standard genetic code. In mammals, TGA is used as a tryptophan codon rather than as a termination codon, whereas AGR (R = A, G) specifies a stop instead of arginine and AUA codes for methionine instead of isoleucine.[3] A modified tRNA wobble base interaction with mRNA codons allows mitochondria to translate all codons with less than the 32 tRNA species required according to Crick's wobble hypothesis. Mitochondrial tRNAs with uridine in the first (wobble) position of the anticodon read all four codons of the four-codon families,[3,4] whereas those containing a chemically modified uridine read both codons of two-codon families with a purine in the third position.[5–7] The methionine codons AUG and AUA of mammalian mitochondria, however, are recognized by a single anticodon, which has 5-formylcytidine in the wobble position.[8] The tRNA carrying this anticodon is thought to be charged either with *N*-formylmethionine to function as initiator of mitochondrial protein synthesis[9] or with methionine for elongation of the polypeptide chain. Two-codon families with a pyrimidine in the third position are decoded by tRNAs with an unmodified guanidine in the wobble position. The altered wobble rules would imply that 23 tRNA species are required to decode mtDNA, however, as mentioned above, in mammals AGR codons indicate a stop and the corresponding tRNA is absent. Hence, the 22 tRNA species encoded by mammalian mtDNA are sufficient to translate all 13 mitochondrial proteins. An overview of the codons and anticodons of mammalian mitochondria is given in Fig. 2.2.

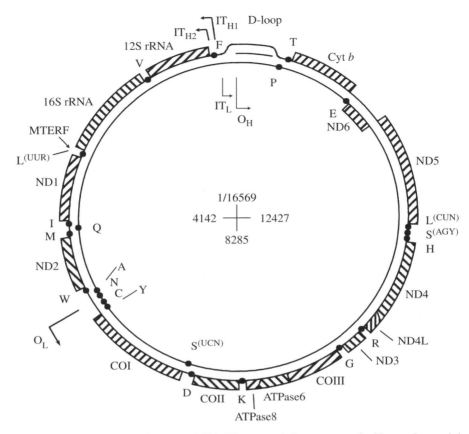

Fig. 2.1 Map of the 16,569-bp human mtDNA. The outer circle represents the H-strand, containing the majority of genes; the inner circle represents the L-strand. The control region (D-loop) is shown as a three-stranded structure. The origins of H-strand (O_H) and L-strand (O_L) replication and the direction of DNA synthesis are indicated by long bent arrows; initiation of transcription sites (IT_L, IT_{H1}, IT_{H2}) and the direction of RNA synthesis are denoted by short arrows. The binding site for the mitochondrial transcription terminator (MTERF) is indicated. The 22 tRNA genes are depicted by dots and the single letter code of the amino acids (isoacceptors for serine and leucine are distinguished by their codon sequence). The genes for the two rRNA species (12S and 16S) and the 13 protein-coding genes are shown as shaded boxes. *ND*, *CO*, and *ATPase* refer to genes coding for subunits of NADH : ubiquinone oxidoreductase, ferrocytochrome-*c* : oxygen oxidoreductase (cytochrome-*c* oxidase), and F_1F_0–ATP synthase, respectively, and Cyt *b* encodes apocytochrome-*b* of ubiquinol : ferricytochrome-*c* oxidoreductase. (Adapted from Ref. [13] with permission.)

Despite having their own genome, mitochondria are not self-supporting entities in the cell. Of the mammalian mitochondrial proteome, only 13 protein subunits of the oxidative phosphorylation complexes are encoded on mtDNA. All other mitochondrial proteins are nuclear-encoded, synthesized in the cytosol (usually as precursors containing an N-terminal presequence for mitochondrial targeting) and are subsequently imported into the organelle. Thus, although mammalian mtDNA contains the genes for a full set of tRNAs and the two

Codon	Anticodon (Amino acid)	Codon	Anticodon (Amino acid)	Codon	Anticodon (Amino acid)	Codon	Anticodon (Amino acid)
UUU	GAA (Phe)	UCU		UAU	GUA (Tyr)	UGU	GCA (Cys)
UUC		UCC		UAC		UGC	
UUA	U*AA (Leu)	UCA	UGA (Ser)	UAA	— (Stop)	UGA	U*CA (Trp)
UUG		UCG		UAG		UGG	
CUU		CCU		CAU	GUG (His)	CGU	
CUC	UAG (Leu)	CCC	UGG (Pro)	CAC		CGC	UCG (Arg)
CUA		CCA		CAA	U*UG (Gln)	CGA	
CUG		CCG		CAG		CGG	
AUU	GAU (Ile)	ACU		AAU	GUU (Asn)	AGU	GCU (Ser)
AUC		ACC	UGU (Thr)	AAC		AGC	
AUA	C*AU (Met)	ACA		AAA	U*UU (Lys)	AGA	— (Stop)
AUG		ACG		AAG		AGG	
GUU		GCU		GAU	GUC (Asp)	GGU	
GUC	UAC (Val)	GCC	UGC (Ala)	GAC		GGC	UCC (Gly)
GUA		GCA		GAA	U*UC (Glu)	GGA	
GUG		GCG		GAG		GGG	

Fig. 2.2 Codons (5′–3′) and anticodons (5′–3′) in mammalian mitochondria. Chemically modified nucleotides in the first (wobble) position of the anticodon are marked with an asterisk.

rRNAs, mitochondrial tRNAs are charged by nuclear-encoded aminoacyl-tRNA synthases and all mammalian mitochondrial ribosomal proteins are imported. Likewise, mtDNA transcription relies on nuclear-encoded factors. How these hybrid mitochondrial transcription and translation systems function is reviewed below.

Transcription of mtDNA

Initiation of transcription

In the 1980s, mainly through the efforts of the laboratories of Attardi and Clayton, the basic mechanism of mitochondrial transcription was solved (reviewed in[10–13]). Human mtDNA transcription start sites and promoter regions were mapped using a variety of techniques. All available data are consistent with the conclusion that there are two major initiation of transcription sites (IT_{H1} and IT_L) situated within 150 bp of one another in the major non-coding region (Fig. 2.3). A promoter element with a pentadecamer consensus sequence motif, 5'-CANACC(G)CC(A)AAAGAYA-3' (N = A, C, G, T; Y = C, T), encompasses the transcription initiation sites (underlined) and is critical for transcription. H-strand transcription starts at nucleotide position 561 (IT_{H1}; numbering according to[14]) located within the H-strand promoter (HSP), whereas the L-strand transcription starts at nucleotide position 407 (IT_L) located within the L-strand promoter (LSP). Enhancer elements located just upstream of the promoter regions are required for optimal transcription (Fig. 2.3). These elements, which were later shown to be binding sites for a transcription factor (mtTFA), exhibit sequence similarity, but only if one element is inverted relative to the other. This suggests that these *cis*-acting enhancers are able to function bidirectionally. Despite their close proximity, IT_{H1} and IT_L are functionally independent. A second putative initiation site for H-strand transcription (IT_{H2}) is located around nucleotide position 638 in the tRNA^{Phe} gene (Fig. 2.3). Its promoter region only shows limited similarity with the pentadecamer consensus sequence and IT_{H2} is thought to be used less frequently for transcription of the H-strand than IT_{H1}.

The RNA polymerase that binds to the HSP and LSP is relatively non-selective in its interaction with DNA. The enzyme has not been purified to homogeneity. Nevertheless, a cDNA predicted to encode the 1230-amino acid residue precursor of human mitochondrial RNA polymerase has been identified by screening of the human Expressed Sequence Tag database (dbEST) with the yeast sequence.[15] The human gene (*POLRMT*) has been mapped to chromosome 19p13.3.[15] Mitochondrial RNA polymerases are homologous to the single subunit

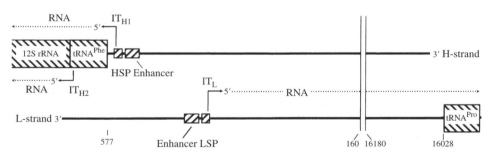

Fig. 2.3 Schematic representation of the initiation of transcription of human mtDNA. The genes encoding 12S rRNA, tRNA^{Phe}, and tRNA^{Pro} are indicated with shaded boxes on the H- and L-strand. Transcription initiation sites and direction of synthesis are indicated by bent arrows, dotted lines represent synthesized RNA. In the D-loop region (the 1118-bp sequence between nucleotides 577 and 16,028), two major transcription initiation sites are present. Initiation of transcription site IT_{H1}, encompassed by the H-strand promoter (HSP), directs the transcription of the H-strand, whereas initiation of transcription site IT_L, encompassed by the L-strand promoter (LSP), directs the transcription of the L-strand. A second, minor initiation of transcription site (IT_{H2}) for H-strand transcription is located in the gene for tRNA^{Phe}, near the boundary with the 12S rRNA gene. Enhancer elements upstream of the HSP and LSP that are known to bind the mitochondrial transcription factor A are indicated. (Adapted from Ref. [13] with permission.)

RNA polymerases of T3, T7, and SP6 bacteriophages, though the amino acid similarity is restricted to the C-terminal half of the mitochondrial enzyme.[15,16] Structural and mutation studies have indicated that this evolutionarily conserved region is important for promoter selectivity and polymerase activity.[17] Recent deletion mutation experiments in yeast suggested that the N-terminal half of mitochondrial RNA polymerases harbour a functional domain, distinct from the polymerase activity, which appears to be required for mtDNA maintenance.[18]

Mitochondrial transcription factor A (mtTFA, also known as TFAM, TCF6, or mtTF1) is an abundant 25-kDa protein that confers promoter selectivity on the polymerase. Human mtTFA has been purified,[19] its cDNA has been cloned[20] and its gene (*TFAM*) assigned to chromosome 10q21.[21] The protein comprises two high mobility group (HMG) domains, separated by a 27-amino acid residue linker and followed by a 25-amino acid residue C-terminal tail. The HMG boxes are DNA binding motifs that are shared with abundant non-histone components of chromatin and with specific regulators of nuclear transcription.[22] The factor binds to the enhancer regions located 12–39 bp upstream of the respective transcription initiation sites, IT_{H1} and IT_L[19,23,24] (Fig. 2.3). Binding at these sites is required for accurate and efficient initiation of transcription. Mutation analysis of mtTFA has indicated that its basic C-terminal tail is important for specific DNA recognition and is essential for high levels of transcription.[25] Both major promoters in human mitochondria are able to function bidirectionally.[26] The asymmetric binding of mtTFA relative to the transcription start site may ensure that transcription proceeds primarily in a unidirectional fashion (Fig. 2.3). Common with many other members of the HMG family of proteins, mtTFA has the capacity to bend and unwind the DNA duplex and to wrap around the distorted DNA strands.[27,28] These mtTFA-induced conformational changes at the promoter sites may facilitate access of the core RNA polymerase to the template for initiation of transcription.

In addition to being a pivotal component of the basal mitochondrial transcription apparatus, mtTFA appears to have an important function in maintenance of mtDNA. Levels of mtTFA vary concomitantly with levels of mtDNA (reviewed in[13,29]). Binding of mtTFA is not restricted to the enhancer elements upstream of the HSP and LSP. The factor is inherently flexible in its recognition of mtDNA sequences[23,27] and is likely to be involved in the formation of various nucleoprotein complexes or even packaging of the entire mtDNA molecule. Heterozygous mtTFA knockout mice exhibit decreased mtDNA levels, whereas homozygous knockout embryos are devoid of mtDNA and die.[30] The depletion of mtDNA in these mice may be caused by the lack of RNA primers that initiate mtDNA replication[10,13,29] or a failure of the mtDNA molecules to adopt their higher-order structure, or both.

Attempts to reconstitute human mtDNA transcription with recombinant mitochondrial RNA polymerase and mtTFA have failed,[31,32] suggesting that at least one additional *trans*-acting factor is necessary. The unsuccessful reconstitution experiments have prompted database searches for human sequences showing homology with a mitochondrial transcription factor cloned in yeast.[33] These screenings resulted in the identification of two additional human mitochondrial transcription factors, mtTFB1 and mtTFB2.[34,35] The genes for mtTFB1 and mtTFB2 (*TFB1M* and *TFB2M*) have been assigned to chromosomes 6q25.1–q25.3 and 1q44, respectively. Both genes show virtually identical patterns of transcription by Northern blot analysis,[35] suggesting co-expression of mtTFB1 and mtTFB2. Nevertheless, each factor on its own can support HSP- and LSP-specific transcription in a pure recombinant *in vitro* system, containing mitochondrial RNA polymerase and mtTFA.[35] Both ~40-kDa factors interact directly with the polymerase, but mtTFB2 is at least tenfold more active in promoting transcription than mtTFB1.[35] Primary sequence comparisons and crystallography data have revealed that the mtTFB class of transcription factors are related to a superfamily of RNA adenine methyl-transferases.[34–36] Remarkably, mtTFB1 has the ability to bind *S*-adenosylmethionine *in vitro*,[34] suggesting that perhaps a functional relationship exists between mtTFBs and this family of RNA modification enzymes.

Elongation and termination of transcription

The L-strand is transcribed as a single polycistronic precursor.[37] Although the HSP can direct transcription of the entire H-strand in a similar fashion, a more complicated model has been postulated by Attardi and co-workers.[38] Exponentially growing HeLa cells synthesize the two mitochondrial rRNA species at a much higher rate than the mRNAs encoded on the H-strand.[39] Attardi and co-workers explain this difference in part by the existence of two functionally distinct transcription events, each starting at a different initiation site for H-strand transcription.[40] According to their dual H-strand transcription initiation model, transcription starts relatively frequent at IT_{H1} (Fig. 2.3) and then terminates at the 3′-end of the 16S rRNA gene (Fig. 2.1). This transcription process is thought to be responsible for synthesis of the bulk of the mitochondrial rRNAs, tRNA^{Phe}, and tRNA^{Val}. In contrast, transcription starting at IT_{H2} (Fig. 2.3) occurs less often, but results in a polycistronic molecule that includes all coding sequences of the H-strand. The existence of two individually controlled, overlapping H-strand transcription units is supported by the findings that ethidium bromide and ATP can modulate the relative H-strand transcription rates of rRNA and mRNA independently.[41,42] Consistent with these observations, ethidium bromide and ATP-dependent modifications in protein–DNA footprints have been revealed upstream of IT_{H1}, which correlate with changes in the rate of rRNA synthesis, but not of mRNA synthesis.[24] Furthermore, a protein–DNA interaction site has been identified upstream of IT_{H2}[24] that could represent the initiation complex. It is, however, not clear how two initiation events occurring less than 100 bp apart can determine the fate of RNA synthesis at the 3′-end of the 16S rRNA gene, more than 2500 nucleotides downstream.

The higher synthesis rate of rRNA compared to mRNA is further explained by an attenuation event at the 16S rRNA/tRNA$^{Leu(UUR)}$ gene boundary. The first indication of early termination of H-strand transcription came from S1 nuclease protection analysis of the 3′-ends of mammalian 16S rRNA molecules.[43,44] These mapping studies revealed that the genomic location of the last template-encoded nucleotide of the majority of 16S rRNA molecules corresponded to the nucleotide immediately adjacent to the 5′-end of the tRNA$^{Leu(UUR)}$ gene, whereas the last nucleotide of the minor types mapped to any position up to 7 nucleotides downstream in the tRNA$^{Leu(UUR)}$ gene sequence. These ragged ends suggest that mature 16S rRNA species are produced by accurate endonucleolytic cleavage of a longer RNA precursor, or by imprecise transcript termination within the tRNA$^{Leu(UUR)}$ gene. Subsequently, a crude protein fraction was isolated from mitochondrial HeLa cell lysates, which in DNase I footprinting studies protected the region immediately downstream of the mtDNA sequence corresponding to *in vivo* produced 3′-ends of 16S rRNA molecules and promoted specific termination of transcription.[45] The footprint comprises a conserved tridecamer sequence motif 5′-TGGCAGAGCCCGG-3′ (L-strand), located within the tRNA$^{Leu(UUR)}$ gene. *In vitro* mutagenesis and transcription experiments have shown that this sequence element is essential and sufficient for directing termination of transcription.[46–48]

The groups of Clayton and Attardi have shown that the mitochondrial protein fraction mediating attenuation of transcription contains polypeptides of around 34 kDa.[47,49] The human cDNA specifying the major polypeptide from this fraction has been cloned[50] and the gene (*MTERF*) has been mapped to chromosome 7q21–q22. This mitochondrial transcription termination factor, termed MTERF[45] or mtTERM,[47] contains three leucine zipper motifs bracketed by two basic domains that are all critical for its specific DNA-binding capacity.[50] The footprint produced by the recombinant protein is similar, but not identical to that produced by the ~34-kDa polypeptide fraction and the recombinant protein is not sufficient to terminate transcription *in vitro*.[50] These observations suggest that an additional component of the ~34-kDa polypeptide fraction is needed for termination activity. The apparent complexity of this system is not surprising, given that it should be able to modulate its activity in response to the cellular demand for mitochondrial rRNAs on one hand, and for mitochondrial tRNAs and mRNAs on the other.

Interestingly, *in vitro* transcription assays with the ~34-kDa fraction have demonstrated that the MTERF-containing complex bound to its mtDNA target site functions bidirectionally and shows an even greater efficiency of termination in the reverse orientation relative to the promoter site.[51] Thus, in addition to an attenuation function for H-strand transcription, the protein complex may halt L-strand transcription at a site where no L-strand-encoded genes are present downstream (Fig. 2.1). The complex induces bending of DNA.[48] It probably stops elongation of transcription by constituting a physical barrier, rather than by a specific interaction with the mitochondrial RNA polymerase, because the complex also mediates termination of transcription by heterologous RNA polymerases.[48]

Processing of primary transcripts

After the RNA polymerase has passed the border region of the 16S rRNA and tRNA$^{Leu(UUR)}$ genes, H-strand transcription appears to be straightforward and is assumed to result in transcription of the entire H-strand.[37] The two rRNA and most of the mRNA coding sequences are immediately contiguous to tRNA sequences (Fig. 2.1). This remarkable genetic arrangement has led to the proposal that the secondary structure of the tRNA sequences function as punctuation marks in the reading of the mtDNA information.[2] Precise endoribonucleolytic excision of the tRNAs from the nascent transcript will concomitantly yield correctly processed rRNAs and, in most cases, correctly processed mRNAs.[2,52] In those cases in which a mRNA terminus cannot be accounted for by tRNA excision, the endoribonuclease may recognize a secondary RNA structure at the border that shares critical features with the cloverleaf configuration of a tRNA.

Excision of mitochondrial tRNAs involves two enzymatic activities. Cleavage at the 5′-end is performed by a mitochondrial RNase P (mtRNase P), which recognizes the secondary structure of tRNA sequences in the nascent RNA. The nuclear and eubacterial counterparts of this enzyme are ribonucleoproteins, but the most extensively studied chloroplast RNase P (from spinach) appears to be composed exclusively of protein.[53] Yeast mtRNase P is comprised of a nuclear-encoded protein and a mtDNA-encoded RNA species.[54,55] The composition of mammalian mtRNase P is controversial. Rossmanith and colleagues claim that mtRNase P in HeLa cells is a protein enzyme,[56,57] whereas Attardi and colleagues claim it is a ribonucleoprotein.[58,59] A mtRNase P with similar properties as the enzyme described by Attardi's group has also been reported to occur in rat liver mitochondria.[60] Attardi's group has shown that mtRNase P from extensively purified HeLa cell mitochondria is a particle with a sedimentation constant of ~17S and, surprisingly, that its 340-nucleotide RNA component is identical in sequence to the H1 RNA component of nuclear RNase P.[59] No information is currently available concerning the protein composition of mammalian mtRNase P.

Nuclear RNase P, which has a similar sedimentation constant as mtRNase P, contains at least seven protein subunits.[61] The nuclear RNase P complex is structurally and functionally related to another RNase, the RNase MRP (mitochondrial RNA processing) complex. Although the two ribozymes have a different RNA moiety, the RNA can be folded into a similar secondary structure.[61] Moreover, nuclear RNase P and RNase MRP share most, if not all, of their protein subunits.[61] RNase MRP has been implicated in 5′-end formation of 5.8S rRNA in the nucleoli, as well as the 5′-end formation of L-strand transcripts that function as primers for H-strand replication in mitochondria.[13,29,61] It is tempting to speculate that mammalian mtRNase P has not only its RNA moiety in common with nuclear RNase P, but also shares some protein subunits with nuclear RNase P and RNase MRP.

Activity of the endoribonuclease catalysing cleavage at the 3′-end of mitochondrial tRNAs has been identified in *in vitro* assays of HeLa cell and rat liver mitochondrial extracts,[56,60,62] but the enzyme's low abundance has hampered its structural characterization. The assays have demonstrated that sequences downstream of the cleavage site are critical for recognition by the 3′-tRNA precursor-processing endonuclease.[62] The enzyme exhibits no detectable activity with intact pre-tRNAs as substrate, but does convert 5′-processed intermediates to mature tRNAs,[56,60,62] suggesting that processing of the 5′-end precedes processing of the 3′-end. The mammalian mitochondrial tRNA$^{Ser(AGY)}$ gene is directly flanked by the genes for tRNA^{His} and tRNA$^{Leu(CUN)}$ (Fig. 2.1). *In vitro* examination of the processing pathway of tRNA$^{Ser(AGY)}$ has suggested that mtRNase P and mitochondrial 3′-tRNA precursor-processing endonuclease recognize only the tRNA^{His} and tRNA$^{Leu(CUN)}$ structures in the precursor molecule and excise these two flanking tRNAs, thereby, as a consequence, releasing the enclosed tRNA$^{Ser(AGY)}$.[63]

Some mammalian mitochondrial tRNA genes seem to overlap. For instance, the human gene for tRNA^{Tyr} seems to share an A residue with the downstream gene for tRNA^{Cys}, such that this nucleotide potentially represents not only the first base of tRNA^{Cys}, but also the discriminator nucleotide of tRNA^{Tyr}. *In vitro* assays with a HeLa cell mitochondrial extract and runoff tRNA^{Tyr}/tRNA^{Cys} precursors as substrate have revealed that tRNA^{Cys} is released in its complete form, whereas tRNA^{Tyr} lacks the nucleotide at the discriminator position.[64] Experiments in which tRNA^{Cys} was partially deleted or completely replaced have indicated that the cleavage reaction represents the activity of the mitochondrial 3′-tRNA precursor-processing endonuclease recognizing the upstream tRNA^{Tyr}.[64] The truncated 3′-end of this tRNA^{Tyr} is then completed in an editing reaction that adds the missing adenyl residue.[64,65]

Post-transcriptional modifications

Several bases of the excised tRNAs are subject to chemical modification.[1,66] This will require the activity of imported enzymes, which have yet to be characterized. The base modifications are important for cloverleaf folding,[67] efficient aminoacylation[68] and proper codon recognition.[5–7] Maturation of the tRNAs is completed by addition of the sequence CCA to their 3′-termini,[56] necessary for the attachment of the amino acid. The CCA-adding enzyme (ATP (CTP)-tRNA-specific nucleotidyltransferase or MtCCA) has been partly purified from bovine liver mitochondria and the protein has been identified by mass spectrometry.[69] Subsequently, the human and murine cDNA sequences have been determined by dbEST searches.[69] The calculated molecular mass of the mature protein is ~47 kDa. The human gene, *MtCCA*, is located on chromosome 3p25.1.[69]

Processing of the polycistronic transcripts on the 5'-side of each tRNA sequence by mtRNase P makes the 3'-ends of the upstream mRNA or rRNA available for adenylation.[2] 12S rRNA is mono-adenylated, while 16S rRNA is polyadenylated by up to 10 residues.[43,44] Messengers carry poly(A) tails of ~55 residues.[70] Adenylation is likely to stabilize the transcripts. A poly(A) polymerizing activity has been identified in rat and bovine mitochondrial extracts.[69,71] Purification of the rat enzyme yielded a protein of 60 kDa,[71] but purification of the bovine enzyme has failed so far, due to instability of the protein.[69] Unlike nuclear mRNAs, mitochondrial mRNAs do not have upstream polyadenylation signals, suggesting that the recognition of the messenger by the mitochondrial poly(A) polymerase is fundamentally different.

The charging of mitochondrial tRNAs with their cognate amino acids is catalysed by nuclear-encoded mitochondrial aminoacyl-tRNA synthetases that are specific for each particular tRNA. Several human mitochondrial aminoacyl-tRNA synthetases have now been cloned and biochemically characterized.[72–76] These studies indicate that although mitochondrial aminoacyl-tRNA synthetases show a high degree of homology to the corresponding bacterial enzymes, there are some striking structural differences. For instance, prokaryotic as well as (eukaryotic) cytosolic phenylalanyl-tRNA synthetases have an $\alpha_2\beta_2$ tetramer structure, whereas their mitochondrial equivalent is a monomer containing three sequence motifs that normally reside in the α subunit and one motif that is commonly present in the β subunit.[72]

The mammalian mitochondrial translation system utilizes two tRNA^{Ser} species, one specific for codons AGY and the other for UCN. In addition, two tRNA^{Leu} species are used, one specific for codons UUR and the other for CUN (Fig. 2.2). Mitochondrial leucyl-tRNA synthetases have not been studied in detail, but tRNA recognition studies of mammalian mitochondrial seryl-tRNA synthetase have demonstrated that a single enzyme is responsible for serylation of both tRNA^{Ser} species.[75,76] This is remarkable, because the two tRNA^{Ser} isoacceptors share no common sequence motifs and are topologically quite distinct, with tRNA$^{Ser(AGY)}$ lacking the entire arm with the dihydrouridine loop.[1]

In order to function as the initiator tRNA during protein synthesis, a fraction of the mitochondrial methionyl-tRNAs pool is converted to *N*-formylmethionyl-tRNA. This is achieved by mitochondrial methionyl-tRNA transformylase. Bovine methionyl-tRNA transformylase has been cloned and characterized.[77] In contrast to *Escherichia coli* methionyl-tRNA transformylase, which uses the C^1A^{72} mismatch in acceptor stem of the RNA moiety as identity element, the 40-kDa bovine enzyme appears to use the aminoacyl moiety for substrate recognition.[78] This may prevent the formylation of other mitochondrial aminoacyl-tRNAs, which share structural features with the acceptor stem of methionyl-tRNA^{Met}.

Mitochondrial protein synthesis

Mitochondrial ribosomes

Mitochondrial ribosomes reside in the matrix of the organelle. In mammals, about half of the ribosomes are associated with the inner mitochondrial membrane.[79] Mitochondrial ribosomes are considered to be prokaryotic in nature for a number of reasons. First, the spectrum of antibiotics inhibiting mitochondrial protein synthesis resembles that of bacteria.[80] Second, mitochondrial ribosomes use *N*-formylmethionyl-tRNA for polypeptide chain initiation.[9] Third, mitochondrial translation initiation and elongation factors are also functional on bacterial ribosomes *in vitro*.[81–84] Nevertheless, the physiochemical properties of mitochondrial ribosomes differ not only considerably from their cytosolic, but also from their bacterial counterparts. Mammalian mitochondrial ribosomes have a remarkably low RNA content, resulting in a low sedimentation coefficient of ~55S.[85–88] The ~39S and ~28S ribosomal subunits contain respectively, the 16S and the 12S rRNA species encoded by mtDNA.[85,86] No 5S rRNA has been detected in animal mitochondrial ribosomes,[85,86] even though this ~120-nucleotide RNA is present in all prokaryotic, chloroplast, and cytosolic ribosomes, as well as mitochondrial ribosomes of higher plants and some algae, where it is encoded by mtDNA.[89] Notwithstanding this, nuclear-encoded 5S rRNA has been found to be tightly associated with highly purified mitochondrial fractions of mammalian cells.[90,91] The number of mitochondrially imported 5S rRNA molecules appears to be comparable with the predicted average number of ribosomes per organelle.[92] Although this does not prove that 5S rRNA is part of the mitochondrial ribosome, the relatively high number of 5S rRNA molecules associated with mitochondria is intriguing. Despite the fact that isolated mitochondria faithfully carry out protein synthesis, an *in vitro* mitochondrial translation system, using only mitochondrial extracts, is not available. Although isolated mitochondrial ribosomes show poly(U)-directed, phenylalanine polymerizing activity,[93] polymerizing activity directed by natural mRNAs has never been demonstrated. In view of these findings, a functional role for nuclear-encoded 5S rRNA in mammalian mitochondrial ribosomes cannot be discounted.

The apparent low RNA content of mammalian mitochondrial ribosomes is compensated by a relatively high protein content and results in a total mass of mitochondrial ribosomes which is higher than that of bacterial ribosomes.[93] Recent progress in protein analysis techniques and genome sequencing has allowed the identification of most, if not all, human mitochondrial ribosomal protein (MRP) sequences.[94–97] The majority of the human MRP genes have been mapped.[98] There are 29 distinct proteins in the small ribosomal subunit the nomenclature of which is discussed by Koc *et al.*[94] Fourteen of these are homologous to proteins of the *E. coli* small ribosomal subunit. The other 15 proteins have no apparent homologues in prokaryotic, chloroplast, or cytosolic ribosomes, but are unique to mitochondrial ribosomes. The human large mitochondrial ribosomal subunit contains 48 different proteins the nomenclature of which is also discussed by Koc *et al.*[97] Twenty-eight of these are homologous to proteins of the *E. coli* large ribosomal subunit, while the remaining 20 proteins are specific to mitochondrial ribosomes. Surprisingly, three sequence variants have been found for one of the proteins of the small mitochondrial ribosomal subunit, MRP-S18.[94] In analogy to bacterial ribosomes, it is likely that each mitochondrial ribosome contains a single copy of MRP-S18. Therefore, the presence of three MRP-S18 isoforms suggests that there is a heterogeneous population of mitochondrial ribosomes, which may have different decoding properties. Another surprising finding is that two proteins of the small ribosomal subunit, MRP-S29 and MRP-S30, were earlier identified as the pro-apoptotic proteins DAP3 and PDCD, respectively.[96,99] These observations implicate mitochondrial ribosomes as a major component in cellular apoptotic signalling pathways.

Initiation of translation

Mammalian mitochondrial mRNAs are devoid of significant upstream untranslated regions[52] and lack a 7-methylguanylate cap structure at their 5′-end.[100] Consequently, unlike prokaryotic messengers, mitochondrial messengers have no leader sequences to facilitate ribosome binding, and a cap recognition and scanning mechanism for directing the ribosome to the initiator codon, as used by cytosolic ribosomes, is also ruled out. The low mitochondrial translation efficiency[101] may in fact be the result of the absence of a 5′-end ribosome recognition site and necessitate the observed abundance of mitochondrial mRNAs compared to nuclear mRNAs,[102,103] to ensure a sufficient level of translation.

In vitro experiments with bovine mitochondrial ribosomes have demonstrated that, in contrast to prokaryotic and cytosolic small ribosomal subunits, the small mitochondrial ribosomal subunit has the ability to bind mRNA tightly in a sequence independent fashion and in the apparent absence of auxiliary initiation factors or initiating *N*-formylmethionyl-tRNA.[104] As judged from the size of the mRNA fragment protected from RNase T_1 digestion, the principal interaction between the small subunit and the RNA takes place over a 30–80-nucleotide stretch,[105,106] but ~400 nucleotides are minimally required for efficient binding.[106] This may explain why the two shortest open reading frames of mammalian mtDNA, *ATPase8* and *ND4L* (<300 nucleotides), are both part of overlapping genes, *ATPase8/ATPase6* and *ND4L/ND4* (Fig. 2.1). Both pairs of overlapping genes result in dicistronic transcripts. Monocistronic messages of *ATPase8* and *ND4L* are possibly too short to interact effectively with the small ribosomal subunit.

Once the small ribosomal subunit is bound to the template mRNA, the subunit is assumed to move towards the initiation codon, mediated by as yet unspecified auxiliary factors.[105] Mitochondrial protein synthesis is considered to follow the classical model of protein synthesis, as described for *E. coli*. Thus, during the first step of mitochondrial protein synthesis, the initiator tRNA will bind to the peptidyl (P) site on the ribosome, while the two other sites for tRNA molecules, the aminoacyl (A) site and the exit (E) site, remain empty. The only initiation factor identified in mammalian mitochondria to date is mitochondrial translation initiation factor 2 (mtIF-2).[82,107] It is a monomeric protein with a molecular mass of ~78 kDa. The cDNA sequence for human mtIF-2 has been determined[108] and the gene (*MTIF2*) has been mapped to chromosome 2p16–p14.[109] Mammalian mtIF-2 is homologous to prokaryotic IF-2 and belongs to the family of GTPases that are molecular switches capable of alternating between an active (mtIF-2 · GTP) and an inactive (mtIF-2 · GDP) conformation. Reminiscent of its bacterial equivalent, mtIF-2 promotes binding of *N*-formylmethionyl-tRNA to the small ribosomal subunit in a GTP and mRNA-dependent reaction. Detailed *in vitro* characterization of bovine mtIF-2 has suggested that mtIF-2 may bind to the small ribosomal subunit prior to its interaction with GTP, but GTP enhances the affinity between mtIF-2 and the small (26S) subunit, and allows *N*-formylmethionyl-tRNA to join the complex.[84,107] Hydrolysis of GTP is thought to facilitate the release of mtIF-2 and the concomitant association of the large (39S) ribosomal subunit to form the 55S initiation complex. GTP hydrolysis appears, however, not to be strictly required for subunit association, because non-hydrolysable analogues of GTP can still promote formation of the initiation complex.[107]

Elongation of translation

The mitochondrial elongation factors (mtEFs) are homologous to the three elongation factors, EF–Tu, EF–Ts and EF–G, found in *E. coli*. All three have been purified from bovine liver mitochondria[81,83] and their cDNAs have been cloned from various mammalian sources, including human.[110–114] The molecular mass of mature human mtEF-Tu is 43 kDa, while that of mtEF-Ts is 31 kDa. The genes for human mtEF-Tu (*TUFM*) and mtEF-Ts (*TSFM*) have been assigned to chromosomes 16p11.2 and 12q13–q14, respectively.[112,115] Interestingly, two human genes and corresponding cDNA sequences have been identified for mtEF-G, gene *EFG*1 located on chromosome 3q35.1–q26.2 and gene *EFG*2 located on chromosome 5q13.[114] The two genes are phylogenetically conserved through evolution.[114] The amino acid sequence identity between the two human ~80-kDa isoforms is only 33 per cent, but some domains are highly conserved. Comparison of Northern blot hybridization results[113,114] suggests that mtEF-G1 and mtEF-G2 are co-expressed in all tissues rather than specifically expressed in different tissues. These data point to complementary roles of mtEF-G1 and mtEF-G2 during elongation of the polypeptide chain.

In *E. coli*, EF–Tu promotes the codon-dependent placement of aminoacyl-tRNA at the A-site of the ribosome. This process requires the formation of the ternary complex, aminoacyl-tRNA · EF-Tu · GTP. After positioning of the correct aminoacyl-tRNA at the A-site, GTP is hydrolysed and EF-Tu · GDP leaves the ribosome. The nucleotide exchange factor, EF-Ts, displaces GDP and is in turn replaced by GTP to form EF-Tu · GTP, which is able to start another round of elongation. Following peptide bond formation catalysed by the large ribosomal subunit, the third factor, EF-G, drives the translocation of the tRNAs at the A and P sites of the ribosome to the P and E sites, respectively. Concomitantly, the mRNA is moved to expose the next codon to the A site. During the last step of the elongation cycle, the deacylated tRNA at the E site is released from the ribosome. Similar to EF-Tu, EF-G is a GTPase that undergoes a cycle in which it alternates between an active state when bound to GTP and an inactive state when bound to GDP.[116]

Although the main features of the elongation cycle in mammalian mitochondria are thought to be similar to those of *E. coli*, there are subtle differences in the manner in which the mtEF-Tu interacts with other components of the translation machinery. A binary complex of mtEF-Tu with its nucleotide exchange factor has been isolated from bovine liver mitochondria.[81] This mtEF-Tu · Ts complex is very stable and, unlike its bacterial equivalent, cannot easily be dissociated by guanine nucleotides.[81] Under experimental conditions, however, the mtEF-Tu · Ts complex will dissociate in the presence of GTP and phenylalanyl-tRNA, resulting in a ternary complex similar to that observed in *E. coli*.[117] Careful evaluation of the equilibrium dissociation constants of bovine mtEF-Tu with its ligands have indicated that the K_{GDP} as well as the K_{GTP} for mtEF-Tu are about two orders of magnitude higher than the dissociation constants of the corresponding complexes formed by *E. coli* EF-Tu.[118] The K_{tRNA} and K_{Ts} for the aminoacyl-tRNA · mtEF-Tu · Ts complex are sixteen-fold and three-fold higher, respectively, than those of the bacterial complex.[119] Even though some dissociation constants governing the elongation cycle are strikingly different in mammalian mitochondria and in *E. coli*, when the concentrations of the various components under *in vivo* conditions are taken into account, calculations indicate that the ternary complex will be the major form of (mt)EF-Tu in both systems.[119] Thus, the bacterial as well as the mitochondrial system appear to be designed to operate under conditions in which the ternary complex is readily available for the translation process.

Resolution of the crystal structure of bovine mtEF-Tu · GDP at 1.94 Å has revealed that the residues of mtEF-Tu directly involved in contacts to GDP are almost identical to those of *E. coli* EF-Tu[120] and are, therefore, unlikely to be responsible for the large difference in affinity for the ligand. The decrease in affinity may, however, be due to an increased mobility of parts of mtEF-Tu around the binding site. The X-ray diffraction data have further indicated that the C-terminal extension of mtEF-Tu, which is not present in bacterial EF-Tu, has structural similarities with DNA recognizing zinc fingers.[120] This suggests that the extension may be involved in RNA binding.

Termination of translation

Termination of protein synthesis requires the action of several auxiliary factors, termed release factors. In *E. coli*, release factor RF1 recognizes the stop codons UAA and UAG, while RF2 recognizes the stop codons UAA and UGA. A third factor, RF3, boosts the activities of RF1 and RF2. Binding of RF1 or RF2 to a stop codon at the A site results in hydrolysis of the bond between the polypeptide chain and the tRNA at the P site. The detached polypeptide leaves the ribosome, followed by the tRNA. mRNA release is mediated by a fourth factor, the ribosome recycling factor (RRF or RF4). Subsequently, the two subunits of the ribosome disassemble and the small ribosomal subunit is set to start a new round of protein synthesis.[121,122]

To date, the organellar equivalents of two release factors have been identified, but biochemical characterization of these factors has been limited. A single release factor of ~39 kDa has been isolated and partially purified from rat mitochondria.[123] It recognizes codons UAA and UAG, but not UGA (which serves as a codon for tryptophan in mammalian mitochondria; Fig. 2.2). Therefore, the factor has been called mtRF-1. Rat mtRF-1 does not recognize the codons AGG or AGA, which are used as terminators in human mitochondria.[14] Rat mitochondria, however, only employ UAA as terminator.[124] Therefore, recognition of the AGG and AGA codons is not necessary in rat mitochondria. A putative human mtRF1 cDNA has been identified by screening of the human dbEST with the *E. coli* RF1 protein sequence.[125] The cDNA is predicted to code for a 52-kDa protein that shows significant sequence homology with mtRF1s of lower eukaryotes. The protein does not carry an obvious N-terminal presequence for mitochondrial targeting. Neither its mitochondrial location nor its activity has been established. The gene for the putative human mtRF1 (*MTRF1*) has been assigned to chromosome 13q14.1–q14.3.[126]

dbEST searches have also revealed human cDNA sequences with homology to *E. coli* RRF.[125] The cDNA is predicted to encode a 29-kDa protein, which like the putative human mtRF1 does not have a clear N-terminal presequence. The mitochondrial location of the protein is by no means proven and its activity has not been verified. The putative human mtRRF shows 25–30 per cent sequence identity to prokaryotic RRFs, but only 19 per cent sequence identity with the possible mtRRF (Fil1p) of the yeast *Saccharomyces cerevisiae*.[125,127] The gene for the putative human mtRRF (*MRRF*) has been mapped to chromosome 9q32–q34.1.[126]

Concluding remarks

Over the past two decades, our understanding of mitochondrial transcription and translation has progressed dramatically. The low abundance of most of the protein factors involved in these processes has long presented serious impediments for biochemical characterization, but advances in proteomic analysis techniques have allowed rapid expansion of our knowledge of mitochondrial proteins. This is most clearly illustrated by the fact that recently, within an exceptionally short time-span, all 79 human mitochondrial ribosomal protein sequences were identified.[94-97] In addition, screening of the human dbEST with protein sequences of transcription or translation factors from prokaryotes or yeast has proven a very fruitful approach. It appears that we are now quickly approaching the point at which the full complement of nuclear-encoding factors critical for mtDNA expression is known. This will have an important impact on the development of diagnostic tools for human mitochondrial diseases. Although the basic mechanisms of mitochondrial transcription and translation are known, further studies aimed at defining the exact roles of all factors involved will be necessary to fully comprehend the often complex relationship between a patient's genotype and clinical phenotype.

Acknowledgements

I thank Siôn L Williams and Paul E Hart for critical reading of the manuscript.

References

1. Wolstenholme DR (1992). Animal mitochondrial DNA: structure and evolution. *Intern. Rev. Cytol.* **141**: 173–216.
2. Ojala D, Montoya J, and Attardi G (1981). tRNA punctuation model of RNA processing in human mitochondria. *Nature* **290**: 470–474.
3. Barrell BG, Anderson S, Bankier AT, *et al.* (1980). Different pattern of codon recognition by mammalian mitochondrial tRNAs. *Proc. Natl Acad. Sci. USA* **77**: 3164–3166.
4. Bonitz SG, Berlani R, Coruzzi G, *et al.* (1980). Codon recognition rules in yeast mitochondria. *Proc. Natl Acad. Sci. USA* **77**: 3167–3170.
5. Heckman JE, Sarnoff J, Alzner-DeWeerd B, Yin S, and RajBhandary UL (1980). Novel features in the genetic code and codon reading patterns in *Neurospora crassa* mitochondria based on sequences of six mitochondrial tRNAs. *Proc. Natl Acad. Sci. USA* **77**: 3159–3163.
6. Martin RP, Sibler A-P, Gehrke CW, *et al.* (1990). 5[[(carboxymethyl)amino]methyl]uridine is found in the anticodon of yeast mitochondrial tRNAs recognizing two-codon families ending in a purine. *Biochemistry* **29**: 956–959.
7. Yasukawa T, Suzuki T, Ishii N, Ohta S, and Watanabe K (2001). Wobble modification defect in tRNA disturbs codon-anticodon interaction in a mitochondrial disease. *EMBO J.* **20**: 4794–4802.
8. Moriya J, Yokogawa T, Wakita K, *et al.* (1994). A novel modified nucleoside found at the first position of the anticodon of methionine tRNA from bovine liver mitochondria. *Biochemistry* **33**: 2234–2239.
9. Galper JB and Darnell JE (1969). The presence of *N*-formyl-methionyl-tRNA in HeLa cell mitochondria. *Biochem. Biophys. Res. Commun.* **34**: 205–214.
10. Clayton DA (1991). Replication and transcription of vertebrate mitochondrial DNA. *Annu. Rev. Cell Biol.* **7**: 453–478
11. Shadel GS and Clayton DA (1993). Mitochondrial transcription initiation. *J. Biol. Chem.* **268**: 16083–16086.
12. Tracy RL and Stern DB (1995). Mitochondrial transcription initiation: promoter structures and RNA polymerases. *Curr. Genet.* **28**: 205–216.
13. Taanman J-W (1999). The mitochondrial genome: structure, transcription, translation and replication. *Biochim. Biophys. Acta* **1410**: 103–123.
14. Anderson S, Bankier AT, Barrell BG, *et al.* (1981). Sequence and organization of the human mitochondrial genome. *Nature* **290**: 457–465.
15. Tiranti V, Savoia A, Forti F, *et al.* (1997). Identification of the gene encoding the human mitochondrial RNA polymerase (h-mtRPOL) by cyberscreening of the Expressed Sequence Tags database. *Hum. Mol. Genet.* **6**: 615–625.

16. Masters BS, Stohl LL, and Clayton DA (1987). Yeast mitochondrial RNA polymerase is homologous to those encoded by bacteriophages T3 and T7. *Cell* **51**: 89–99.
17. Gardner LP, Mookhtiar KA, and Cloeman JE (1997). Initiation, elongation, and processivity of carboxyl-terminal mutants of T7 RNA polymerase. *Biochemistry* **36**: 2908–2918.
18. Wang Y and Shadel GD (1999). Stability of the mitochondria genome requires an amino-terminal domain of yeast mitochondrial RNA polymerase. *Proc. Natl Acad. Sci. USA* **96**: 8046–8051.
19. Fisher RP and Clayton DA (1988). Purification and characterization of human mitochondrial transcription factor 1. *Mol. Cell Biol.* **8**: 3496–3509.
20. Parisi M and Clayton DA (1991). Similarity of human mitochondrial transcription factor 1 to high mobility group proteins. *Science* **252**: 965–969.
21. Tiranti V, Rossi E, Ruiz-Carrillo A, *et al.* (1995). Chromosomal localization of mitochondrial transcription factor A (TCF6), single-stranded DNA-binding protein (SSBP), and endonuclease G (ENDOG), three human housekeeping genes involved in mitochondrial biogenesis. *Genomics* **25**: 559–564.
22. Grosschedl R, Giese K, and Pagel J (1994). HMG domain proteins: architectural elements in the assembly of nucleoprotein structures. *Trends Genet.* **10**: 94–99.
23. Ghivizzani SC, Madsen CS, Nelen MR, Ammini CV, and Hauswirth WW (1994). In organello footprint analysis of human mitochondrial DNA: human mitochondrial transcription factor A interactions at the origin of replication. *Mol. Cell. Biol.* **14**: 7717–7730.
24. Micol V, Fernández-Silva P, and Attardi G (1997). Functional analysis of *in vivo and in organello* footprinting of HeLa cell mitochondrial DNA in relationship to ATP and ethidium bromide effects on transcription. *J. Biol. Chem.* **272**: 18896–18904.
25. Dairaghi DJ, Shadel GS, and Clayton DA (1995). Addition of a 29 residue carboxy-terminal tail converts a simple HMG box-containing protein into a transcriptional activator. *J. Mol. Biol.* **249**: 11–28.
26. Chang DD, Hixson JE, and Clayton DA (1988). Minor transcription initiation events indicate that both human mitochondrial promoters function bidirectionally. *Mol. Cell. Biol.* **6**: 294–301.
27. Fisher RP, Lisowsky T, Parisi MA, and Clayton DA (1992). DNA wrapping and bending by a mitochondrial high mobility group-like transcriptional activator protein. *J. Biol. Chem.* **267**: 3358–3367.
28. Diffley JFX and Stillman B (1991). DNA binding properties of an HMG1-related protein from yeast mitochondria. *J. Biol. Chem.* **267**: 3368–3374.
29. Shadel GS and Clayton DA (1997). Mitochondrial DNA maintenance in vertebrates. *Annu. Rev. Biochem.* **66**: 409–435.
30. Larsson N-G, Wang J, Wilhelmsson H, *et al.* (1998). Mitochondrial transcription factor A is necessary for mtDNA maintenance and embryogenesis in mice. *Nat. Genet.* **18**: 231–236.
31. Nam S-C and Kang C (2001). Expression of cloned cDNA for the human mitochondrial RNA polymerase in *Escherichia coli* and purification. *Protein Expr. Purif.* **21**: 485–491.
32. Prieto-Martín A, Montoya J, and Martínez-Azorín F (2001). A study on the human mitochondrial RNA polymerase activity points to existence of a transcription factor B-like protein. *FEBS Lett.* **503**: 51–55.
33. Lisowsky T and Michaelis G (1988). A nuclear gene essential for mitochondrial replication suppresses a defect of mitochondrial transcription in *Saccharomyces cerevisiae*. *Mol. Gen. Genet.* **214**: 218–223.
34. McCulloch V, Seidel-Rogol BL, and Shadel GS (2002). A human mitochondrial transcription factor is related to RNA adenine methyltransferases and binds S-adenosylmethionine. *Mol. Cell. Biol.* **22**: 1116–1125.
35. Falkenberg M, Gaspari M, Rantanen A, Trifunovic A, Larsson, N-G, and Gustafsson CM (2002). Mitochondrial transcription factors B1 and B2 activate transcription of human mtDNA. *Nat. Genet.* **31**: 289–294.
36. Schubot FD, Chen CJ, Rose JP, Dailey TA, Dailey HA, and Wang BC (2001). Crystal structure of the transcription factor sc-mtTFB offers insights into mitochondrial transcription. *Protein Sci.* **10**: 1980–1988.

37. Murphy WI, Attardi B, Tu C, and Attardi G (1975). Evidence for complete symmetrical transcription *in vivo* of mitochondrial DNA in HeLa cells. *J. Mol. Biol.* **99**: 809–814.
38. Montoya J, Gaines GL, and Attardi G (1983). The pattern of transcription of the human mitochondrial rRNA genes reveals two overlapping transcription units. *Cell* **34**: 151–159.
39. Gelfand R and Attardi G (1981). Synthesis and turnover of mitochondrial ribonucleic acid in HeLa cells: the mature ribosomal and messenger ribonucleic acid species are metabolically unstable. *Mol. Cell. Biol.* **1**: 497–511.
40. Montoya J, Christianson T, Levens D, Rabinowitz M, and Attardi G (1982). Identification of initiation sites for heavy-strand and light-strand transcription in human mitochondrial DNA. *Proc. Natl Acad. Sci. USA* **79**: 7195–7199.
41. Gaines G and Attardi G (1984). Intercalating drugs and low temperatures inhibit synthesis and processing of ribosomal RNA in isolated human mitochondria. *J. Mol. Biol.* **172**: 451–466.
42. Gaines G, Rossi C, and Attardi G (1987). Markedly different ATP requirements for rRNA synthesis and mtDNA light strand transcription *versus* mRNA synthesis in isolated human mitochondria. *J. Biol. Chem.* **262**: 1907–1915.
43. Dubin DT, Montoya J, Timko KD, and Attardi G (1982). Sequence analysis and precise mapping of the 3′ ends of HeLa cell mitochondrial ribosomal RNAs. *J. Mol. Biol.* **157**: 1–19.
44. Van Etten RA, Bird JW, and Clayton DA (1983). Identification of the 3′-ends of the two mouse mitochondrial ribosomal RNAs. *J. Biol. Chem.* **258**: 10104–10110.
45. Kruse B, Narasimhan N, and Attardi G (1989). Termination of transcription in human mitochondria: identification and purification of a DNA binding protein factor that promotes termination. *Cell* **58**: 391–397.
46. Christianson TW and Clayton DA (1988). A tridecamer DNA sequence supports human mitochondrial RNA 3′-end formation *in vitro*. *Mol. Cell. Biol.* **8**: 4502–4509.
47. Hess JF, Parisi MA, Bennett JL, and Clayton DA (1991). Impairment of mitochondrial transcription termination by a point mutation associated with the MELAS subgroup of mitochondrial encephalomyopathies. *Nature* **351**: 236–239.
48. Shang J and Clayton DA (1994). Human mitochondrial transcription termination exhibits RNA polymerase independence and biased bipolarity *in vitro*. *J. Biol. Chem.* **269**: 29112–29120.
49. Daga A, Micol V, Hess D, Aebersold R, and Attardi G (1993). Molecular characterization of the transcription termination factor from human mitochondria. *J. Biol. Chem.* **268**: 8123–8130.
50. Fernandez-Silva P, Martinez-Azorin F, Micol V, and Attardi G (1997). The human mitochondrial transcription termination factor (mTERF) is a multizipper protein but binds to DNA as a monomer, with evidence pointing to intramolecular leucine zipper interactions. *EMBO J.* **16**: 1066–1079.
51. Christianson TW and Clayton DA (1986). *In vitro* transcription of human mitochondrial DNA: accurate termination requires a region of DNA sequence that can function bidirectionally. *Proc. Natl Acad. Sci. USA* **83**: 6277–6281.
52. Montoya J, Ojala D, and Attardi G (1981). Distinctive features of the 5′-terminal sequences of the human mitochondrial mRNAs. *Nature* **290**: 465–470.
53. Frank DN and Pace NR (1998). Ribonuclease P: unity and diversity in a tRNA processing ribozyme. *Annu. Rev. Biochem.* **67**: 153–180.
54. Miller DL and Martin NC (1983). Characterisation of the yeast mitochondrial locus necessary for tRNA biosynthesis: DNA sequence analysis and identification of a new transcript. *Cell* **34**: 911–917.
55. Dang YL and Martin NC (1993). Yeast mitochondrial RNase P. *J. Biol. Chem.* **268**: 19791–19796.
56. Rossmanith W, Tullo A, Potuschak T, Karwan R, and Sbisà E (1995). Human mitochondrial tRNA processing. *J. Biol. Chem.* **270**: 12885–12891.
57. Rossmanith W and Karwan RM (1998). Characterization of human mitochondrial RNase P: novel aspects in tRNA processing. *Biochem. Biophys. Res. Commun.* **247**: 234–241.
58. Doersen C-J, Guerrer-Takada C, Altman S, and Attardi G (1985). Characterization of an RNase P activity from HeLa cell mitochondria. *J. Biol. Chem.* **260**: 5942–5949.

59. Puranam RS and Attardi G (2001). The RNase P associated with HeLa cell mitochondria contains an essential RNA component identical in sequence to that of the nuclear RNase P. *Mol. Cell. Biol.* **21**: 548–561.

60. Manam S and Van Tuyle GC (1987). Separation and characterization of 5'- and 3'-tRNA processing nucleases from rat liver mitochondria. *J. Biol. Chem.* **262**: 10272–10279.

61. Van Eenennaam H, Jarrous N, Van Venrooij WJ, and Pruijn GJM (2000). Architecture and function of the human endonucleases RNase P and RNase MRP. *IUBMB Life* **49**: 265–272.

62. Levinger L, Jacobs O, and James M (2001). *In vitro* 3'-end endonucleolytic processing defect in a human mitochondrial tRNA$^{Ser(UCN)}$ precursor with the U7445C substitution, which causes non-syndromic deafness. *Nucleic Acids Res.* **29**: 4334–4340.

63. Rossmanith W (1997). Processing of human mitochondrial tRNA$^{Ser(AGY)}$: a novel pathway in tRNA biosynthesis. *J. Mol. Biol.* **265**: 365–371.

64. Reichert A, Rothbauer U, and Mörl M (1998). Processing and editing of overlapping tRNAs in human mitochondria. *J. Biol. Chem.* **273**: 31977–31984.

65. Reichert A and Mörl M (2000). Repair of tRNAs in metazoan mitochondria. *Nucleic Acids Res.* **28**: 2043–2048.

66. Sprinzl M, Horn C, Brown M, Loudovitch A, and Steinberg S (1998). Compilation of tRNA sequences and sequences of tRNA genes. *Nucleic Acids Res.* **26**: 148–153.

67. Helm M, Giegé R, and Florentz C (1999). A Watson–Crick base-pair-disrupting methyl group (m^{1}A9) is sufficient for cloverleaf folding of human mirochondrial tRNA^{Lys}. *Biochemistry* **38**: 13338–13346.

68. Degoul F, Brulé H, Cepanec C, Helm M, Marsac C, Leroux, J-P, Griegé R, and Florentz C (1998). Isoleucylation properties of native human mitochondrial tRNA^{Ile} and tRNA^{Ile} transcriptis. *Hum. Mol. Genet.* **7**: 347–354.

69. Nagaike T, Suzuki T, Tomari Y, *et al.* (2001). Identification and characterization of mammalian mitochondrial tRNA nucleotidyltransferases. *J. Biol. Chem.* **276**: 40041–40049.

70. Ojala D and Attardi G (1974). Identification and partial characterization of multiple discrete polyadenylic acid containing RNA components coded for by HeLa cell mitochondrial DNA. *J. Mol. Biol.* **82**: 151–174.

71. Rose KM, Morris HP, and Jacob ST (1975). Mitochondrial poly(A) polymerase from poorly differentiated hepatoma: purification and characteristics. *Biochemistry* **14**: 1025–1032.

72. Bullard JM, Cai Y-C, Demeler B, and Spremulli LL (1999). Expression and characterization of a human mitochondrial phenylalanyl-tRNA synthetase. *J. Mol. Biol.* **288**: 567–577.

73. Bullard JM, Cai Y-C, and Spremulli LL (2000). Expression and characterization of the human mitochondrial leucyl-tRNA synthetase. *Biochim. Biophys. Acta* **1490**: 245–258.

74. Jørgensen R, Søgaard TMM, Rossing AB, Martensen PM, and Justesen J (2000). Identification and characterization of human mitochondrial tryptophanyl-tRNA synthetase. *J. Biol. Chem.* **275**: 16820–16826.

75. Yokogawa T, Shimada N, Takeuchi N, *et al.* (2000). Characterization and tRNA recognition of mammalian mitochondrial seryl-tRNA synthetase. *J. Biol. Chem.* **275**: 19913–19920.

76. Shimada N, Suzuki T, and Watanabe K (2001). Dual mode recognition of two isoacceptor tRNAs by mammalian mitochondrial seryl-tRNA synthetase. *J. Biol. Chem.* **276**: 46770–46778.

77. Takeuchi N, Kawakami M, Omori A, Ueda T, Spremulli LL, and Watanabe K (1998). Mammalian mitochondrial methionyl-tRNA transformylase from bovine liver. *J. Biol. Chem.* **273**: 15085–15090.

78. Taneuchi N, Vail L, Panvert M, *et al.* (2001). Recognition of tRNAs by methionyl-tRNA transformylase from mammalian mitochondria. *J. Biol. Chem.* **276**: 20064–20068.

79. Liu M and Spremulli L (2000). Interaction of mammalian mitochondrial ribosomes with the inner membrane. *J. Biol. Chem.* **275**: 29400–29406.

80. Borst P and Grivell LA (1971). Mitochondrial ribosomes. *FEBS Lett.* **13**: 73–88.

81. Schwartzbach CJ and Spremulli LL (1989). Bovine mitochondrial protein synthesis elongation factors *J. Biol. Chem.* **264**: 19125–19131.
82. Liao H-X and Spremulli LL (1990). Identification and initial characterization of translational initiation factor 2 from bovine mitochondria. *J. Biol. Chem.* **265**: 13618–13622.
83. Chung HKJ and Spremulli LL (1990). Purification and characterization of elongation factor G from bovine liver mitochondria. *J. Biol. Chem.* **265**: 21000–21004.
84. Ma J and Spremulli LL (1996). Expression, purification, and mechanistic studies of bovine mitochondrial translational initiation factor 2. *J. Biol. Chem.* **271**: 5805–5811.
85. Attardi G and Ojala D (1971). Mitochondrial ribosomes in HeLa cells. *Nat. New Biol.* **229**: 133–136.
86. Brega A and Vesco C (1971). Ribonucleoprotein particles involved in HeLa mitochondrial protein synthesis. *Nat. New Biol.* **229**: 136–139.
87. Hamilton, MG and O'Brien TW (1974). Ultracentrifugal characterization of the mitochondrial ribosome and subribosomal particles of bovine liver: molecular size and composition. *Biochemistry* **13**: 5400–5403.
88. Patel VB, Cunningham CC, and Hantgan RR (2001). Physiochemical properties of rat liver mitochondrial ribosomes. *J. Biol. Chem.* **276**: 6739–6746.
89. Lang, BF, Goff LJ, and Gray MW (1996). A 5 S rRNA gene is present in the mitochondrial genome of the protist *Reclinomonas americana* but is absent from red algal mitochondrial DNA. *J. Mol. Biol.* **261**: 607–613.
90. Yoshionari S, Koike T, Yokogawa T, *et al.* (1994). Existence of nuclear-encoded 5S-rRNA in bovine mitochondria. *FEBS Lett.* **338**: 137–142.
91. Magalhães PJ, Andreu AL, and Schon EA (1998). Evidence for the presence of 5S rRNA in mammalian mitochondria. *Mol. Biol. Cell* **9**: 2375–2382.
92. Entelis NS, Kolesnikova OA, Dogan S, Martin RP, and Tarassov IA (2001). 5S rRNA and tRNA import into human mitochondria. *J. Biol. Chem.* **276**: 45642–45653.
93. Cahill A, Baio DL, and Cunningham CC (1995). Isolation and characterization of rat liver mitochondrial ribosomes. *Anal. Biochem.* **232**: 47–55.
94. Koc EC, Burkhart W, Blackburn K, Moseley A, and Spremulli LL (2001). The small subunit of the mammalian mitochondrial ribosome. *J. Biol. Chem.* **276**: 19363–19374.
95. Suzuki T, Terasaki M, Takemoto-Hori C, *et al.* (2001). Structural compensation for the deficit of rRNA with proteins in the mammalian mitochondrial ribosome. *J. Biol. Chem.* **276**: 21724–21736.
96. Suzuki T, Terasaki M, Takemoto-Hori C, *et al.* (2001). Proteomic analysis of the mammalian mitochondrial ribosome. *J. Biol. Chem.* **276**: 33181–33195.
97. Koc EC, Burkhart W, Blackburn K, *et al.* (2001). The large subunit of the mammalian mitochondrial ribosome. *J. Biol. Chem.* **276**: 43958–43969.
98. Kenmochi N, Suzuki T, Uechi T, *et al.* (2001). The human mitochondrial ribosomal protein genes: mapping of 54 genes to the chromosomes and implications for human disorders. *Genomics* **77**: 65–70.
99. Koc EC, Ranasinghe A, Burkhart W, *et al.* (2001). A new face on apoptosis: death-associated protein 3 and PDCD9 are mitochondrial ribosomal proteins. *FEBS Lett.* **492**: 166–170.
100. Gromann K, Amairic F, Crews S, and Attardi G (1978). Failure to detect "cap" structures in mitochondrial DNA-coded poly(A)-containing RNA from HeLa cells. *Nucleic Acids Res.* **5**: 637–651.
101. Cantatore P, Flagella Z, Fracasso F, Lezza AMS, Gadaleta MN, and de Montalvo A (1987). Synthesis and turnover rates of four rat liver mitochondrial RNA species. *FEBS Lett.* **213**: 144–148.
102. Van den Bogert C, De Vries H, Holtrop M, Muus P, Dekker HL, Van Galen MJM, Bolhuis PA, and Taanman J-W (1993). Regulation of the expression of mitochondrial proteins: relationship between mtDNA copy number and cytochrome-*c* oxidase activity in human cells and tissues. *Biochim. Biophys. Acta* **1144**: 177–183.

103. Garstka HL, Fäcke M, Escribano JR, and Wiesner RJ (1994). Stoichiometry of mitochondrial transcripts and regulation of gene expression by mitochondrial transcription factor A. *Biochem. Biophys. Res. Commun.* **200**: 619–626.

104. Liao H-X and Spremulli LL (1989). Interaction of bovine mitochondrial ribosomes with messenger RNA. *J. Biol. Chem.* **264**: 7518–7522.

105. Denslow ND, Michaels GS, Montoya J, Attardi G, and O'Brien TW (1989). Mechanism of mRNA binding to bovine mitochondrial ribosomes. *J. Biol. Chem.* **264**: 8328–8338.

106. Liao H-X and Spremulli LL (1990). Effects of length and mRNA secondary structure on the interaction of bovine mitochondrial ribosomes with messenger RNA. *J. Biol. Chem.* **265**: 11761–11765.

107. Liao H-X and Spremulli LL (1991). Initiation of protein synthesis in animal mitochondria. *J. Biol. Chem.* **266**: 20714–20719.

108. Ma L and Spremulli LL (1995). Cloning and sequence analysis of the human mitochondrial translational initiation factor 2 cDNA. *J. Biol. Chem.* **270**: 1859–1865.

109. Bonner DS, Wiley JE, and Farwell MA (1998). Assignment of the human mitochondial translational initiation factor 2 gene (*MTIF2*) to human chromosome 2 bands p16–p14 by *in situ* hybridization and with somatic cell hybrids. *Cytogenet. Cell Genet.* **83**: 80–81.

110. Wells J, Henkler F, Leversha M, and Koshy R (1995). A mitochondrial elongation factor-like protein is over-expressed in tumours and differentially expressed in normal tissues. *FEBS Lett.* **358**: 119–125.

111. Xin H, Woriax V, Burkhart W, and Spremulli LL (1995). Cloning and expression of mitochondrial translational elongation factor Ts from bovine and human liver. *J. Biol. Chem.* **270**: 17243–17249.

112. Ling M, Merante F, Chen H-S, Duff C, Duncan AMV, and Robinson BH (1997). The human mitochondrial elongation factor tu (EF-Tu) gene: cDNA sequence, genomic localization, genomic structure, and identification of a pseudogene. *Gene* **197**: 325–336.

113. Gao J, Yu L, Zhang P, *et al.* (2001). Cloning and characterization of human and mouse mitochondrial elongation factor G, *GFM* and *Gfm*, and mapping of *GFM* to human chromosome 3q25.1–q26.2. *Genomics* **74**: 109–114.

114. Hammarsund M, Wilson W, Corcoran M, *et al.* (2001). Identification and characterization of two novel human mitochondrial elongation factor genes, *hEFG2* and *hEFG1*, phylogenetically conserved through evolution. *Hum. Genet.* **109**: 542–550.

115. Vernon JL, Burr PC, Wiley JE, and Farwell MA (2000). Assignment of the mitochondrial translation elongation factor Ts gene (*TSFM*) to human chromosome 12 bands q13→q14 by *in situ* hybridization and with somatic cell hybrids. *Cytogenet. Cell Genet.* **89**: 145–146.

116. Nierhaus KH (1996). An elongation factor turn-on. *Nature* **379**: 491–492.

117. Woriax VL, Bullard JM, Ma L, Yokogawa T, and Spremulli LL (1997). Mechanistic studies of the translational elongation cycle in mammalian mitochondria. *Biochim. Biophys. Acta* **1352**: 91–101.

118. Cai Y-C, Bullard JM, Thompson NL, and Spremulli LL (2000). Interaction of mammalian mitochondrial elongation factor EF-Tu with guanine nucleotides. *Protein Sci* **9**: 1791–1800.

119. Cai Y-C, Bullard JM, Thompson NL, and Spremulli LL (2000). Interaction of mitochondrial elongation factor Tu with aminoacyl-tRNA and elongation factor Ts. *J. Biol. Chem.* **275**: 20308–20314.

120. Andersen GR, Thirup S, Spremulli LL, and Nyborg J (2000). High resolution crystal structure of bovine mitochondrial EF-Tu in complex with GDP. *J. Mol. Biol.* **297**: 421–436.

121. Nakamura Y, Ito K, and Isaksson LA (1996). Emerging understanding of translation. *Cell* **87**: 147–150.

122. Janosi L, Mottagui-Tabar S, Isaksson LA, *et al.* (1998). Evidence for *in vivo* ribosome recycling, the fourth step in protein biosynthesis. *EMBO J.* **17**: 1141–1151.

123. Lee CC, Timms KM, Trotman CNA, and Tate WP (1987). Isolation of a rat mitochondrial release factor: accommodation of the genetic code for termination. *J. Biol. Chem.* **262**: 3548–3552.

124. Gadaleta G, Pepe G, De Candia G, Quagliariello C, Sbisà E, and Saccone C (1989). The complete nucleotide sequence of the *Rattus norvegicus* mitochondrial genome: cryptic signals revealed by comparative analysis between vertebrates. *J. Mol. Evol.* **28**: 497–516.
125. Zhang Y and Spremulli LL (1998). Identification and cloning of human mitochondrial translational release factor 1 and the ribosome recycling factor. *Biochim. Biophys. Acta* **1443**: 245–250.
126. Hansen LL, Jorgensen R, and Justesen J (2000). Assignment of the human mitochondrial translational release factor 1 (*MTRF1*) to chromosome 13q14.1–q14.3 and of the human mitochondrial recycling factor (*MRRF*) to chromosome 9q32–q34.1 with radiation hybrid mapping. *Cytogenet. Cell Genet.* **88**: 91–92.
127. Kanai T, Takeshita S, Atomi H, Umemura K, Ueda M, and Tanaka A (1998). A regulatory factor, Fil1p, involved in derepression of the isocitrate lyase gene in *Saccharomyces cerevisiae*. *Eur. J. Biochem.* **256**: 212–220.

3 Mitochondrial biogenesis

Carla M Koehler

The chapter focuses on the intensively studied area of protein import into mitochondria and protein maturation within mitochondria. Existing knowledge relies heavily on work done in yeast; recent identification of diseases that result when these processes are disrupted is providing valuable insights into human mitochondrial biogenesis.

Introduction

The mitochondrion contains approximately 1000 proteins. Of these mitochondrial proteins, 3–32,[1] depending on the organism, are coded by the mitochondrial genome. The remainder are translated in the cytosol and imported into mitochondria to one of four locations, the outer membrane, the intermembrane space, the inner membrane, or the matrix (Fig. 3.1). A precursor protein destined for the mitochondrion thus contains targeting as well as sorting information, and the mitochondrion has developed an elaborate translocation machinery that mediates

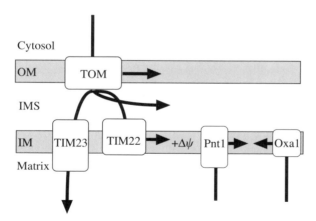

Fig. 3.1 Protein import and export pathways in the mitochondrion. Cytosolic proteins are imported through the translocase of the outer membrane (TOM) and then, depending upon their destination, remain in the outer membrane (OM), intermembrane space (IMS), or engage the translocases of the inner membrane (TIM). Precursors with a typical amino-terminal targeting sequence generally utilize the TIM23 complex, whereas proteins that reside in the inner membrane (IM), often lacking a targeting sequence, utilize the TIM22 complex. Mitochondrial encoded proteins may be exported to the inner membrane via Oxa1 and Pnt1. Pathways are depicted schematically by arrows. See text for details.

protein import and export. The TOM (translocase of the outer membrane) complex mediates protein translocation across the outer membrane and insertion of outer membrane proteins. The inner membrane contains the TIM23 (translocase of inner membrane) complex for the translocation of proteins that reside predominantly in the matrix and intermembrane space and the TIM22 complex for translocation of many inner membrane proteins (the nomenclature of the mitochondrial protein transport systems has been unified such that proteins are named Tom or Tim corresponding to translocase of outer membrane and inner membrane, respectively, followed by the number indicating the component's molecular weight).[2] The mitochondrion also contains at least two protein export pathways for inner membrane proteins generally coded on the mitochondrial genome. Assembly of protein complexes is mediated by processing peptidases that remove targeting sequences and a battery of chaperones that guide protein folding. A protein surveillance system is present to regulate the assembly and degradation of protein complexes.

Much of what is understood about mitochondrial biogenesis has been learned through studies in the model systems *Saccharomyces cerevisiae* and *Neurospora crassa*. *S. cerevisiae* is amenable to genetics and biochemistry, while *N. crassa* is amenable to biochemistry. By comparing components identified in *S. cerevisiae* and *N. crassa*, a picture has emerged in which the translocation systems are homologous. Indeed, as additional genomes are sequenced, the mitochondrial protein translocation systems among animals, plants and fungi appear highly conserved; hence, results from initial studies in model organisms have provided valuable insights into the mechanism of mitochondrial biogenesis in mammalian systems.

Fundamental principles of mitochondrial protein import

The mitochondrial outer membrane contains abundant porin, a large protein pore that allows the passage of various small metabolites by simple diffusion. In contrast, the inner membrane must maintain an electrochemical gradient and therefore be ion impermeable. The inner membrane contains, in addition to the enzymes of oxidative phosphorylation, a large family of carrier proteins that mediate the transport of metabolites.

Mitochondrial proteins generally are imported post-translationally from the cytosol and are kept in an import-competent state by chaperones.[3–5] Most soluble proteins of the matrix and some proteins of the inner membrane and intermembrane space have an amino-terminal extension of 20–50 amino acid residues, with a range of 10–80 residues,[6] which is generally cleaved after import. Other precursors do not contain an amino-terminal targeting sequence; rather the targeting information resides within the mature protein.[7] This group includes outer membrane proteins, and some intermembrane space and inner membrane proteins. Regardless of the targeting sequence, all precursors are recognized by receptors of the TOM complex and then pass through the TOM channel.[8,9] Translocation requires that the precursors must be at least partially unfolded.[10]

After crossing the outer membrane through the TOM channel, the precursor is directed to either the TIM23 or TIM22 translocase of the inner membrane. Proteins with a presequence are imported via the TIM23 complex,[11] which forms a tightly regulated channel across the inner membrane. The membrane potential ($\Delta\psi$) across the inner membrane is a requisite for translocation across the inner membrane,[12] while an ATP-dependent translocation motor drives import to completion.[13–15] Mitochondrial heat shock protein 70 (mHsp70) serves as the molecular motor. The matrix contains a mitochondrial processing peptidase (MPP) that cleaves the presequence,[16] and the protein folds into its active form, possibly with the assistance of chaperones such as mHsp70, Hsp60, and Hsp10.[13,17,18] Proteins destined for the inner membrane such as the metabolic carriers and import components are directed through the aqueous intermembrane space by the small Tim proteins to the TIM22 complex.[19–22] The TIM22 complex mediates insertion into the inner membrane in a $\Delta\psi$-dependent manner.

Mitochondrial targeting signals

A classic mitochondrial targeting signal is an amino-terminal cleavable presequence that functions as a matrix targeting signal. Based on studies focused on the import of synthetic fusion proteins between a mitochondrial targeting sequence and a passenger protein, the presequence contains all the information for targeting, membrane translocation, and often sorting.[6] The presequence is an amphipathic alpha-helix in which one side is positively charged and the opposite face is hydrophobic. It was thought that the hydrophobic surface would interact with the membrane while the hydrophilic surface would be important for recognition by receptors. However, recent NMR studies suggest that the hydrophobic side binds in a shallow groove of the import receptor Tom20[23] and the positively charged side binds to negative charges on the periphery. Because the membrane potential $\Delta\psi$ (negative on the matrix side) directs the presequence across the inner membrane by an electrophoretic effect, the net positive charge of the presequence is important.[12]

Although the majority of presequences for matrix proteins are cleaved, a few exceptions exist. The mitochondrial chaperone Hsp10 and the ribosomal protein Nam9 are synthesized with a presequence that is not cleaved.[24,25] The DNA helicase, Hmi1, has a targeting sequence at its carboxy terminus.[26] Unlike mitochondrial precursors that are translocated in an amino- to carboxy-terminal direction, Hmi1 seemingly is translocated in reverse orientation, indicating that mitochondrial protein translocation is highly adaptive.

For proteins with destinations other than the matrix, variations on the presequence mediate sorting. In general, a hydrophobic segment generally follows the targeting sequence. The hydrophobic sorting signal, referred to as a 'stop-transfer' sequence, causes a specific arrest of the precursor in the membrane.[27] There are 4 general categories. First, the bipartite presequence is used to sort some proteins such as cytochrome b_2 and cytochrome c_1 to the intermembrane space and inner membrane, respectively.[27] A positively charged matrix-targeting sequence is followed by a 'stop-transfer' hydrophobic segment that arrests in the TIM23 complex. The 'stop-transfer' sequence is related to the signals found in bacterial and eukaryotic secretory proteins. The sorting sequences are cleaved at the outer surface of the inner membrane by the intermembrane space processing peptidase, Imp1–Imp2.[28] Second, some inner membrane proteins such as subunit Va of cytochrome oxidase have a cleavable presequence and a hydrophobic membrane anchor sequence in the mature part of the protein.[29] Third, some outer membrane proteins contain a non-cleavable presequence, followed by a long hydrophobic stretch. Of this group, NADH: cytochrome b_5 reductase arrests in the TOM complex owing to this hydrophobic stretch. Other outer membrane proteins are inserted at the carboxy-terminus; insertion of these proteins is believed to occur post-translationally as the C-terminus carries the targeting information. In the last group, some inner membrane proteins contain an internal targeting signal that consists of a membrane-spanning domain followed by a positively charged segment. Interestingly, this internal signal is postulated to form a hairpin—loop structure in the inner membrane.[30]

Still other mitochondrial proteins do not contain any obvious targeting information at the amino terminus, although it is assumed that targeting and sorting information is located within the mature part of the protein. Examples in this class are those of the mitochondrial carrier family, and the inner membrane import components Tim17, Tim22, and Tim23.[31–33] The mitochondrial carrier family has 3 dozen members in yeast,[34] including the ADP/ATP carrier (AAC), the phosphate carrier (P_iC) and the dicarboxylate carrier. These proteins are made up of a tripartite repeat consisting of two membrane spanning domains separated by a hydrophilic loop. As a result, the protein contains three to six internal targeting segments, distributed throughout the length of the protein.[31,32] In contrast to cleavable presequences, these internal signals do not always contain charged amino acid residues and a consensus sequence has not been identified. Similarly, the import component Tim23 contains several targeting and sorting signals including hydrophobic transmembrane domains and positively charged loops.[33,35] Indeed, the diversity of targeting information among mitochondrial proteins reflects the diverse protein import pathways.

Cytosolic chaperones

Through studies with various translational systems including wheat germ extract, reticulocyte lysate, and yeast extracts, a handful of cytosolic chaperones have been identified. However, most chaperones seemingly have a general role in keeping precursors in an import-competent state rather than specifically directing precursors to mitochondria. Two such chaperones are cytosolic Hsp70 and Ydj1, a farnesylated yeast homologue of bacterial DnaJ.[36,37] Mitochondrial precursors were found to accumulate in the cytosol of yeast strains in which the abundance of Hsp70 was decreased.[36] Similarly, transport of secretory proteins to the endoplasmic reticulum was defective, confirming that Hsp70 functions as a general chaperone. Specifically, Hsp70 has been shown to bind to synthetic prepeptides as well as the surface of mitochondria.[38] An allele of *Ydj*1 was identified in a screen for mutants (*mas*5) that displayed defects in growth and mitochondrial protein import.[39] Because the bacterial *DnaJ* acts with *DnaK*, *Ydj*1 may assist cytosolic Hsp70 to cycle on and off unfolded precursors. Recently, the nascent polypeptide-associated complex (NAC) has been identified in both genetic and biochemical schemes as a component that may promote co-translational import. NAC was originally identified in mammalian cell extracts as a ribosome-associated factor that interacts with nascent polypeptides.[40] NAC was purified from yeast cytosol as a component that stimulated the import of the precursor malate dehydrogenase in nascent chain-ribosome complexes.[41] In yeast, disruption of either of the genes encoding the subunits of the NAC heterodimer caused defects in protein targeting to the mitochondria, in particular the steady-state level of fumarase was reduced.[42]

Two cytosolic chaperones however have been identified that seemingly are specific for mitochondrial protein import. Mitochondrial import stimulation factor (MSF) was purified using affinity chromatography with an immobilized prepeptide[43] and presequence binding factor (PBF) was purified based on its ability to stimulate import of a purified precursor.[37] PBF binds precursors in a presequence-dependent manner and stimulates protein import, perhaps by cooperating with cytosolic Hsp70. MSF is a heterodimer that stimulates the import of a wide variety of precursors, including those without presequences. MSF has two activities: It forms stable complexes with precursors and binds to receptors Tom37 and Tom70 and promotes unfolding of precursors through ATP hydrolysis.[44] Interestingly, MSF is a member of the 14-3-3 protein family; these proteins are present in virtually all organisms, but the yeast homologs do not facilitate protein import.[45]

The outer membrane translocase

Whether the precursor protein has been released from the ribosome, or remains in the process of translation, the precursor interacts with the receptors of the TOM complex to initiate translocation across the mitochondrial outer membrane (Fig. 3.2). There are eight subunits of the TOM complex in *Saccharomyces cerevisiae* (Fig. 3.2).[46] Receptors include Tom20 and Tom22, which are highly conserved in fungi and animals, and Tom70 and Tom37.[8,47] The translocation channel consists of Tom40 and the small Tom proteins, Tom5, Tom6, and Tom7.[48,49] The stable Tom core complex is approximately 400 kDa.[46] In yeast, the pore-forming Tom40 and multifunctional receptor Tom22 are essential for viability.[50]

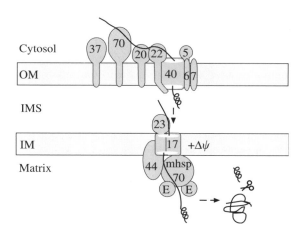

Fig. 3.2 Protein import pathway for precursors that contain a typical amino-terminal presequence. This pathway is mediated by the Tim17/Tim23 complex and an associated ATP-driven protein transport motor on the inner face of the inner membrane. As a precursor with an amino-terminal basic matrix-targeting signal (helical line) emerges from the TOM complex, it binds to an acidic Tim23 domain in the intermembrane space and thereby induces transient docking of the TOM- and the Tim17/Tim23 system. In the presence of a membrane potential $\Delta\psi$, the presequence passes through the inner membrane. The ATP-drive translocation motor consisting of mitochondrial Hsp70, the nucleotide exchange factor mitochondrial GrpE (E) and the membrane anchor Tim44 drives translocation to completion. In the matrix, the matrix processing protease (scissors) removes the matrix-targeting sequence and a battery of chaperones may aid in folding to generate the mature protein. See text for further details. OM, IMS, IM: outer membrane, intermembrane space, inner membrane, respectively.

Tom20 preferentially binds to precursors with amino-terminal presequences and then passes the precursor to Tom22. The Tom20 consists of a soluble cytosolic domain that is anchored to the membrane by an amino-terminal transmembrane domain.[51] The cytosolic domain contains a single tetratricopeptide repeat motif, a 34-residue motif implicated in protein–protein interactions,[52] and specifically binds to mitochondrial precursors.[31] Recently, the first NMR structural studies have revealed the interaction between Tom20 and the presequence.[23] Tom20 contains 4 α-helices that form a stable structure with a shallow hydrophobic groove flanked by hydrophilic residues at the periphery. The presequence peptide is bound to Tom20 in an α-helical structure, with the hydrophobic amino acids sitting in the groove and the hydrophilic residues oriented to the aqueous solvent. In addition, Tom20 recognizes internal targeting signals of precursors without a presequence, but Tom20 mostly likely is serving as an intermediate to pass the precursor from Tom70 to Tom22.[31]

In contrast, Tom70 preferentially binds to the β-subunit of the F_1-ATPase, and precursors with internal targeting sequences such as members of the mitochondrial carrier family through hydrophobic interactions as well as with cytosolic chaperones.[53] Like Tom20, Tom70 contains a large cytosolic domain with tetratricopeptide repeats, anchored to the membrane by an amino-terminal transmembrane domain.[53] Several Tom70 dimers bind simultaneously to one carrier protein, potentially preventing aggregation before subsequent passage to Tom22.[54,55] Yeast mitochondria also have a related protein, Tom72. Although its specific role has not been defined, Tom72 may mediate interactions between mitochondria and the cytoskeleton.[56,57]

Tom22 is a multifunctional organizer of the TOM complex. Tom22 is essential for viability; however, one particular yeast strain was identified that could grow slowly without the protein,[48] which helped to confirm the diverse functions of Tom22. Tom22 contains domains on both sides of the outer membrane, with the amino-terminus forming a large cytosolic domain and the carboxy-terminus forming a small domain in the intermembrane space.[58,59] Both domains are negatively charged and mediate the import of precursors through the TOM complex to the TIM complexes. In fact, Tom22 serves as a convergence point for precursors that initially bind to either Tom20 or Tom70.[58–60] And the transmembrane domain maintains association between the individual Tom40 channels; Tom22 also seems to regulate the gating activity of the Tom40 channels.[48]

Tom37 originally was identified in a screen for yeast mutants defective in phospholipid biosynthesis.[61] Subsequent biochemical and genetic studies indicated that Tom37 associated with Tom70 and deletion of *TOM37* resulted in decreased *in vitro* import of a set of precursors that are imported preferentially via Tom70.[61] However, Tom37 was recently shown to exhibit characteristics of a peripheral membrane protein and its specific role in protein import remains to be defined.[60,62] The human homolog metaxin has similar properties. Metaxin was identified serendipitously because of its chromosomal location between thrombospondin 3 and glucocerebrosidase.[63] During studies on thrombospondin 3, metaxin was identified because it is essential for the survival of the post-implantation mouse embryo. Overexpression of metaxin in mammalian cells decreased the import of preproteins, suggesting it may function as a receptor.[64] Metaxin however is not a central component of the Tom complex, but does form a complex with a related cytosolic protein metaxin 2.[65] The early embryonic lethal phenotype of mice lacking metaxin demonstrates that efficient import of proteins into mitochondria is critical for development and the identification of metaxin 2 indicates that the import pathway in mammalian systems may be more complex than fungi.

The TOM pore

The Tom40 is the core component of the TOM complex and is essential for viability in yeast. Tom40 is a β-barrel protein containing eight membrane-spanning domains and probably forms a dimer. Recently, it has been reconstituted in lipid vesicles and shown to be a cationic-specific channel.[66] In another *tour de force*, the TOM complex has been purified from *Neurospora crassa* mitochondria with a hexahistidine-tagged Tom22.[49] Electron microscopy and image reconstruction experiments revealed that the complex is 138 Å wide, containing up to two pores with an internal diameter of 20 Å. The purified TOM complex was reconstituted into lipid vesicles and shown to be both voltage-gated and cation-selective.[67] The current model proposes that a single channel is formed by two Tom40 molecules and that a complete TOM complex contains two to three channels.[47,67] In addition to forming the pore, Tom40 contains binding sites for precursors.

The TOM pore also contains three small TOM proteins, Tom5, Tom6, and Tom7. Tom5 acts as a receptor particularly for the small Tim proteins of the intermembrane space.[68] Tom6 and Tom7 are involved with the TOM complex assembly and disassembly.[69] Tom6 promotes assembly of Tom22 with Tom40. In yeast mutants lacking Tom6, the destabilized Tom complex is dissociated into 100-kDa units, each containing a Tom40 dimer.[48,69] In contrast, Tom7 mediates dissociation and thereby a lateral release of precursors into the outer membrane. Sorting of proteins, such as porin, is inhibited strongly in mitochondria lacking Tom7.[69,70]

How do proteins pass through the Tom complex? Other than the release of precursors from cytosolic chaperones, an ATP requirement has not been shown. Instead, the 'acid chain hypothesis' predicts that increased affinity for negatively charged domains on the receptors on the outer membrane and then the inner membrane, followed by Tim23 in the intermembrane space, may serve as a driving force for import.[71,72] However, hydrophobic interactions also are important in precursor recognition,[73] suggesting that a combination of binding interactions facilitates transport across the outer membrane.

TIM23 import pathway

The mitochondrial membrane has various translocons to mediate protein import. Precursors with an amino-terminal targeting presequence follow the 'general import pathway' (Fig. 3.2)[74,75]; their import is mediated by the Tim17/Tim23 complex (designated TIM23 complex) and the translocation motor consisting of Tim44, mitochondrial Hsp70, and the nucleotide exchange factor mitochondrial GrpE. This translocation is dependent upon the presence of a membrane potential ($\Delta\psi$) and generally requires ATP hydrolysis by mHsp70 on the matrix side for unidirectional translocation. The TIM23 complex acts independently of the TOM complex although the two can be reversibly asssociated while a precuror is in transit.[76] During transient association, the super TOM-TIM23 complex is approximately 600 kDa.[77] All components of the TIM23 translocase are essential for viability in *S. cerevisiae*. The TIM23 complex of the inner membrane thus is a complicated machine with broad similarities to the *Sec* machinery of *E. coli* and the endoplasmic reticulum.

In contrast to the outer membrane, the inner membrane is necessarily ion impermeable. The TIM channel must therefore be highly regulated during opening to prevent ion leakage and to accommodate a peptide chain in transit.[78] The TIM23 channel of the inner membrane is comprised of two related proteins, Tim17 and Tim23.[11,79–81] The size of this channel is approximately 22 Å as shown by studies in which particles of different sizes have been attached to precursors. Both Tim17 and Tim23 proteins are essential for viability, but one can not substitute for the other. While Tim17 seems to function only in channel formation, Tim23 is a multifunctional protein, similar to Tom22. Tim17 and Tim23 have four putative membrane spanning domains, and Tim23 contains a negatively charged domain in the intermembrane space that recognizes precursors taking the general import route. Tim17 and Tim23 are partner proteins in a 90 kDa complex but associate transiently with the translocation motor.[77] Tim23 has been proposed to form a dimer in the absence of a membrane potential such that the import channel is closed;[82] binding of the Tim23 intermembrane space domain to the precursor then triggers dimer dissociation, allowing the precursor to pass through the import channel. An intriguing observation also is that the amino-terminal domain of Tim23 inserts into the outer membrane and tethers both membranes.[83] However, specific binding to the TOM complex has not been identified so the relevance to protein import is not clear.

Initiation of translocation across the inner membrane depends on the membrane potential $\Delta\psi$, which is negative on the matrix side. The positively charged presequence passes across the inner membrane because of the electrophoretic effect of the membrane potential.[84] For the completion of translocation, the matrix-sided components, Tim44, mHsp70, and mGrpE function as the ATP-dependent translocation motor.[13,85] Tim44 is stably associated with the inner membrane but is mainly exposed at the matrix side. Mitochondrial Hsp70 has three domains: an amino-terminal ATPase domain, a central peptide-binding domain, and a shorter carboxy-terminal segment.[86,87] The interaction with Tim44 is dependent on the ATPase domain and is stabilized by the other two domains.[88] After the initial $\Delta\psi$–driven translocation of the amino-terminal targeting sequence, mHsp70 is required for the translocation of the remainder of the precursor across the inner membrane.[89,90] The co-chaperone mGrpE is a matrix protein homologous to the nucleotide exchange factor GrpE of bacteria.[13,91] mGrpE interacts with mHsp70 bound to a precursor and promotes the reaction cycle of mHsp70, thereby allowing nucleotide release.[92]

Two models, still under much debate, have been proposed to explain the role of mHsp70 in protein import. The Brownian rachet model proposes that mHsp70 binds passively to trap the precursor as it emerges on the matrix side through spontaneous fluctuations. The bound mHsp70 then blocks diffusion back into the channel.[93–95] The motor model is based on the experimental observation that Hsp70s undergo conformational changes in an ATP-dependent manner.[96,97] Since mHsp70 binds to both the incoming precursor and Tim44, an ATP-dependent conformational change could directly create a pulling force at the amino-terminus of the precursor. If this action were repeated in an ATP-dependent cycle, mHsp70 could function as a motor, pulling the precursor into the matrix in a mechanism similar to myosin functions in muscle contraction.[98,99] Recent studies indicate that both mechanisms cooperate in protein translocation.[15,100,101] For loosely folded precursors, the Brownian ratchet model could be sufficient to trap proteins. However, for precursors with tightly folded domains, the pulling action of mHsp70 would be requisite to complete translocation. Folded protein domains undergo spontaneous fluctuations that can lead to complete or partial unfolding. Thus, partial trapping by mHsp70 would be sufficient for import of precursors when their spontaneous unfolding is complete. However, ATP-dependent conformational changes of mHsp70 would be required to harness smaller fluctuations of folded domains and provide additional energy to overcome the activation barrier required for complete unfolding.[102] Indeed, recent studies with mitochondria from wild-type and mHsp70 mutant strains provided evidence that a single mechanism is not sufficient to explain the role of mHsp70 in import.[15,100] The mitochondria carry a mutant mHsp70 that efficiently holds precursors but is impaired in binding to Tim44. The mutant mitochondria efficiently import loosely folded precursors but are impaired in the import of folded domains and do not function in pulling. Thus, both holding and active pulling cooperate.

After translocation into the matrix, the imported proteins fold into their active conformations. The diverse nature of the imported proteins is reflected by the array of folding helpers, including mHsp70, the Hsp60–Hsp10 system, and the peptidyl-prolyl *cis/trans* isomerases (PPIases). Different precursors have different requirements for assistance in protein folding.[18] Mitochondrial Hsp70 cooperates with co-chaperone Mdj1, the homolog of bacterial DnaJ, to mediate folding in the matrix.[13,92] The Hsp60–Hsp10 system is homologous to the prokaryotic GroEL–GroES complex. Hsp60 promotes productive folding of proteins by enclosing them in a central cavity that is covered by Hsp10.[17] The mode of action of Hsp60 is based on detailed analysis of the bacterial system.[103] Interestingly, Hsp60 deficiency was observed in fibroblasts from a patient with mitochondrial encephalomyopathy,[104] and it was proposed to be the primary cause of mitochondrial dysfunction, however, no gene defect has been identified.[105] PPIases catalyze the *cis/trans* isomerization of peptide bonds preceding a prolyl residue;[106] isomerization is slow in the absence of PPIases and is a rate-limiting step in protein folding. The mitochondrial PPIase can bind to the immunosuppressive drug cyclosporin A and is hence termed cyclophilin 20 (corresponding to its apparent molecular weight).[107,108]

To date, additional proteins in this TIM machinery have been identified, but their specific role in protein import has not been determined. Tim11 was identified because of its intimate association with the Tim channel.[109] Studies with a cytochrome b_2 arrested translocation intermediate and a crosslinker with a short spacer arm crosslinked Tim11 with very high specificity. Further studies revealed it as the γ-subunit of ATP synthase and imply it acts as an ATPase assembly factor.[110] Studies by Endo and colleagues, based on the presence of site-specific crosslinks with a mitochondrial precursor with a classical targeting sequence, have revealed other proteins that also might play a role in import.[111] Of these, a 50-kDa protein is identified as a potential new import component.[111]

The proteolytic system of the mitochondrion

Mitochondrial biogenesis depends on a complex proteolytic system. Components include the processing peptidases in the matrix and intermembrane space and the ATP-dependent proteases in the inner membrane and matrix. In contrast to the protein import components, the proteolytic system is highly conserved, including homology with prokaryotic proteases. In yeast, the proteolytic system operates predominantly during starvation conditions for the non-selective degradation of mitochondrial proteins, but also is important for assembly of protein complexes and for presequence cleavage.[112,113] Mitochondrial peptidases are divided into three groups: processing peptidases, oligopeptidases and ATP-dependent proteases.

Processing peptidases are present in the mitochondrial matrix and intermembrane space for the cleavage of presequences. The mitochondrial processing peptidase (MPP) is located in the matrix and is responsible for the first processing: removal of the presequence.[114] The heterodimeric Zn^{2+}−metallopeptidase consists of two subunits and is essential for viability in yeast.[115] The α-MPP subunit recognizes and binds to the presequence followed by cleavage via the β-MPP subunit.[116] Maturation of some matrix and intermembrane space proteins depends on a second processing step. A subset of matrix proteins undergoes an additional processing step by the mitochondrial intermediate peptidase (MIP).[117] After MPP cleavage, MIP cleaves off amino-terminal octapeptides from some matrix proteins, including iron-utilizing proteins and components of the electron transport chain, the tricarboxylic acid cycle, and the mitochondrial genetic machinery.[118,119] The physiological relevance of MIP processing remains to be elucidated. The intermembrane space contains the inner membrane protease (IMP),[120] which is homologous to eubacterial and eukaryotic signal peptidases.[121] IMP is composed of two related subunits with non-overlapping substrate specificities; both subunits are integral membrane proteins and expose their catalytic sites to the intermembrane space.[28] After processing in the matrix by MPP, IMP cleaves off the remainder of the bipartite signal sequence from proteins such as cytochrome b_2 and cytochrome c_1.

In contrast to the specific proteolytic events mediated by the processing peptidases, ATP-dependent proteases mediate the complete turnover of mitochondrial proteins. These proteases are located in the matrix and the inner membrane and are evolved from prokaryotic ancestors.[113,122] Interestingly, these proteases have two functions: they degrade non-assembled and misfolded polypeptides and act as chaperones to mediate the assembly of protein complexes that are crucial for mitochondrial function.[113,122] The matrix proteases are the Lon/Pim1 protease and the Clp-like proteases. The Lon protease has an ATPase domain characteristic of Walker-type P-loop ATPases.[123,124] Substrates of Lon include non-assembled polypeptides, subunits of the F_1F_0–ATP synthase and ribosomal proteins.[123,124] Yeast mitochondria lacking the Lon protease accumulate inclusion bodies that most likely contain aggregated proteins and accumulate extensive mutations in mitochondrial DNA. Interestingly, the Lon protease has been shown to bind single-stranded DNA in a site-specific manner suggesting that Lon might play a direct role in mitochondrial DNA metabolism.[125] The Clp proteases have been identified in mammalian mitochondria but are absent in lower eukaryotes, including yeast.[126] The Clp proteases form hetero-oligomeric complexes with ATPase and proteolytic subunits.[127] These proteases unfold misfolded polypeptides allowing either refolding by other chaperone systems, or if associated with a proteolytic subunit, their degradation.

The inner membrane is rich in proteins and has its own quality control system that consists of two ATP-dependent proteases, termed AAA proteases (for ATPases associated with a variety of cellular activities).[128–130] They expose their catalytic sites to opposite membrane surfaces, the *m*atrix or *i*ntermembrane space side and are termed *m*- and *i*-AAA proteases, respectively. A proteolytic domain is present at the carboxy-terminus while the amino-terminus anchors the protease to the membrane. Mutant yeast strains lacking the *i*-AAA protease lose respiratory competence at elevated temperature and accumulate mitochondria with a punctate, non-reticulated morphology.[131–133] Turnover of mitochondria by the vacuole is increased resulting in an increased rate of mitochondrial DNA escape.[131] The only identified substrate of the *i*-AAA is a subunit of cytochrome oxidase but others likely exist.[62,131] In yeast, the m-AAA protease is composed of two subunits, Yta10 (Afg3) and Yta12 (Rca1).[62, 134,135] Substrates consist of non-assembled subunits of the respiratory complexes and of the F_1F_0-ATP synthase.[136,137] The m-AAA protease is essential for the maintenance of oxidative phosphorylation. Two orthologs of yeast *m*-AAA protease subunits have been identified in humans.[138] Mutation in one, paraplegin, causes an autosomal recessive form of hereditary spastic paraplegia.[138] Deficiencies in oxidative phosphorylation were observed in these cells, similar to defects observed in yeast. One would expect additional diseases to be linked to a defect in the mitochondrial proteolytic system.

What is the fate of the degraded proteins? Proteolysis of non-assembled mitochondrially coded proteins by AAA proteases results in the formation of a heterogeneous array of peptides and free amino acids within the mitochondria.[139] The degraded products are exported from the mitochondrial matrix by a mitochondrial ABC (ATP-binding cassette) transporter, Mdl1, to the intermembrane space.[140] Mdl1 is a half-type ABC protein that is similar to the transporter associated with antigen presentation in higher eukaryotic cells, which transports peptides into the lumen of the endoplasmic reticulum.[141] The degraded products then exit to the cytosol by passive diffusion, via porin or possibly the TOM complex. The physiological role of peptide export is not known. Interestingly, peptides derived from mitochondrially coded membrane proteins have been detected at the cell surface of mammalian cells, where they are presented by class I MHC molecules. It has been postulated that the mitochondrially coded minor histocompatability antigens are generated by AAA proteases in the mitochondria and then released to the cytosol, from where they enter the conventional class I antigen presentation pathway.[62,142] Alternatively, the exported peptides may be involved in signalling pathways between the mitochondrion and the nucleus.[143]

TIM22 import pathway

Many inner membrane proteins lack a cleavable targeting sequence, carrying instead their targeting and sorting information within the 'mature' part of the polypeptide chain. This category of proteins includes at least 34 members of the yeast mitochondrial carrier family[34] which span the inner membrane six times, as well as the TIM, components. The mechanism by which these inner membrane proteins cross the hydrophilic intermembrane space and then insert correctly into the inner membrane only has been elucidated recently; a new protein import pathway (designated TIM22) that acts specifically on inner membrane proteins has been identified (Fig. 3.3).[20–22,144–146] Components in this pathway are located in the mitochondrial inner membrane and intermembrane space.

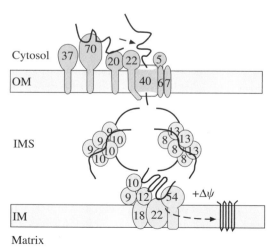

Fig. 3.3 Import of proteins into the mitochondrial inner membrane. As the precursor emerges from the TOM complex, it binds to the Tim9/Tim10 or Tim8/Tim13 complex of the intermembrane space. The bound precursor is then usually delivered to an insertion complex composed of Tim10, Tim12, Tim18, Tim22, and Tim54 that catalyses the membrane potential ($\Delta\psi$)-dependent insertion of the precursor into the inner membrane. See text for details.

A family of small proteins in the mitochondrial intermembrane space mediates import of inner membrane proteins across the intermembrane space.[20,21,144–146] Five proteins, Tim8, Tim9, Tim10, Tim12, and Tim13 have been identified in the yeast intermembrane space, while similar complements are present in other metazoans. The amino acid sequences of the small Tim proteins are 25 per cent identical and 50 per cent similar to each other. They also share a 'twin CX_3C' motif, in which two cysteine residues are separated by three amino acids and each cysteine block is separated from the other by 11–16 amino acids.[145] This motif is reminiscent of a canonical zinc finger, but with a longer spacer. Recombinant Tim10- and Tim12 fusion proteins bind zinc, and interaction between Tim10 and AAC is inhibited by zinc chelators,[20] suggesting that the small Tim proteins bind zinc and that zinc binding is required for their function *in vivo*.

The proteins Tim10 and Tim12 were the first two components of the intermembrane space to mediate protein import.[20,21] Fractionation of yeast mitochondria showed that most of Tim10 was located in the soluble intermembrane space whereas Tim12 was peripherally bound to the outer surface of the inner membrane. Both proteins could be crosslinked chemically to a partly imported AAC precursor, indicating that they interact directly with the imported protein. However, the different intramitochondrial locations of Tim10 and Tim12 reflect their different functions in the import pathway. Inactivation or depletion of Tim12 did not interfere with import of AAC into the intermembrane space, but prevented insertion of AAC into the inner membrane. In contrast, inactivation or depletion of Tim10 blocked import of AAC, P_iC, and Tim22 across the outer membrane. Thus, Tim10 functions before Tim12, probably by binding the incoming precursor as it emerges from the TOM complex.

The Tim9 was identified as a partner protein with Tim10 through genetic and biochemical approaches.[144,146] Most of Tim9 is located in the mitochondrial intermembrane space as a soluble 70 kDa complex containing approximately equimolar amounts of the Tim9 and Tim10;[144,146] the remainder is present in the 300 kDa insertion complex. A single serine → cysteine mutation in Tim9 allowed the protein to suppress the temperature-sensitive mutation in Tim10.[144]

The other two yeast proteins related to Tim10 and Tim12, Tim8 and Tim13,[145] were found in the intermembrane space as a distinct 70 kDa complex that could be separated from the Tim9/Tim10 complex by ion exchange chromatography.[145] Deletion of Tim8 or Tim13, alone or in combination, had no notable effect on cell growth and did not significantly affect import of AAC or P_iC into isolated mitochondria. However, deletion of Tim8 in combination with a temperature-sensitive Tim10 mutation was lethal.[145] Studies with a broader spectrum of precursors in strains lacking Tim8 or Tim13 revealed that Tim8/Tim13 mediated import of Tim23.[35,147,148] Thus the Tim8/Tim13 complex most likely works in parallel with the Tim9/Tim10 complex by mediating the import of a subset of integral inner membrane proteins.

The specific route taken by the substrate to reach the inner membrane is still uncertain. One possibility is that the small Tim complexes act as chaperone-like molecules to guide the precursor across the aqueous intermembrane space, yielding a soluble intermediate in which the precursor is bound to the 70 kDa complexes in the intermembrane space. This model is supported by import studies with temperature-sensitive *tim*10 and *tim*12 mutants, and by the fact that an AAC translocation intermediate bound to Tim10 in intact mitochondria is protected from added protease.[21,144] It predicts a transient complex in which Tim9/Tim10 or Tim8/Tim13 are bound directly to the precursor. Equally plausible is a model in which the 70-kDa complexes form a link between the TOM and the TIM complexes. In this model, the precursor is not released into the intermembrane space, but binds to the small Tim proteins as it emerges from the TOM complex. Further transfer to the Tim22/Tim54 complex could then occur without release into the intermembrane space. This model is supported by the recent finding that an AAC translocation intermediate is partially degraded by added protease.[32] It predicts a transient complex in which the TOM complex as well as the small Tim proteins are bound to the precursor.

Tim22, an essential inner membrane protein, was the first component of the inner membrane complex identified, based on homology to Tim17 and Tim23.[19] Surprisingly, depletion of Tim22 did not affect the general import pathway but inhibited the insertion of inner membrane proteins, particularly those of the carrier family. Although the new protein seemed to participate in mitochondrial import, it was not part of the well-characterized Tim17/Tim23 complex. Rather, Tim22 was recovered from detergent-solubilized mitochondria in a separate high molecular weight complex.[19] A second component, Tim54, was identified through a two hybrid interaction with the mitochondrial outer membrane protein Mmm1.[22] Subsequent analysis revealed that Tim54 is an integral inner membrane protein and partners with Tim22. Inactivation of Tim54 in a temperature-sensitive *tim*54 mutant inhibited import of AAC into isolated mitochondria.[22]

Tim18 was recently identified because it interacted genetically with a temperature-sensitive *tim*54 mutant[149] and co-immunoprecipitated with Tim54.[150] Tim18 is an integral inner membrane protein that is 40 per cent identical to Sdh4, the membrane anchor of succinate dehydrogenase.[151] Tim18, Tim22, and Tim54 with the tiny Tim proteins of the intermembrane space form a 300-kDa complex. While a direct role in protein import has not been established, Tim18 may regulate assembly of the 300-kDa complex because depletion of Tim18 yielded a functional complex of 250 kDa.[149,150]

Defective protein import: a novel type of mitochondrial disease

Humans contain at least six homologues of the small Tim proteins found in the yeast mitochondrial intermembrane space. One of these homologue had already been termed deafness–dystonia peptide (DDP1) because its loss results in the severe X-linked Mohr–Tranebjaerg syndrome, characterized by deafness, dystonia, muscle weakness, dementia, and blindness.[152,153]

DDP1 is most similar to yeast Tim8 and, when expressed in monkey or yeast cells, is located in mitochondria.[145] Mohr–Tranebjaerg syndrome is thus almost certainly a new type of mitochondrial disease caused by a defective protein import system of mitochondria. Loss of DDP1 function probably lowers the mitochondrial abundance of some inner membrane proteins that are critical for the function, development or maintenance of the sensorineural and muscular systems in mammals. The findings in yeast suggest that DDP1 functions as a complex with related partner proteins, perhaps with hTim13. As mutations in DDP1 partner proteins may also be deleterious, and as all potential partner proteins are autosomally encoded, non-X-linked diseases with symptoms resembling those of Mohr–Tranebjaerg syndrome may well have a related etiology. Further, the link between a mitochondrial import defect and a neurodegenerative disease may provide insights into the molecular basis of other more frequent neurological diseases such as Parkinsonism that have been correlated with mitochondrial dysfunction.

Protein export pathways

Recent studies in protein export pathways for mitochondrially coded proteins have revealed new membrane components. While the topology of mitochondrial export resembles that of bacterial secretion, yeast lacks a detectable homologue of the bacterial Sec translocase.[154] However, at least two pathways have been identified for protein export from the matrix to the inner membrane (Fig. 3.1). Oxa1 is a nuclear-coded inner membrane protein that mediates export of amino- and carboxy-tails of the mitochondrially coded precursor cytochrome *c* oxidase subunit II (Cox2) and also plays a role in ATP synthase formation.[155,156] Oxa1 interacts directly with nascent mitochondrially synthesized polypeptides.[156] However, its precise role in membrane insertion is not clear because *oxa*1 mutants can be suppressed by mutations in the nuclear gene coding the cytochrome c_1 subunit of the bc_1 complex.[155] This suppression suggests that the conserved Oxa1 function can be bypassed in the membrane insertion process. Interestingly, Oxa1p has homologs in bacteria, YidC,[157] and chloroplasts, termed ALB3 in *Arabidopsis thaliana*.[158] YidC is essential for *E. coli* viability and mediates the membrane insertion of Sec-independent proteins,[157] while ALB3 is an essential protein mediating integration of the light harvesting chlorophyll-binding protein into thylakoid membranes.[158] Recently, a second protein Mba1 with overlapping functions has been identified that seemingly functions independently of Oxa1. Mba1 also mediates the export of mitochondrial translation products and nuclear-coded proteins that are conservatively sorted.[159]

A third export component, Pnt1, has been identified in an elegant genetic screen to identify yeast mutants defective for the export of mitochondrially coded proteins.[160] Pnt1 is an integral inner membrane protein facing into the matrix that mediates export of the carboxy-terminus of Cox2. However, its precise role in export has not been determined because deletion of *pnt1* in *S. cerevisiae* did not impair Cox2 processing. Deletion of the *PNT1* orthologue from *Kluyveromyces lactis*, KlPNT1, resulted in a non-respiratory phenotype, absence of cytochrome oxidase activity, and a defect in the assembly of KlCox2 that appears to be due to a block of carboxy-tail export. Thus, it may be possible that Oxa1 and Pnt1 have overlapping functions in *S. cerevisiae*. The *PNT1* was, previously identified as a gene that caused resistance to the antimicrobial drug pentamidine.[161] Given the coordination that must be required to assemble the large respiratory complexes of the inner membrane, additional components probably are required.

Perspectives

Biogenesis of the various import components itself is complicated, with individual subunits using different pathways.[68] Tim54 is imported via Tim9/Tim10[148] and inserted into the inner membrane through the TIM23 machinery,[68] whereas Tim22 is imported via the TIM22 complex.[21,68,146] Import of the small Tim proteins bypasses the Tim import machinery altogether, requiring Tom5, but no membrane potential.[68] The complex interplay between the different machineries may ensure coordinated regulation of the assembly of the mitochondrial protein import systems.

The recent discoveries of new import components and new import pathways reveal how little is known about mitochondrial biogenesis, particularly the inner membrane, but also suggest that the answers to these questions will lead to exciting insights into this complicated biological process in normal and disease states.

References

1. Gray MW, Burger G, and Lang BF (1999). Mitochondrial evolution. *Science* **283**: 1476–1481.
2. Pfanner N, Douglas MG, Endo T, Hoogenraad NJ, Jensen RE, Meijer M, *et al.* (1996). Uniform nomenclature for the protein transport machinery of the mitochondrial membranes. *Trends Biochem. Sci.* **21**: 51–52.
3. Pfanner N. Protein sorting: Recognizing mitochondrial presequences. *Curr. Biol.* **10**: R415–R415
4. Neupert W (1997). Protein import into mitochondria. *Ann. Rev. Biochem.* 863–917
5. Schatz G and Dobberstein B (1996). Common principles of protein translocation across membranes. *Science* **271**: 1519–1526.
6. Hurt EC, Pesold-Hurt B, and Schatz G (1984). The amino-terminal region of an imported mitochondrial precursor polypeptide can direct cytoplasmic dihydrofolate reductase into the mitochondrial matrix. *EMBO J.* **3**: 3149–3156
7. Pfanner N, Hoeben P, Tropschug M, and Neupert W (1987). The carboxyl-terminal two-thirds of the ADP/ATP carrier polypeptide contains sufficient information to direct translocation into mitochondria. *J. Biol. Chem.* **262**: 14851–14854.
8. Söllner T, Rassow J, Wiedmann M, Schlossmann J, Keil P, Neupert W, *et al.* (1992). Mapping of the protein import machinery in the mitochondrial outer membrane by crosslinking of translocation intermediates. *Nature* **355**: 84–87.
9. Bolliger L, Junne T, Schatz G, and Lithgow T (1995). Acidic receptor domains on both sides of the outer membrane mediate translocation of precursor proteins into yeast mitochondria. *EMBO J.* **14**: 6318–6326.
10. Eilers M and Schatz G (1986). Binding of a specific ligand inhibits import of a purified precursor protein into mitochondria. *Nature* **322**: 228–232.
11. Ryan KR and Jensen RE (1993). Mas6p can be cross-linked to an arrested precursor and interacts with other proteins during mitochondrial protein import. *J. Biol. Chem.* **268**: 23743–23746.
12. Martin J, Mahlke K, and Pfanner N (1991). Role of an energized inner membrane in mitochondrial protein import: $\Delta\psi$ drives the movement of presequences. *J. Biol. Chem.* **266**: 18051–18057.
13. Kang PJ, Ostermann J, Shilling J, Neupert W, Craig EA, and Pfanner N (1990). Requirement for hsp70 in the mitochondrial matrix for translocation and folding of precursor proteins. *Nature* **348**: 137–143.
14. Horst M, Oppliger W, Feifel B, Schatz G, and Glick BS (1996). The mitochondrial protein import motor: dissociation of mitochondrial hsp70 from its membrane anchor requires ATP binding rather than ATP hydrolysis. *Protein Sci.* **5**: 759–767.
15. Voos W, von Ahsen O, Muller H, Guiard B, Rassow J, and Pfanner N (1996). Differential requirement for the mitochondrial Hsp70-Tim44 complex in unfolding and translocation of preproteins. *EMBO J.* **15**: 2668–2677.
16. Hawlitschek G, Schneider H, Schmidt B, Tropschug M, Hartl FU, and Neupert W (1988). Mitochondrial protein import: identification of processing peptidase and of PEP, a processing enhancing protein. *Cell* **53**: 795–806.
17. Ostermann J, Horwich AL, Neupert W, and Hartl FU (1989). Protein folding in mitochondria requires complex formation with hsp60 and ATP hydrolysis. *Nature* **341**: 125–130.
18. Rospert S, Looser R, Dubaquie Y, Matouschek A, Glick BS, and Schatz G (1996). Hsp60-independent protein folding in the matrix of yeast mitochondria. *EMBO J.* **15**: 764–774.
19. Sirrenberg C, Bauer MF, Guiard B, Neupert W, and Brunner M (1996). Import of carrier proteins into the mitochondrial inner membrane mediated by Tim22. *Nature* **384**: 582–585.
20. Sirrenberg C, Endres M, Folsch H, Stuart RA, Neupert W, and Brunner M (1998). Carrier protein import into mitochondria mediated by the intermembrane proteins Tim10/Mrs11 and Tim12/Mrs5. *Nature* **391**: 912–915.

21. Koehler CM, Jarosch E, Tokatlidis K, Schmid K, Schweyen RJ, and Schatz G (1998). Import of mito-chondrial carriers mediated by essential proteins of the intermembrane space. *Science* **279**: 369–373.

22. Kerscher O, Holder J, Srinivasan M, Leung RS, and Jensen RE (1997). The Tim54p-Tim22p com-plex mediates insertion of proteins into the mitochondrial inner membrane. *J. Cell Biol.* **139**: 1663–1675.

23. Abe YTS, Muto T, Mihara K, Nishikawa S-I, Endo T, *et al.* (2000). Structural basis of presequence recognition by the mitochondrial presequence receptor Tom20. *Cell* **100**: 551–560.

24. Rospert S, Junne T, Glick BS, and Schatz G (1993). Cloning disruption of the gene encoding yeast mitochondrial chaperonin 10, the homolog of E. coli groES. *FEBS Lett.* **335**: 358–360.

25. Dmochowska A, Konopinska A, Krzymowska M, Szczesniak B, and Boguta M (1995). The NAM9-1 suppressor mutation in a nuclear gene encoding ribosomal mitochondrial protein of Saccharomyces cerevisiae. *Gene* **162**: 81–85.

26. Lee CM, Sedman J, Neupert W, and Stuart RA (1999). The DNA helicase, Hmi1p, is transported into mitochondria by a C-terminal cleavable targeting signal. *J. Biol. Chem.* **274**: 20937–20942.

27. Glick BS, Brandt A, Cunningham K, Muller S, Hallberg RL, and Schatz G (1992). Cytochromes c1 and b2 are sorted to the intermembrane space of yeast mitochondria by a stop-transfer mechanism. *Cell* **69**: 809–822.

28. Nunnari J, Fox TD, and Walter P (1993). A mitochondrial protease with two catalytic subunits of nonoverlapping specificities. *Science* **262**: 1997–2004.

29. Gartner F, Voos W, Querol A, Miller BR, Craig EA, Cumsky MG, *et al.* (1995). Mitochondrial import of subunit Va of cytochrome c oxidase characterized with yeast mutants. *J. Biol. Chem.* **270**: 3788–3795.

30. Folsch H, Guiard B, Neupert W, and Stuart RA (1996). Internal targeting signal of the BCS1 protein: a novel mechanism of import into mitochondria. *EMBO J.* **15**: 479–487.

31. Brix J, Rudiger S, Bukau B, Schneider-Mergener J, and Pfanner N (1999). Distribution of binding sequences for the mitochondrial import receptors Tom20, Tom22, and Tom70 in a presequence-carrying preprotein and a non-cleavable preprotein. *J. Biol. Chem.* **274**: 16522–16530.

32. Endres M, Neupert W, and Brunner M (1999). Transport of the ADP/ATP carrier of mitochondria from the TOM complex to the TIM22.54 complex. *EMBO J.* **18**: 3214–3221.

33. Davis AJ, Ryan KR, and Jensen RE (1998). Tim23p contains separate and distinct signals for tar-geting to mitochondria and insertion into the inner membrane. *Mol. Biol. Cell* **9**: 2577–2593.

34. Palmieri F, Bisaccia F, Capobianco L, Dolce V, Fiermonte G, Iacobazzi V, *et al.* (1996). Mitochondrial metabolite transporters. *Biochim. Biophys. Acta* **1275**: 127–132.

35. Paschen SA, Rothbauer U, Kaldi K, Bauer MF, Neupert W, and Brunner M (2000). The role of the TIM8–13 complex in the import of Tim23 into mitochondria. *EMBO J.* **19**: 6392–6400.

36. Deshaies RJ, Koch BD, Werner-Washburne M, Craig EA, and Schekman R (1988). A subfamily of stress proteins facilitates translocation of secretory and mitochondrial precursor polypeptides. *Nature* **332**: 800–805.

37. Murakami H, Pain D, and Blobel G (1988). 70-kD heat shock-related protein is one of at least two distinct cytosolic factors stimulating protein import into mitochondria. *J. Cell. Biol.* **107**: 2051–2057.

38. Lithgow T, Ryan M, Anderson RL, Hoj PB, and Hoogenrad NJ (1993). A constitutive form of heat-shock protein 70 is located in the outer membranes of mitochondria from rat liver. *FEBS Lett.* **332**: 277–281.

39. Attencio DP and Yaffe MP (1992). MAS5, a yeast homolog of DnaJ involved in mitochondrial pro-tein import. *Mol. Cell. Biol.* **12**: 283–291.

40. Wiedmann B, Sakai H, Davis TA, and Wiedmann M (1994). A protein complex required for signal-sequence-specific sorting and translocation. *Nature* **370**: 434–437.

41. Fünfschilling U and Rospert S (1999). Nascent polypeptide-associated complex stimulates protein import into yeast mitochondria. *Mol. Biol. Cell* **10**: 3289–3299.

42. George R, Beddoe T, Landl K, and Lithgow T (1998). The yeast nascent polypeptide-associated complex initiates protein targeting to mitochondria *in vivo. Proc. Natl Acad. Sci. USA* **95**: 2296–2301.

43. Mihara K and Omura T (1996). Cytosolic factors in mitochondrial protein import. *Experientia* **52**: 1063–1068.

44. Komiya T, Hachiya N, Sakaguchi M, Omura T, and Mihara K (1994). Recognition of mitochondria-targeting signals by a cytosolic import stimulation factor, MSF. *J. Biol. Chem.* **269**: 30893–30897.

45. Roberts RL, Mosch HU, and Fink GR (1997). 14-3-3 proteins are essential for RAS/MAPK cascade signaling during pseudohyphal development in S. cerevisiae. *Cell* **89**: 1055–1065.

46. Dekker PJ, Muller H, Rassow J, and Pfanner N (1996). Characterization of the preprotein translocase of the outer mitochondrial membrane by blue native electrophoresis. *Biol. Chem.* **377**: 535–538.

47. Ahting U, Thun C, Hegerl R, Typke D, Nargang FE, Neupert W, *et al.* (1999). The TOM core complex: the general protein import pore of the outer membrane of mitochondria. *J. Cell Biol.* **147**: 959–968.

48. van Wilpe S, Ryan MT, Brix J, Maarse AC, Meisinger C, Brix J, *et al.* (1999). Tom22 is a multifunctional organizer of the mitochondrial preprotein translocase. *Nature* **401**: 485–489.

49. Künkele KP, Heins S, Dembowski M, Nargang FE, and Benz R, Thieffry M, *et al.* (1998). The preprotein translocation channel of the outer membrane of mitochondria. *Cell* **93**: 1009–1019.

50. Baker KP and Schatz G (1991). Mitochondrial proteins essential for viability mediate protein import into yeast mitochondria. *Nature* **349**: 205–208.

51. Söllner T, Griffiths G, Pfaller R, Pfanner N, and Neupert W (1989). MOM19, an import receptor for mitochondrial precursor proteins. *Cell* **59**: 1061–1070.

52. Ramage L, Junne T, Hahne K, Lithgow T, and Schatz G (1993). Functional cooperation of mitochondrial protein import receptors in yeast. *EMBO J.* **12**: 4115–4123.

53. Hines V, Brandt A, Griffiths G, Horstmann H, Brutsch H, and Schatz G (1990). Protein import into yeast mitochondria is accelerated by the outer membrane protein MAS70. *EMBO J.* **9**: 3191–3200.

54. Wiedemann N, Pfanner N, and Ryan MT (2001). The three modules of ADP/ATP carrier cooperate in receptor recruitment and translocation into mitochondria. *EMBO J.* **20**: 951–960.

55. Brix J, Ziegler GA, Dietmeier K, Schneider-Mergener J, Schulz GE, and Pfanner N (2000). The mitochondrial import receptor Tom70: identification of a 25 kDa core domain with a specific binding site for preproteins. *J. Mol. Biol.* **303**: 479–488.

56. Bömer U, Pfanner N, and Dietmeier K (1996). Identification of a third yeast mitochondrial Tom protein with tetratrico peptide repeats. *FEBS Lett.* **382**: 153–158.

57. Schlossmann J, Lill R, Neupert W, and Court DA (1996). Tom71, a novel homologue of the mitochondrial preprotein receptor Tom70. *J. Biol. Chem.* **271**: 17890–17895.

58. Lithgow T, Junne T, Suda K, Gratzer S, and Schatz G (1994). The mitochondrial outer membrane protein Mas22p is essential for protein import and viability of yeast. *Proc. Natl Acad. Sci. USA* **91**: 11973–11977.

59. Kiebler M, Keil P, Schneider H, van der Klei IJ, Pfanner N, and Neupert W (1993). The mitochondrial receptor complex: a central role of MOM22 in mediating preprotein transfer from receptors to the general insertion pore. *Cell* **74**: 483–492.

60. Ryan MT, HM, and Pfanner N (1999). Functional Staging of ADP/ATP Carrier Translocation across the Outer Mitochondrial Membrane. *J. Biol. Chem.* **274**: 20619–20627.

61. Gratzer S, Lithgow T, Bauer RE, Lamping E, Paltauf F, Kohlwein SD, *et al.* (1995). Mas37p, a novel receptor subunit for protein import into mitochondria. *J. Cell Biol.* **129**: 25–34.

62. Hachiya N, Mihara K, Suda K, Horst M, Schatz G, and Lithgow T (1995). Reconstitution of the initial steps of mitochondrial protein import. *Nature* **376**: 705–709.

63. Armstrong LC, Komiya T, Bergman BE, Mihara K, and Bornstein P (1997). Metaxin is a component of a preprotein import complex in the outer membrane of the mammalian mitochondrion. *J. Biol. Chem.* **272**: 6510–6518.

64. Abdul KM, Terada K, Yano M, Ryan MT, Streimann I, Hoogenraad NJ, *et al.* (2000). Functional analysis of human metaxin in mitochondrial protein import in cultured cells and its relationship with the Tom complex. *Biochem. Biophys. Res. Comm.* **276**: 1028–1034.

65. Armstrong LC, Saenz AJ, and Bornstein P (1999). Metaxin 1 interacts with metaxin 2, a novel related protein associated with the mammalian mitochondrial outer membrane. *J. Cell. Biochem.* **74**: 11–22.

66. Hill K, Model K, Ryan MT, Dietmeier K, Martin F, Wagner R, *et al.* (1998). Tom40 forms the hydrophilic channel of the mitochondrial import pore for preproteins. *Nature* **395**: 516–521.

67. Künkele KP, Juin P, Pompa C, Nargang FE, Henry JP, Neupert W, *et al.* (1998). The isolated complex of the translocase of the outer membrane of mitochondria. Characterization of the cation-selective and voltage-gated preprotein-conducting pore. *J. Biol. Chem.* **273**: 31032–31039.

68. Kurz M, Martin H, Rassow J, Pfanner N, and Ryan MT (1999). Biogenesis of Tim proteins of the mitochondrial carrier import pathway: Differential targeting mechanisms and crossing over with the main import pathway. *Mol. Biol. Cell* **10**: 2461–2474.

69. Dekker PJ, Ryan MT, Brix J, Muller H, Honlinger A, and Pfanner N (1998). Preprotein translocase of the outer mitochondrial membrane: molecular dissection and assembly of the general import pore complex. *Mol. Cell. Biol.* **18**: 6515–6524.

70. Krimmer TDR, Ryan MT, Meisinger C, Kassenbrock CK, Blachly-Dyson E, *et al.* (2001). Biogenesis of porin of the outer mitochondrial membrane involves an import pathway via receptors and the general import pore of the TOM complex. *J. Cell Biol.* **2001**: 289–300.

71. Schatz G (1997). Just follow the acid chain. *Nature* **388**: 121–122.

72. Komiya T, Rospert S, Koehler C, Looser R, Schatz G, and Mihara K (1998). Interaction of mito-chondrial targeting signals with acidic receptor domains along the protein import pathway: evi-dence for the 'acid chain' hypothesis. *EMBO J.* **17**: 3886–3898.

73. Brix J, Dietmeier K, and Pfanner N (1997). Differential recognition of preproteins by the purified cytsolic domains of the mitochondrial import receptors Tom20, Tom22, and Tom70. *J. Biol. Chem.* **272**: 20730–20735.

74. Pfanner N and Meijer M (1997). The Tom and Tim machine. *Curr. Biol.* **7**: 100–103.

75. Horst M, Azem A, Schatz G, and Glick BS (1997). What is the driving force for protein import into mitochondria? *Biochim. Biophys. Acta* **1318**: 71–78.

76. Horst M, Hilfiker-Rothenfluh S, Oppliger W, and Schatz G (1995). Dynamic interaction of the pro-tein translocation systems in the inner and outer membranes of yeast mitochondria. *EMBO J.* **14**: 2293–2297.

77. Dekker PJ, Martin F, Maarse AC, Bomer U, Muller H, Guiard B, *et al.* (1997). The Tim core com-plex defines the number of mitochondrial translocation contact sites and can hold arrested prepro-teins in the absence of matrix Hsp70-Tim44. *EMBO J.* **16**: 5408–5419.

78. Schwartz MP and Matouschek A (1999). The dimensions of the protein import channel in the outer and inner mitochondrial membranes. *Proc. Natl Acad. Sci. USA* **98**: 13086–13090.

79. Ryan KR, Menold MM, Garrett S, and Jensen RE (1994). SMS1, a high-copy suppressor of the yeast mas6 mutant, encodes an essential inner membrane protein required for mitochondrial protein import. *Mol. Biol. Cell* **5**: 529–538.

80. Maarse AC, Blom J, Keil P, Pfanner N, and Meijer M (1994). Identification of the essential yeast protein MIM17, an integral mitochondrial inner membrane protein involved in protein import. *FEBS Lett.* **349**: 215–221.

81. Dekker PJ, Keil P, Rassow J, Maarse AC, Pfanner N, and Meijer M (1993). Identification of MIM23, a putative component of the protein import machinery of the mitochondrial inner mem-brane. *FEBS Lett.* **330**: 66–70.

82. Bauer MF, Sirrenberg C, Neupert W, and Brunner M (1996). Role of Tim23 as voltage sensor and presequence receptor in protein import into mitochondria. *Cell* **87**: 33–41.

83. Donzeau M, Kaldi K, Adam A, Paschen S, Wanner G, Guiard B, *et al.* (2000). Tim23 links the inner and outer mitochondrial membranes. *Cell* **101**: 401–412.

84. Geissler A, Krimmer T, Bomer U, Guiard B, Rassow J, and Pfanner N (2000). Membrane potential-driven protein import into mitochondria. The sorting sequence of cytochrome b₂ modulates the delta Ψ-dependence of translocation of the matrix-targeting sequence. *Mol. Biol. Cell* **11**: 3977–3991.

85. Craig EA, Kramer J, Shilling J, Werner-Washburne M, Holmes S, Kosic-Smithers J, *et al.* (1989). SSC1, an essential member of the yeast HSP70 multigene family, encodes a mitochondrial protein. *Mol. Cell. Biol.* **9**: 3000–3008.

86. Hartl FU (1996). Molecular chaperones in cellular protein folding. *Nature* **381**: 571–579.

87. Bukau B and Horwich AL (1998). The Hsp70 and Hsp60 chaperone machines. *Cell* **92**: 351–366.

88. Krimmer T, Rassow J, Kunau WH, Voos W, and Pfanner N (2000). The mitochondrial protein import motor: the ATPase domain of matrix Hsp70 is crucial for binding to Tim44, while the peptide binding domain and the carboxy-terminal segment play a stimulatory role. *Mol. Cell. Biol.* **20**: 5879–5887.

89. Gambill BD, Voos W, Kang PJ, Miao B, Langer T, Craig EA, *et al.* (1993). A dual role for mitochondrial heat shock protein 70 in membrane translocation of preproteins. *J. Cell. Biol.* **123**: 109–117.

90. Kronidou NG, Oppliger W, Bolliger L, Hannavy K, Glick BS, Schatz G, *et al.* (1994). Dynamic interaction between Isp45 and mitochondrial hsp70 in the protein import system of the yeast mitochondrial inner membrane. *Proc. Natl Acad. Sci. USA* **91**: 12818–12822.

91. Bolliger L, Deloche O, Glick BS, Georgopoulos C, Jeno P, Kronidou N, *et al.* (1994). A mitochondrial homolog of bacterial GrpE interacts with mitochondrial hsp70 and is essential for viability. *EMBO J.* **13**: 1998–2006.

92. Voos W, Gambill BD, Laloraya S, Ang D, Craig EA, and Pfanner N (1994). Mitochondrial GrpE is present in a complex with hsp70 and preproteins in transit across membranes. *Mol. Cell. Biol.* **14**: 6627–6634.

93. Neupert W, Hartl FU, Craig EA, and Pfanner N (1990). How do polypeptides cross the mitochondrial membranes? *Cell* **63**: 447–450.

94. Ungermann C, Guiard B, Neupert W, and Cyr DM (1996). The delta psi- and Hsp70/MIM44-dependent reaction cycle driving early steps of protein import into mitochondria. *EMBO J.* **15**: 735–744.

95. Gaume B, Klaus C, Ungermann C, Guiard B, Neupert W, and Brunner M (1998). Unfolding of preproteins upon import into mitochondria. *EMBO J.* **17**: 6497–6507.

96. Shi L, Kataoka M, and Fink AL (1996). Conformational characterization of DnaK and its complexes by small-angle X-ray scattering. *Biochemistry* **35**: 3297–3308.

97. von Ahsen O, Voos W, Henninger H, and Pfanner N (1995). The mitochondrial protein import machinery. Role of ATP in dissociation of the Hsp70.Mim44 complex. *J. Biol. Chem.* **270**: 29848–29853.

98. Glick BS (1995). Can hsp70 proteins act as force generating motors? *Cell* **80**: 11–14.

99. Pfanner N and Meijer M (1995). Protein sorting. Pulling in the proteins. *Curr. Biol.* **5**: 132–135.

100. Voisine C, Craig EA, Zufall N, von Ahsen O, Pfanner N, and Voos W (1999). The protein import motor of mitochondria: unfolding and trapping of preproteins are distinct and separable functions of matrix Hsp70. *Cell* **97**: 565–574.

101. Huang S, Ratliff KS, Schwartz MP, Spenner JM, and Matouschek A (1999). Mitochondria unfold precursor proteins by unraveling them from their N-termini. *Nat. Struct. Biol.* **6**: 1132–1138.

102. Matouschek A, Pfanner N, and Voos W (2000). Protein unfolding by mitochondria: The Hsp70 motor. *EMBO Reports* **1**: 404–410.

103. Fenton WA, Weissman JS, and Horwich AL (1996). Putting a lid on protein folding: structure and function of the co-chaperonin, GroES. *Chem. Biol.* **3**: 157–161.

104. Briones P, Vilaseca MA, Ribes A, Vernet A, Lluch M, Cusi V, *et al.* (1997). A new case of multiple mitochondrial enzyme deficiencies with decreased amount of heat shock protein 60. *J. Inherit. Metab. Dis.* **20**: 569–577.

105. Huckriede A, Heikema A, Wilschut J, and Agsteribbe E (1996). Transient expression of a mitochondrial precursor protein. A new approach to study mitochondrial protein import in cells of higher eukaryotes. *Eur. J. Biochem.* **237**: 288–294.

106. Schmid FX (1993). Prolyl isomerases: enzymatic catalysis of slow protein-folding reactions. *Annu. Rev. Biophys. Biomol. Struct.* **22**: 123–143.

107. Rassow J, Mohrs K, Koidl S, Barthelmess IB, Pfanner N, and Tropschug M (1995). Cyclophilin 20 is involved in mitochondrial protein folding in cooperation with molecular chaperones Hsp70 and Hsp60. *Mol. Cell. Biol.* **15**: 2654–2662.

108. Matouschek A, Rospert S, Schmid K, Glick BS, and Schatz G (1995). Cyclophilin catalyzes protein folding in yeast mitochondria. *Proc. Natl Acad. Sci. USA* **92**: 6319–6323.

109. Tokatlidis K, Junne T, Moes S, Schatz G, Glick BS, and Kronidou N (1996). Translocation arrest of an intramitochondrial sorting signal next to Tim11 at the inner-membrane import site. *Nature* **384**: 585–588.

110. Arnold I, Pfeiffer K, Neupert W, Stuart RA, and Schagger H (1998). Yeast mitochondrial F1F0–ATP synthase exists as a dimer: identification of three dimer-specific subunits. *EMBO J.* **17**: 7170–7178.

111. Kanamori T, Nishikawa S, Shin I, Schultz PG, and Endo T (1997). Probing the environment along the protein import pathways in yeast mitochondria by site-specific photocrosslinking. *Proc. Natl Acad. Sci. USA* **94**: 485–490.

112. Rep M and Grivell LA (1996). The role of protein degradation in mitochondrial function and biogenesis. *Curr. Genet.* **30**: 367–380.

113. Langer T and Neupert W (1996). Regulated protein degradation in mitochondria. *Experientia* **52**: 1069–1076.

114. Geli V, Yang MJ, Suda K, Lustig A, and Schatz G (1990). The MAS-encoded processing protease of yeast mitochondria. Overproduction and characterization of its two nonidentical subunits. *J. Biol. Chem.* **265**: 19216–19222.

115. Witte C, Jensen RE, Yaffe MP, and Schatz G (1988). MAS1, a gene essential for yeast mitochondrial assembly, encodes a subunit of the mitochondrial processing protease. *EMBO J.* **7**: 1439–1447.

116. Luciano P and Geli V (1996). The mitochondrial processing peptidase: function and specificity. *Experientia* **52**: 1077–1082.

117. Isaya G, Kalousek F, Fenton WA, and Rosenberg LE (1991). Cleavage of precursors by the mitochondrial processing peptidase requires a compatible mature protein or an intermediate octapeptide. *J. Cell Biol.* **113**: 65–76.

118. Kalousek F, Isaya G, and Rosenberg LE (1992). Rat liver mitochondrial intermediate peptidase (MIP): purification and initial characterization. *EMBO J.* **11**: 2803–2809.

119. Isaya G, Miklos D, and Rollins RA (1994). *MIP1*, a new yeast gene homologous to the rat mitochondrial intermediate peptidase gene, is required for oxidative metabolism in *Saccharomyces cerevisiae*. *Mol. Cell. Biol.* **14**: 5603–5616.

120. Schneider A, Behrens M, Scherer P, Pratje E, Michaelis G, and Schatz G (1991). Inner membrane protease I, an enzyme mediating intramitochondrial protein sorting in yeast. *EMBO J.* **10**: 247–254.

121. Dalbey RE, Lively MO, Bron S, and van Dijl JM (1997). The chemistry and enzymology of the type I signal peptidase. *Protein Sci.* **6**: 1129–1138.

122. Suzuki CK, Rep M, Maarten van Dijl J, Suda K, Grivell LA, and Schatz G (1997). ATP-dependent proteases that also chaperone protein biogenesis. *Trends Biochem. Sci.* **22**: 118–123.

123. Suzuki CK, Suda K, Wang N, and Schatz G (1994). Requirement for the yeast gene LON in intramitochondrial proteolysis and maintenance of respiration. *Science* **264**: 891.

124. Wagner I, Arlt H, van Dyck L, Langer T, and Neupert W (1994). Molecular chaperones cooperate with PIM1 protease in the degradation of misfolded proteins in mitochondria. *EMBO J.* **13**: 5135–5145.

125. Fu GK and Markovitz DM (1998). The human Lon protease binds to mitochondrial promoters in a single-stranded, site-specific, strand-specific manner. *Biochemistry* **37**: 1905–1909.

126. Bross P, Andresen BS, Knudsen I, Kruse TA, and Gregersen N (1995). Human ClpP protease: cDNA sequence, tissue-specific expression and chromosomal assignment of the gene. *FEBS Lett.* **377**: 249–252.

127. Gottesman S, Maurizi MR, and Wickner S (1997). Regulatory subunits of energy-dependent proteases. *Cell* **91**: 435–438.

128. Patel S and Latterich M (1998). The AAA team: related ATPases with diverse functions. *Trends Cell. Biol.* **8**: 65–71.

129. Beyer A (1997). Sequence analysis of the AAA protein family. *Protein Sci.* **6**: 2043–2058.

130. Leonhard K, Herrmann JM, Stuart RA, Mannhaupt G, Neupert W, and Langer T (1996). AAA proteases with catalytic sites on opposite membrane surfaces comprise a proteolytic system for the ATP-dependent degradation of inner membrane proteins in mitochondria. *EMBO J.* **15**: 4218–4229.

131. Weber ER, Hanekamp T, and Thorsness PE (1996). Biochemical and functional analysis of the YME1 gene product, an ATP and zinc-dependent mitochondrial protease from S. cerevisiae. *Mol. Biol. Cell* **7**: 307–317.

132. Thorseness PE, White KH, and Fox TD (1993). Inactivation of *YME1*, a member of the ftsH-SEC18-PAS1-CDC48 family of putative ATPase-encoding genes, causes increased escape of DNA from mitochondria in *Saccharomyces cerevisiae. Mol. Cell. Biol.* **13**: 54118–55426.

133. Campbell CL, Tanaka N, White KH, and Thorsness PE (1994). Mitochondrial morphological and functional defects in yeast caused by *yme1* are suppressed by mutation of a 26S protease subunit homologue. *Mol. Biol. Cell* **5**: 899–905.

134. Guelin E, Rep M, and Grivell LA (1994). Sequence of the AFG3 gene encoding a new member of the FstH/Yme1/Tma subfamily of the AAA-protein family. *Yeast* **10**: 1389–1394.

135. Tauer R, Mannhaupt G, Schnall R, Pajic A, Langer T, and Feldmann H (1994). Yta10p, a member of a novel ATPase family in yeast, is essential for mitochondrial function. *FEBS Lett.* **353**: 197–200.

136. h'Arlt H, Tauer R, Feldmann H, Neupert W, and Langer T (1996). The YTA10–12 complex, an AAA protease with chaperone-like activity in the inner membrane of mitochondria. *Cell* **85**: 875–885.

137. Guelin E, Rep M, and Grivell LA (1996). Afg3p, a mitochondrial ATP-dependent metalloprotease, is involved in the degradation of mitochondrially-encoded Cox1, Cox3, Cob, Su6, Su8, and Su9 subunits of the inner membrane complexes III, IV and V. *FEBS Lett.* **381**: 42–46.

138. Casari G, De Fusco M, Ciarmatori S, Zeviani M, Mora M, Fernandez P, *et al.* (1998). Spastic paraplegia and OXPHOS impairment caused by mutations in paraplegin, a nuclear-encoded mitochondrial metalloprotease. *Cell* **93**: 973–983.

139. Desautels M and Goldberg AL (1982). Liver mitochondria contain an ATP-dependent, vanadate-sensitive pathway for the degradation of proteins. *Proc. Natl Acad. Sci. USA* **79**: 1869–1873.

140. Young L, Leonhard K, Tatsuta T, Trowsdale J, and Langer T (2001). Role of the ABC transporter Mdl1 in peptide export from mitochondria. *Science* **291**: 2135–2138.

141. Elliott T, Young L, Leonhard K, Tatsuta T, Trowsdale J, and Langer T (1997). Transporter associated with antigen processing between mitochondria and their cellular environment. *Adv. Immunol.* **65**: 47–109.

142. Lindahl KF, Byers DE, Dabhi VM, Hovik R, Jones EP, Smith GP, *et al.* (1997). H2-M3, a full-service class Ib histocompatibility antigen. *Annu. Rev. Immunol.* **15**: 851–879.

143. Hallstrom TC and Moye-Rowley WS (2000). Multiple signals from dysfunctional mitochondria activate the pleiotropic drug resistance pathway in Saccharomyces cerevisiae. *J. Biol. Chem.* **275**: 37347–37356.

144. Koehler CM, Merchant S, Oppliger W, Schmid K, Jarosch E, Dolfini L, *et al.* (1998). Tim9p, an essential partner subunit of Tim10p for the import of mitochondrial carrier proteins. *EMBO J.* **17**: 6477–6486.

145. Koehler CM, Leuenberger D, Merchant S, Renold A, Junne T, and Schatz G (1999). Human deafness dystonia syndrome is a mitochondrial disease. *Proc. Natl Acad. Sci. USA* **96**: 2141–2146.

146. Adam A, Endres M, Sirrenberg C, Lottspeich F, Neupert W, and Brunner M (1999). Tim9, a new component of the TIM22.54 translocase in mitochondria. *EMBO J.* **18**: 313–319.

147. Davis AJ, Sepuri NB, Holder J, Johnson AE, and Jensen RE (2000). Two intermembrane space TIM complexes interact with different domains of Tim23p during its import into mitochondria. *J. Cell Biol.* **150**: 1271–1282.

148. Leuenberger D, Bally NA, Schatz G, and Koehler CM (1999). Different import pathways through the mitochondrial intermembrane space for inner membrane proteins. *EMBO J.* **17**: 4816–4822.

149. Kerscher O, Sepuri NB, and Jensen RE (2000). Tim18p is a new component of the Tim54p-Tim22p translocon in the mitochondrial inner membrane. *Mol. Biol. Cell* **11**: 103–116.

150. Koehler CM, Murphy MP, Bally N, Leuenberger D, Oppliger W, Dolfini L, *et al.* (2000). Tim18p, a novel subunit of the inner membrane complex that mediates protein import into the yeast mitochondrial inner membrane. *Mol. Cell. Biol.* **20**: 1187–1193.

151. Oyedotun KS and Lemire BD (1997). The carboxyl terminus of the Saccharomyces cerevisiae succinate dehydrogenase membrane subunit, SDH4p, is necessary for ubiquinone reduction and enzyme stability. *J. Biol. Chem.* **272**: 31382–31388.

152. Tranebjaerg L, Schwartz C, Eriksen H, Andreasson S, Ponjavic V, Dahl A, *et al.* (1995). A new X linked recessive deafness syndrome with blindness, dystonia, fractures, and mental deficiency is linked to Xq22. *J. Med. Genet.* **32**: 257–263.

153. Jin H, May M, Tranebjaerg L, Kendall E, Fontan G, Jackson J, *et al.* (1996). A novel X-linked gene, DDP, shows mutations in families with deafness (DFN-1), dystonia, mental deficiency and blindness. *Nat. Genet.* **14**: 177–180.

154. Glick BS and Von Heijne G (1996). Saccharomyces cerevisiae mitochondria lack a bacterial-type sec machinery. *Protein Sci.* **5**: 2651–2652.

155. Hamel P, Lemaire C, Bonnefoy N, Brivet-Chevillotte P, and Dujardin G (1998). Mutations in the membrane anchor of yeast cytochrome c_1. compensate for the absence of Oxa1p and generate carbonate-extractable forms of cytochrome c_1. *Genetics* **150**: 601–611.

156. Hell K, Herrmann J, Pratje E, Neupert W, and Stuart RA (1997). Oxa1p mediates the export of the N- and C-termini of pCoxII from the mitochondrial matrix to the intermembrane space. *FEBS Lett.* **418**: 367–370.

157. Samuelson JC, Chen M, Jiang F, Moller I, Wiedmann M, Kuhn A, *et al.* (2000). YidC mediates membrane protein insertion in bacteria. *Nature* **406**: 637–641.

158. Sundberg E, Slagter JG, Fridborg I, Cleary SP, Robinson C, and Coupland G (1997). ALBINO3, an Arabidopsis nuclear gene essential for chloroplast differentiation, encodes a chloroplast protein that shows homology to proteins present in bacterial membranes and yeast mitochondria. *Plant Cell* **9**: 717–730.

159. Preuss M, Leonhard K, Hell K, Stuart RA, Neupert W, and Herrmann JM (2001). Mba1, a novel component of the mitochondrial protein export machinery of the yeast Saccharomyces cerevisiae. *J. Cell Biol.* **153**: 1085–1096.

160. He S and Fox TD (1999). Mutations affecting a yeast mitochondrial inner membrane protein, pnt1p, block export of a mitochondrially synthesized fusion protein from the matrix. *Mol. Cell. Biol.* **19**: 6598–6607.

161. Ludewig G and Staben C (1994). Characterization of the *PNT1* pentamidine resistance gene of *Saccharomyces cerevisiae*. *Antimicrob. Agents Chemotherap.* **38**: 2850–285.

4 Oxidative phosphorylation: an overview

Mårten Wikström

Mitochondria are intracellular organelles characteristic of all eukaryotic cells. They are the sole site of oxidative phosphorylation, a process where free energy from aerobic cell respiration is converted into adenosine triphosphate (ATP), the major energy currency of the cell. In aerobic cells oxidative phosphorylation is the major mechanism of ATP formation and is hence of key importance for their survival. There is compelling evidence for the view that mitochondria evolved from aerobic bacteria in an endosymbiotic process some 2–3 billion years ago.[1,2] Larger anaerobic cells engulfed the aerobic bacteria, followed over time by sequential transfer of most of their genes to the developing nucleus of the host cell. Present day mitochondria retain a bacterial-like ribosome, and circular DNA molecules that encode gene products, which despite their small number have fundamental metabolic functions. These functions relate to the key role of mitochondria in the energy metabolism of eukaryotic cells.

This chapter aims to give a broad overview of the process of oxidative phosphorylation, and does not therefore always cite original work. Instead, several specialist review articles have been cited to help those readers who require a more detailed and comprehensive picture.

General structure of the mitochondrion

The size and shape of mitochondria vary between different tissues, as do their number per cell. Yet, the basic structure remains essentially the same. An outer membrane encompasses the organelle, and presumably arose from the cell membrane of the ancient endosymbiont host. The lipid composition of the outer membrane is indeed similar to that of the plasma membrane. From a bioenergetic point of view it is important to note that the outer membrane is relatively permeable to metabolites as well as to small molecules, in part due to the presence of porins.

The inner membrane is very different, deriving from the cell membrane of the engulfed aerobic bacterium. It is usually highly convoluted into *cristae* structures which maximizes its surface area, and it contains membrane proteins to about 70 per cent by weight. This highly unusual membrane lacks cholesterol and uniquely contains the negatively charged phospholipid cardiolipin. The inner membrane is by itself quite impermeable to most molecules, including small ions, which is one of the keys to its bioenergetic function. Metabolites, such as adenosine diphosphate (ADP), inorganic phosphate (P_i), some citric acid cycle intermediates, and ions, such as Ca^{2+}, may penetrate only by means of specific proteinaceous *carrier molecules* or *transporters* in the membrane. The exception is gas molecules, such as O_2 and CO_2, and some other generally uncharged hydrophobic substances, which readily penetrate due to their apolar character. A specific example is various weak organic acids that penetrate the membrane both in the uncharged acid form and in the dissociated anionic form due to effective delocalization of the charge.[3,4] This property renders such compounds to be *uncoupling agents*: by catalysing proton transfer across the membrane they dissipate the *proton-motive force* and maximize the rate of respiration without synthesis of ATP.

The inner membrane is the site of oxidative phosphorylation. It contains the protein complexes constituting the so-called *respiratory chain*, as well as the *H⁺–ATP synthase*, the key enzyme of oxidative synthesis of ATP. However, it also contains several other membrane proteins, such as a plethora of metabolite and ion carriers that link the metabolism of the cytoplasm with that of the inner mitochondrial space, the *matrix*. The number of mitochondria per cell is not necessarily the relevant bioenergetic parameter, due to the variation in mitochondrial size, but rather the amount of inner mitochondrial membrane per cell. The abundance of proteins in the inner membrane can be approximated from the inner membrane area (ca. 40 m^2 per g of protein for rat liver mitochondria)[5] and the concentration of some of the most abundant proteins, cytochrome *c* oxidase and the H⁺–ATP synthase (each ca. 0.14 $\mu mol/g$ of protein in rat liver mitochondria). Therefore, on the average, a square of membrane surface of ca. 38 nm × 38 nm will contain 10 monomers of each of these proteins (Fig. 4.1), *plus* five cytochrome bc_1 monomers (Complex III), one copy of Complex I, 80 ubiquinone molecules, 12 cytochromes *c*, and several thousand phospholipid molecules.[6] This protein density per membrane area is roughly similar in heart muscle,[7] but in heart some 70 per cent of the cytosol is occupied by mitochondria.

The matrix space inside the inner membrane may best be described as a gel due to the very high concentration of proteins and other macromolecules, including, for example, the enzymes of the Krebs' cycle and fatty acid oxidation. The usually very narrow *intermembrane space* between the inner and the outer membrane is also the site of specific enzymes.[8]

The thermodynamic basis of oxidative phosphorylation

Oxidative phosphorylation is the synthesis of ATP from ADP and inorganic phosphate (P_i) driven by the free energy from oxidation of foodstuffs by molecular oxygen. Primary processing of foodstuffs encompasses a large number of enzymatic reactions of intermediary metabolism before the main oxidative reactions can begin. The oxidation of fatty acids, for example, yields the activated two-carbon unit acetyl coenzyme A (AcCoA) and causes reduction of oxidized nicotinamide adenine dinucleotide (NAD⁺) and flavin adenine dinucleotide (FAD) in the mitochondrion. The reduced forms of these cofactors, NADH and $FADH_2$, may be directly oxidized by the respiratory chain, but the high-energy electrons of the acetyl group in AcCoA are first transformed into NADH and $FADH_2$ by the reactions of Krebs' tricarboxylic acid cycle, with production of CO_2. It is noteworthy that all these enzymatic reactions occur within the matrix space inside the mitochondrion.

Oxidation of NADH to NAD⁺ ($E_{m,7} = -0.32$ V) by O_2 to form water ($E_{m,7} = 0.815$ V) is a highly exergonic reaction, that is, it is spontaneous ('downhill') from a thermodynamic viewpoint (but not necessarily rapid), and releases energy that may be captured by linking the reaction to an endergonic ('uphill') process. Otherwise, the energy would be lost as heat. The standard free energy change of the reaction at pH 7 can be calculated from $\Delta E_{m,7}$, the difference between the midpoint potentials of the two redox couples,

$$\Delta G'_o = -nF\Delta E_{m,7} \qquad (1)$$

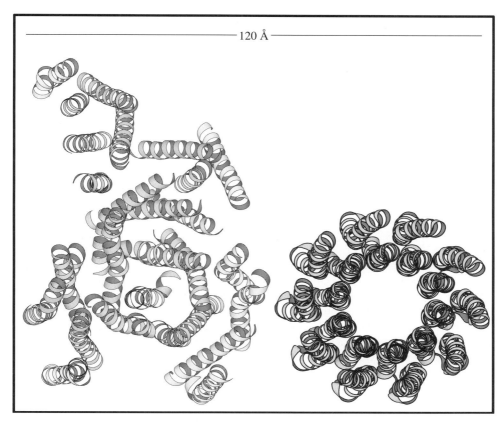

Fig. 4.1 Packing density of Complex IV and H⁺–ATP synthase in the inner mitochondrial membrane. A square of 120×120 Å of the inner membrane contains, on the average, one monomer each of cytochrome *c* oxidase (left) and the H⁺–ATP synthase complex (right). In both, the structures within the membrane are depicted based on the crystal structures.[32,48] Cytochrome *c* oxidase includes subunits I (blue), II (green) and III (red) plus helices from nuclear-encoded subunits (light blue). For the H⁺–ATP synthase only the ring of 10 *c*-subunits forming the major structure of the membranous F_0 is shown (see text). These two structures already occupy about 50% of the 120×120 Å membrane area, which must still accommodate all the other proteins of the inner membrane. (See Plate 1.)

where *n* is the number of redox equivalents transferred in the reaction and *F* is the Faraday (ca. 23 kcal/Vmol). Thus, the standard free energy change for the *driving* reaction in oxidative phosphorylation, the oxidation of NADH by O_2, is ca. -26.1 kcal/mol when expressed on a one-electron basis (the standard electrochemical convention), or -52.2 kcal/mol when expressed per mole of oxygen atoms reduced (or per mole of NADH oxidized). It should be recalled, however, that the actual free energy change at pH = 7 ($\Delta G'$) depends not only on $\Delta G'_0$ but also on the concentrations of the reactants and products. $\Delta G'_0$ is the free energy change at standard conditions, [NADH] = [NAD⁺] and $[O_2] \sim 1$ mM (pH = 7). The physiological O_2 concentration in tissues is considerably lower (ca. 5–15 μM),[9] which makes the actual redox potential (E_h) of the O_2/H_2O couple ca. 30 mV lower than the $E_{m,7}$ value. On the other hand, the physiological $NADH/NAD^+$ ratio in the mitochondrion is usually significantly higher than unity, which in turn tends to make the E_h of this redox couple lower than the $E_{m,7}$. Therefore, in this case the actual $\Delta G'$ for the driving redox reaction may not differ much from the value of $\Delta G'_o$.

The standard free energy change ($\Delta G'_o$) at pH = 7 of the *driven* reaction, ATP synthesis from ADP and P_i, is ca. 8 kcal/mol.[10] However, in the living cell the actual free energy of ATP synthesis (ΔG_p; also called phosphorylation potential),

$$\Delta G_p = \Delta G'_o + RT \ln([ATP]/[ADP][P_i]) \tag{2}$$

(where R is the gas constant, 1.98 cal/degreemol, and T is the absolute temperature) is much higher (up to a maximum of ca. 16 kcal/mol) due to the high $ATP/ADP \cdot P_i$ ratio that is usually maintained in the physiological steady state.

Oxidative phosphorylation with NADH-linked substrates may then, overall, be written as

$$NADH + H^+ + \tfrac{1}{2} O_2 + mADP + mP_i \rightarrow NAD^+ + H_2O + mATP \tag{3}$$

where the *driving* reaction is coupled to the *driven* reaction. Here, m is the number of ATP molecules produced per oxygen atom reduced, or the so-called P/O ratio. This ratio is a measure of the extent of *coupling* between the two partial reactions, which may be determined experimentally as the ratio of fluxes of ATP synthesis and O_2 consumption. Alternatively, it may be estimated from the 'jump' in O_2 consumption upon adding a known small amount of ADP to respiring mitochondria (ADP/O ratio).[11] However, as we shall see below, the coupling between the redox reactions of the respiratory chain and ATP synthesis is not as direct as eqn. (3) might suggest.

The chemiosmotic theory

Peter Mitchell proposed the chemiosmotic theory of oxidative phosphorylation in 1961[11,13] and this theory has held up very well on the physiological, though not entirely on the mechanistic level. The chemiosmotic theory explains the means by which ATP synthesis is driven at the expense of the energy produced by the redox reactions of the respiratory chain. This can briefly be summarized as the *central dogma of membrane bioenergetics*, namely

$$\text{Redox reactions} \rightarrow \Delta\mu_{H^+} \rightarrow \text{ATP}$$

where $\Delta\mu_{H^+}$, the electrochemical proton gradient (or the *protonmotive force*) across the inner mitochondrial membrane, provides the thermodynamic link between the driving and the driven reactions of the respiratory chain and the ATP synthase, respectively. This means that the redox reactions primarily generate $\Delta\mu_{H^+}$ by being coupled to the translocation of protons across the membrane. The synthesis of ATP, in turn, can occur only at the expense of subsequent downhill proton translocation in the opposite direction driven by $\Delta\mu_{H^+}$, which is consumed in the process.

The electrochemical proton gradient ($\Delta\mu_{H^+}$) is the sum of two terms, the electrical membrane potential ($\Delta\psi$) and the pH gradient across the membrane (ΔpH), so that

$$\Delta\mu_{H^+} = \Delta\psi + 2.3 \, (RT/F) \cdot \Delta\text{pH} \tag{4}$$

where F is the Faraday constant (ca. 23 kcal/Vmol), and applying the usual convention where $\Delta\psi$ has its positive pole in the intermembrane space (C-phase) and the negative in the matrix (M-phase), and ΔpH being defined as pH_M *minus* pH_C. At room temperature the term 2.3 RT/F has a value of ca. 60 mV, and therefore eqn. (4) is often approximated as

$$\Delta\mu_{H^+} \sim \Delta\psi + 60 \cdot \Delta pH \tag{5}$$

where both $\Delta\mu_{H^+}$ and $\Delta\psi$ are expressed in millivolts. Finally, the Gibbs free energy change corresponding to the transfer of n protons across $\Delta\mu_{H^+}$ may be obtained from

$$\Delta G = n \cdot F \cdot \Delta\mu_H{}^+$$

The respiratory chain and cell respiration

The respiratory chain is a functional notion, which implies that oxidation of NADH by O_2 takes place in a chain-like, sequential manner catalysed by three protein complexes bound to the inner mitochondrial membrane (Fig. 4.2), namely, NADH: ubiquinone oxidoreductase (Complex I), ubiquinol: ferricytochrome c oxidoreductase (Complex III, or the cytochrome bc_1 complex), and ferrocytochrome c: O_2 oxidoreductase (Complex IV, cytochrome c oxidase,

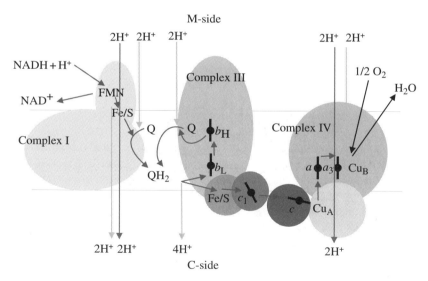

Fig. 4.2 Respiratory chain. Schematic representation of the three complexes of the mitochondrial respiratory chain, and the additional redox carriers ubiquinone (Q) and cytochrome c (c). The function is drawn on a two-equivalent (two-electron) basis (oxidation of NADH; reduction of $\frac{1}{2}O_2$). Note that Complex III requires *two* turnovers to achieve this (cf. Fig. 4.3). The redox centres are marked as follows. Complex I: flavin mononucleotide (FMN), several iron–sulphur centres (Fe/S); Complex III: two haems, b_H and b_L, the Rieske iron–sulphur centre (Fe/S), and cytochrome c_1; Complex IV: two copper centres, Cu_A and Cu_B, and the two haem groups haem a and haem a_3. Blue arrows (protons) denote proton transfers directly linked to the redox chemistry; red arrows (protons) denote proton translocation. (See Plate 2.)

or cytochrome aa$_3$). In addition, ubiquinone (a hydrophobic substituted benzoquinone residing within the lipid membrane) and cytochrome *c* participate as redox carriers that functionally 'bridge' Complexes I and III, and III and IV, respectively. Reducing equivalents (i.e. electrons or hydrogen atoms) are transferred sequentially through this 'chain', until they reach O$_2$ at the active site of Complex IV, where dioxygen is reduced to water. Cell respiration is thus a continuous flux of redox equivalents from substrates to molecular oxygen. Apart from the function of the respiratory complexes as oxidoreductases, they also have another important common function, namely, the ability to conserve a large fraction of the free energy of the redox reactions for ATP synthesis. In this respect, they differ from Complex II (succinate–ubiquinone oxidoreductase), which was earlier considered part of the respiratory chain mainly due to its association to the inner membrane. However, Complex II has no capability of energy conservation, and belongs functionally to the Krebs' cycle enzymes, where it catalyses the oxidation of succinate to fumarate with transfer of the reducing equivalents to ubiquinone.[15] The association of Complex II to the inner membrane is due to the electron acceptor—ubiquinone—which resides there. Complex II shares this feature with other auxiliary enzymes that use ubiquinone as the electron acceptor, such as α-glycerophosphate dehydrogenase and some other FAD-containing enzymes oxidizing fatty acid. Thus, oxidation of these metabolites bypasses Complex I by delivering the reducing equivalents directly to ubiquinone.

Protonmotive function of the respiratory chain complexes

Complexes I, III, and IV have in common a protonmotive function which implies that part of the free energy of the respective redox reaction is converted into $\Delta\mu_{H^+}$ in accordance with the central dogma of bioenergetics. In part, this conversion occurs by Mitchell's original *redox loop* principle, the basis of which is directionality of the hydrogen and electron transfer steps of the oxidoreduction reactions with respect to the membrane (Fig. 4.2, blue arrows). This may be exemplified by the situation in Complex IV where the binuclear haem a_3–Cu$_B$ site of O$_2$ reduction receives the electrons from cytochrome *c* on the C-side of the membrane, whereas the protons required for O$_2$ reduction to water arrive at the site from the M-side. Thus, some of the elemental redox reactions are themselves orientated relative to the membrane in such a way that redox function creates charge separation ($\Delta\psi$) as well as a pH gradient (ΔpH) across it. In addition, however, Complex IV and probably Complex I (but not Complex III) function as proton pumps (Fig. 4.2, red arrows), which implies true translocation of protons coupled to the redox chemistry of the complex, a function not anticipated in Mitchell's original theory. For example, in the case of Complex IV the proton-pumping function doubles the extent of energy conservation: twice as many electrical charges are translocated across the membrane per electron transferred than would be the case with the orientated redox chemistry alone.

Complex I[14,16,17]

Complex I is by far the largest respiratory chain complex. It contains more than 40 different subunits of which seven hydrophobic proteins are encoded in mtDNA and are thought to make up much of the membrane domain of this complex. An extrinsic domain on the M-side of the membrane contains most of the redox cofactors, one oxidized flavin mononucletide (FMN) molecule and more than six iron–sulphur centres (Fe/S). Complex I is the only member of the respiratory chain for which there is so far no high-resolution structure. Electron microscopic studies have shown that the molecule is L-shaped,[18] presumably with one domain within the membrane, and the other protruding towards the M-phase. The FMN cofactor is at the site of oxidation of NADH, but the subsequent arrangement of the iron–sulphur centres and their role in electron transfer is largely unknown. One higher potential Fe/S centre, N2, is thought to function at the terminal ubiquinone reduction site. The mechanism of proton translocation is also obscure but an $H^+/2e^-$ ratio of 4 is reasonably well established. In Fig. 4.2 this ratio has been rationalized by assuming (arbitrarily) that there is pumping of two protons per pair of electrons (red arrows) and by ascribing the remaining proton translocation to the redox loop principle (blue arrows).

Complex III[14,19,20]

The cytochrome bc_1 complex of bovine heart mitochondria is a dimer with 11 subunits per monomer. The catalytic core, however, consists of only three protein subunits: the membrane-embedded cytochrome b with two haem groups (b_L and b_H; for low and high potential, respectively) spans the membrane and places the two haems close to the C- and the M-side, respectively. The Rieske Fe/S protein and cytochrome c_1 are both anchored to the membrane by single membrane-spanning α-helices (only these subunits are shown schematically in Fig. 4.2), and present their redox centres close to the C-side. Two large subunits (the 'core proteins') extend towards the M-phase but these are missing in bacterial bc_1 complexes. These latter proteins are likely to function as peptidases, that is, a function unrelated to the proton-motive redox function of the complex. The other subunits of the mitochondrial complex are relatively small in size, of basically unknown function, and they also have no counterpart in bacterial bc_1. This resembles the situation for both Complexes I and IV, where the mitochondrial enzymes have a considerable number of 'supernumerary' subunits in addition to those known to be responsible for the protonmotive redox function, and homologues of which are found in the corresponding complexes from aerobic bacteria.

One of the keys to the protonmotive function of Complex III is the bifurcation in the pathway of ubiquinol oxidation (Fig. 4.3). In this process, one of the two electrons of ubiquinol is transferred to the high-potential part of the chain and the other to cytochrome b.[21,22] Ubiquinol was originally envisaged as the reductant of cytochrome b while the ubisemiquinone formed in this reaction was suggested to reduce haem c_1, because the ubisemiquinone intermediate was thought to be a relatively stable species.[21] Today, however, the opposite order of events is thought to be the case with a very unstable semiquinone intermediate.

The second key is the cycling of the electron delivered from ubiquinol to cytochrome b back to reduce ubiquinone at another site in the Complex, as proposed by Mitchell in his protonmotive Q-cycle mechanism.[22,23] In this mechanism, which was subsequently revised by Crofts *et al.*,[24] ubiquinol is oxidized in a bifurcated fashion at the so-called centre o in the complex, near the C-side of the membrane, a site that binds specific inhibitors such as myxothiazol and stigmatellin. One of the two electrons is transferred to the high-potential Fe/S centre of the Rieske protein, and further to O_2 via cytochromes c_1, c and Complex IV. The other electron is delivered to the low-potential haem b (b_L) from which it is transferred across the membrane to the high-potential haem b_H and to ubiquinone bound to a second binding-site i near the inside (M-side) of the membrane. This latter site specifically binds antimycin, one of the classical inhibitors of the respiratory chain, which displaces ubiquinone

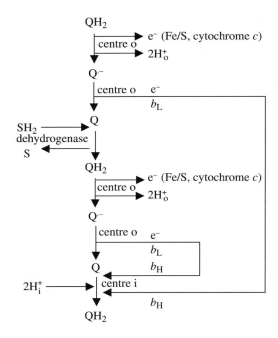

Fig. 4.3 The protonmotive ubiquinone cycle (Q cycle; see text).

from the site. Two-electron reduction of ubiquinone to ubiquinol at site i completes the Q cycle, which is depicted in Fig. 4.3. Note that the full Q cycle involves oxidation of *two* ubiquinol molecules at site o, reduction of one ubiquinone molecule at site i, and reduction of another ubiquinone molecule by hydrogenated substrate (e.g. by NADH via Complex I or by succinate via Complex II).

The Q-cycle mechanism is protonmotive due to the bifurcated oxidation of ubiquinol at site o, the sidedness of the ubiquinone oxidation and reduction sites relative to the membrane, and the transmembrane arrangement of the *b*-type haem groups. Since the redox partners of ubiquinone at the two sites are electron carriers, protons will be taken up from the M-side on reduction of quinone at centre i, and released to the C-side on oxidation of quinol at centre o. This amounts to net translocation of *two* protons (two electrical charge equivalents) across the membrane per electron *pair* transferred, even though the protons move electroneutrally across as hydrogen atoms in the form of ubiquinol, and despite the release of *four* protons per $2e^-$ on the C-side (Figs 4.2 and 4.3). The two protons released in excess of the two protons translocated may be thought of as having been derived from the hydrogenated substrate in the M-phase, and having been translocated electroneutrally across the membrane as hydrogen atoms. Moreover, the release of these 'extra' protons into the C-phase on oxidation of ubiquinol at centre o has little thermodynamic implication because they do not contribute to generation of $\Delta\psi$. They also do not contribute significantly to ΔpH due to the very large volume and buffering power of the C-phase (equivalent to the cytoplasm), relative to that of the M-phase. For this reason, the ΔpH component of the protonmotive force is by and large due to proton withdrawal from the M-phase and the resulting rise of pH in this phase. In the Q cycle, the protonmotive movement of charge across the membrane thus occurs by electron transfer along the haem groups of cytochrome *b*, and not by proton translocation as such.

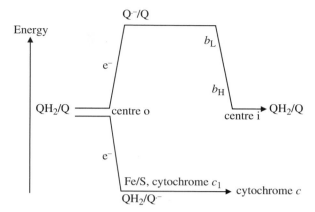

Fig. 4.4 Energetics of the Q cycle (see text).

Though somewhat more complicated than a classical Mitchellian redox loop, the proton-motive function of the Q cycle hence follows exactly the redox loop principle of orientated redox reactions in the membrane.

From a thermodynamic viewpoint the oxidation of ubiquinol at centre o may be likened to a disproportionation of the initial redox energy level of the two-electron redox couple QH_2/Q; one of the two electrons attains a high potential due to equilibration with the high-potential part of the chain—ultimately the O_2/H_2O couple. At the expense of this, the other electron attains a low potential by which it can drive reduction of the *b*-type haem groups, and more important, drive negative electric charge across the membrane to create $\Delta\psi$ (Fig. 4.4).

The crystal structure of Complex III from a number of different species has been solved[25–28] and they are consistent with the Q-cycle mechanism. However, the structures have revealed a most unexpected feature, namely, that the position of the Fe/S centre varies depending on the state of the complex. Thus, this centre can be close to cytochrome c_1 (to which it donates electrons), or close to centre o from where it receives electrons, or attain intermediate positions. This indicates that movement of the Fe/S domain may be an intrinsic part of the catalytic cycle of the bc_1 complex.[26,29] The membrane anchor of the Rieske protein has a hinge structure, which allows movement of the head region that contains the Fe/S centre. Such domain movement of the high-potential acceptor of electrons from centre o may be essential to secure the bifurcated path of quinol oxidation and thus to prevent both electrons of ubiquinol from being transferred to cytochrome *c*, which would destroy the proton-motive function. At the same time, this mechanism may ensure fast electron transfer from quinol to the Fe/S centre, as well as from the latter to haem c_1.[20]

Complex IV[14,30,31]

Complex IV from higher eukaryotes is a cytochrome *c* oxidase that consists of 13 different subunits per monomer; the enzyme is thought to be present as a dimer in the inner mitochondrial membrane although the reason for this is unknown as the monomer appears to be fully functional. The three largest subunits form the catalytic core of cytochrome *c* oxidase, the X-ray structure of which is available both for the mitochondrial[32] and for the bacterial enzyme.[33] These three subunits are encoded by mtDNA and their homologues are found in most respiratory oxidases from prokaryotes. The ten nuclear subunits of the mitochondrial enzyme surround the catalytic core in a 'protective' fashion;[32] some of them may be regulatory[34] and this field is an interesting example of the largely unknown cooperative function of nuclear and mitochondrial genes and gene products.

Subunit I contains three of the four redox centres of cytochrome c oxidase: one low-spin haem called haem a, and a binuclear O_2-reduction site with haem a_3 and a copper ion (Cu_B) next to it. These three centres reside at a similar depth, about one-third into the membrane domain from the C-side (Fig. 4.2) whereas the fourth centre, a bimetallic copper site (Cu_A) is part of a hydrophilic domain of subunit II that protrudes into the aqueous C-domain. Cytochrome c binds to this last domain and donates electrons—one at a time—into the enzyme. Electron transfer takes place via Cu_A and haem a into the O_2-binding site. Subunit III consists of seven hydrophobic transmembrane helices in the mitochondrial enzyme, but contains no redox cofactors. Deletion of its gene results in poor or incomplete assembly of the complex, but removal of this subunit after assembly has little effect on the protonmotive redox function. Subunit III has been proposed to participate in the channelling of O_2 from the membrane into the enzyme's active site.[35]

The protonmotive function of Complex IV is based on two principles. One is the Mitchellian redox loop: the electrons for reduction of O_2 arrive into the haem a_3/Cu_B site from cytochrome c on the C-side of the membrane, whereas the protons required for the formation of water in this reaction are taken from the opposite M-side. This directionality of the redox reaction leads to translocation of four electrical charge equivalents across the membrane per O_2 molecule reduced, as well as to generation of ΔpH. However, in addition to this, the enzyme couples the redox reaction to net translocation of four H^+ from the M- to the C-side of the membrane per O_2 reduced;[36] by this *proton-pumping* function the efficiency of transducing redox energy to protonmotive force is doubled; the efficiency is twice that of Complex III and similar to that of Complex I, despite the fact that the number of protons released per electron on the C-side is only one half of the number for Complex III.

Since the binuclear O_2-reduction site receives one electron at the time, it forms intermediate states during the catalytic cycle. The two-electron reduced ferrous/cuprous site reacts with O_2 to initially form an O_2-adduct, Compound A (Fig. 4.5).[37] The rate of this reaction is diffusion-limited, the rate constant being of the order of 10^8 M^{-1} s^{-1} at room temperature. In accordance with this, spectroscopic data have shown that Compound A is formed with a time constant of ca. 8 µs at 1 mM O_2. However, the binding of O_2 to the site is weak ($K_d \sim 0.3$ mM) and the operational high oxygen affinity (a low Michaelis constant of ca. 0.1 µM) is instead due to effective 'trapping' of the O_2 to the site by fast electron transfer.[37,38] If there are no electrons available in haem a or Cu_A, Compound A decays in ca. 0.17 ms to form the so-called P_M state of the binuclear centre. This reaction is of particular interest because the bound O_2 molecule is effectively reduced here in a four-electron step into the equivalent of two 'water molecules'. This reaction includes two-electron oxidation of the ferrous haem a_3 into the ferryl state (Fe[IV] = O), and one-electron oxidation of Cu_B into the cupric form, presumably with a bound hydroxide ligand (Cu[II]–OH). The fourth electron is probably donated by a conserved tyrosine residue in the site yielding a neutral tyrosine radical.[39] In this way, the cofactors within the active site of the enzyme receive the oxidizing power of the O_2/H_2O couple in a single step, the resulting two 'deprotonated water molecules' being represented by the oxide ion bound to the ferryl haem iron and the hydroxide ion bound to the

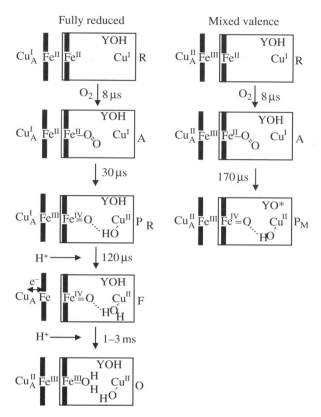

Fig. 4.5 Intermediates described in the reaction of fully reduced and 'mixed valence' cytochrome *c* oxidase with O_2. The rectangle symbolizes the binuclear centre of O_2 reduction with haem a_3 and Cu_B, plus the conserved tyrosine residue (YOH) that may form the neutral tyrosine radical (YO*). The Cu_A and haem a centres are drawn on the left of the rectangle.

copper (Fig. 4.5). Notably, the conversion of Compound A into P_M is not associated with any net proton uptake,[40] nor with translocation of charge across the dielectric.[41] This means that no conservation of energy in the form of $\Delta\mu_{H^+}$ has yet occured. Now the stage is set for exergonic electron transfer from the donor side (cytochrome *c*) via Cu_A and haem *a* to the high-potential electron acceptors generated in the haem a_3/Cu_B site, and this is coupled to formation of $\Delta\mu_{H^+}$.

At the present time there is some controversy with respect to which partial reactions in the catalytic cycle that are linked to proton-pumping.[42–44] On the basis of equilibrium thermo-dynamic work it was thought originally that all proton translocation would be associated with the oxidative phase of the catalytic cycle (Fig. 4.5).[45] However, more recent kinetic work has revealed that oxidation of the fully reduced enzyme by O_2 is linked to pumping of only two protons.[43] However, this reaction appeared to generate a metastable ferric/cupric state of the binuclear site, which if immediately re-reduced yielded pumping of the remaining two protons. Otherwise this metastable state decays into the relaxed ferric/cupric state O the subsequent reduction of which is no longer associated with proton-pumping.[43] The molecular basis for this phenomenon is not yet known, but it might be a means of regulating the proton-pumping efficiency of Complex IV.

The H$^+$–ATP synthase[14,46,47]

This remarkable enzyme, sometimes also called Complex V, is the smallest machine known. Basically, it consists of two parts: a trimeric orange-like structure of α and β subunits (F_1) containing the catalytic sites for ATP synthesis and protruding far into the M-phase, and a membrane unit (F_0) which catalyses proton translocation. F_1 and F_0 are linked by the important coupling subunit γ that is attached to F_0 via other small subunits, and reaches all the way into the centre of the trimeric F_1 unit (Fig. 4.6). One important key to function is the fact that the bent γ subunit imposes asymmetry among the three catalytic $\alpha\beta$ interfaces in F_1, rendering them all different in structure as well as in their property of binding adenine nucleotides (AdNs) and P_i. The crystallographic elucidation of the structure of F_1 (and subsequently of a less detailed structure of the F_0F_1 complex;[48]) by John Walker and his collaborators[49] provided the basis and the keys to the function of this enzyme. The mitochondrial F_0 unit consists of a disk of 10 hydrophobic c-subunits, each of which contains a glutamic acid residue within the membrane domain; F_0 of some bacterial and chloroplast F_1F_0 complexes may contain a different number of c-subunits. The F_0 unit also contains subunits a and b which are important in proton translocation as well as in providing a stator linking the edge of F_0 to the $\alpha\beta$ unit of F_1.

The F_1F_0 complex functions as a rotatory machine where the protonmotive force propels the c-subunit disk into rotation around an axis perpendicular to the membrane plane, which makes the attached γ-subunit rotate as well, around its long axis. Due to its asymmetry this subunit continuously forces changes in the structure of the three catalytic $\alpha\beta$ interfaces, between so-called 'tight', 'open' and 'loose' conformations. When in the 'loose' conformation the interface readily binds ADP and P_i. When transformed into the 'tight' conformation (by a 120° turn of the disk and of γ) ADP and P_i spontaneously react, expelling a water molecule, to form ATP within the site. This is possible thermodynamically because in this latter state the formed ATP is very tightly bound relative to ADP and P_i. Finally, upon

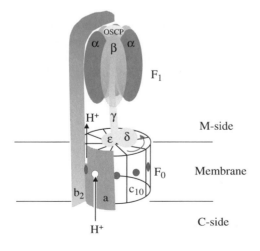

Fig. 4.6 H$^+$–ATP synthase (see text). The proton electrochemical gradient is thought to cause rotation of the disk within F_0 consisting of the c subunits, whereby the attached δ, ϵ, and γ subunits rotate as well. Axial rotation of the latter within the catalytic $\alpha_3\beta_3$ unit (F_1) leads to synthesis of ATP. (See Plate 3.)

a further 120° turn, this site becomes 'open' and releases ATP into the surrounding medium. The same sequence of events occurs simultaneously at the two other interfaces, so that at each point in time one is in the 'loose', one in the 'tight', and one in the 'open' state. This type of *binding change mechanism* was first proposed by Paul Boyer based on elegant kinetic studies with isotopically labelled phosphate and water, and he indeed suggested that a rotatory movement might be the basis for such a mechanism.[50] The proof for such movement came from the ingenious studies by Yoshida *et al.* who visualized ATP hydrolysis-linked rotatory motion of the γ subunit by attaching it artificially to a long fluorescence-labelled rod of actin.[51] Note, that in these experiments the ATP synthase works in a direction opposite to the normal physiological one.

The disk consisting of the *c*-subunits is thought to be set in motion by a mechanism first suggested by Wolfgang Junge *et al.*,[52] and depicted schematically in Fig. 4.6. The glutamic residue of the particular *c*-subunit 'in position' at the single a-subunit at the disk's periphery is protonated from the C-side of the membrane via a proton-conducting path, and driven by the protonmotive force across the membrane. This renders the *c*-subunit uncharged and therefore 'soluble' in the membrane phospholipids, whereby the ring moves to remove the glutamic acid from contact with the a-subunit into contact with membrane lipids. This movement, in turn, places the glutamate of the next c-subunit in a position to be protonated, and so on until the *c*-subunit with a protonated glutamic acid reaches another position near the a-subunit, where a proton-conducting pathway leads to the M-side of the membrane. The protonmotive force now drives the proton off the glutamic acid, and the formed glutamate can be reprotonated from the C-side in the next position of the disk. Interestingly, the three-fold symmetry of the F_1 domain does not match the ten-fold symmetry of the disk of *c*-subunits. This means that 10 protons are normally transferred across the membrane to produce a full 360° rotation and the formation of 3 molecules of ATP, which yields a non-integer H^+/ATP ratio of 3.33. This, in turn, implies that there must be some rotational elasticity in the γ-subunit to overcome the symmetry mismatch between F_0 and F_1, a property that may well render the rotatory motion more smooth energetically than it might otherwise be if the two structures were symmetrically matched.

Above, we have mainly considered the action of the F_0F_1 complex in the physiologically most relevant direction—the synthesis of ATP. However, the complex also readily catalyses the reverse reaction, that is, the hydrolysis of ATP to ADP and P_i (ATPase activity). In fact, this spontaneous activity is dominating under conditions where there is no protonmotive force across the membrane; ATP hydrolysis by membranous F_0F_1 creates $\Delta\mu_{H^+}$ rather than consumes it and the rotatory motion is reversed in direction.

Transport of ADP/ATP and P_i

For some aspects of the overall process of oxidative phosphorylation it is important to distinguish between the two components of $\Delta\mu_{H^+}$. Due to the orientation of the catalytic sites in F_1 of the H^+–ATP synthase towards the M-phase, this is where the substrates of the enzyme, ADP and P_i, must be available and where ATP is produced, although most of the ATP will be required to drive energy-dependent reactions in the cytoplasm, producing ADP and P_i in that space. A plausible reason for this apparent inconsistency (why is the ATP synthase not orientated in the opposite direction?) is related to the origin of the mitochondrion as an aerobic bacterium, where ATP was obviously to be produced within the cell. For this reason the mitochondria of eukaryotic cells needed to develop unique transport systems in the inner membrane for ATP/ADP and for P_i. The adenine nucleotide translocator[53] is an exchange carrier (AdN carrier) that exchanges ADP for ATP (and vice versa) and which is specific for the ADP^{3-} and ATP^{4-} ionic forms of these nucleotides. The physiologically essential export of ATP from the M- to the C-phase, and concomitant import of ADP, will therefore be an *electrogenic* process equivalent to moving one positive charge from the C-phase to the M-phase. It follows that the adenine nucleotide transport will be goverened by the $\Delta\psi$ across the membrane, and that part of the energy from respiration will be used for ADP import into the mitochondrion, and ATP export. In this way, respiration (via the protonmotive force and nucleotide transport) drives the phosphorylation potential (eqn. (2)) of the cytosol to a higher value than it is in the mitochondrial matrix. On the other hand, the transport of P_i across the membrane is an *electroneutral* process[53] that is catalysed by a carrier protein that is structurally related to the AdN carrier.[54] Note that both the AdN and the phosphate carrier are products of nuclear genes, and that a defect in either will compromise oxidative phosphorylation. The P_i transport can be thought of either as a co-transport of $H_2PO_4^-$ and H^+ (*symporter*), as a counter-exchange of $H_2PO_4^-$ against OH^- (*antiporter*), or even as transport of phosphoric acid as such (H_3PO_4; *uniporter*). Import of P_i into the M-phase is therefore coupled to the import of 'a proton without its charge', and will hence be driven by the ΔpH component of $\Delta\mu_{H^+}$, but will be insensitive to the membrane potential. The transport of other metabolites and ions on specific carriers across the inner mitochondrial membrane is coupled to either the membrane potential, to ΔpH, or to both (i.e. to $\Delta\mu_{H^+}$). More generally, it may be concluded that the central dogma of membrane bioenergetics presented above is an oversimplification: the $\Delta\mu_{H^+}$ produced by respiration is not only used for the synthesis of ATP, but also to drive transport of important metabolites and ions across the inner mitochondrial membrane.

Stoichiometry of oxidative phosphorylation

From the above description of the respiratory chain and the H^+–ATP synthase we conclude that 10, 6, and 4 charge equivalents are maximally translocated across the inner mitochondrial membrane per consumed oxygen atom (H^+/O ratio) upon oxidation of NADH, succinate (ubiquinol), and cytochrome *c*, respectively, while the number of H^+ translocated across F_0 to produce one ATP should be 3.33 on average. Taking into account the protonmotive function of the AdN translocator and the P_i carrier, 4.33 H^+ would have to be translocated into the mitochondrion to produce one ATP molecule in the cytoplasm. Dividing the H^+/O ratios with the latter H^+/ATP ratio yields maximal P/O ratios of 2.3, 1.39, and 0.92 for oxidation of NADH, succinate, and cytochrome c, respectively. This is much less than the classical ratios of 3, 2, and 1 that are still widely found in textbooks although the main reasons for this difference were aptly discussed by Hinkle *et al.* 10 years ago.[11] These workers argued for an H^+/ATP ratio of 4 (including ATP and P_i transport), yielding maximal P/O ratios of 2.5, 1.5, and 1.0. However, the very recent observation of 10 c-subunits in the F_0 portion of the ATP synthase, the rotatory mechanism of this enzyme, and its three $\alpha\beta$ subunit interfaces would argue for the slightly higher H^+/ATP ratio and therefore for the slightly lower maximal P/O ratios quoted above. However, the discrepancy between these latter ratios and those measured by Hinkle *et al.* is less than 10 per cent and thus probably not significant. Finally, it should be stressed that these P/O ratios are the maximum ratios possible in the light of present knowledge, assuming no protonic leaks across the membrane, as well as 100 per cent coupling between electrons and protons in the respiratory chain complexes, as well as between protons and ATP in the H^+–ATP synthase. The close correspondence between these theoretical ratios and those measured experimentally suggests that such protonic or electronic 'leaks' are usually very small in normal mitochondria undergoing oxidative phosphorylation, which is thus a highly efficient means of energy transduction.

Acknowledgements

This work was supported by grants from The Sigrid Juselius Foundation, University of Helsinki, and the Academy of Finland (program 44895). I am grateful to Dr Liisa Laakkonen for producing Fig. 4.1.

References

1. Margulis L (1970). In: *Origins of Eukaryotic Cells.* New Haven and London: Yale University Press.
2. Raven PH (1970). *Science* **169**: 641–646.
3. Skulachev VP, Sharaff AA, and Liberman EA (1967). *Nature* **216**: 718–719.
4. Skulachev VP (1999). In: *Frontiers of Cellular Bioenergetics* (eds Papa *et al.*), New York: Kluwer Academic/Plenum Publishers, pp. 89–118.
5. Mitchell P (1966). *Chemiosmotic Coupling in Oxidative and Photosynthetic Phosphorylation,* Bodmin, UK: Glynn Research Ltd.
6. Wikström M and Saraste M (1984). In: *Bioenergetics* (ed. L Ernster), Amsterdam and New York: Elsevier Science, pp. 49–94.
7. Klingenberg M (1967). In: *Mitochondrial Structure and Compartmentation* (eds E Quagliariello *et al.*), Bari, Italy: Adriatica Editrice, pp. 124–125.
8. Ernster L and Kuylenstierna B (1969). In: *Mitochondria, Structure and Function, FEBS Symposium Vol. 17* (eds L Ernster and Z Drahota), London & New York: Academic Press, pp. 5–31.
9. Wittenberg BA and Wittenberg JB (1989). *Annu. Rev. Physiol.* **51**: 857–878.
10. Rosing J and Slater EC (1972). *Biochim. Biophys. Acta* **267**: 275–290.
11. Hinkle PC, Kumar AA, Resetar A, and Harris DL (1991). *Biochemistry* **30**: 3576–3582.
12. Mitchell P (1961). *Nature* **191**: 144–148.
13. Nicholls DG and Ferguson SJ (1992). Bioenergetics 2, London: Academic Press.
14. Saraste M (1999). *Science* **283**: 1488–1493.
15. Lancaster CRD and Kröger A (2000). *Biochim. Biophys. Acta* **1459**: 422–431.
16. Ohnishi T, Sled VS, Yano T, Yagi T, Burbaev DS, and Vinogradov AD (1998). *Biochim. Biophys. Acta* **1365**: 301–308.
17. Brandt U (1997). *Biochim. Biophys. Acta* **1318**: 79–91.
18. Gunebaut V, Mills D, Weiss H, and Leonard KR (1996). *J. Mol. Biol.* **265**: 409–418.
19. Berry EA, Guergova-Kuras M, Huang L, and Crofts AR (2000). *Annu. Rev. Biochem.* **69**: 1005–1075.
20. Darrouzet E, Moser CM, Dutton PL, and Daldal F (2001). *TIBS* **26**: 445–451.
21. Wikström MKF and Berden JA (1972). *Biochim. Biophys. Acta* **283**: 403–420.
22. Mitchell P (1975). *FEBS Lett.* **59**: 137–139.
23. Mitchell P (1976). *J. Theor. Biol.* **62**: 327–367.
24. Crofts AR, Meinhardt SW, Jones KR, and Snozzi M (1983). *Biochim. Biophys. Acta* **723**: 202–218.

25. Xia D, Yu C-A, Kim H, Jia-Zhi Xia J-Z, Kachurin AM, Zhang L, Yu L, and Deisenhofer J (1997). *Science* **277**: 60–66.
26. Zhang Z, Huang L-S, Shulmeister VM, Chi Y-I, Kim K-K, Hung L-W, Crofts AR, Berry EA, and Kim S-H (1998). *Nature* **392**: 677–684.
27. Iwata S, Lee JW, Okada K, Lee JK, Iwata M, Rasmussen B, Link TA, Ramaswamy S, and Jap BK (1998). *Science* **281**: 64–71.
28. Hunte C, Koepke J, Lange C, Rossmanith T, and Michel H (2000). *Structure* **8**: 669–684.
29. Crofts AR, Guergova-Kuras M, Huang L-S, Kuras R, Zhang Z, and Berry EA (1999). *Biochemistry* **38**: 15791–15806.
30. Babcock GT and Wikström M (1992). *Nature* **356**: 301–309.
31. Babcock GT (1999). *Proc. Natl Acad. Sci. USA* **96**: 12971–12973.
32. Tsukihara T, Aoyama H, Yamashita E, Tomizaki T, Yamaguchi H, Shinzawa-Itoh K, Nakashima R, Yaono R, and Yoshikawa S (1996). *Science* **272**: 1136–1144.
33. Iwata S, Ostermeier C, Ludwig B, and Michel H (1995). *Nature* **376**: 660–669.
34. Kadenbach B, Napiwotzki J, Frank V, Arnold S, Exner S, and Hüttemann M (1998). *J. Bioenerg. Biomembr.* **30**: 25–33.
35. Riistama S, Puustinen A, García-Horsman A, Iwata S, Michel H, and Wikström M (1996). *Biochim. Biophys. Acta* **1275**: 1–4.
36. Wikström M (1977). *Nature* **266**: 271–273.
37. Chance B, Saronio C, and Leigh JS (1975). *J. Biol. Chem.* **250**: 9226–9237.
38. Verkhovsky MI, Morgan JE, Puustinen A, and Wikström M (1996). *Nature* **380**: 268–270.
39. Proshlyakov DA, Pressler MA, DeMaso C, Leykam JF, DeWitt DL, and Babcock GT (2000). *Science* **290**: 1588–1591.
40. Mitchell R, Mitchell P, and Rich PR (1992). *Biochim. Biophys. Acta* **811**: 188–191.
41. Jasaitis A, Verkhovsky MI, Morgan JE, Verkhovskaya ML, and Wikström M (1999). *Biochemistry* **38**: 2697–2706.
42. Michel H (1999). *Biochemistry* **38**: 15129–15140.
43. Verkhovsky MI, Jasaitis A, Verkhovskaya ML, Morgan JE, and Wikström M (1999). *Nature* **400**: 480–483.
44. Wikström M (2000). *Biochemistry* **39**: 3515–3519.
45. Wikström M (1989). *Nature* **338**: 776–778.
46. Pedersen PL (ed.) (2000). *J. Bioenerg. Biomembr.* **32**: 423–546.
47. Weber J and Senior AE (2000). *Biochim. Biophys. Acta* **1458**: 300–309.
48. Stock D, Leslie AGW, and Walker JE (1999). *Science* **286**: 1700–1705.
49. Abrahams JP, Leslie AGW, Lutter R, and Walker JE (1994). *Nature* **370**: 621–628.
50. Boyer PD (1993). *Biochim. Biophys. Acta* **1140**: 215–250.
51. Noji H, Yasufda R, Yoshida M, and Kinosita K Jr (1997). *Nature* **386**: 299–302.
52. Junge W, Lill H, and Engelbrecht S (1997). *Trends Biochem. Sci.* **22**: 420–423.
53. Krämer R, and Palmieri F (1992). In: *Molecular Mechanisms in Bioenergetics* (ed. L Ernster), Amsterdam: Elsevier, pp. 359–384.
54. Palmieri F and Van Ommen B (1999). In: *Frontiers of Cellular Bioenergetics* (eds S Papa *et al.*), New York: Kluwer Academic/Plenum Publishers, pp. 489–519.

Section II   Pathological mutations of mitochondrial DNA

5 Clinical aspects of mitochondrial encephalomyopathies

T Pulkes and MG Hanna

Introduction

Human diseases caused by impaired respiratory chain function have been increasingly recognized in recent years.[1–13] Although neurological diseases are the commonest consequence of such respiratory chain dysfunction, it is now apparent that virtually any tissue in the body can be affected (see Table 5.1). This is perhaps unsurprising when one considers the central role of the respiratory chain in normal cell and tissue function. The neurological diseases associated with respiratory chain impairment are collectively known as the mitochondrial encephalomyopathies, a term which reflects the common involvement of both the central nervous system (CNS) and skeletal muscle in these patients. Normal respiratory chain function is dependent on an elaborate interplay between the mitochondrial genome and the nuclear genome. It follows that human mitochondrial diseases are genetically heterogeneous. Early genetic mitochondrial research focussed upon the smaller mitochondrial genome (mtDNA). This has proved to be a rich source of mutations that cause human mitochondrial disease. To date, over a hundred separate primary pathogenic mutations in mtDNA have been described in association with a bewildering array of clinical phenotypes. More recently, the first nuclear genes associated with mitochondrial disease have been reported.

A common histochemical feature in the skeletal muscle biopsies taken from many patients with mitochondrial encephalomyopathies is the so-called 'ragged red fibre (RRF)'. This represents an abnormal proliferation of mitochondria at the level of single muscle fibres.[1] This is best seen on transverse section using the modified Gomori trichrome stain which has affinity for mitochondria (see front cover). The presence of significant numbers of RRFs in a muscle biopsy is a strong indicator that there is dysfunction of the respiratory chain, which is likely to be the cause of the patient's disease. Indeed, most clinicians practising in this area of medicine would regard the presence of RRFs as one of the 'gold standard' diagnostic tests for a mitochondrial encephalomyopthy. Indeed, various authors recognized the association between the RRFs, mitochondrial respiratory chain dysfunction, and human neurological diseases long before any genetic defect was discovered.[1,2]

As long ago as 1962, Luft et al. described the first case of a mitochondrial myopathy in a patient with non-thyroidal hypermetabolism with mild weakness (Luft's disease).[3] The morphological abnormalities were limited to skeletal muscle with abnormal accumulations of mitochondria in subsarcolemmal and intermyofibrillar spaces,[4] typical of RRFs.[5] Elegant biochemical studies in this patient revealed a disturbance of respiratory chain function. Although Luft's disease was the first description of a mitochondrial myopathy, only two such cases have

Table 5.1 Clinical features of mitochondrial encephalomyopathies

Neurological features	Non-neurological features
Muscle	Heart
External ophthalmoplegia	Cardiac conduction block
Limb weakness and wasting	Cardiomyopathy
Exercise intolerance	
Muscle pain	Endocrinopathy
Rhabdomyolysis	Diabetes mellitus
Myoglobinuria	Hypoparathyroidism
	Hypothyroidism
Central nervous system	Growth hormone deficiency
Ataxia	Delayed puberty
Myoclonus	Irregular menses
Stroke-like episodes	Infertility
Seizures	Hirsutism
Mental retardation or dementia	
Leukodystrophy	Hematological
Parkinsonism	Sideroblastic anaemia
Dystonia	Pancytopenia
Chorea	Acanthocytosis
Migraine headache	
Optic neuropathy	Liver
Pigmentary retinopathy	Hepatic failure
Sensorineural hearing loss	
Vestibular dysfunction	Pancreas
	Pancreatic exocrine deficiency
Peripheral nervous system	
Sensorimotor neuropathy	Renal
	Renal tubular acidosis
	Bartter-like syndrome
	Gastrointestinal tract
	Intestinal pseudo-obstruction
	Dysmotility
	Dermatological
	Lipomas

been reported to date and the molecular basis of the disorder remains a mystery.[6] Although the presence of the RRF is very good evidence of mitochondrial disease, the converse is not true. Hence, the absence of RRFs does not preclude mitochondrial disease. In current specialist practice, the diagnosis of human mitochondrial disease relies on a range of modalities including clinical assessment, muscle biopsy, histochemical and biochemical analysis, and DNA analysis (mainly mtDNA at the time of writing).

This review will focus chiefly upon the clinical aspects of the commonest human disease phenotypes associated with mutations in mtDNA and respiratory chain dysfunction.

Neurological presentations of respiratory chain disease

Neurological diseases caused by respiratory chain dysfunction exhibit considerable clinical heterogeneity. They may affect predominantly the peripheral nervous system or the brunt of the disease may fall upon the CNS. Combinations of peripheral and CNS involvement are not uncommon. Generally, the prognosis worsens with the degree of CNS involvement. Some of these diseases are remarkably selective; for example, only affecting the optic nerve or the auditory nerve in isolation. The neurological mitochondrial diseases have recently been shown to be an important cause of morbidity and mortality in the general population.[15]

Chronic progressive external ophthalmoplegia (CPEO)

Kearns–Sayre syndrome (KSS)

Chronic progressive external ophthalmoplegia is one of the most common clinical manifestations of mitochondrial disease. This disorder that is slowly progressive usually begins in late childhood or in adolescence, although onset after 40 can occasionally be seen. Ptosis and ophthalmoplegia (limitation of eye movement) are the initial clinical features and may be followed by limb weakness, fatigue, or exercise intolerance. The limitation of eye movements is usually in all directions of gaze. Diplopia (double vision) is not usually present. Opthalmoplegia rarely cause symptoms until it is nearly total when the patient may have to turn the head to look to either side. The ptosis may be asymmetrical initially and may progress to complete occlusion of the pupil. Limb weakness, when present, is mainly proximal and mild. Patients often have limitation of daily activities due to exercise intolerance rather than weakness.[13] Life expectancy is not usually reduced in uncomplicated CPEO.

Kearns–Sayre syndrome is a more serious disorder in which CPEO is one feature. Strictly, it is defined by the development of CPEO and pigmentary degeneration of the retina before the age of 20 years. In addition, one or more of the following should be present: cardiac conduction block, cerebellar ataxia, or increased protein in cerebrospinal fluid (CSF; >1 g/l). Other features which are variably present include short stature, sensory neural hearing loss, vestibular dysfunction, and impaired intellectual function. The ptosis and ophthalmoplegia are as described above. The pigmentary retinal degeneration can be visualized on ophthalmoscopic examination as a fine, diffuse, hypo and hyperpigmentation of the retina. It is mostly in the central retinal region and is described as a 'salt and pepper' appearance. It rarely causes severe impairment of visual acuity or visual field defects.[10] Cardiac conduction block can cause syncopal attacks, congestive heart failure, or cardiac arrest. In contrast to CPEO, the prognosis in KSS is poor. Most patients die in the third or fourth decade.[16]

Over the past 10 years there have been many reports of patients with phenotypes intermediate between isolated CPEO and full-blown KSS. For example, there are cases of CPEO with pigmentary retinopathy but no other features of KSS. Clinically, there is a spectrum of disease severity ranging from isolated 'benign' CPEO through to severe and often fatal KSS.[17] The commonest mtDNA defect associated with phenotypes ranging from CPEO to KSS is the single large-scale deletion.[14] There is some evidence to suggest that the severity of the phenotype relates to the proportion of the deleted mtDNA molecule and its tissue distribution.[17]

Most CPEO patients harbouring a single large-scale rearrangement of mtDNA are sporadic cases without any family history. Single large deletions are not generally found in other family members of sporadic CPEO and KSS patients.[18,19] In one family, a mother and her son harboured single large deletions, However, their deletions were different in size and location suggesting that maternal transmission was not the explanation.[20] The absence of family history in the vast majority of CPEO/KSS cases has, in part, led to the view that large-scale

Table 5.2 MtDNA point mutations associated with CPEO

Gene	MtDNA mutation	Reference
*tRNA*Leu(UUR)	A3243G	21
*tRNA*Ile	T4274C	142
	T4285C	143
	G4309A	144
*tRNA*Asn	A5692G	145
	G5703A	146
*tRNA*Leu(CUN)	T12311C	147
	G12315A	22

Abbreviations: tRNA = transfer RNA, Leu = Leucine, Ile = Isoleucine, Asn = Asparagine.

rearrangements of mtDNA may be somatic mutational events followed by clonal expansion.[19] Although most CPEO patients harbour single mtDNA deletions, a minority harbour point mutations in mtDNA. Approximately 15 per cent of CPEO patients harbour the A3243G point mutation which more commonly associates with the MELAS phenotype. The A3243G mutation is in the mitochondrial transfer RNA (tRNA) leucine(UUR) (tRNALeu(UUR)) gene which is inherited by maternal transmission.[21] At least seven other mtDNA point mutations have been reported in association with CPEO; each mutation being identified in a single case or family (Table 5.2). One of the mutations, a G12315A mutation in the tRNALeu(CUN) gene was identified in a sporadic patient with CPEO, sensorineural hearing loss and a pigmentary retinopathy. The mutation was only present in muscle and was not present in several other tissues including skeletal myoblasts. This suggested rapid segregation of mutant mtDNA during embryogenic development and a low probability of transmission to offspring.[22]

Multiple deletions of the mtDNA have been identified in families with autosomal dominant CPEO (see Chapter 9).

Isolated skeletal myopathy

Although limb muscle weakness is commonly associated with other clinical features of mitochondrial encephalomyopathies, such weakness not infrequently is the sole clinical manifestation. The age of onset of such cases ranges from late childhood to adult life. Patients typically exhibit a slowly progressive course. It commonly associates with exercise intolerance and exertional fatigue which limit the patient's functional capacity. A small proportion of patients with the 'chronic fatigue syndrome' turn out to have isolated mitochondrial myopathy.[23] Ocassionally, the presentation may be more dramatic with muscle pain and rhabdomyolysis resulting in myoglobinuria.[24,25]

Isolated mitochondrial myopathy is genetically heterogeneous and has been described in association with large-scale single deletions and point mutations in both transfer RNA gene and protein-coding genes (Table 5.3). Many of the patients harbouring pont mutations exhibit maternal inheritance. However, we recently described sporadic patients harbouring point mutations in the cytochrome *b* gene. These point mutations exhibited interesting characteristics. They appeared to represent somatic mutations occurring in skeletal muscle and were not detected in other tissues such as blood.[23,26]

Table 5.3 MtDNA mutations associated with mitochondrial myopathies

Gene	MtDNA mutation	Phenotypes	Ref.
tRNA[Leu(UUR)]	A3243G	Myopathy	48
	A3251G	Myopathy/sudden death	148
*ND*1	7bp-inversion	Myopathy/exercise intolerance	149
*ND*4	G11832A	Exercise intolerance	26
Cyt b	G14846A	Exercise intolerance	23
	G15059A	Exercise intolerance	150
	G15084A	Exercise intolerance	23
	G15168A	Exercise intolerance	23
	24bp-del, G15498A	Exercise intolerance	23
	G15615A	Exercise intolerance	151
	G15723A	Exercise intolerance	23
	G15762A	Myopathy	152
COX II	T7587C	Myopathy/ataxia/deafness	153
COX III	T7671C	Myopathy	154
	15-bp del	Exercise intolerance	155

Abbreviations: ND = NADH dehydrogenase, COX = cytochrome oxidase, bp = base pairs, del = deletion.

Myoclonic epilepsy with ragged red fibres (MERRF)

This is one of the well-recognized predominantly CNS mitochondrial diseases. The association between progressive myoclonic epilepsy and RRFs was first observed by Tsaris *et al.* in 1973.[27] Subsequently, Fukuhara *et al.* described two further patients with myoclonic epilepsy associated with RRFs and suggested that this is a distinctive mitochondrial encephalomyopathy syndrome. They proposed the acronym MERRF.[11] Four other progressive myoclonic epilepsy syndromes including Unverricht–Lundborg disease (Baltic myoclonus), Lafora-body disease, sialidosis, and neuronal lipofuscinosis, enter into the differential diagnosis. However, unlike these other progressive myoclonic epilepsy syndromes, MERRF usually exhibits maternal inheritance. The age of onset varies widely form childhood up to 50-years old. Early age of onset often correlates with a more severe clinical course leading to death in adulthood.[28]

MERRF is characterized by myoclonus, seizures, and cerebellar ataxia often in association with mild limb myopathy. The myoclonus is usually stimulus-sensitive that is, sensitive to action, noise, or photic stimuli. Seizures may be tonic-clonic, focal, absence, or atonic types. Associated features which are often present include dementia, optic neuropathy, sensorineural hearing loss, ophthalmoplegia, peripheral neuropathy, foot deformity, and lipomas.[17,29] These associated features are clinical clues in the differential diagnosis of progressive myoclonic ataxia. Retinitis pigmentosa, stroke-like episodes, diabetes mellitus (DM), and chronic pancreatitis are less common additional features.[30–33] Although the full syndrome is quite characteristic, there can be quite marked clinical heterogeneity with in families. Electrophysiological features are variable and there are no features to distinguish cases of mitochondrial disease from other causes of progressive myoclonic epilepsy.[34] Neuropathology reveals neuronal loss and gliosis affecting the dentate nuclei of the cerebellum, the globus pallidus, the posterior columns, and the spinocerebellar tracts of the spinal cord. Abnormal mitochondria have been observed in the cells of the cerebellar cortex and of the dentate nuclei.[35,36] The pathological changes of Leigh's syndrome (LS) are found in some patients with very severe phenotypes.[36,37] Skeletal muscle biopsy typically reveals RRFs, even in patients with little clinical limb muscle weakness and is therefore a very useful diagnostic test.

Approximately 80 per cent of cases of MERRF are associated with the A8344G mutation in the mitochondrial tRNA^{Lys} gene.[38,39] Significant clinical heterogeneity is often observed in large MERRF families harbouring the A8344G mutation. There is a significant correlation between the proportion of mutant mtDNA in blood and both clinical severity, and age of onset. Unlike large-scale rearrangements, all mothers of affected offspring harbour the A8344G mutant mtDNA. Symptomatic mothers are more likely to have affected offspring than asymptomatic mothers.[28] The MERRF is also associated with other tRNA^{Lys} point mutations including T8356C and G8363A mutations. The 7472C-insertion (7472insC) mutation in the tRNA$^{Ser(UCN)}$ gene has been identified in five families with myoclonus, ataxia, seizures, sensorineural hearing loss, and myopathy, a phenotype very similar to the MERRF phenotype.[39–42] In contrast to patients harbouring theA8344G mutation, the published patients harbouring 7472insC mutation do not have RRFs on the skeletal muscle biopsies, rather, the majority of muscle fibres exhibit a decrease in cytochrome oxidase (COX) activity. However, we have recently identified the 7472insC mutation in a MERRF family with typical RRFs (unpublished data).

Mitochondrial encephalopathy, lactic acidosis, and stroke-like episodes (MELAS)

This is an important predominantly CNS mitochondrial disease in which a major feature is stroke-like episodes which can be fatal.

In 1975, Schapira *et al.* first described a syndrome associated with stroke-like episodes, lactic acidaemia, and RRFs.[43] The acronym MELAS was subsequently introduced by Pavlakis to characterize a distinctive group of patients who had young onset stroke-like episodes and lactic acidosis.[12] Hirano *et al.* reviewed 69 MELAS cases and proposed the following invariant criteria for a diagnosis of MELAS: (i) stroke-like episode before age 40 (ii) encephalopathy characterized by seizures, dementia, or both and (iii) lactic acidosis, RRF, or both. The diagnosis may be considered secure if there are also at least two of the following: normal early development, recurrent headache, or recurrent vomiting.[44] It is notable that MELAS patients with mental retardation (indicating impaired early development) or first stroke-like episode after age 40 are occasionally observed suggesting the diagnosis of MELAS should be considered at any age in the presence of consistent clinical and imaging features.[45,46]

The stroke-like episodes frequently do not conform to a single vascular territory as is the case for the commonest type of strokes in the population, ischaemic strokes. MELAS strokes commonly affect parieto-ocipital areas resulting in hemianopia or cortical blindness. Complete recovery is uncommon. Usually, patients have some residual deficits and progressive encephalopathy following the stroke-like episodes leading to dementia and premature death.[47,48] The stroke-like episodes are often accompanied by migrainous type headache, recurrent vomiting, and seizures. Seizures may be focal, for example, focal motor seizures are not uncommon. Secondary generalized seizures or myoclonic seizures are also described. Other common additional features include short stature, sensorineural hearing loss, and DM.

Myopathy, cardiomyopathy, optic neuropathy, cerebellar features, sensorimotor axonal neuropathy, gastrointestinal pseudo-obstruction, and nephropathy are less commonly associated features.[12,48,49]

The commonest mtDNA defect associated with MELAS was identified simultaneously by two Japanese groups, Goto *et al.*[50] and Kobayashi *et al.* in 1990.[51] This is the A3243G mutation in the tRNA[Leu(UUR)]gene and is identified in over 80 per cent of MELAS cases.[50] Families harbouring the A3243G mutation usually exhibit a maternal inheritance pattern. The A3243G mutation may associate with marked clinical heterogeneity even in the same family. It is of interest that less than half of the patients harbouring the A3243G mutation exhibit MELAS.[15,52] Other clinical syndromes associated with the A3243G mutation include CPEO, diabetes and deafness, myopathy or MERRF.[22,48] The precise factors underlying such clinical diversity, which is more marked than for the A8344G mutation, remain unclear. The proportion of the mutant mtDNA, the tissue distribution of mutant mtDNA, the threshold effect, and nuclear and mitochondrial DNA backgrounds have all been invoked. Recently, we provided evidence to suggest that a polymorphism, A12308G, in the mitochondrial tRNA[Leu(CUN)] increased the risk of developing stroke-like episodes in patients harbouring the A3243G mutation.[52]

Other less common mtDNA mutations associated with MELAS including T3271C mutation in tRNA[Leu(UUR)] gene[53] and G13513 in the ND5 gene[54] (Table 5.4). The majority of MELAS patients harbouring T3271C mutation are Japanese although it has been reported in two Caucasian families.[55,56] The G13513A mutation appears to be the second commonest cause of MELAS in the United Kingdom and is part of our DNA diagnostic screening test in MELAS patients.[57] The G13513A mutation has also been identified in MELAS cases in other countries in Europe and in North America suggesting that it may be common in Caucasians.[54,58,59]

Table 5.4 MtDNA mutations associated with MELAS

Gene	MtDNA mutation	Reference
	Single large deletion	156
	Large scale tandem duplication	157
tRNA[Leu(UUR)]	A3243G	50, 51
	A3252G	158
	A3260G	159
	T3271C	53
	T3291C	160
tRNA[Phe]	G583A	45
tRNA[Val]	G1642A	161
tRNA[Cys]	A5814G	162
COX III	T9957C	163
ND5	G13513A	54
	A13514G	59

Abbreviations: tRNA = transfer RNA, Leu = leucine, Phe = phenylalanine, Val = valine, Cys = cysteine, COX = cytochrome oxidase, ND = NADH dehydrogenase.

Leber's hereditary optic neuropathy (LHON)

This mitochondrial disease is generally confined to the optic nerve and is an important cause of blindness in otherwise normal people, especially males.

The LHON has been recognized as a distinctive syndrome causing subacute bilateral visual loss for over a hundred years.[60] The LHON is characterized by acute or subacute severe bilateral visual loss commonly in young males, which may develop simultaneously or more commonly sequentially. The time interval between affected eyes averages 8 weeks and the duration of progression of visual loss in each eye is usually over a period of 1–6 weeks.[61,62] Although its commonest age at onset is between 11–30 years of age, patients outside of this age range are not uncommon. In the pedigree analysis of 85 LHON families by Harding *et al.*, onset of the first visual symptom ranged from age 6 to 62 years.[63] Patients often complain of fogging or blurring corresponding to centrocaecal scotoma. An enlarged blind spot and loss of central vision are usually evident on examination. The visual acuity generally falls to counting fingers. In only 5 per cent of patients is the loss milder than this—down to a visual acuity of 6/60 or better.[61] Pain on eye movement, around the affected eye or Uhthoff's phenomenon is an uncommon feature, which may help to distinguish acute LHON from acute optic neuritis in multiple sclerosis (MS) on clinical grounds. The pupils usually exhibit a slow symmetrical response to light, although a relative afferent pupillary defect is common at early stage when one eye is predominantly affected.[64]

Fundoscopy generally shows optic disc swelling, telangiectatic vessels in the peripapillary retinal nerve fibre layer, and tortuousity of the retinal arteries in the early stage. Although retinal microangiopathy is not detected in over one-third of patients examined within 3 months of visual loss, these characteristic fundoscopic features may remain for several months after the onset of visual loss. Optic disc pallor may be first seen as early as 1 month from the onset of visual loss and is universal by 6 months. Optic disc or retinal haemorrhage is an uncommon presentation.[61] The severity of the fundoscopic changes correlate with the stage of disease, being the most marked during the acute phase of visual loss.[65] Asymptomatic members of LHON families may also have varying degrees of microangiopathy in the fundi but nerve fibre layer abnormalities are not seen.[66] The vascular abnormalities in asymptomatic family members of the LHON patients are suggested to be a sign of developing acute visual loss.[67] Fluorescein angiography rarely shows leakage.[68]

In the early stage, visual evoked potentials (VEPs) exhibit delayed latency, are desynchronized, and are reduced in amplitude. They tend to be less prolonged in latency and smaller amplitude compared to VEPs recorded in patients with demyelinating optic neuritis. VEPs are usually absent in patients with severe visual loss of long duration.[69]

Magnetic resonance imaging (MRI) scans of optic nerves within 4 months of onset of visual loss are often normal. High signal of the affected optic nerves on the MRI scans is commonly shown after 4 months.

Most patients with LHON have no associated neurological problems but there are studies reporting MRI brain abnormalities and additional clinical features. For example, one study of brain MRI scans of LHON females who also had a MS-like illness and who harboured the G11778A mutation, showed multiple white matter abnormalities predominantly involving the periventricular area. These findings are sometimes observed in females without MS-like illness harbouring the G11778A mutation. In those females with an MS-like illness, the clinical, immunological, and MRI features are indistinguishable from those of MS. The higher prevalence of MS-like illness associated with LHON than in general populations suggests that these observations do not occur coincidentally.[70] Brain MRI scans of males are generally normal.[61,71]

Almost all LHON patients harbour one of three common mtDNA point mutations in the mitochondrial complex I subunit genes including G3460A in ND1 gene, G11778A in ND4 gene, and T14484C in ND6 gene.[63] The G11778A mutation is the commonest cause of LHON.[72] The patients harbouring the T14484C have better prognosis for some visual recovery compared to patients harbouring the G3460A or G11778A mutations. In contrast to MELAS and MERRF mutations, LHON mutations are often homoplasmic in blood and other tissues. Although most families exhibit a maternal inheritance pattern, about one-third of the patients do not have a family history of visual impairment. Even in LHON families in which all maternal relatives contain homoplasmic proportions of a pathogenic mutation, males are much more commonly clinically affected than females. The excess of affected males was suggested to be due to an X-linked visual loss susceptibility locus (VLSL) by Bu *et al.*[73] and Vilkki *et al.* in 1991.[74] Although this genetic finding has not been confirmed by other groups,[75–78] pedigree analysis does support the existence of X-linked VLSL gene as an explanation for the male excess.[63]

Sensorineural hearing loss

Sensorineural hearing loss is a common associated feature in many of the mitochondrial encephalomyopathy phenotypes such as MELAS, MERRF, or KSS. Indeed, if a patient with a complex CNS disease also has deafness, this is regarded as clue to the investigating clinician that the patient may have a mitochondrial disease. However, mitochondrial sensorineural deafness in isolation without any other neurological features is relatively recently recognized. Initial observations in several families exhibiting maternal inheritance of susceptibility to antibiotic-induced ototoxicity provided the first evidence that isolated deafness might be a mitochondrial disease phenotype.[79,80] Prezant *et al.* proposed that the mitochondrial ribosomal RNA (rRNA) may be a candidate gene due to the similarity of the aminoglycosides binding site of the 16S rRNA of *Escherichia coli (E. coli)* and a region of the human mitochondrial 12S rRNA.[81] They described four families with aminoglycoside-induced and non-syndromic sensorineural deafness in association with a A1555G mutation in the 12S rRNA.[81] Surprisingly, the A1555G mutation has been shown to be a common cause of late-onset familial non-syndromic sensorineural deafness in Spain accounting for 27 per cent of the familial cases.[82] The high prevalence of A1555G mutation in Spain is not caused by a founder effect.[83] A study in Japan revealed that the A1555G accounts for over 3 per cent of all patients with sensorineural hearing loss in an auditory out patient clinic and that one-third of these cases had previously had aminoglycosides injections.[84] Typically, patients with the 1555 mutation have late-onset bilateral gradually progressive sensorineural hearing loss. However, age at onset of less than 2 years is reported. The age at onset varies widely within individual families although most patients develop symptoms before 40 years of age. Hearing loss is both spontaneous or may follow exposure to aminoglycosides treatment. It usually affects high frequencies at the beginning. Hearing loss is often mild unless it is aminoglycosides-induced, in which case it is generally associated with acute deafness a few weeks after receiving aminoglycosides treatment.[82,85]

Families with maternally inherited sensorineural hearing loss are also described in association with A7445G, T7511C, and 7472insC mutations in the tRNA$^{Ser(UCN)}$ gene.[86–88] The clinical features are similar to the A 1555G mutation but the A7445G and T7511C mutations have not been reported in association with aminoglycoside-induced deafness. Families harbouring the 7472insC mutation may also exhibit other neurological features including ataxia, myoclonus, seizures, and polyneuropathy.[40,89]

Neurogenic muscle weakness, ataxia, and retinitis pigmentosa (NARP)

The NARP was originally described in a maternally inherited family with a variable combination of retinitis pigmentosa, ataxia, neurogenic muscle weakness, developmental delay, seizures, dementia, optic atrophy, and sensory neuropathy by Holt *et al*.[90] This group identified a heteroplasmic T8993G mutation in the mitochondrial ATP synthase subunit 6 (ATPase 6) gene in all studied family members. The more severe clinical phenotypes and the earlier age at onset cases correlated with higher proportions of the mutant mtDNA in blood. This correlation was supported by 44 subsequent reports.[91,92] Individuals with levels of mutant mtDNA less than 70 per cent are usually asymptomatic or are mildly affected. The NARP often associates with proportions of mutant mtDNA in muscle or blood between 70 and 90 per cent. Patients harbouring proportions of mutant mtDNA above 90 per cent generally develop one of the most severe and frequently lethal phenotypes of LS.[93,94] Some studies have indicated that the proportions of the T8993G mutant mtDNA in different tissues are generally homogeneous in contrast to tRNA gene mutations where large differences in mutant load are reported.[94,95] For these reasons, molecular diagnosis of the T8993G and in particular prenatal diagnosis is considered to be more reliable than for other mtDNA mutations such as those in tRNA genes (see Chapter 16 for further discussion of prenatal diagnosis).[96,97]

In contrast to KSS, the retinopathy in NARP patients is often typical of retinitis pigmentosa. Fundoscopy reveals clumps of pigment and bone corpuscle formation in both retinae leading to constricted visual fields or blindness. Gait and limb ataxia of cerebellar type is prominent and there is usually cerebellar atrophy on brain scan. Limb weakness is often mild and may be obscured by limb ataxia. Axonal sensory neuropathy may involve any sensory modalities and tendon reflexes are absent. Muscle biopsies do not show the typical histochemical evidence of mitochondrial myopathy such as RRFs or absence of COX activity.[90] Instead, the muscle biopsy simply shows changes of denervation of muscle as a consequence of the neuropathy. The combination of the described clinical features in association with maternal transmission are therefore important clues for the diagnosis which can be confirmed by mtDNA analysis.

Leigh's Syndrome (LS)

In 1951, Leigh first described a child who died from subacute severe encephalomyelopathy with striking and distinctive neuropathological abnormalities mainly involving the thalamus, basal ganglia, and brainstem.[98] The LS is one of the most common mitochondrial encephalomyopathies in infancy. It is a devastating disorder associated with a range of neurological signs including psychomotor retardation, optic atrophy, ophthalmoplegia, ptosis, nystagmus, ataxia, tremor, dystonia, pyramidal signs, and abnormal breathing. Definite diagnosis depends on either characteristic neuroimaging or the postmortem neuropathological features of bilateral symmetrical spongiform lesions localized especially in the thalamus, basal ganglia, and brainstem. These findings are microscopically associated with cystic cavitation, demyelination, vascular proliferation, and gliosis.[99] The onset of LS is often in the first year of life, however juvenile or adult-onset LS is occasionally described.[100,101]

Although the first genetic defect identified is in the ATPase 6 gene of the mtDNA, theT8993G mutation,[102,103] LS is more commonly inherited as an autosomal recessive trait than as a maternally inherited trait, that is to say, it is the result of a mutation(s) in nuclear DNA, and is discussed in detail in Chapter 10.[104] Interestingly, autosomal recessive LS families frequently have either isolated Complex IV (cytochrome *c* oxidase COX), or Complex I (NADH–ubiquinone reductase) deficiency or less commonly Complex II (succinic–ubiquinone reductase) deficiency. Recently, nuclear genes encoding important mitochondrial proteins have been identified in some families with autosomal LS. The X-linked recessive families with a defect of pyruvate dehydrogenase complex (PDHC), which does not affect the respiratory chain directly, also exhibit LS.[105]

Mutant nuclear genes associated with LS include the flavoprotein gene of complex II, and the *SURF*-1 gene involved in COX assembly, which accounts for 75 per cent of LS with COX deficiency. Mutations in other COX assembly genes, *SCO*1 and *SCO*2 have subsequently been identified in patients with severe infantile encephalopathy. In contrast to patients harbouring *SURF*-1 mutations who generally have LS, patients harbouring *SCO*2 mutations often exhibit hypertrophic cardiomyopathy and have a severe encephalomyopathy which resembles LS but without the characteristic neuropathological features of LS.[106] In contrast, a *SCO*1 mutation, described in two brothers with neonatal-onset hepatic failure, ketoacidotic coma, and encephalopathy, proved fatal within 2 months of birth. LS with Complex I deficiency accounts for almost 20 per cent of LS cases, the mutations identified to date are located in nuclear-encoded Complex I genes. Two affected families exhibited autosomal recessive LS with typical neuropathological findings.

Sensory ataxic neuropathy, dysarthia, ophthamoparesis (SANDO)

When the peripheral nervous system bears the brunt of a mitochondrial disease, skeletal muscle rather than peripheral nerve is most likely to be affected. However, recently, cases have been reported in which the dominant presenting symptom is a severe peripheral neuropathy.

Four sporadic patients from North America developed a distinct clinical syndrome presenting with severe sensory ataxic neuropathy, dysarthia, and late-onset progressive external ophthalmoplegia. Fadic *et al.* proposed the acronym SANDO and identified multiple deletions in the mtDNA in all patients. The most prominent feature is sensory ataxic neuropathy and ophthalmoplegia often developing after the age of 30. Migraine and depression were also common in these cases. Nerve conduction studies showed a predominantly sensory axonal neuropathy. Muscle biopsies generally reveal RRF with or without COX-deficient fibres.[107]

Non-neurological features

Non-neurological clinical features may associate with primary mtDNA disorders (Table 5.1). When present they often accompany neurological phenotypes rather than presenting as the sole manifestation. For example, short stature and DM in MELAS, cardiomyopathy in KSS, or lipomatosis with MERRF. Sometimes, these associated non-neurological features may be an important determinant of the prognosis, for example, premature death in KSS is often due to cardiac conduction disturbance and cardiomyopathy. There is also now considerable evidence that shows that isolated non-neurological involvement can be the sole manifestation of mitochondrial disease, for example, isolated cardiomyopathy. In the next section, we focus on some of the important non-neurological features often associated with mitochondrial encephalomyopathies.

Heart

Cardiac manifestations are relatively common presentations of mitochondrial encephalomyopathies and can be fatal. The common cardiac features are both conduction defects and cardiomyopathy. One study investigated cardiac manifestations in 17 patients with classical mitochondrial phenotypes (6 CPEO, 3 KSS (single large deletions), 5 MELAS (A3243G), and 3 MERRF (A8344G)). Of these, 3 patients with KSS had cardiac conduction defects, 2 of 3 MERRF patients had significant cardiomyopathy and 2 of 5 patients with MELAS had symmetrical left ventricular hypertrophy.[108] Hypertrophic cardiomyopathy is occasionally described in LS (T8993C).[109]

Maternally inherited isolated hypertrophic cardiomyopathy is genetically heterogeneous. It has been described in association with several mtDNA point mutations including A1555G in the 12S rRNA gene, A3243G in the tRNA[Leu(UUR)] gene, A4295G and A4300G in the tRNA[Ile] gene, A8296G and G8363A in the tRNA[Lys] gene, G15423A in the cytochrome *b* gene, and some sporadic cases with mtDNA depletion.[110–117]

Dilated cardiomyopathy is less common than the hypertrophic type. It has been described in patients with MELAS and MERRF.[108,118] Familial isolated 'idiopathic' dilated cardiomyopathy is described in association with mtDNA multiple deletions and a point mutation, T12297C in the tRNA[Leu(CUN)] gene.[118,119]

Endocrine

DM is commonly associated with A3243G (MELAS) mutation. This mutation is also described in families with maternally inherited isolated DM and deafness.[28] Rearrangements of mtDNA are also often associated with type II diabetes, in particular partial duplications.[120–122] Moreover, a common mtDNA variant present in 9 per cent of the UK population appears to be a predisposing factor in some forms of multigenic type II diabetes.[123] Patients with mitochondrial encephalomyopathy often have short stature, which has sometimes been shown to be associated with deficient growth hormone secretion.[124] Other less common endocrine involvements are shown in Table 5.1.

Bone marrow

Pearson's syndrome is a fatal infantile disorder characterized by refractory sideroblastic anaemia, thrombocytopenia, neutropenia, and pancreatic exocrine dysfunction. Bone marrow pathology is characterized by remarkable vacuolization of erythroid and myeloid precursors, haemosiderosis, and ringed sideroblasts.[125] Additional features include renal tubular acidosis and hepatic failure. It has been described in association with mtDNA large-scale rearrangements such as single large deletions and less commonly with deletion-duplication.[126,127] Most patients die at young age, however some patients who have survived have been observed to subsequently develop KSS.[128,129] A variant of Pearson's syndrome associated with a single large mtDNA deletion has been reported. The patient developed congenital hypoplastic anaemia, renal tubulopathy, DM, and cerebral atrophy. She subsequently developed progressive external ophthalmoplegia and KSS.[130] These observations suggest that Pearson's syndrome and KSS represent a clinical continuum caused by single deletions and that the different phenotypes may be determined by variation in mutant load.

A form of sideroblastic anaemia has also been described in families harbouring mtDNA mutations (namely the A8344G mutation and multiple deletions of mtDNA),[131,132] and with a mutation in a putative mitochondrial iron transporter gene (ABC7).[133]

Gastrointestinal tract

Mitochondrial neurogastrointestinal encephalomyopathy (MNGIE)

The MNGIE is a unique autosomal recessive multisystem disorders associated with multiple deletions or partial depletion of mtDNA (see also Chapter 9). It is characterized by gastrointestinal dysmotility, cachexia, ptosis, progressive external ophthalmoplegia, polyneuropathy, and leukoencephalopathy on brain MRI.[134,135] Onset may vary from 5 months to 43 years of age although the majority of patients have experienced symptoms before 20 years of age. Patients often died in the forth decade. Almost half of the patients develop gastrointestinal symptoms as the initial manifestation. Opthalmoplegia is also a common initial presentation.

Gastrointestinal features are the most prominent clinical features including borborygmi, abdominal pain and cramps, diarrhoea, early satiety, nausea/vomiting, diverticulosis, pseudo-obstruction, gastroparesis, and dysphagia. Cachexia is another prominent feature, but despite the apparent muscle atrophy, muscle strength is well maintained.[136]

Neurological symptoms are often mild. Peripheral neuropathy affecting both motor and sensory nerves leading to glove-stocking sensory loss and mild distal limb weakness is frequent. Patients occasionally have debilitating weakness. Hearing loss is observed in almost half of the patients. Pigmentary retinopathy and mental retardation are rare. Nerve conduction studies are invariably consistent with demyelinating neuropathy but it sometimes also shows additional features compatible with axonal neuropathy. Electromyography sometimes shows myogenic pattern in addition to more common neuropathic features. Increased CSF protein is observed in most patients. Brain MRI generally reveals diffuse leukoencephalopathy. It there may well be no clinical manifestation attributable to the leukoencephalopathy, such as pyramidal signs or dementia. COX-deficient muscle fibres are invariably observed and almost two-third of patients have RRF on muscle biopsy.[136]

Treatment

The development of more effective treatments for patients with mitochondrial diseases remains one of the most important research challenges in this field. At present, there is no genetic therapy or other therapy which has been shown to have a clinically significant impact on the natural history or molecular pathogenesis of these disease. However, there are many practical measures the clinicians can institute to improve the quality of life for patients.

Advice about avoiding situations which may prompt lactic acidosis such as excessive exertion or alcohol is important in certain cases. Prompt treatment of lactic acidosis if it occurs may be life saving. Control of seizures with anticonvulsant medication, although avoiding valproate, is important. Other medications which are often considered include coenzyme Q_{10}, carnitine, riboflavin, and thiamine. However, these are only usually effective if the patient has been demonstrated to have a specific deficiency of one or other of these factors. Many clinicians in this area offer patients a trial of coenzyme Q_{10} if fatigue is a prominent symptom, although clinical trials have not proven its effectiveness. Acute stroke-like episodes have been reported to be rapidly improved by steroid treatment.[43,137]

Practical aids such as hearing aids and ptosis props can be very valuable. Surgical intervention such as ptosis surgery or cochlea implant surgery both have an important place in carefully selected patients. The services of a neurorehabilitation team are often invaluable to patients with significant CNS or peripheral nervous system involvement and should be offered in all such cases. Screening for non-neurological tissue involvement is important; for example, we routinely arrange cardiac evaluation in all mitochondrial patients.

Understandably, patients wish to know the risks of transmitting their disease. Genetic counselling is therefore a very important part of management. However, except for single large-scale rearrangements which are sporadic, genetic counselling for other types of mtDNA mutations is presently problematic because of the absence of reliable recurrence risks (however see also Chapter 16).

Recent research has provided evidence that therapeutic muscle damage or certain types of exercise programmes may reduce the proportion of mutant mtDNA in skeletal muscle. This would be expected to result in improved respiratory chain function and therefore clinical function. Although encouraging, further work is need before true clinical benefit to patients is proven.[22,138–141]

Acknowledgements

Our research is supported by the Medical Research Council (UK) and the Brain Research Trust.

References

1. Engel WK (1962). The essentiality of histo- and cytochemical studies of skeletal muscle in the investigation of neuromuscular disease. *Neurology* **12**: 778–794.
2. Engel WK and Cunningham GG (1963). Rapid examination of muscle tissue. An improved trichrome method for fresh-frozen biopsy sections. *Neurology* **13**: 919–923.
3. Luft R, Ikkos D, Palmieri G, Ernster L, and Afzelius B (1962). A case of severe hypermetabolism of nonthyroid origin with a defect in the maintainance of mitochondrial respiratory control- A correlated clinical, biochemical, and morphological study. *J. Clin. Invest.* **41**: 1776–1804.
4. Haydar NA, Conn HL, Jr., Afifi A, Wakid N, Ballas S, and Fawaz K (1971). Severe hypermetabolism with primary abnormality of skeletal muscle mitochondria. *Ann. Intern. Med.* **74**(4): 548–558.
5. Engel WK (1967). Muscle biopsies in neuromuscular diseases. *Pediatr. Clin. North Am.* **14**(4): 963–995.

6. DiMauro S, Bonilla E, Lee CP, Schotland DL, Scarpa A, Conn H, Jr., *et al.* (1976). Luft's disease. Further biochemical and ultrastructural studies of skeletal muscle in the second case. *J. Neurol. Sci.* **27**(2): 217–232.

7. Drachman DA, Ophthalmoplegia plus (1968). The neurodegenerative disorders associated with progressive external ophthalmoplegia. *Arch. Neurol.* **18**(6): 654–674.

8. Olson W, Engel WK, Walsh GO, and Einaugler R (1972). Oculocraniosomatic neuromuscular disease with 'ragged-red' fibers. *Arch. Neurol.* **26**(3): 193–211.

9. Morgan-Hughes JA and Mair WGP (1973). Atypical muscle mitochondria in oculoskeletal myopathy. *Brain* **96**: 215–224.

10. Berenberg RA, Pellock JM, DiMauro S, Schotland DL, Bonilla E, Eastwood A, *et al.* (1977). Lumping or splitting? 'ophthalmoplegia plus' or Kearns–Sayre syndrome? *Ann. Neurol.* **1**: 37–54.

11. Fukuhara N, Tokiguchi S, Shirakawa K, and Tsubaki T (1980). Myoclonus epilepsy associated with ragged-red fibres (mitochondrial abnormalities): disease entity or a syndrome? Light-and electron-microscopic studies of two cases and review of literature. *J. Neurol. Sci.* **47**(1): 117–133.

12. Pavlakis SG, Phillips PC, DiMauro S, De Vivo DC, and Rowland LP (1984). Mitochondrial myopathy, encephalopathy, lactic acidosis, and strokelike episodes: a distinctive clinical syndrome. *Ann. Neurol.* **16**(4): 481–488.

13. Petty RK, Harding AE, and Morgan-Hughes JA (1986). The clinical features of mitochondrial myopathy. *Brain* **109**(Pt 5): 915–938.

14. Holt IJ, Harding AE, and Morgan-Hughes JA (1988). Deletions of muscle mitochondrial DNA in patients with mitochondrial myopathies. *Nature* **331**(6158): 717–719.

15. Chinnery PF, Johnson MA, Wardell TM, Singh-Kler R, Hayes C, Brown DT, *et al.* (2000). The epidemiology of pathogenic mitochondrial DNA mutations. *Ann. Neurol.* **48**(2): 188–193.

16. DiMauro S and Bonilla E (1997). Mitochondrial encephalomyopathies. In: RN Rosenberg, SB Prusiner, S DiMauro, and RL Barchi (eds) *The Molecular and Genetics Basis of Neurological Disease*. Boston: Butterworth-Heinemann, pp. 201–235.

17. Hammans SR and Morgan-Hughes JA (1994). Mitochondrial myopathies: clinical features, investigation, treatment and genetic counselling. In: *Mitochondrial Disorders in Neurology* (eds AHV Schapira and S DiMauro), Oxford: Butterworth-Heinemann, pp. 49–74.

18. Moraes CT, DiMauro S, Zeviani M, Lombes A, Shanske S, Miranda AF, *et al.* (1989). Mitochondrial DNA deletions in progressive external ophthalmoplegia and Kearns-Sayre syndrome. *N. Engl. J. Med.* **320**(20): 1293–1299.

19. Zeviani M, Gellera C, Pannacci M, Uziel G, Prelle A, Servidei S, *et al.* (1990). Tissue distribution and transmission of mitochondrial DNA deletions in mitochondrial myopathies. *Ann. Neurol.* **28**(1): 94–97.

20. Ozawa T, Yoneda M, Tanaka M, Ohno K, Sato W, Suzuki H, *et al.* (1988). Maternal inheritance of deleted mitochondrial DNA in a family with mitochondrial myopathy. *Biochem. Biophys. Res. Commun.* **154**(3): 1240–1247.

21. Moraes CT, Ciacci F, Silvestri G, Shanske S, Sciacco M, Hirano M, *et al.* (1993). Atypical clinical presentations associated with the MELAS mutation at position 3243 of human mitochondrial DNA. *Neuromuscul. Disord.* **3**(1): 43–50.

22. Fu K, Hartlen R, Johns T, Genge A, Karpati G, and Shoubridge EA (1996). A novel heteroplasmic tRNAleu(CUN) mtDNA point mutation in a sporadic patient with mitochondrial encephalomyopathy segregates rapidly in skeletal muscle and suggests an approach to therapy. *Hum. Mol. Genet.* **5**(11): 1835–1840.

23. Andreu AL, Hanna MG, Reichmann H, Bruno C, Penn AS, Tanji K, *et al.* (1999). Exercise intolerance due to mutations in the cytochrome b gene of mitochondrial DNA. *N. Engl. J. Med.* **341**(14): 1037–1044.

24. Chinnery PF, Johnson MA, Taylor RW, Lightowlers RN, and Turnbull DM (1997). A novel mitochondrial tRNA phenylalanine mutation presenting with acute rhabdomyolysis. *Ann. Neurol.* **41**(3): 408–410.

25. Karadimas CL, Greenstein P, Sue CM, Joseph JT, Tanji K, Haller RG, *et al.* (2000). Recurrent myoglobinuria due to a nonsense mutation in the COX I gene of mitochondrial DNA. *Neurology* **55**(5): 644–649.

26. Andreu AL, Tanji K, Bruno C, Hadjigeorgiou GM, Sue CM, Jay C, *et al.* (1999). Exercise intolerance due to a nonsense mutation in the mtDNA ND4 gene. *Ann. Neurol.* **45**(6): 820–823.

27. Tsaris P, Engel WK, and Kark P (1973). Familial myoclonic epilepsy syndrome associated with skeletal muscle mitochondrial abnormalities. *Neurology* **23**: 408.

28. Hammans SR, Sweeney MG, Brockington M, Lennox GG, Lawton NF, Kennedy CR, *et al.* (1993). The mitochondrial DNA transfer RNA(Lys)A → G(8344) mutation and the syndrome of myoclonic epilepsy with ragged red fibres (MERRF). Relationship of clinical phenotype to proportion of mutant mitochondrial DNA. *Brain* **116** (Pt 3): 617–632.

29. Rosing HS, Hopkins LC, Wallace DC, Epstein CM, and Weidenheim K (1985). Maternally inherited mitochondrial myopathy and myoclonic epilepsy. *Ann. Neurol.* **17**(3): 228–237.

30. Morgan-Hughes JA, Hayes DJ, Clark JB, Landon DN, Swash M, Stark RJ, *et al.* (1982). Mitochondrial encephalomyopathies: biochemical studies in two cases revealing defects in the respiratory chain. *Brain* **105** (Pt 3): 553–582.

31. Toyono M, Nakano K, Kiuchi M, Imai K, Suzuki H, Shishikura K, *et al.* (2001). A case of MERRF associated with chronic pancreatitis. *Neuromuscul. Disord.* **11**(3): 300–304.

32. Austin SA, Vriesendorp FJ, Thandroyen FT, Hecht JT, Jones OT, and Johns DR (1998). Expanding the phenotype of the 8344 transfer RNAlysine mitochondrial DNA mutation. *Neurology* **51**(5): 1447–1450.

33. Byrne E, Trounce I, Dennett X, Gilligan B, Morley JB, and Marzuki S (1988). Progression from MERRF to MELAS phenotype in a patient with combined respiratory complex I and IV deficiencies. *J. Neurol. Sci.* **88**(1–3): 327–337.

34. So N, Berkovic S, Andermann F, Kuzniecky R, Gendron D, and Quesney LF (1989). Myoclonus epilepsy and ragged-red fibres (MERRF). 2. Electrophysiological studies and comparison with other progressive myoclonus epilepsies. *Brain* **112** (Pt 5): 1261–1276.

35. Fukuhara N (1991). MERRF: a clinicopathological study. Relationships between myoclonus epilepsies and mitochondrial myopathies. *Rev. Neurol.* (Paris) **147**(6–7): 476–479.

36. Berkovic SF, Carpenter S, Evans A, Karpati G, Shoubridge EA, Andermann F, *et al.* (1989). Myoclonus epilepsy and ragged-red fibres (MERRF). 1. A clinical, pathological, biochemical, magnetic resonance spectrographic and positron emission tomographic study. *Brain* **112** (Pt 5): 1231–1260.

37. Sweeney MG, Hammans SR, Duchen LW, Cooper JM, Schapira AH, Kennedy CR, *et al.* (1994). Mitochondrial DNA mutation underlying Leigh's syndrome: clinical, pathological, biochemical, and genetic studies of a patient presenting with progressive myoclonic epilepsy. *J. Neurol. Sci.* **121**(1): 57–65.

38. Hammans SR, Sweeney MG, Brockington M, Morgan-Hughes JA, and Harding AE (1991). Mitochondrial encephalopathies: molecular genetic diagnosis from blood samples. *Lancet* **337**(8753): 1311–1313.

39. Silvestri G, Ciafaloni E, Santorelli FM, Shanske S, Servidei S, Graf WD, *et al.* (1993). Clinical features associated with the A → G transition at nucleotide 8344 of mtDNA ('MERRF mutation'). *Neurology* **43**(6): 1200–1206.

40. Tiranti V, Chariot P, Carella F, Toscano A, Soliveri P, Girlanda P, *et al.* (1995). Maternally inherited hearing loss, ataxia and myoclonus associated with a novel point mutation in mitochondrial tRNASer(UCN) gene. *Hum. Mol. Genet.* 1995; **4**(8): 1421–1427.

41. Jaksch M, Klopstock T, Kurlemann G, Dorner M, Hofmann S, Kleinle S, *et al.* (1998). Progressive myoclonus epilepsy and mitochondrial myopathy associated with mutations in the tRNA(Ser(UCN)) gene. *Ann. Neurol.* **44**(4): 635–640.

42. Schuelke M, Bakker M, Stoltenburg G, Sperner J, and von Moers A (1998). Epilepsia partialis continua associated with a homoplasmic mitochondrial tRNA(Ser(UCN) mutation. *Ann. Neurol.* **44**(4): 700–704.

43. Shapira Y, Cederbaum SD, Cancilla PA, Nielsen D, and Lippe BM (1975). Familial poliodystrophy, mitochondrial myopathy, and lactate acidemia. *Neurology* **25**(7): 614–621.

44. Hirano M, Ricci E, Koenigsberger MR, Defendini R, Pavlakis SG, DeVivo DC, *et al.* (1992). Melas: an original case and clinical criteria for diagnosis. *Neuromuscul. Disord.* **2**(2): 125–135.

45. Hanna MG, Nelson IP, Morgan-Hughes JA, and Wood NW (1998). MELAS: a new disease associated mitochondrial DNA mutation and evidence for further genetic heterogeneity. *J. Neurol. Neurosurg. Psychiatry* **65**(4): 512–517.

46. Damian MS, Seibel P, Reichmann H, Schachenmayr W, Laube H, Bachmann G, *et al.* (1995). Clinical spectrum of the MELAS mutation in a large pedigree. *Acta. Neurol. Scand.* **92**(5): 409–415.

47. Goto Y, Horai S, Matsuoka T, Koga Y, Nihei K, Kobayashi M, *et al.* (1992). Mitochondrial myopathy, encephalopathy, lactic acidosis, and stroke-like episodes (MELAS): a correlative study of the clinical features and mitochondrial DNA mutation. *Neurology* **42**(3 Pt 1): 545–550.

48. Hammans SR, Sweeney MG, Hanna MG, Brockington M, Morgan-Hughes JA, and Harding AE (1995). The mitochondrial DNA transfer RNALeu(UUR) A → G(3243) mutation. A clinical and genetic study. *Brain* **118** (Pt 3): 721–734.

49. Ciafaloni E, Ricci E, Shanske S, Moraes CT, Silvestri G, Hirano M, *et al.* (1992). MELAS: clinical features, biochemistry, and molecular genetics. *Ann. Neurol.* **31**(4): 391–398.

50. Goto Y, Nonaka I, and Horai S (1990). A mutation in the tRNA(Leu)(UUR) gene associated with the MELAS subgroup of mitochondrial encephalomyopathies. *Nature* **348**(6302): 651–653.

51. Kobayashi Y, Momoi MY, Tominaga K, Momoi T, Nihei K, Yanagisawa M, *et al.* (1990). A point mutation in the mitochondrial tRNA(Leu)(UUR) gene in MELAS (mitochondrial myopathy, encephalopathy, lactic acidosis and stroke-like episodes). *Biochem. Biophys. Res. Commun.* **173**(3): 816–822.

52. Pulkes T, Sweeney MG, and Hanna MG (2000). Increased risk of stroke in patients with the A12308G polymorphism in mitochondria. *Lancet* **356**(9247): 2068–2069.

53. Goto Y, Nonaka I, and Horai S (1991). A new mtDNA mutation associated with mitochondrial myopathy, encephalopathy, lactic acidosis and stroke-like episodes (MELAS). *Biochim. Biophys. Acta.* **1097**(3): 238–240.

54. Santorelli FM, Tanji K, Kulikova R, Shanske S, Vilarinho L, Hays AP, *et al.* (1997). Identification of a novel mutation in the mtDNA ND5 gene associated with MELAS. *Biochem. Biophys. Res. Commun.* **238**(2): 326–328.

55. Marie SK, Goto Y, Passos-Bueno MR, Zatz M, Carvalho AA, Carvalho M, *et al.* (1994). A Caucasian family with the 3271 mutation in mitochondrial DNA. *Biochem. Med. Metab. Biol.* **52**(2): 136–139.

56. Tarnopolsky MA, Maguire J, Myint T, Applegarth D, and Robinson BH (1998). Clinical, physiological, and histological features in a kindred with the T3271C melas mutation. *Muscle. Nerve.* **21**(1): 25–33.

57. Pulkes T, Eunson L, Patterson V, Siddiqui A, Wood NW, Nelson IP, *et al.* (1999). The mitochondrial DNA G13513A transition in ND5 is associated with a LHON/MELAS overlap syndrome and may be a frequent cause of MELAS. *Ann. Neurol.* **46**(6): 916–919.

58. Penisson-Besnier I, Reynier P, Asfar P, Douay O, Sortais A, Dubas F, *et al.* (2000). Recurrent brain hematomas in MELAS associated with an ND5 gene mitochondrial mutation. *Neurology* **55**(2): 317–318.

59. Corona P, Antozzi C, Carrara F, D'Incerti L, Lamantea E, Tiranti V, *et al.* (2001). A novel mtDNA mutation in the ND5 subunit of complex I in two MELAS patients. *Ann. Neurol.* **49**(1): 106–110.

60. von Graefe A (1858). Ein Ungewöhnlicher fall von hereditäre amaurose. *Arch. für. Ophthalmol.* **4**: 266–268.

61. Riordan-Eva P, Sanders MD, Govan GG, Sweeney MG, Da Costa J, and Harding AE (1995). The clinical features of Leber's hereditary optic neuropathy defined by the presence of a pathogenic mitochondrial DNA mutation. *Brain* **118** (Pt 2): 319–337.

62. Newman NJ, Lott MT, and Wallace DC (1991). The clinical characteristics of pedigrees of Leber's hereditary optic neuropathy with the 11778 mutation. *Am. J. Ophthalmol.* **111**(6): 750–762.

63. Harding AE, Sweeney MG, Govan GG, and Riordan-Eva P (1995). Pedigree analysis in Leber hereditary optic neuropathy families with a pathogenic mtDNA mutation. *Am. J. Hum. Genet.* **57**(1): 77–86.

64. Harding AE and Sweeney MG (1994). Leber's hereditary optic neuropathy. In: *Mitochondrial disorders in Neurology* (eds AHV Schapira and S DiMauro), Oxford: Butterworth-Heinemann, pp. 181–198.

65. Nikoskelainen E, Hoyt WF, and Nummelin K (1983). Ophthalmoscopic findings in Leber's hereditary optic neuropathy. II. The fundus findings in the affected family members. *Arch. Ophthalmol.* **101**(7): 1059–1068.

66. Nikoskelainen E, Hoyt WF, and Nummelin K (1982). Ophthalmoscopic findings in Leber's hereditary optic neuropathy. I. Fundus findings in asymptomatic family members. *Arch. Ophthalmol.* **100**(10): 1597–1602.

67. Nikoskelainen E (1985). The clinical findings in Leber's hereditary optic neuroretinopathy. Leber's disease. *Trans. Ophthalmol. Soc. UK* **104** (Pt 8): 845–852.

68. Nikoskelainen E, Hoyt WF, Nummelin K, and Schatz H (1984). Fundus findings in Leber's hereditary optic neuroretinopathy. III. Fluorescein angiographic studies. *Arch. Ophthalmol.* **102**(7): 981–989.

69. Carroll WM and Mastaglia FL (1979). Leber's optic neuropathy: a clinical and visual evoked potential study of affected and asymptomatic members of a six generation family. *Brain* **102**(3): 559–580.

70. Horvath R, Abicht A, Shoubridge EA, Karcagi V, Rozsa C, Komoly S, *et al.* (2000). Leber's hereditary optic neuropathy presenting as multiple sclerosis-like disease of the CNS. *J. Neurol.* **247**(1): 65–67.

71. Harding AE, Sweeney MG, Miller DH, Mumford CJ, Kellar-Wood H, Menard D, *et al.* (1992). Occurrence of a multiple sclerosis-like illness in women who have a Leber's hereditary optic neuropathy mitochondrial DNA mutation. *Brain* **115** (Pt 4): 979–989.

72. Wallace DC, Singh G, Lott MT, Hodge JA, Schurr TG, Lezza AM, *et al.* (1988). Mitochondrial DNA mutation associated with Leber's hereditary optic neuropathy. *Science* **242**(4884): 1427–1430.

73. Bu XD and Rotter JI (1991). X chromosome-linked and mitochondrial gene control of Leber hereditary optic neuropathy: evidence from segregation analysis for dependence on X chromosome inactivation. *Proc. Natl Acad. Sci. USA* **88**(18): 8198–8202.

74. Vilkki J, Ott J, Savontaus ML, Aula P, and Nikoskelainen EK (1991). Optic atrophy in Leber hereditary optic neuroretinopathy is probably determined by an X-chromosomal gene closely linked to DXS7. *Am. J. Hum. Genet.* **48**(3): 486–491.

75. Sweeney MG, Davis MB, Lashwood A, Brockington M, Toscano A, and Harding AE (1992). Evidence against an X-linked locus close to DXS7 determining visual loss susceptibility in British and Italian families with Leber hereditary optic neuropathy. *Am. J. Hum. Genet.* **51**(4): 741–748.

76. Chalmers RM, Davis MB, Sweeney MG, Wood NW, and Harding AE (1996). Evidence against an X-linked visual loss susceptibility locus in Leber hereditary optic neuropathy. *Am. J. Hum. Genet.* **59**(1): 103–108.

77. Carvalho MR, Muller B, Rotzer E, Berninger T, Kommerell G, Blankenagel A, *et al.* (1992). Leber's hereditary optic neuroretinopathy and the X-chromosomal susceptibility factor: no linkage to DXs7. *Hum. Hered.* **42**(5): 316–320.

78. Juvonen V, Vilkki J, Aula P, Nikoskelainen E, and Savontaus ML (1993). Reevaluation of the linkage of an optic atrophy susceptibility gene to X-chromosomal markers in Finnish families with Leber hereditary optic neuroretinopathy (LHON). *Am. J. Hum. Genet.* **53**(1): 289–292.

79. Hu DN, Qui WQ, Wu BT, Fang LZ, Zhou F, Gu YP, *et al.* (1991). Genetic aspects of antibiotic induced deafness: mitochondrial inheritance. *J. Med. Genet.* **28**(2): 79–83.

80. Higashi K (1989). Unique inheritance of streptomycin-induced deafness. *Clin. Genet.* **35**(6): 433–436.

81. Prezant TR, Agapian JV, Bohlman MC, Bu X, Oztas S, Qiu WQ, *et al.* (1993). Mitochondrial ribosomal RNA mutation associated with both antibiotic- induced and non-syndromic deafness. *Nat. Genet.* **4**(3): 289–294.

82. Estivill X, Govea N, Barcelo E, Badenas C, Romero E, Moral L, *et al.* (1998). Familial progressive sensorineural deafness is mainly due to the mtDNA A1555G mutation and is enhanced by treatment of aminoglycosides. *Am. J. Hum. Genet.* **62**(1): 27–35.

83. Torroni A, Cruciani F, Rengo C, Sellitto D, Lopez-Bigas N, Rabionet R, *et al.* (1999). The A1555G mutation in the 12S rRNA gene of human mtDNA: recurrent origins and founder events in families affected by sensorineural deafness. *Am. J. Hum. Genet.* **65**(5): 1349–1358.

84. Usami S, Abe S, Akita J, Namba A, Shinkawa H, Ishii M, *et al.* (2000). Prevalence of mitochondrial gene mutations among hearing impaired patients. *J. Med. Genet.* **37**(1): 38–40.

85. Usami S, Abe S, Kasai M, Shinkawa H, Moeller B, Kenyon JB, *et al.* (1997). Genetic and clinical features of sensorineural hearing loss associated with the 1555 mitochondrial mutation. *Laryngoscope* **107**(4): 483–490.

86. Reid FM, Vernham GA, and Jacobs HT (1994). A novel mitochondrial point mutation in a maternal pedigree with sensorineural deafness. *Hum. Mutat.* **3**(3): 243–247.

87. Sue CM, Tanji K, Hadjigeorgiou G, Andreu AL, Nishino I, Krishna S, *et al.* (1999). Maternally inherited hearing loss in a large kindred with a novel T7511C mutation in the mitochondrial DNA tRNA(Ser(UCN)) gene. *Neurology* **52**(9): 1905–1908.

88. Verhoeven K, Ensink RJ, Tiranti V, Huygen PL, Johnson DF, Schatteman I, *et al.* (1999). Hearing impairment and neurological dysfunction associated with a mutation in the mitochondrial tRNASer(UCN) gene. *Eur. J. Hum. Genet.* **7**(1): 45–51.

89. Ensink RJ, Verhoeven K, Marres HA, Huygen PL, Padberg GW, ter Laak H, *et al.* (1998). Early-onset sensorineural hearing loss and late-onset neurologic complaints caused by a mitochondrial mutation at position 7472. *Arch. Otolaryngol. Head. Neck. Surg.* **124**(8): 886–891.

90. Holt IJ, Harding AE, Petty RK, and Morgan-Hughes JA (1990). A new mitochondrial disease associated with mitochondrial DNA heteroplasmy. *Am. J. Hum. Genet.* **46**(3): 428–433.

91. Tatuch Y, Pagon RA, Vlcek B, Roberts R, Korson M, and Robinson BH (1994). The 8993 mtDNA mutation: heteroplasmy and clinical presentation in three families. *Eur. J. Hum. Genet.* **2**(1): 35–43.

92. Makela-Bengs P, Suomalainen A, Majander A, Rapola J, Kalimo H, Nuutila A, *et al.* (1995). Correlation between the clinical symptoms and the proportion of mitochondrial DNA carrying the 8993 point mutation in the NARP syndrome. *Pediatr. Res.* **37**(5): 634–639.

93. Santorelli FM, Shanske S, Macaya A, DeVivo DC, and DiMauro S (1993). The mutation at nt 8993 of mitochondrial DNA is a common cause of Leigh's syndrome. *Ann. Neurol.* **34**(6): 827–834.

94. Uziel G, Moroni I, Lamantea E, Fratta GM, Ciceri E, Carrara F, *et al.* (1997). Mitochondrial disease associated with the T8993G mutation of the mitochondrial ATPase 6 gene: a clinical, biochemical, and molecular study in six families. *J. Neurol. Neurosurg. Psychiatry* **63**(1): 16–22.

95. Ciafaloni E, Santorelli FM, Shanske S, Deonna T, Roulet E, Janzer C, *et al.* (1993). Maternally inherited Leigh syndrome. *J. Pediatr.* **122**(3): 419–422.

96. Harding AE, Holt IJ, Sweeney MG, Brockington M, and Davis MB (1992). Prenatal diagnosis of mitochondrial DNA8993 T–G disease. *Am. J. Hum. Genet.* **50**(3): 629–633.

97. Dahl HH, Thorburn DR, and White SL (2000). Towards reliable prenatal diagnosis of mtDNA point mutations: studies of nt8993 mutations in oocytes, fetal tissues, children and adults. *Hum. Reprod.* **15** (Suppl. 2): 246–255.

98. Leigh D (1951). Subacute necrotizing encephalomyelopathy in an infant. *J. Neurol. Neurosurg. Psychiatry* **14**: 216–221.

99. DiMauro S, Hirano M, Bonilla E, Moraes CT, and Schon EA (1994). Cytochrome oxidase deficiency: progress and problems. In: *Mitochondrial Disorders in Neurology* (eds AHV Schapira and S. DiMauro), Oxford: Butterworth-Heinemann, 91–115.

100. Santorelli FM, Mak SC, Vazquez-Memije E, Shanske S, Kranz-Eble P, Jain KD, *et al.* (1996). Clinical heterogeneity associated with the mitochondrial DNA T8993C point mutation. *Pediatr. Res.* **39**(5): 914–917.

101. Nagashima T, Mori M, Katayama K, Nunomura M, Nishihara H, Hiraga H, *et al.* (1999). Adult Leigh syndrome with mitochondrial DNA mutation at 8993. *Acta Neuropathol. (Berl)* **97**(4): 416–422.

102. Tatuch Y, Christodoulou J, Feigenbaum A, Clarke JT, Wherret J, Smith C, *et al.* (1992). Heteroplasmic mtDNA mutation (T–G) at 8993 can cause Leigh disease when the percentage of abnormal mtDNA is high. Am *J. Hum. Genet.* **50**(4): 852–858.

103. Shoffner JM, Fernhoff PM, Krawiecki NS, Caplan DB, Holt PJ, Koontz DA, *et al.* (1992). Subacute necrotizing encephalopathy: oxidative phosphorylation defects and the ATPase 6 point mutation. *Neurology* **42**(11): 2168–2174.

104. DiMauro S and De Vivo DC (1996). Genetic heterogeneity of Leigh syndrome. *Ann. Neurol.* **40**: 5–7.

105. Rahman S, Blok RB, Dahl HH, Danks DM, Kirby DM, Chow CW, *et al.* (1996). Leigh syndrome: clinical features and biochemical and DNA abnormalities. *Ann. Neurol.* **39**(3): 343–351.

106. Sue CM, Karadimas C, Checcarelli N, Tanji K, Papadopoulou LC, Pallotti F, *et al.* (2000). Differential features of patients with mutations in two COX assembly genes, SURF-1 and SCO2. *Ann. Neurol.* **47**(5): 589–595.

107. Fadic R, Russell JA, Vadanarayanan VV, Lehar M, Kuncl RW, and Johns DR (1997). Sensory ataxic neuropathy as the presenting feature of a novel mitochondrial disease. *Neurology* **49**: 239–245.

108. Anan R, Nakagawa M, Miyata M, Higuchi I, Nakao S, Suehara M, *et al.* (1995). Cardiac involvement in mitochondrial diseases. A study on 17 patients with documented mitochondrial DNA defects. *Circulation* **91**(4): 955–961.

109. Marin-Garcia J, Ananthakrishnan R, Korson M, Goldenthal MJ, and Perez-Atayde A (1996). Cardiac mitochondrial dysfunction in Leigh syndrome. *Pediatr. Cardiol.* **17**(6): 387–389.

110. Silvestri G, Bertini E, Servidei S, Rana M, Zachara E, Ricci E, *et al.* (1997). Maternally inherited cardiomyopathy: a new phenotype associated with the A to G AT nt.3243 of mitochondrial DNA (MELAS mutation). *Muscle Nerve* **20**(2): 221–225.

111. Santorelli FM, Tanji K, Manta P, Casali C, Krishna S, Hays AP, *et al.* (1999). Maternally inherited cardiomyopathy: an atypical presentation of the mtDNA 12S rRNA gene A1555G mutation. *Am. J. Hum. Genet.* **64**(1): 295–300.

112. Santorelli FM, Mak SC, El Schahawi M, Casali C, Shanske S, Baram TZ, *et al.* (1996). Maternally inherited cardiomyopathy and hearing loss associated with a novel mutation in the mitochondrial tRNA(Lys) gene (G8363A). *Am. J. Hum. Genet.* **58**(5): 933–939.

113. Merante F, Tein I, Benson L, and Robinson BH (1994). Maternally inherited hypertrophic cardiomyopathy due to a novel T-to-C transition at nucleotide 9997 in the mitochondrial tRNA(glycine) gene. *Am. J. Hum. Genet.* **55**(3): 437–446.

114. Merante F, Myint T, Tein I, Benson L, and Robinson BH (1996). An additional mitochondrial tRNA(Ile) point mutation (A-to-G at nucleotide 4295) causing hypertrophic cardiomyopathy. *Hum. Mutat.* **8**(3): 216–222.

115. Casali C, D'Amati G, Bernucci P, DeBiase L, Autore C, Santorelli FM, *et al.* (1999). Maternally inherited cardiomyopathy: clinical and molecular characterization of a large kindred harboring the A4300G point mutation in mitochondrial deoxyribonucleic acid. *J. Am. Coll. Cardiol.* **33**(6): 1584–1589.

116. Valnot I, Kassis J, Chretien D, de Lonlay P, Parfait B, Munnich A, *et al.* (1999). A mitochondrial cytochrome b mutation but no mutations of nuclearly encoded subunits in ubiquinol cytochrome c reductase (complex III) deficiency. *Hum. Genet.* **104**(6): 460–466.

117. Marin-Garcia J, Ananthakrishnan R, Goldenthal MJ, Filiano JJ, and Perez-Atayde A (1997). Cardiac mitochondrial dysfunction and DNA depletion in children with hypertrophic cardiomyopathy. *J. Inherit. Metab. Dis.* **20**(5): 674–680.

118. Grasso M, Diegoli M, Brega A, Campana C, Tavazzi L, and Arbustini E (2001). The mitochondrial DNA mutation T12297C affects a highly conserved nucleotide of tRNA(Leu(CUN)) and is associated with dilated cardiomyopathy. *Eur. J. Hum. Genet.* **9**(4): 311–315.

119. Suomalainen A, Paetau A, Leinonen H, Majander A, Peltonen L, and Somer H (1992). Inherited idiopathic dilated cardiomyopathy with multiple deletions of mitochondrial DNA. *Lancet* **340**(8831): 1319–1320.

120. Poulton J, Deadman ME, and Gardiner RM (1989). Duplications of mitochondrial DNA in mitochondrial myopathy. *Lancet* **1**(8632), 236–240.

121. Ballinger SW, Shoffner JM, Gebhart S, Koontz DA, and Wallace DC (1994). Mitochondrial diabetes revisited. *Nat. Genet.* **7**: 458–459 (letter).

122. Dunbar DR, Moonie PA, Swingler RJ, Davidson D, Roberts R, and Holt IJ (1993). Maternally transmitted partial direct tandem duplication of mitochondrial DNA associated with diabetes mellitus. *Hum. Mol. Genet.* **2**: 1619–1624.

123. Poulton J (1998). Does a common mitochondrial DNA polymorphism underlie susceptibility to diabetes and the thrifty genotype? *Trends Genet.* **10**, 387–389.

124. Yorifuji T, Kawai M, Momoi T, Sasaki H, Furusho K, Muroi J, *et al.* (1996). Nephropathy and growth hormone deficiency in a patient with mitochondrial tRNA(Leu(UUR)) mutation. *J. Med. Genet.* **33**(7): 621–622.

125. Pearson HA, Lobel JS, Kocoshis SA, Naiman JL, Windmiller J, Lammi AT, *et al.* (1979). A new syndrome of refractory sideroblastic anemia with vacuolization of marrow precursors and exocrine pancreatic dysfunction. *J. Pediatr.* **95**(6): 976–984.

126. Rotig A, Colonna M, Bonnefont JP, Blanche S, Fischer A, Saudubray JM, *et al.* (1989). Mitochondrial DNA deletion in Pearson's marrow/pancreas syndrome. *Lancet* **1**(8643): 902–903.

127. Superti-Furga A, Schoenle E, Tuchschmid P, Caduff R, Sabato V, DeMattia D, *et al.* (1993). Pearson bone marrow-pancreas syndrome with insulin-dependent diabetes, progressive renal tubulopathy, organic aciduria and elevated fetal haemoglobin caused by deletion and duplication of mitochondrial DNA. *Eur. J. Pediatr.* **152**(1): 44–50.

128. McShane MA, Hammans SR, Sweeney M, Holt IJ, Beattie TJ, Brett EM, *et al.* (1991). Pearson syndrome and mitochondrial encephalomyopathy in a patient with a deletion of mtDNA. *Am. J. Hum. Genet.* **48**(1): 39–42.

129. Simonsz HJ, Barlocher K, and Rotig A (1992). Kearns–Sayre's syndrome developing in a boy who survived pearson's syndrome caused by mitochondrial DNA deletion. *Doc. Ophthalmol.* **82**(1–2): 73–79.

130. Majander A, Suomalainen A, Vettenranta K, Sariola H, Perkkio M, Holmberg C, *et al.* (1991). Congenital hypoplastic anemia, diabetes, and severe renal tubular dysfunction associated with a mitochondrial DNA deletion. *Pediatr. Res.* **30**(4): 327–330.

131. Casademont J, Barrientos A, Cardellach F, Rotig A, Grau JM, Montoya J, *et al.* (1994). Multiple deletions of mtDNA in two brothers with sideroblastic anemia and mitochondrial myopathy and in their asymptomatic mother. *Hum. Mol. Genet.* **3**(11): 1945–1949.

132. Wang YL, Choi HK, Aul C, Gattermann N, and Heinisch J (1999). The MERRF mutation of mitochondrial DNA in the bone marrow of a patient with acquired idiopathic sideroblastic anemia. *Am. J. Hematol.* **60**(1): 83–84.

133. Allikmets R, Raskind WH, Hutchinson A, Schueck ND, Dean M, and Koeller DM (1999). Mutation of a putative mitochondrial iron transporter gene (ABC7) in X- linked sideroblastic anemia and ataxia (XLSA/A). *Hum. Mol. Genet.* **8**(5): 743–749.

134. Bardosi A, Creutzfeldt W, DiMauro S, Felgenhauer K, Friede RL, Goebel HH, *et al.* (1987). Myo-, neuro-, gastrointestinal encephalopathy (MNGIE syndrome) due to partial deficiency of cytochrome-c-oxidase. A new mitochondrial multisystem disorder. *Acta. Neuropathol. (Berl.)* **74**(3): 248–258.

135. Hirano M, Silvestri G, Blake DM, Lombes A, Minetti C, Bonilla E, *et al.* (1994). Mitochondrial neurogastrointestinal encephalomyopathy (MNGIE): clinical, biochemical, and genetic features of an autosomal recessive mitochondrial disorder. *Neurology* **44**(4): 721–727.

136. Nishino I, Spinazzola A, Papadimitriou A, Hammans S, Steiner I, Hahn CD, *et al.* (2000). Mitochondrial neurogastrointestinal encephalomyopathy: an autosomal recessive disorder due to thymidine phosphorylase mutations. *Ann. Neurol.* **47**(6): 792–800.

137. Gubbay SS, Hankey GJ, Tan NT, and Fry JM (1989). Mitochondrial encephalomyopathy with corticosteroid dependence. *Med. J. Aust.* **151**(2): 100–103.

138. Weber K, Wilson JN, Taylor L, Brierley E, Johnson MA, Turnbull DM, *et al.* (1997). A new mtDNA mutation showing accumulation with time and restriction to skeletal muscle. *Am. J. Hum. Genet.* **60**(2): 373–380.

139. Clark KM, Bindoff LA, Lightowlers RN, Andrews RM, Griffiths PG, Johnson MA, *et al.* (1997). Reversal of a mitochondrial DNA defect in human skeletal muscle. *Nat. Genet.* **16**(3): 222–224.

140. Taivassalo T, Fu K, Johns T, Arnold D, Karpati G, and Shoubridge EA (1999). Gene shifting: a novel therapy for mitochondrial myopathy. *Hum. Mol. Genet.* **8**(6): 1047–1052.

141. Taivassalo T, Shoubridge EA, Chen J, Kennaway NG, DiMauro S, Arnold DL, *et al.* (2001). Aerobic condition in patients with mitochondrial myopathies: physiological, biochemical, and genetic effects. *Ann. Neurol.*

142. Chinnery PF, Johnson MA, Taylor RW, Durward WF, and Turnbull DM (1997). A novel mitochondrial tRNA isoleucine gene mutation causing chronic progressive external ophthalmoplegia. *Neurology* **49**(4): 1166–1168.

143. Silvestri G, Servidei S, Rana M, Ricci E, Spinazzola A, Paris E *et al.* (1996). A novel mitochondrial DNA point mutation in the tRNA(Ile) gene is associated with progressive external ophtalmoplegia. *Biochem. Biophys. Res. Commun.* **220**(3): 623–627.

144. Franceschina L, Salani S, Bordoni A, Sciacco M, Napoli L, Comi GP, *et al.* (1998). A novel mitochondrial tRNA(Ile) point mutation in chronic progressive external ophthalmoplegia. *J. Neurol.* **245**(11): 755–758.

145. Seibel P, Lauber J, Klopstock T, Marsac C, Kadenbach B, and Reichmann H (1994). Chronic progressive external ophthalmoplegia is associated with a novel mutation in the mitochondrial tRNA(Asn) gene. *Biochem. Biophys. Res. Commun.* **204**(2): 482–489.

146. Moraes CT, Ciacci F, Bonilla E, Jansen C, Hirano M, Rao N, *et al.* (1993). Two novel pathogenic mitochondrial DNA mutations affecting organelle number and protein synthesis. Is the tRNA(Leu(UUR)) gene an etiologic hot spot? *J. Clin. Invest.* **92**(6): 2906–2915.

147. Hattori Y, Goto Y, Sakuta R, Nonaka I, Mizuno Y, and Horai S (1994). Point mutations in mitochondrial tRNA genes: sequence analysis of chronic progressive external ophthalmoplegia (CPEO). *J. Neurol. Sci.* **125**(1): 50–55.

148. Sweeney MG, Bundey S, Brockington M, Poulton KR, Winer JB, and Harding AE (1993). Mitochondrial myopathy associated with sudden death in young adults and a novel mutation in the mitochondrial DNA leucine transfer RNA(UUR) gene. *Q. J. Med.* **86**(11): 709–713.

149. Musumeci O, Andreu AL, Shanske S, Bresolin N, Comi GP, Rothstein R, *et al.* (2000). Intragenic Inversion of mtDNA: A New Type of Pathogenic Mutation in a Patient with Mitochondrial Myopathy. *Am. J. Hum. Genet.* **66**(6): 1900–1904.

150. Andreu AL, Bruno C, Dunne TC, Tanji K, Shanske S, Sue CM, *et al.* (1999). A nonsense mutation (G15059A) in the cytochrome b gene in a patient with exercise intolerance and myoglobinuria. *Ann. Neurol.* **45**(1): 127–130.

151. Dumoulin R, Sagnol I, Ferlin T, Bozon D, Stepien G, and Mousson B (1996). A novel gly290asp mitochondrial cytochrome b mutation linked to a complex III deficiency in progressive exercise intolerance. *Mol. Cell. Probes* **10**(5): 389–391.

152. Andreu AL, Bruno C, Shanske S, Shtilbans A, Hirano M, Krishna S, *et al.* (1998). Missense mutation in the mtDNA cytochrome b gene in a patient with myopathy. *Neurology* **51**(5): 1444–1447.

153. Clark KM, Taylor RW, Johnson MA, Chinnery PF, Chrzanowska-Lightowlers ZM, Andrews RM, *et al.* (1999). An mtDNA mutation in the initiation codon of the cytochrome C oxidase subunit II gene results in lower levels of the protein and a mitochondrial encephalomyopathy. *Am. J. Hum. Genet.* **64**(5): 1330–1339.

154. Rahman S, Taanman JW, Cooper JM, Nelson I, Hargreaves I, Meunier B, *et al.* (1999). A missense mutation of cytochrome oxidase subunit II causes defective assembly and myopathy. *Am. J. Hum. Genet.* **65**(4): 1030–1039.

155. Keightley JA, Hoffbuhr KC, Burton MD, Salas VM, Johnston WS, Penn AM, *et al.* (1996). A microdeletion in cytochrome c oxidase (COX) subunit III associated with COX deficiency and recurrent myoglobinuria. *Nat. Genet.* **12**(4): 410–416.

156. Campos Y, Garcia-Silva T, Barrionuevo CR, Cabello A, Muley R, and Arenas J (1995). Mitochondrial DNA deletion in a patient with mitochondrial myopathy, lactic acidosis, and stroke-like episodes (MELAS) and Fanconi's syndrome. *Pediatr. Neurol.* **13**(1): 69–72.

157. Poulton J, Deadman ME, and Gardiner RM (1989). Tandem direct duplications of mitochondrial DNA in mitochondrial myopathy: analysis of nucleotide sequence and tissue distribution. *Nucleic. Acids. Res.* **17**(24): 10223–10229.

158. Morten KJ, Cooper JM, Brown GK, Lake BD, Pike D, and Poulton J (1993). A new point mutation associated with mitochondrial encephalomyopathy. *Hum. Mol. Genet.* **2**(12): 2081–2087.

159. Nishino I, Komatsu M, Kodama S, Horai S, Nonaka I, and Goto Y (1996). The 3260 mutation in mitochondrial DNA can cause mitochondrial myopathy, encephalopathy, lactic acidosis, and strokelike episodes (MELAS). *Muscle Nerve* **19**(12): 1603–1604.

160. Goto Y, Tsugane K, Tanabe Y, Nonaka I, and Horai S (1994). A new point mutation at nucleotide pair 3291 of the mitochondrial tRNA(Leu(UUR)) gene in a patient with mitochondrial myopathy, encephalopathy, lactic acidosis, and stroke-like episodes (MELAS). *Biochem. Biophys. Res. Commun.* **202**(3): 1624–1630.

161. Taylor RW, Chinnery PF, Haldane F, Morris AA, Bindoff LA, Wilson J, *et al.* (1996). MELAS associated with a mutation in the valine transfer RNA gene of mitochondrial DNA. *Ann. Neurol.* **40**(3): 459–462.

162. Manfredi G, Schon EA, Bonilla E, Moraes CT, Shanske S, and DiMauro S (1996). Identification of a mutation in the mitochondrial tRNA(Cys) gene associated with mitochondrial encephalopathy. *Hum. Mutat.* **7**(2): 158–163.

163. Manfredi G, Schon EA, Moraes CT, Bonilla E, Berry GT, Sladky JT, *et al.* (1995). A new mutation associated with MELAS is located in a mitochondrial DNA polypeptide-coding gene. *Neuromuscul. Disord.* **5**(5): 391–398.

6 Rearrangements of mitochondrial DNA

Eric A Schon

Mitochondrial transmission

A unique feature of mammalian mitochondria is that they are inherited exclusively from the mother.[1] Even though sperm mitochondria enter the oocyte at fertilization, they are destroyed early in development,[2] and only the mitochondrial DNAs (mDNAs) contributed by the oöcyte repopulate the foetus.

There are hundreds or even thousands of mitochondria in each cell, with each organelle containing an average of 5 mtDNAs.[3] Thus, in mitochondrial disorders due to mutations in mtDNA, instead of one or two mutated alleles (as in classic Mendelian disorders), there can be thousands of mutated alleles in a typical cell. In other words, these mitochondrial diseases follow the rules of population, not Mendelian genetics.

Both mitochondrial division and mtDNA replication are unrelated to the cell cycle or to the timing of nuclear DNA replication. Thus, a dividing cell has the potential to donate a variable number of organelles and genomes to its daughter cells, a phenomenon termed *mitotic segregation*. This process becomes important clinically if a patient is *heteroplasmic*, that is, he or she harbours two populations of mtDNA—normal mtDNAs and mutated mtDNAs causing a mitochondrial disease. Because of mitotic segregation, the phenotypic expression of a pathogenic mtDNA mutation may vary both in time (during development or over the course of a life-span) and in space (among tissues or cells). Segregation of mtDNAs need not always be random, as active selection can either eliminate or concentrate a population of mutant mtDNAs in certain cells and tissues. Taken together, the effects of heteroplasmy, mitotic segregation, and selection can combine to generate a respiratory chain deficiency in some tissues but not in others, but this will occur only if the number of mutant mtDNAs exceeds a certain *threshold*, which varies from tissue to tissue depending upon their energy requirements. Skeletal muscle and brain are among those tissues with the highest energy requirements, which is why many (but certainly not all) mitochondrial disorders are encephalomyopathies.

Our ability to study the relationship between mtDNA genotype and phenotype is severely hampered by the fact that there are currently no methods available to introduce exogenous mtDNA into mammalian mitochondria. Fortunately, a 'backdoor' approach to solving this problem has been developed, in which exogenous mitochondria (containing their own mtDNAs) are introduced into human cell lines containing mitochondria that have been depleted of their own endogenous mtDNA (called ρ^0 cells, using the nomenclature established for yeast).[4] Because the ρ^0 line is auxotrophic for pyrimidines and pyruvate (due to the loss of a functional respiratory chain), one can select for the repopulation of the cells by exogenous mtDNA based on complementation of the metabolic defects with the exogenous mitochondria (and their mtDNAs). This cytoplasmic hybrid (cybrid) technology is a powerful tool to study pathogenic mtDNA mutations *in vitro*.

Diseases associated with large-scale rearrangements of mtDNA

Sporadic mtDNA deletions

Progressive external ophthalmoplegia (PEO) is a disorder of skeletal muscle characterized by paralysis of the extraocular muscles.[5] A notable clinical feature of PEO is ptosis (droopy eyelids), due to weakness of the levator muscles that hold up the eyelids. In skeletal muscle biopsies from patients with PEO, one can observe massive proliferation of mitochondria in a subset of fibres (usually type I),—known as *ragged-red fibres*, or RRF—upon histochemical staining with Gomori trichrome[6] or by histochemistry to reveal succinate dehydrogenase (SDH) activity. Typically, RRF are devoid of respiratory chain activity, based on the lack of histochemical stain for cytochrome *c* oxidase (COX) activity.[7] Moreover, these COX-negative regions are distributed segmentally along the muscle fibres (i.e. the COX-negative region is flanked by COX-positive regions on either side). The density of RRF observed in cross-sections of muscle increases during the progression of the disease;[8] in other words, the size of the ragged-red region, when viewed longitudinally, expands steadily and inexorably.

Because PEO is essentially a pure myopathy, the disease, while debilitating, is usually not life-threatening. However, PEO can also be part of a much more severe, and ultimately fatal, multisystem disorder called Kearns–Sayre syndrome (KSS).[9,10] Clinically, KSS is defined by the triad of onset before age 20, PEO, and pigmentary retinopathy, plus at least one of the following: cerebellar ataxia, heart block, and cerebrospinal fluid (CSF) protein content above 100 mg/dl. Other common but nonspecific features include endocrine abnormalities (e.g. diabetes, hypoparathyroidism, short stature), neurosensory hearing loss, and dementia. In both KSS and PEO, biochemical studies of muscle often show multiple respiratory chain enzyme defects, especially COX deficiency.

Historically, both PEO and KSS were difficult to classify, because most patients were sporadic (i.e. mothers and siblings of the proband were unaffected). However, following a landmark paper published in 1988 by John Morgan-Hughes and his colleagues,[11] it was found that large-scale partial deletions of mtDNA (Δ-mtDNAs) were present in patients with either sporadic PEO or sporadic KSS.[12–14] The same Δ-mtDNAs seen in PEO and KSS are also present in an early-onset sporadic haematopoetic disorder called Pearson's marrow/pancreas syndrome (PS),[15,16] which is characterized by sideroblastic anaemia and exocrine pancreatic dysfunction. The anaemia is often fatal despite blood transfusion therapy.[15] The few patients who survive Pearson syndrome (PS) later develop KSS.[17]

In PEO, KSS, and PS, the Δ-mtDNAs can be detected by Southern blot hybridization analysis: linearization of total DNA with a restriction enzyme that cuts only once in the mitochondrial genome (e.g. *Pvu*II; see Fig. 6.2), followed by hybridization with a mtDNA-specific probe, reveals a single population of mtDNAs migrating more rapidly in the electrophoretic gel than do the linearized full-length (i.e. 16.6-kb) normal mtDNAs. The size and location of the deletion, and the proportion of Δ-mtDNA, differ among patients and, to a first approximation, do not appear to correlate to the severity or the presentation of the disease. Since 1988, more than 200 different deletions have been identified in KSS/PEO/PS patients, and all patients have been heteroplasmic (with up to 80 per cent Δ-mtDNA) in affected tissues. Although the deleted species found in any one patient is unique, one particular deletion, that removes 4977 bp of mtDNA between the ATPase 8 and the ND5 genes (see Fig. 6.1), has been found in about one-third of all patients, and has therefore been called the 'common' deletion.[18,19]

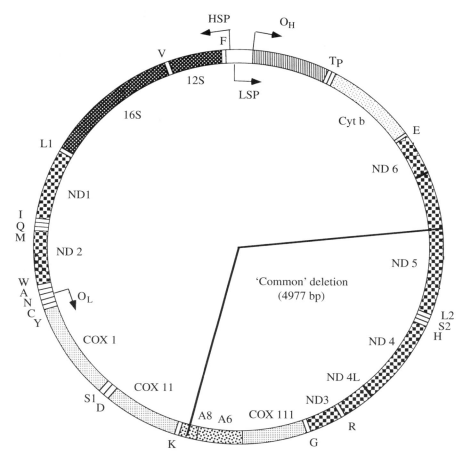

Fig. 6.1 Map of the human mitochondrial genome, showing the 13 polypeptide-coding genes and 24 protein synthesis genes (12S and 16S rRNAs, and 22 tRNAs [1-letter amino acid code]). The location of the 4977-bp segment of mtDNA that is removed in the 'common deletion' found in sporadic KSS, PEO, and PS is also indicated (see Fig. 6.2).

The fact that only a single species of Δ-mtDNA is found in any one patient with sporadic PEO or KSS implies that the population of Δ-mtDNAs is a clonal expansion of a single mutation event occurring early in oögenesis or embryogenesis.[20] Besides explaining why the deletions in each patient appear to be clonal, this hypothesis would also explain why these diseases are sporadic. Support for this idea comes from the observation that extremely low levels of mtDNA rearrangements have been found in the oocytes of normal women.[21–24] Human oocytes contain between 100,000 and 600,000 mtDNAs,[21,25,26] of which approximately 1000 will eventually repopulate the foetus. If a single rearranged mtDNA somehow managed to slip through this bottleneck and enter the foetus, it would explain why these diseases are sporadic, why they are so rare, and why the rearrangements are clonal.

Following fertilization, there is no mtDNA replication until the blastocyst stage of development, when germ layer differentiation begins. One can easily imagine how a few rearranged

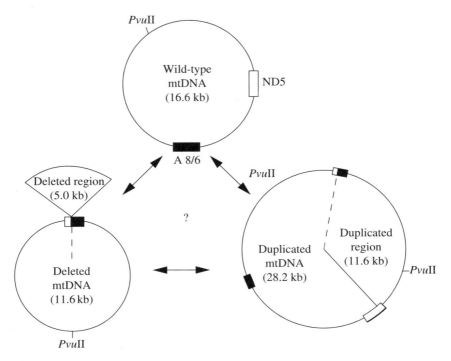

Fig. 6.2 A typical large-scale mtDNA rearrangement (the 'common deletion' [pie-shaped protruding pie segment], which removes 4977 bp between ATPase 8 [solid box] and ND5 [open box]), illustrating the relationship between the partially-deleted and the corresponding partially-duplicated molecules. Note that the deletion breakpoint (dashed line) is the same in both molecules. Note also that the *Pvu*II site located at nt-2650 on the mitochondrial genome is present once in the wt- and the Δ-mtDNA, but is present twice in the dup-mtDNA.

mtDNAs present at or immediately following the blastocyst stage could segregate in a highly skewed fashion among the germ layer cells or their progeny. In this scenario, mutated mtDNAs entering all the germ layers would result in KSS (which is a multisystem disorder), whereas segregation to muscle would result in PEO.[20] In the case of PS, the haematopoetic lineage would be the predominant, but not excusive, recipient of mutated mtDNAs.

The hypothesis of clonality implies that a single rearranged molecule present in the oocyte or the embryo will multiply to become the trillions of Δ-mtDNAs found in the patients. It is currently unknown how this selective amplification of Δ-mtDNAs occurs. It may be merely that the Δ-mtDNAs 'out-replicate' the wild-type mtDNAs (wt-mtDNAs) because they are smaller, but this hypothesis has a few problems. First, the few experiments addressing this issue imply that this is not the case.[27,28] Moreover, the turnover of mitochondria in muscle is on the order of weeks,[29] while the replication of mtDNA takes about 2 h. It is therefore not clear what proliferative advantage would be conferred by cutting the replication time down to 1 h in a Δ-mtDNA that were half the size of a wt-mtDNA. Finally, the amplification of mtDNAs is intimately connected to the proliferation of the organelles in which they reside. It may be that respiratory insufficiency causes the entire organelle to divide wildly, and as the mitochondria multiply, so too do the mutations. In other words, the proliferation of the mtDNAs may be secondary to the proliferation of the organelles, with the deleted mtDNAs merely 'passengers along for the ride'.[30]

Even though each deletion removes a different set of mitochondrial genes, all KSS patients have fundamentally the same presentation and features, as do all PEO and PS patients. How can we reconcile the relative uniformity of clinical presentation with the wide variation in the regions of the genome that are deleted? The answer to this question relates to the fact that the 22 transfer RNA (tRNA) genes are not clustered on the mtDNA, but rather are distributed around the genome (see Fig. 6.1). Although the deleted mtDNAs are transcribed into RNA in the usual way, those processed transcripts encoding polypepides (i.e. the mRNAs) are not translated, because the deletions remove essential tRNAs that are required for protein synthesis.[31–39] Thus, it does not matter where the deletion resides, as long as even one tRNA gene is deleted, and in fact, every documented pathogenic deletion in KSS and PEO removes at least one tRNA gene.

The 'deleted tRNA hypothesis' implies that mRNAs are not translated correctly because the organelle is lacking the subset of tRNAs located within the deletion. However, in a heteroplasmic population of deleted and wt-mtDNAs, the wt-mtDNAs ought to be able to complement the translational deficiency by providing those tRNAs that are missing from the Δ-mtDNA, assuming, of course, that both mtDNA species reside within the same organelle. In fact, such complementation can indeed occur. For example, cybrids containing mitochondria from a patient with a large-scale deletion produced the expected 'fusion protein' encoded by the mRNA straddling the deletion breakpoint, but only when the proportion of wt-mtDNAs in the cybrids was above approximately 20–30 per cent.[34] Genetic and functional complementation, and even homologous recombination between mtDNAs, have also been inferred from a number of studies,[40–49] but the frequency of mtDNA recombination events in the absence of selection is probably quite low.[43]

If complementation can occur, why are many muscle fibres in KSS/PEO patients devoid of any observable respiratory chain function? The most reasonable answer is that respiratorily-deficient fibres are unable to complement function because there are essentially no wt-mtDNAs present within organelles in the RRFs—in other words, mitochondria in COX-negative RRFs are, to all intents and purposes, 'homoplasmic deleted'. Muscle fibres containing homoplasmic levels of Δ-mtDNAs have been observed morphologically, using 'single-fibre PCR' and *in-situ* hybridization methods.[31,36,50] The absence of wt-mtDNAs in these RRF, however, begs the question as to why little or no complementation is observed between COX-negative RRFs and the adjacent COX-positive regions in the muscle fibre that contain large amounts (or even a majority) of wt-mtDNAs. In other words, why does not complementation occur in the 'mixing zone' at the boundaries of RRF and non-RRF? In fact, such mixing can probably occur,[36,45] but for unknown reasons—perhaps related to the regulation of interorganellar fusion and fission, and to the intracellular mobility of individual mitochondria[51]—it does not occur frequently enough to prevent the inexorable growth of the RRFs.[8,43] The recent generation of a 'transmitochondrial' mouse harbouring heteroplasmic mtDNA deletions,[52] which is the first authentic animal model of any mtDNA-related disease, should help resolve this question.

Sporadic mtDNA duplications

Not long after the discovery of Δ-mtDNAs in sporadic KSS, it was found that some patients harboured large-scale partial mtDNA duplications (dup-mtDNAs), and furthermore, that duplicated and deleted mtDNAs coexisted in these patients.[53–56] Moreover, in these 'triplasmic' patients (i.e. containing wt-, dup-, and Δ-mtDNAs), the two rearranged species are topologically related: the dup-mtDNA can be thought of as being composed of a wt-mtDNA and a Δ-mtDNA arranged head-to-tail (Fig. 6.2). Thus, the only novel sequence in the dup-mtDNA as compared to wt-mtDNA is located at the boundary of the duplicated region, which is identical to the boundary in the corresponding Δ-mtDNA. This finding implies the two rearranged molecules are generated through a common mechanism, or that one may be derived from the other.[28,50,57–60]

The importance of dup-mtDNAs in the generation of Δ-mtDNAs, from both a mechanistic and clinical standpoint, has been underestimated, mainly for technical reasons. As noted above, Δ-mtDNAs are usually detected as a second band on Southern blots of *Pvu*II-digested mtDNA, migrating more rapidly in the gel than does the wt-mtDNA. The *Pvu*II cuts only once in the mtDNA, at mtDNA nucleotide position 2650, located in the 'minor arc' between O_H and O_L that is rarely (but not always[35]) deleted in patients (Fig. 6.2). Thus, cleavage with this enzyme usually cannot distinguish a deletion from a duplication, because a dup-mtDNA will contain *two Pvu*II sites, separated by a distance corresponding to the size of a simple deletion. Similarly, because the breakpoint spanning a deletion is identical to that spanning the junction where the duplicated segment of mtDNA is inserted into the wild-type sequence, amplification of the mtDNA spanning the deletion breakpoint and the duplication junction by polymerase chain reaction (PCR) will yield identical PCR products, rendering the two indistinguishable. In sum, it is quite likely that many dup-mtDNAs were overlooked.[61–63]

Deletions of mtDNA are pathogenic because they invariably remove at least one tRNA gene. Duplications of mtDNA, on the other hand, are not lacking any tRNAs (if anything, some genes are present in excess), and it is noteworthy that cells harbouring high levels of dup-mtDNAs do not have obvious phenotypic abnormalities.[39,50,57] This does not mean that dup-mtDNAs have no phenotypic consequences. For example, a particular dup-mtDNA in a patient may result in a functionally deleterious 'fusion gene' generated at the rearrangement breakpoint; there may be interacting nuclear factors;[57] or, more likely, the duplicated species will eventually recombine to yield a wt-mtDNA and the corresponding deleted species, which is pathogenic.[28] If the population of recombined Δ-mtDNAs segregates in such a way that it predominates in cells, clinical consequences will then ensue. This was shown in a patient who had a late-onset myopathy associated with approximately 50 per cent wt-mtDNA, 48 per cent dup-mtDNA, and only 2 per cent Δ-mtDNA: essentially all the Δ-mtDNAs were concentrated in the patient's RRFs, whereas the wt- and dup-mtDNAs were present in the 'COX-normal' fibres.[50]

Sporadic large-scale rearrangements of mtDNA in normal human ageing

Tissues from normal individuals, and especially long-lived tissues with high oxidative requirements, such as brain and muscle, contain Δ-mtDNAs that are similar, and in many cases identical, to those found in great abundance in patients with sporadic PEO, KSS, and PS. However, rather than harbouring a single deleted species, ageing individuals harbour numerous deleted species,[64,65] each presumably the result of an individual somatic mutation event. The deletions found in normal individuals are present in extremely low amounts, detectable only by PCR, and accumulate during ageing, in an exponential fashion.[66]

As with the authentic rearrangement disorders, both deleted and duplicated mtDNAs have been detected in normal ageing.[67,68] Since dup-mtDNAs are 'less' pathogenic than Δ-mtDNAs, one therefore cannot conclude that the presence of rearranged mtDNAs in aged tissues, in whatever quantity, has pathological consequences without a more detailed understanding of the molecules' topologies.

Maternally inherited duplications

Although dup-mtDNAs arise sporadically in KSS and PEO, they can also be transmitted maternally. Interestingly, the clinical phenotypes associated with these inherited large-scale mtDNA rearrangements do not include 'complete' KSS. Rather, the patients show some of the features of the syndrome, such as cerebellar ataxia, renal tubulopathy, and diabetes mellitus (DM);[69] myopathy, PEO, and diabetes;[70] and diabetes and deafness.[71] The diabetes, which is a frequent symptom found in KSS patients,[72,73] is usually the late-onset type II, non-insulin-dependent, form.[69–71,74] Notably, these patients usually do not have the symptoms of KSS, and although dup-mtDNAs are present in muscle, RRF are not.

Maternally inherited deletions

The data regarding the maternal transmissability of Δ-mtDNAs are conflicting. There was an early report of maternal transmission of Δ-mtDNA from mother with PEO to her daughter, who also had PEO, but the two deletions were different.[75] In a second report, a mother with KSS clearly did not pass her deletion to her daughter,[76] but a mother with PEO apparently did transmit the deletion to her son.[77] Finally, a patient with cyclic vomiting syndrome was reported to harbour a large-scale deletion with evidence of maternal history.[78]

Since, it is difficult to distinguish between a deletion and the corresponding duplication, reports of the transmission of Δ-mtDNAs without strong evidence eliminating the possibility of the presence of a dup-mtDNA should be treated with caution. It is clear, however, that in the one known mouse model of mtDNA rearrangements.[52] The Δ-mtDNAs can indeed be 'transmitted' (in the sense that mother and child harbour the same deleted species), and we have also found evidence that the same can occur in humans (our unpublished data). However, in each of these cases it is unknown if the transmitted molecule is truly a deletion, as it is also possible that the deleted species passes through the germ line via a transiently generated duplicated intermediate. Finally, some reports of inheritance of Δ-mtDNA in a child[79] may actually reflect the analysis of low levels of age-related Δ-mtDNAs in the mother generated via somatic mutation, and are not authentic transmission at all.

Small-scale rearrangements of mtDNA

A few small-scale deletions have also been described, but essentially none of them deleted tRNA genes and none was associated with sporadic KSS or PEO. It is true that four relatively large deletions, ranging in size from 0.5 to 2.0 kb, also did not remove tRNA genes, but these rearrangements were present in patients with familial PEO and numerous other large-scale deletions.[80,81]

Regarding microdeletions, one has been found to be a neutral polymorphism that appears to have originated among people of Polynesian origin. The deletion removes one of two tandem 9-bp repeats in the 3′-untranslated region of the *COXII* gene (*COXII* is the only gene with a 3′-UTR).[82] A patient with motor neuron disease had a deletion of 1 of 2 tandem repeats, 5 bp in length, located within the *COXI* gene, resulting in a frameshift.[83] A patient with recurrent myoglobinuria and COX deficiency harboured a heteroplasmic mtDNA microdeletion of only 15 bp located within the *COXIII* gene that removed five in-frame amino acids from the polypeptide.[84] This deletion was flanked by two 7-bp direct repeats. An unusual rearrangement was recently described, in which a patient with a pure myopathy and isolated complex I deficiency had an intragenic inversion of 7 bp that caused an in-frame substitution of three amino acids.[85] Notably, the inverted region was flanked by 7-bp perfect *inverted* repeat.

Maternal inheritance of a heteroplasmic, small-scale mtDNA rearrangement has also been described, in a sporadic KSS patient who harboured a typical large-scale deletion plus an unrelated tandem duplication of a 265-bp segment of non-coding mtDNA located in the D-loop region.[86] The duplication, but not the deletion, was present in the patient's clinically normal mother, implying that the duplication was not pathogenic.[86,87] While it is clear that this mini-duplication, and others like it, are present in normal individuals[88] the issue of pathogenicity is nevertheless controversial, as the 265-bp duplication,[89] as well as a 204-bp duplication also located in the D-loop,[90] have been found in patients with mitochondrial diseases.

Some regions in the D-loop are particularly unstable, including a polypyrimidine stretch around nt-310 that is C-rich.[91] The region containing the 265-bp duplication is also unstable, as triplications of this element have also been observed,[57,60,89] and a similar situation results in systematic and permanent D-loop heteroplasmy in bats[92] and rabbits.[93]

Concluding remarks

The exact mechanism by which mtDNA deletions are generated is unknown. However, analysis of the rather considerable number of rearranged mtDNAs reported in the literature since 1988, coupled with the results from a number of experiments performed *in vitro*,[30,39,51,55,67,68,70,78,94,95] allow for some educated guesses. More than one-third of all reported deletions are flanked precisely by direct repeats 4 bp in length or greater (unpublished data). These have been called 'class I' deletions,[30] in order to distinguish them from 'class II' deletions, which are flanked by perfect or imperfect direct repeats in an imprecise manner (about a third of all deletions) or have no obvious sequence homologies at the boundaries of the breakpoints (the remaining one-third).[30] Interestingly, of those deletions with no obvious flanking repeats (or with those flanked by repeats less than 4 bp in length, which we consider to be present merely by coincidence), about half contained strings of polypurines or polypyrimidines in the region of the breakpoint, which have the potential to form 'bent DNA'.[96]

Taken together, the data imply that mtDNA rearrangements are the result of homologous recombination events, but it is not clear if these events are primarily due to legitimate recombination (e.g. crossing-over at a homologous region) or illegitimate recombination (e.g. slipped mispairing).[95,97,98] Either type of event could cause a deletion directly, or a deletion could arise as the result of an intramolecular recombination event from a pre-existing duplication.[39,68,70]

However they arise, the identification and analysis of mitochondrial DNA rearrangements in human pathologies has shed light not only on the aetiology and pathogenesis of a major subgroup of mitochondrial disorders, but has also provided insight into basic questions regarding the generation and maintenance of the mitochondrial genome.

Acknowledgements

This work was supported by grants from the US National Institutes of Health (NS28828, NS39854, and HD32062) and the Muscular Dystrophy Association.

References

1. Giles RE, Blanc, H, Cann, HM, and Wallace, DC (1980). Maternal inheritance of human mitochondrial DNA. *Proc. Natl Acad. Sci. USA* **77**: 6715–6719.
2. Kaneda H, Hayashi J-I, Takahama S, Taya C, Fischer Lindahl K, and Yonekawa H (1995). Elimination of paternal mitochondrial DNA in intraspecific crosses during early mouse embryogenesis. *Proc. Natl Acad. Sci. USA* **92**: 4542–4546.
3. Satoh M and Kuroiwa T (1991). Organization of multiple nucleoids and DNA molecules in mitochondria of a human cell. *Exp. Cell Res.* **196**: 137–140.
4. King MP and Attardi G (1989). Human cells lacking mtDNA: repopulation with exogenous mitochondria by complementation. *Science* **246**: 500–503.
5. Rowland LP, Hays AP, DiMauro S, DeVivo DC, and Behrens M (1983). Diverse clinical disorders associated with morphological abnormalities of mitochondria. In: *Mitochondrial Pathology in Muscle Diseases* (eds C Cerri and G Scarlato), Padua: Piccin Editore, pp. 141–158.
6. Engel WK and Cunningham CG (1963). Rapid examination of muscle tissue: an improved trichrome stain method for fresh-frozen biopsy sections. *Neurology* **13**: 919–923.
7. Bonilla E, Sciacco M, Tanji K, Sparaco M, Petruzzella V, and Moraes CT (1992). New morphological approaches to the study of mitochondrial encephalomyopathies. *Brain Pathol.* **2**: 113–119.
8. Larsson NG, Holme E, Kristiansson B, Oldfors A, and Tulinius M (1990). Progressive increase of the mutated mitochondrial DNA fraction in Kearns–Sayre syndrome. *Pediatr. Res.* **28**: 131–136.
9. Kearns TP and Sayre GP (1958). Retinitis pigmentosa, external ophthalmoplegia, and complete heart block. *Arch. Ophthalmol.* **60**: 280–289.
10. Berenberg RA, Pellock JM, DiMauro S, Schotland DL, Bonilla E, Eastwood A, Hays A, Vicale CT, Behrens M, Chutorian A, and Rowland LP (1977). Lumping or splitting? 'Ophthalmoplegia plus' or Kearns–Sayre syndrome? *Ann. Neurol.* **1**: 37–43.
11. Holt IJ, Harding AE, and Morgan-Hughes JA (1988). Deletions of mitochondrial DNA in patients with mitochondrial myopathies. *Nature* **331**: 717–719.
12. Lestienne P and Ponsot G (1988). Kearns–Sayre syndrome with muscle mitochondrial DNA deletion. *Lancet* **1**: 885 (letter).
13. Zeviani M, Moraes CT, DiMauro S, Nakase H, Bonilla E, Schon EA, and Rowland LP (1988). Deletions of mitochondrial DNA in Kearns–Sayre syndrome. *Neurology* **38**: 1339–1346.
14. Moraes CT, DiMauro S, Zeviani M, Lombes A, Shanske S, Miranda AF, Nakase H, Bonilla E, Wernec LC, Servidei S, Nonaka I, Koga Y, Spiro A, Brownell KW, Schmidt B, Schotland DL, Zupanc MD, DeVivo DC, Schon EA, and Rowland LP (1989). Mitochondrial DNA deletions in Progressive External Ophthalmoplegia and Kearns–Sayre syndrome. *N. Engl. J. Med.* **320**: 1293–1299.
15. Pearson HA, Lobel JS, Kocoshis SA, Naiman JL, Windmiller J, Lammi AT, Hoffman R, and Marsh JC (1979). A new syndrome of refractory sideroblastic anemia with vacuolization of marrow precursors and exocrine pancreatic dysfunction. *J. Pediatr.* **95**: 976–984.
16. Rötig A, Cormier V, Koll F, Mize CE, Saudubray J-M, Veerman A, Pearson HA, and Munnich A (1991). Site-specific deletions of the mitochondrial genome in the Pearson marrow-pancreas syndrome. *Genomics* **10**: 502–504.
17. McShane MA, Hammans SR, Sweeney M, Holt IJ, Beattie TJ, Brett EM, and Harding AE (1991). Pearson syndrome and mitochondrial encephalomyopathy in a patient with a deletion of mtDNA. *Am. J. Hum. Genet.* **48**: 39–42.

18. Schon EA, Rizzuto R, Moraes CT, Nakase H, Zeviani M, and DiMauro S (1989). A direct repeat is a hotspot for large-scale deletions of human mitochondrial DNA. *Science* **244**: 346–349.

19. Mita S, Rizzuto R, Moraes CT, Shanske S, Arnaudo E, Fabrizi G, Koga Y, DiMauro S, and Schon EA (1990). Recombination via flanking direct repeats is a major cause of large-scale deletions of human mitochondrial DNA. *Nucleic Acids Res.* **18**: 561–567.

20. Schon EA, Bonilla E, Miranda AF, and DiMauro S (1991). Molecular biology of mitochondrial diseases. In: *Molecular Genetic Approaches to Neuropsychiatric Disease* (eds J. Brosius and R. Fremeau), San Diego: Academic Press, pp. 57–80.

21. Chen X, Prosser R, Simonetti S, Sadlock J, Jagiello G, and Schon EA (1995). Rearranged mito-chondrial genomes are present in human oocytes. *Am. J. Hum. Genet.* **57**: 239–247.

22. Keefe DL, Niven-Fairchild T, Powell S, and Buradagunta S (1995). Mitochondrial deoxyribo-nucleic acid deletions in oocytes and reproductive aging in women. *Fertil. Steril.* **64**: 577–583.

23. Brenner CA, Wolny YM, Barritt JA, Matt DW, Munne S, and Cohen J (1998). Mitochondrial DNA deletion in human oocytes and embryos. *Mol. Hum. Reprod.* **4**: 887–892.

24. Reynier P, Chretien MF, Savagner F, Larcher G, Rohmer V, Barriere P, and Malthiery Y (1998). Long PCR analysis of human gamete mtDNA suggests defective mitochondrial maintenance in spermatozoa and supports the bottleneck theory for oocytes. *Biochem. Biophys. Res. Commun.* **252**: 373–377.

25. Reynier P, May-Panloup P, Chretien MF, Morgan CJ, Jean M, Savagner F, Barriere P, and Malthiery Y (2001). Mitochondrial DNA content affects the fertilizability of human oocytes. *Mol. Hum. Reprod.* **7**: 425–429.

26. Steuerwald N, Barritt JA, Adler R, Malter H, Schimmel T, Cohen J, and Brenner CA (2000). Quantification of mtDNA in single oocytes, polar bodies and subcellular components by real-time rapid cycle fluorescence monitored PCR. *Zygote* **8**: 209–215.

27. Moraes CT and Schon EA (1995). Replication of a heteroplasmic population of normal and partially-deleted human mitochondrial genomes. In: *Progress in Cell Research, Vol. 5* (eds F Palmieri, S Papa, C Saccone, and MN Gadaleta), Amsterdam: Elsevier, pp. 209–215.

28. Tang Y, Manfredi G, Hirano M, and Schon EA (2000). Maintenance of human rearranged mtDNAs in long-term-cultured transmitochondrial cell lines. *Mol. Biol. Cell* **11**: 2349–2358.

29. Menzies RA, Gold PH (1971). The turnover of mitochondria in a variety of tissues of young adult and aged rats. *J. Biol. Chem.* **246**: 2425–2429.

30. Schon EA. Mitochondrial genetics and disease (2000). *Trends Biochem. Sci.* **25**: 555–560.

31. Mita S, Schmidt B, Schon EA, DiMauro S, and Bonilla E (1989). Detection of 'deleted' mitochon-drial genomes in cytochrome *c* oxidase-deficient muscle fibers of a patient with Kearns–Sayre syndrome. *Proc. Natl Acad. Sci. USA* **86**: 9509–9513.

32. Nakase H, Moraes CT, Rizzuto R, Lombes A, DiMauro S, and Schon EA (1990). Transcription and translation of deleted mitochondrial genomes in Kearns–Sayre syndrome: implications for patho-genesis. *Am. J. Hum. Genet.* **46**: 418–427.

33. Shoubridge EA, Karpati G, and Hastings KEM (1990). Deletion mutants are functionally dominant over wild-type mitochondrial genomes in skeletal muscle fiber segments in mitochondrial disease. *Cell* **62**: 43–49.

34. Hayashi J-I, Ohta S, Kikuchi A, Takemitsu M, Goto Y-i, and Nonaka I (1991). Introduction of disease-related mitochondrial DNA deletions into HeLa cells lacking mitochondrial DNA results in mitochondrial dysfunction. *Proc. Natl Acad. Sci. USA* **88**: 10614–10618.

35. Moraes CT, Andreetta F, Bonilla E, Shanske S, DiMauro S, and Schon EA (1991). Replication-competent human mitochondrial DNA lacking the heavy-strand promoter region. *Mol. Cell. Biol.* **11**: 1631–1637.

36. Moraes CT, Ricci E, Petruzzella V, Shanske S, DiMauro S, Schon EA, and Bonilla E (1992). Molecular analysis of the muscle pathology associated with mitochondrial DNA deletions. *Nat. Genet.* **1**: 359–367.

37. Sancho S, Moraes CT, Tanji K, and Miranda AF (1992). Structural and functional mitochondrial abnormalities associated with high levels of partially deleted mitochondrial DNAs in somatic cell hybrids. *Somat. Cell Mol. Genet.* **18**: 431–442.

38. Sciacco M, Bonilla E, Schon EA, DiMauro S, and Moraes CT (1994). Distribution of wild-type and common deletion forms of mtDNA in normal and respiration-deficient muscle fibers from patients with mitochondrial myopathy. *Hum. Mol. Genet.* **3**: 13–19.

39. Tang Y, Schon EA, Wilichowski E, Vazquez-Memije ME, Davidson E, and King MP (2000). Rearrangements of human mitochondrial DNA (mtDNA): new insights into the regulation of mtDNA copy number and gene expression. *Mol. Biol. Cell* **11**: 1471–1485.

40. Awadalla P, Eyre-Walker A, and Smith JM (1999). Linkage disequilibrium and recombination in hominid mitochondrial DNA. *Science* **286**: 2524–2525.

41. Bakker A, Barthelemy C, Frachon P, Chateau D, Sternberg D, Mazat JP, and Lombes A (2000). Functional mitochondrial heterogeneity in heteroplasmic cells carrying the mitochondrial DNA mutation associated with the MELAS syndrome (mitochondrial encephalopathy, lactic acidosis, and strokelike episodes). *Pediatr. Res.* **48**: 143–150.

42. Davidson M, Zhang L, Koga Y, Schon EA, and King MP (1995). Genetic and functional complementation of deleted mitochondrial DNA. *Neurology* **45**: A831.

43. Enriquez JA, Cabezas-Herrera J, Bayona-Bafaluy MP, and Attardi G (2000). Very rare complementation between mitochondria carrying different mitochondrial DNA mutations points to intrinsic genetic autonomy of the organelles in cultured human cells. *J. Biol. Chem.* **275**: 11207–11215.

44. Hagelberg E, Goldman N, Lio P, Whelan S, Schiefenhovel W, Clegg JB, and Bowden DK (1999). Evidence for mitochondrial DNA recombination in a human population of island Melanesia. *Proc. R. Soc. Lond. B Biol. Sci.* **266**: 485–492.

45. Hammans SR, Sweeney MG, Holt IJ, Cooper JM, Toscano A, Clark JB, Morgan-Hughes JA, and Harding AE (1992). Evidence for intramitochondrial complementation between deleted and normal mitochondrial DNA in some patients with mitochondrial myopathy. *J. Neurol. Sci.* **107**: 87–92.

46. Oliver N and Wallace DC (1982). Assignment of two mitochondrially-synthesized polypeptides to human mitochondrial DNA and their use in the study of intracellular mitochondrial interaction. *Mol. Cell. Biol.* **2**: 30–41.

47. Sobreira C, King MP, Davidson M, Schon EA, and Miranda AF (1996). In vitro restoration of respiratory chain function by genetic complementation of two nonoverlapping mitochondrial DNA deletions in postmitotic muscle. *Neurology* **46**: A420–A421.

48. Takai D, Inoue K, Goto Y-i, Nonaka I, and Hayashi JI (1997). The interorganellar interaction between distinct human mitochondria with deletion mutant mtDNA from a patient with mitochondrial disease and with HeLa mtDNA. *J. Biol. Chem.* **272**: 6028–6033.

49. Takai D, Isobe K, and Hayashi JI (1999). Transcomplementation between different types of respiration-deficient mitochondria with different pathogenic mutant mitochondrial DNAs. *J. Biol. Chem.* **274**: 11199–11202.

50. Manfredi G, Vu T, Bonilla E, Schon EA, DiMauro S, Arnaudo E, Zhang L, Rowland LP, and Hirano M (1997). Association of myopathy with large-scale mitochondrial DNA duplications and deletions: which is pathogenic? *Ann. Neurol.* **42**: 180–188.

51. Yaffe MP (1999). The machinery of mitochondrial inheritance and behavior. *Science* **283**: 1493–1497.

52. Inoue K, Nakada K, Ogura A, Isobe K, Goto Y, Nonaka I, and Hayashi JI (2000). Generation of mice with mitochondrial dysfunction by introducing mouse mtDNA carrying a deletion into zygotes. *Nat. Genet.* **26**: 176–181.

53. Poulton J, Deadman ME, and Gardiner RM (1989). Tandem direct duplications of mitochondrial DNA in mitochondrial myopathy: analysis of nucleotide sequence and tissue distribution. *Nucleic Acids Res.* **17**: 10223–10229.

54. Poulton J, Deadman ME, Bindoff L, Morten K, Land J, and Brown G (1993). Families of mtDNA rearrangements can be detected in patients with mtDNA deletions: duplications may be a transient intermediate form. *Hum. Mol. Genet.* **2**: 23–30.

55. Poulton J, Morten KJ, Marchington D, Weber K, Brown KG, Rötig A, and Bindoff L (1995). Duplications of mitochondrial DNA in Kearns–Sayre syndrome. *Muscle Nerve* (3 Suppl.): S154–S158.

56. Brockington M, Alsanjari N, Sweeney MG, Morgan-Hughes JA, Scaravilli F, and Harding AE (1995). Kearns–Sayre syndrome associated with mitochondrial DNA deletion or duplication: a molecular genetic and pathological study. *J. Neurol. Sci.* **131**: 78–87.

57. Holt IJ, Dunbar DR, and Jacobs HT (1997). Behaviour of a population of partially duplicated mitochondrial DNA molecules in cell culture: segregation, maintenance and recombination dependent upon nuclear background. *Hum. Mol. Genet.* **6**: 1251–1260.

58. Schon EA, Bonilla E, and DiMauro S (1997). Mitochondrial DNA mutations and pathogenesis. *J. Bioenerg. Biomembr.* **29**: 131–149.

59. Tengan CH, Kiyomoto BH, Rocha MS, Tavares VL, Gabbai AA, and Moraes CT (1998). Mitochondrial encephalomyopathy and hypoparathyroidism associated with a duplication and a deletion of mitochondrial deoxyribonucleic acid. *J. Clin. Endocrinol. Metab.* **83**: 125–129.

60. Tengan CH and Moraes CT (1998). Duplication and triplication with staggered breakpoints in human mitochondrial DNA. *Biochim. Biophys. Acta* **1406**: 73–80.

61. Does more lead to less

62. Fromenty B, Carrozzo R, Shanske S, and Schon EA (1997). High proportions of mtDNA duplications in patients with Kearns–Sayre syndrome occur in the heart. *Am. J. Med. Genet.* **71**: 443–452.

63. Fromenty B, Manfredi G, Sadlock J, Zhang L, King MP and Schon EA (1996). Efficient and specific amplification of identified partial duplications of human mitochondrial DNA by long PCR. *Biochim. Biophys. Acta* **1308**: 222–230.

64. Chen X, Simonetti S, DiMauro S, and Schon EA (1993). Accumulation of mitochondrial DNA deletions in organisms with various lifespans. *Bull. Mol. Biol. Med.* **18**: 57–66.

65. Zhang C, Baumer A, Maxwell RJ, Linnane AW, and Nagley P (1992). Multiple mitochondrial DNA deletions in an elderly human individual. *FEBS Lett.* **297**: 34–38.

66. Simonetti S, Chen X, DiMauro S, and Schon EA (1992). Accumulation of deletions in human mitochondrial DNA during normal aging: analysis by quantitative PCR. *Biochim. Biophys. Acta* **1180**: 113–122.

67. Kajander OA, Rovio AT, Majamaa K, Poulton J, Spelbrink JN, Holt IJ, Karhunen PJ, and Jacobs HT (2000). Human mtDNA sublimons resemble rearranged mitochondrial genomes found in pathological states. *Hum. Mol. Genet.* **9**: 2821–2835.

68. Bodyak ND, Nekhaeva E, Wei JY, and Khrapko K (2001). Quantification and sequencing of somatic deleted mtDNA in single cells: evidence for partially duplicated mtDNA in aged human tissues. *Hum. Mol. Genet.* **10**: 17–24.

69. Rötig A, Bessis J-L, Romero N, Cormier V, Saudubray J-M, Narcy P, Lenoir G, Rustin P, and Munnich A (1992). Maternally inherited duplication of the mitochondrial genome in a syndrome of proximal tubulopathy, diabetes mellitus, and cerebellar ataxia. *Am. J. Hum. Genet.* **50**: 364–370.

70. Dunbar DR, Moonie PA, Swingler RJ, Davidson D, Roberts R, and Holt IJ (1993). Maternally transmitted partial direct tandem duplication of mitochondrial DNA associated with diabetes mellitus. *Hum. Mol. Genet.* **2**: 1619–1624.

71. Ballinger SW, Shoffner JM, Gebhart S, Koontz DA, and Wallace DC (1994). Mitochondrial diabetes revisited. *Nat. Genet.* **7**: 458–459 (letter).

72. Tanabe Y, Miyamoto S, Kinoshita Y, Yamada K, Sasaki N, Makino E, and Nakajima H (1988). Diabetes mellitus in Kearns–Sayre syndrome. *Eur. Neurol.* **28**: 34–38.

73 Majander A, Suomalainen A, Vettenranta K, Sariola H, Perkkio M, Holmberg C, and Pihko H (1991). Congenital hypoplastic anemia, diabetes, and severe renal dysfunction associated with a mitochondrial deletion. *Pediatr. Res.* **30**: 327–330.

74. Superti-Furga A, Schoenle E, Tuchschmid P, Caduff R, Sabato V, deMattia D, Gitzelmann R, and Steinmann B (1993). Pearson bone marrow-pancreas syndrome with insulin-dependent diabetes, progressive renal tubulopathy, organic aciduria, and elevated fetal haemoglobin caused by deletion and duplication of mitochondrial DNA. *Eur. J. Pediatr.* **152**: 44–50.

75. Ozawa T, Yoneda M, Tanaka M, Ohno K, Sato W, Suzuki H, Nishikimi M, Yamamoto M, Nonaka I, and Horai S (1988). Maternal inheritance of deleted mitochondrial DNA in a family with mitochondrial myopathy. *Biochem. Biophys. Res. Commun.* **154**: 1240–1247.

76. Larsson NG, Eiken HG, Boman H, Holme E, Oldfors A, and Tulinius MH (1992). Lack of transmission of deleted mtDNA from a woman with Kearns–Sayre syndrome to her child. *Am. J. Hum. Genet.* **50**: 360–363.

77. Bernes SM, Bacino C, Prezant TR, Pearson MA, Wood TS, Fournier P, and Fischel-Ghodsian N (1993). Identical mitochondrial DNA deletion in mother with progressive external ophthalmoplegia and son with Pearson marrow-pancreas syndrome. *J. Pediatr.* **123**: 598–602.

78. Boles RG and Williams JC (1999). Mitochondrial disease and cyclic vomiting syndrome. *Dig. Dis. Sci.* **44**: 103S–107S.

79. Akaike M, Kawai H, Kashiwagi S, Kunishige M, and Saito S (1995). A case of Kearns–Sayre syndrome whose asymptomatic mother had abnormal mitochondria in skeletal muscle. *Rinsho Shinkeigaku* **35**: 190–194.

80. Yuzaki M, Ohkoshi N, Kanazawa I, Kagawa Y, and Ohta S (1989). Multiple deletions in mitochondrial DNA at direct repeats of non-D-Loop regions in cases of familial mitochondrial myopathy. *Biochem. Biophys. Res. Commun.* **164**: 1352–1357.

81. Kawashima S, Ohta S, Kagawa Y, Yoshida M, and Nishizawa M (1994). Widespread tissue distribution of multiple mitochondrial DNA deletions in familial mitochondrial myopathy. *Muscle Nerve* **17**: 741–746.

82. Wrischnik LA, Higuchi RG, Stoneking M, Erlich HA, Arnheim N, and Wilson AC (1987). Length mutations in human mitochondrial DNA: direct sequencing of enzymatically amplified DNA. *Nucleic Acids Res.* **15**: 529–542.

83. Comi GP, Bordoni A, Salani S, Franceschina L, Sciacco M, Prelle A, Fortunato F, Zeviani M, Napoli L, Bresolin N, Moggio M, Ausenda CD, Taanman J-W, and Scarlato G (1998). Cytochrome *c* oxidase subunit I microdeletion in a patient with motor neuron disease. *Ann. Neurol.* **43**: 110–116.

84. Keightley JA, Hoffbuhr KC, Burton MD, Salas VM, Johnston WSW, Penn AMW, Buist NRM, and Kennaway NG (1996). A microdeletion in cytochrome *c* oxidase (COX) subunit III associated with COX deficiency and recurrent myoglobinuria. *Nat. Genet.* **12**: 410–416.

85. Musumeci O, Andreu AL, Shanske S, Bresolin N, Comi GP, Rothstein R, Schon EA, and DiMauro S (2000). Intragenic inversion of mtDNA: a new type of pathogenic mutation in a patient with mitochondrial myopathy. *Am. J. Hum. Genet.* **66**: 1900–1904.

86. Brockington M, Sweeney MG, Hammans SR, Morgan-Hughes JA, and Harding AE (1993). A tandem duplication in the D-loop of human mitochondrial DNA is associated with deletions in mitochondrial myopathies. *Nat. Genet.* **4**: 67–71.

87. Hao H, Manfredi G, Clayton DA, and Moraes CT (1997). Functional and structural features of a tandem duplication of the human mtDNA promoter region. *Am. J. Hum. Genet.* **60**: 1363–1372.

88. Wei YH, Pang CY, You BJ, and Lee HC (1996). Tandem duplications and large-scale deletions of mitochondrial DNA are early molecular events of human aging process. *Ann. NY Acad. Sci.* **786**: 82–101.

89. Manfredi G, Servidei S, Bonilla E, Shanske S, Schon EA, DiMauro S, and Moraes CT (1995). High levels of mitochondrial DNA with an unstable 260-bp duplication in a patient with a mitochondrial myopathy. *Neurology* **45**: 762–768.

90. Bouzidi MF, Poyau A, and Godinot C (1998). Co-existence of high levels of a cytochrome b mutation and of a tandem 200 bp duplication in the D-loop of muscle human mitochondrial DNA. *Hum. Mol. Genet.* **7**: 385–391.

91. Torroni A, Lott MT, Cabell MF, Chen YS, Lavergne L, and Wallace DC (1994). mtDNA and the origin of Caucasians: identification of ancient Caucasian-specific haplogroups, one of which is prone to a recurrent somatic duplication in the D-loop region. *Am. J. Hum. Genet.* **55**: 760–776.

92. Wilkinson GS and Chapman AM (1991). Length and sequence variation in evening bat D-loop mtDNA. *Genetics* **128**: 607–617.

93. Casane D, Dennebouy N, de Rochambeau H, Mounolou JC, and Monnerot M (1994). Genetic analysis of systematic mitochondrial heteroplasmy in rabbits. *Genetics* **138**: 471–480.

94. Hayashi JI, Gotoh O, Tagashira Y, Tosu M, and Sekiguchi T (1981). Analysis of mitochondrial DNA species in interspecific hybrid somatic cells using restriction endonucleases. Identification of recombinant mtDNA molecules. *Exp. Cell Res.* **131**: 458–462.

95. Blok RB, Thorburn DR, Thompson GN, and Dahl HH (1995). A topoisomerase II cleavage site is associated with a novel mitochondrial DNA deletion. *Hum. Genet.* **95**: 75–81.

96. Lyamichev VI, Mirkin SM, and Frank-Kamenetskii MD (1986). Structures of homopurine-homopyrimidine tract in superhelical DNA. *J. Biomol. Struct. Dyn.* **3**: 667–669.

97. Shoffner JM, Lott MT, Voljavec AS, Soueidan SA, Costigan DA, and Wallace DC (1989). Spontaneous Kearns–Sayre/chronic external ophthalmoplegia plus syndrome associated with a mitochondrial DNA deletion: a slip-replication model and metabolic therapy. *Proc. Natl Acad. Sci. USA* **86**: 7952–7956.

98. Ville-Ferlin T, Dumoulin R, Stepien G, Matha V, Bady B, Flocard F, Carrier H, Mathieu M, and Mousson B (1995). Fine mapping of randomly distributed multiple deletions of mitochondrial DNA in a case of chronic progressive external ophthalmoplegia. *Mol. Cell. Probes* **9**: 207–214.

7 Pathological mutations affecting mitochondrial protein synthesis

Howard T Jacobs

Introduction

Just as in yeast, mitochondrial DNA mutations in humans can be classified into three broad categories: point mutations affecting protein-coding genes (designated *mit*⁻ in yeast), point mutations affecting the protein synthetic apparatus (*syn*⁻ in yeast), and large deletions. Large deletions in yeast, a class of mtDNA mutants designated ρ⁻, are represented as long, tandem repeats of the non-deleted segment of mtDNA. Large deletions of mtDNA in humans are somewhat different, in that they do not generate multicopy tandemized products, although dimers of the non-deleted region can often be detected, and trimers and higher order multimers may also be present at a lower level. The terms *mit*⁻, *syn*⁻, and ρ⁻ are not commonly used in reference to human mtDNA mutations, but they are nevertheless useful conceptual categories.

This chapter will deal with the *syn*⁻ class of mutation that has been found in pathological states in humans (Fig. 7.1). After a brief survey of the specific mutations that have been reported, together with some details of the clinical phenotypes associated with them, the main focus of the chapter will be on mechanistic studies aimed at understanding how they produce cellular and physiological defects that can manifest as serious disease. Pathological mtDNA mutations have been known for over a decade, yet our mechanistic understanding of them remains remarkably rudimentary. In fact, the findings of different researchers are often contradictory, and one is left with the feeling that some rather fundamental points might, thus far, have escaped our attention. This should be a sobering counter-balance to the euphoria associated with the completion of the human genome sequence. Genome sequencing will undoubtedly lead to an explosion of data, identifying numerous unsuspected sequence polymorphisms and haplotypes with phenotypic significance in relation to disease. But if the example of mitochondrial DNA is a reasonable guide, many decades of painstaking investigations in model systems will be required before we can hope to reach a mechanistic understanding of their pathophysiological significance.

This chapter will also deal only in a brief or superficial way with aspects of mtDNA mutations covered elsewhere in this book: the issue of heteroplasmy and of segregation of mtDNA genotypes during development (see Chapter 15), the mechanisms by which pathological mutations are generated and propagated in the germ line (Chapter 17), the epidemiology and clinical details of mitochondrial disease (Chapters 17 and 5), and mutations of the *mit*⁻ class. The latter primarily affect only one mitochondrial protein, resulting in a usually rather

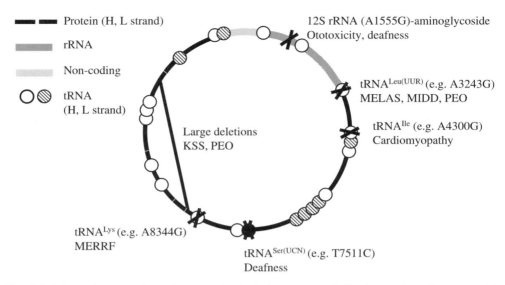

Fig. 7.1 Schematic map of the human mitochondrial genome, indicating major, disease-causing mtDNA mutations affecting genes of the translation system. Codon recognition groups indicated for serine and leucine tRNAs.

narrowly definable clinical phenotype (Chapter 8), but this may nevertheless overlap some features found in patients carrying syn^-- or ρ^--like mutations. The reader is also referred to the chapters dealing with the mitochondrial protein synthetic apparatus itself (Chapter 2).

Pathological mutations of mtDNA affecting protein synthesis

Human mitochondrial DNA (Fig. 7.1) contains, in addition to the 13 structural genes encoding OXPHOS subunits, 24 genes encoding essential RNA components of the translational apparatus, namely two ribosomal and 22 transfer RNAs.[1] In theory, mutations in any of these could cause a complete loss, or at least a severe dysfunction of mitochondrial protein synthesis, affecting all or almost all of the 13 mtDNA-encoded polypeptides. In addition, more subtle mutations in these genes can be envisaged, which might have an effect limited to the synthesis of one or just a few mtDNA-encoded polypeptides. Deletions mutations would be expected to be of the most severe class, since loss of any of the above 24 genes would entail a complete cessation of protein synthesis and loss of all four enzyme complexes to which mtDNA-encoded polypeptides contribute. However, these severe phenotypes would of course entail lethality, were it not for the possibility of heteroplasmy. The most functionally drastic mutations are therefore always found in the heteroplasmic state, raising the complication that the level and tissue distribution of mutant mtDNA can play a role in expression of the clinical phenotype. At more modest levels of heteroplasmy, even drastic mutations can have a subtle phenotypic effect. Conversely, functionally mild mutations that can segregate to homoplasmy in the germ line without compromising early development might nevertheless have a profound effect in some specific tissues.

Transfer RNA mutations

By far the most widely studied class of mtDNA point mutations are those affecting single tRNA genes. At the present time, mutations in 19 of the 22 human mitochondrial tRNA genes have been reported in association with disease, although not every one has been validated by mechanistic studies, or by large-scale epidemiological analysis.[2] Four specific tRNAs have received the most attention, namely those for lysine, for the leucine UUR codon group, for isoleucine and for the serine UCN codon group. Many researchers have suggested that these particular tRNAs, especially leucine (UUR), and to a lesser extent tRNA[Lys], might be hotspots for pathological mutations,[3–5] although much of the bias may have come inadvertently from investigators themselves, who have searched more vigorously for pathological mutations affecting these particular genes, following the earliest reports. It may also be biased by the specific phenotypes that have so far been recognized as 'mitochondrial', which may indeed be associated with defects in these particular tRNA genes more than others. There might, for example, be other clinical phenotypes that have been largely overlooked, which are predominantly associated with mutations in other tRNA genes of mtDNA. Implicit in this statement is the rather remarkable observation that mutations in each tRNA gene seems to be associated with a rather specific clinical phenotype or set of clinical phenotypes. For example, tRNA[Ile] mutations are predominantly found in patients with maternally inherited cardiomyopathy, whereas tRNA[Ser(UCN)] mutations are most common in patients with sensorineural deafness. Even where the same organs are involved, the affected cell type and exact clinical phenotype can be quite different, as nicely shown by eye pathologies associated, respectively, with the A3243G mutation in tRNA[Leu(UUR)] (pigmentary retinopathy) and the A8344G mutation in tRNA[Lys] (optic atrophy).[6] This specificity continues even down to the level of the individual mutation, where different mutations in the same tRNA gene, notably the much-studied tRNA[Leu(UUR)], are found in association with distinct pathological phenotypes. This observation strongly hints at the mechanistic complexity that will be discussed in the next section.

The first mitochondrial tRNA point mutation shown to be associated with human disease was the A8344G substitution in the gene for tRNA[Lys].[7] This heteroplasmic mutation was found to segregate matrilineally with the so-called MERRF syndrome, characterized by myoclonic epilepsy, in combination with ragged red muscle fibres, the histopathological feature diagnostic for mitochondrial myopathy, hence the acronym. MERRF is a complex disorder, commonly including also sensorineural deafness and sometimes bilateral, benign lipoma as additional features. Other mutations in the same tRNA gene, notably at np 8356,[8] have been found in cases of an essentially indistinguishable disease (Fig. 7.2(a)). The A8344G mutation is located in the so-called TΨC loop of the tRNA, although in this particular tRNA, as in many others encoded in mtDNA, the canonical sequence TΨC is not, in fact, present. The mutation at np 8356 affects the base-paired stem of the TΨC arm. One of the goals of the mechanistic studies that will be described in the later sections of this chapter is to understand why this particular combination of features, involving notably myoclonic epilepsy, results from a specific dysfunction of mitochondrial tRNA[Lys].

The second pathological tRNA mutation to be discovered, A3243G in the gene for tRNA[Leu(UUR)],[9] has also become one of the most intensively studied, from several points of view. One major reason for interest in this mutation, apart from its relatively high prevalence[3,10] and the numerous potential effects that have been studied at the molecular level, is the fact that unlike A8344G and, in fact, most other mitochondrial mutations of the

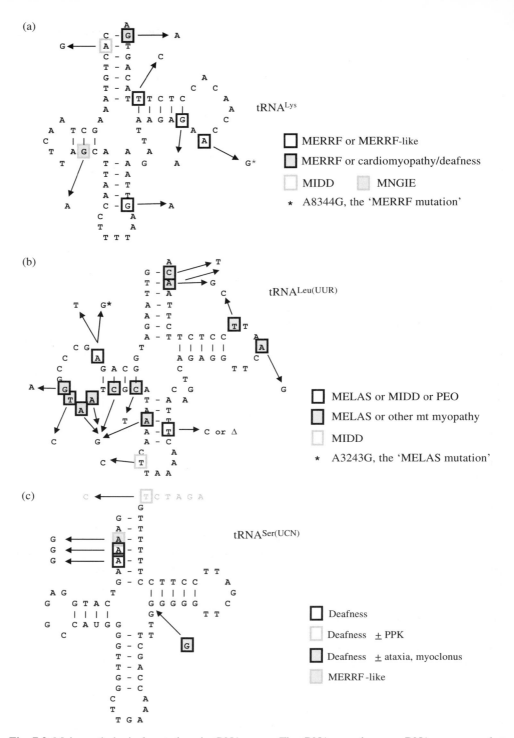

Fig. 7.2 Major pathological mutations in tRNA genes. The tRNAs are shown as DNA sequences, but folded as the conventional clover-leaf secondary structures. (a) tRNA^{Lys}, (b) tRNA^{Leu(UUR)}, (c) tRNA^{Ser(UCN)}. PPK—palmoplantar keratoderma.

syn⁻ class, its clinical phenotype is extremely variable. Much debate has centred on whether A3243G is really found in association with a continuous spectrum of disease or alternatively with 3 or 4 very specific and distinct disorders. Of particular importance from the viewpoint of the geneticist, is the question of whether all of the different phenotypes are found in a given maternal pedigree with the mutation, or whether each affected family tends to exhibit a particular clinical phenotype. A second question is the degree to which the overall severity and type of clinical picture is primarily influenced by heteroplasmy level and distribution. On both questions there is no clear consensus, and few truly systematic investigations have been attempted to address them. These questions will be returned to below.

Broadly, the clinical phenotypes associated with the A3424G mutation can be classified into one of four categories. The original syndromic disorder in which the mutation was found is described by the acronym MELAS (mitochondrial encephalomyopathy, lactic acidosis, and stroke-like episodes), and the mutation is hence often loosely described as 'the MELAS mutation'. However, this is misleading for two reasons. Firstly, some other mtDNA mutations,[2] not all of them even in tRNA–leu(UUR), can also give a MELAS or MELAS-like phenotype. Secondly, the majority of patients with the A3243G mutation have one of the other categories of clinical phenotype associated with the mutation. These are usually described by the terms 'diabetes and/or deafness', often expanded to the acronymic maternally inherited diabetes plus deafness (MIDD), and PEO (progressive external ophthalmoplegia), namely paralysis of the external eye muscles that can sometimes affect skeletal muscle more widely, manifesting as ptosis, generalized muscle weakness and exercise intolerance[4,11] (see van den Ouweland *et al.*, 1992 and Moraes *et al.*, 1993 for the first reports of the A3243G mutation in patients with these more restricted disorders). The fourth diagnostic category is really a catchall for an expanding range of clinical phenotypes that fit neither into the conventional definition of MELAS, nor into the accepted definitions of MIDD or PEO. These include patients with kidney disease, with cardiomyopathy, various kinds of neuropathy, or endocrinopathies other than diabetes.

Many different factors have been proposed to modify the effect of the A3243G mutation, leading to this clinical variability, but none has been clearly demonstrated to act in such a fashion *in vivo*. A strong candidate for involvement is mtDNA haplotype, that is, the combination of other sequence polymorphisms found in mtDNA of the given individual or family, which may include some that are present heteroplasmically at a low level and may have thus escaped detection. This concept is supported by at least one, albeit extreme example of a suppressor mutation of A3243G, which arose in cell culture.[12] Although the specific suppressor mutation has not been found in any patient or family with A3243G, it does provide a clear example of how the phenotype associated with a mitochondrial tRNA gene mutation can be drastically modified by the rest of the mtDNA sequence.

Nuclear genotype has also been proposed to influence the expression of the mutation in some way, and a role also cannot be excluded for environmental and epigenetic modifiers. Any of these may act by promoting a non-random segregation of mutant and wild-type mtDNAs in different tissues, an idea supported by studies of patient-derived mtDNA transferred to different nuclear backgrounds by cybridization,[13] a technique that will be discussed in more detail in the following sections. The level[14,15] and tissue-distribution[16] of heteroplasmy are also undoubted factors affecting the clinical outcome, and there is evidence that this tissue variation in heteroplasmy is under genetic control.[17] Even the degree to which mutant mtDNAs are distributed homogeneously within single cells may be a factor.[18]

One reason for the considerable doubt surrounding these issues is that the exact pathogenic mechanism of the mutation remains to be elucidated, as will be discussed in detail in a succeeding section. A fuller understanding of how the mutation impairs mitochondrial protein synthesis would sharpen the search for interacting factors.

Evidence has accumulated implicating no fewer than 15 other mutations in tRNA^Leu(UUR) in human disease. It should be pointed out that the pathological nature of these mutations is more clearly established in some cases than in others. Nevertheless, the majority has been shown to co-segregate with disease in multiple maternal pedigrees, and to result in a clear dysfunction of mitochondrial metabolism and/or protein synthesis when transferred to a control nuclear background by cybridization. All are found in the heteroplasmic state. The disorders associated with these mutations usually include some form of muscle disease, but cardiomyopathy is sometimes found in addition to skeletal myopathy. Mutations at np 3260 and np 3271 are usually associated with a MELAS-like disease, but detailed epidemiological data are scarce, therefore it remains possible that most or all of these mutations are found in patients whose clinical manifestations overlap those of A3243G patients, and that there is in fact just a continuum of clinical phenotypes representing 'mitochondrial tRNA^Leu(UUR) disease'.

The pathological mutations affecting this tRNA map in many different regions of the molecule, although some may lie relatively close in the three-dimensional structure of the tRNA, a fact which may not be obvious from the conventional clover-leaf secondary structure in which tRNAs are usually drawn (Fig. 7.2(b)). The location of these mutations does not, however, give any obvious clue as to the molecular mechanism(s) of pathogenesis. None has been mapped, for example, to the anticodon loop.

Mutations affecting a third tRNA, dedicated to the UCN serine codon group, are prominently associated with syndromic disorders in which sensorineural deafness appears to be the predominant feature (Fig. 7.2(c)). Most of these mutations differ from those in tRNA^Lys or tRNA^Leu(UUR) in that clinically affected individuals are typically homoplasmic for the mutation, or else have a very high level of heteroplasmy for it. This has lead to the view that these mutations are phenotypically less severe. Many cases of true non-syndromic hearing impairment also appear to be associated with mutations in mitochondrial tRNA^Ser(UCN). Intriguingly, the spectrum of other phenotypes reported in the case of each mutation affecting tRNA^Ser(UCN) are quite specific. The A7445G mutation, for example, is associated, in most affected individuals, with palmoplantar keratoderma (thickening of the skin on the soles of the feet and palms of the hands) in addition to hearing loss, whereas the additional clinical features diagnostic for the 7472 insC mutation can include ataxia and myoclonus. Mutations in the aminoacyl stem of tRNA^Ser(UCN) can manifest either as non-syndromic deafness, or else as a MEREF-like disease.

Ribosomal RNA mutations

Only one ribosomal RNA mutation in mtDNA has been convincingly demonstrated to play a role in human disease, namely the A1555G in small subunit (12S) rRNA gene, associated with both aminoglycoside-induced and non-syndromic deafness.[19] Considering the interest that its discovery aroused, plus the fact that pathological mutations in mitochondrial tRNA mutations are so numerous, it is highly surprising that no other proven pathological rRNA mutations have come to light, although some other mutations in the 12S rRNA gene are probably involved in other cases of the disorder.[20] The np 1555 maps to a phylogenetically conserved and a functionally well-characterized domain of the small subunit rRNA. In affected pedigrees the mutation is always, or almost always found in the homoplasmic state. The mutation is predicted to alter the secondary structure of the 12S rRNA molecule, lengthening a base-paired stem by one nucleotide pair.[21] This is believed to render the structure more like that of bacterial small subunit rRNAs in a region of the molecule that plays a key role in both translational fidelity and interaction of the ribosome with aminoglycoside antibiotics such as streptomycin. This is of crucial interest, because in most well-studied cases, expression of the clinical phenotype associated with this mutation, namely acute-onset sensorineural deafness, is associated with treatment of the patient with aminoglycoside antibiotics.

The A1555G mutation appears to be relatively common in Asia and in Spain and perhaps also Hispanic populations in the Americas. Few reports of the mutation have come from Northern Europe. Although this may reflect genuine population differences, an alternative explanation is the fact that aminoglycoside usage may vary widely between these regions. Aminoglycosides are widely prescribed in Asia. In some other countries where the association has been picked up, aminoglycosides may have been widely available without prescription. This could explain cases that have come to light from non-Asian populations, affecting individuals without a documented history of aminoglycoside therapy.[19,22,23] Nuclear genotype has also been proposed as an modifier, and a candidate locus has been identified on chromosome 8.[24]

Pathological nuclear mutations affecting mitochondrial translation

Apart from the nuclear mutations that adversely affect mitochondrial DNA (see Chapter 9), one might presume there to be a large category of nuclear gene mutations that have phenotypes similar to those of the *mit⁻* or *syn⁻* classes of mtDNA mutations. Stretching the yeast analogy, there are many hundreds of such mutants in yeast, designated *pet⁻* (nuclear mutations with the classic 'petite' phenotype), and several hundred nuclear genes are required to maintain the mitochondrial translation system of humans, so any of these could be targets for mutations that may give a clinical phenotype similar to those of mtDNA *syn⁻* mutants. Indeed, there are many examples of patients with phenotypic features overlapping those of syndromic disorders of mtDNA, such as MELAS,[3,25] in some instances lacking the ragged red fibres that indicate mitochondrial proliferation, considered the hallmark of mtDNA involvement. There are certainly many more patients with unexplained hearing loss or diabetes who do not have any identified pathological mtDNA mutation, but whose primary pathology may result from defects in the machinery of mitochondrial protein synthesis. However, no case of human disease has yet been attributed to a nuclear gene defect affecting the mitochondrial translation system.

A few rare examples of nuclear gene defects more akin to *mit⁻* mutants of mtDNA have come to light (i.e. affecting structural components of the respiratory chain), but the only clear examples of pathological nuclear mutations affecting mitochondrial biosynthesis are those affecting assembly or import (see Chapters 3 and 10).

Although assembly may be intimately linked to translation in mitochondria, pathological mutations specifically affecting the more narrowly defined translational apparatus (ribosomal proteins, aminoacyl-tRNA synthetases, translation factors, or biosynthetic enzymes needed for rRNA and tRNA maturation) remain unknown. This puzzling absence may originate from trivial, methodological causes: individuals with combinations of 'mitochondrial' symptoms such as diabetes, retinopathy, seizures, myopathy, or hearing loss, and who belong to large pedigrees showing clear-cut maternal inheritance of the phenotype, are usually evaluated intensively from the viewpoint of identifying the causal mtDNA mutation. The large database of sequenced mtDNA polymorphisms, combined with the fact that pathological mutations are frequently heteroplasmic, means that with current technology it is a relatively straightforward matter to identify a pathological mtDNA mutation.

Family studies of other such individuals often reveal no evidence of (maternal) inheritance of the disorder, in which case they are considered unlikely candidates for mitochondrial transmission, and not studied further unless there is clear evidence of consanguinity. The presumption has been that even if the etiology of their disorder might be mitochondrial, in the absence of more extensive family data, proving the pathogenicity of a new mutation is going to be very difficult, therefore the only thing that is usually checked is the absence of the 'common' mtDNA mutations, such as A3243G, A1555G, or a clonal mtDNA rearrangement. Autosomal recessive inheritance, which is the obvious alternative explanation, is not usually pursued, due to the inherent difficulties of carrying out a linkage study in small pedigrees, with variable phenotypes, overlapping other complex disorders. Only rare cases of obvious consanguinity are likely to receive proper analysis, and perhaps it is simply the case that none has yet been investigated fruitfully.

Since the symptomology characteristic of mitochondrial disease overlaps that of many common heterogeneous or complex disorders (e.g. hearing impairment, cardiomyopathy, diabetes) a more fruitful strategy may be to focus on these, in the hope that some genes contributing to these phenotypes may prove to be of the *pet⁻* class. However, this prediction has not thus far been supported, in studies of one such disorder, non-syndromic sensorineural hearing impairment. Approximately 50–100 nuclear genes are likely to be involved in the various types of this disorder, and to date about 15 of them have been identified.[26] However, none has yet proven to have a mitochondrial function. Amongst the remaining 35–85 candidates, many *pet⁻* mutants may yet lurk, but it is also possible that the auditory phenotype of greatest mitochondrial relevance, that is, autosomal dominant adult-onset hearing loss, has not yet received much attention. The pathological involvement of nuclear genes for the mitochondrial translational apparatus could also be obscured by nuclear–mitochondrial interactions, leading to superficially uninterpretable inheritance patterns.

Mechanistic studies of mtDNA mutations affecting protein synthesis

The phenomena described in the preceding sections prompt many questions regarding pathogenic mechanisms, both at the level of the individual cell, of the affected tissue and of the organism as a whole. In principle, we can consider several rather distinct potential effects of a *syn⁻* mutation at the cellular level.

Factors influencing expression of a syn⁻ mutation

A mutation in a component of the mitochondrial protein synthetic machinery may be viewed as having a strictly quantitative effect: not enough mitochondrial proteins would be made, leading to a deficiency of polypeptides essential for bioenergetic function. A mutation with a quantitative effect might also make too much rather than too little product, although this hypothesis is usually not considered. A quantitative effect on protein synthesis might be specific rather than generalized: in other words, not enough of something in particular might be made, rather than not enough of everything. A further scenario would be that the effects of a mutation are qualitative rather than quantitative, that is, that in addition to the correct or usual products, one or more additional products are made which do not have the correct structure, and in some way act detrimentally.

The fact that different *syn⁻* mutations do not manifest with identical clinical phenotypes indicates that we must consider all of the above hypotheses in regard to any given mutation, and a single mutation may conceivably manifest generalized or specific quantitative or even qualitative effects on protein synthesis in different tissues or individuals. This may apply, for example, to the case of the A3243G mutation, whose clinical phenotype is so variable. However, it may also apply to other mutations whose phenotypic features are more uniform, such as those in tRNA^{Lys}, where there is nevertheless a considerable phenotypic overlap with some other mtDNA mutations of the *syn⁻* class.

The clinical phenotype of 'mitochondrial translational disease' can in principle be influenced by a variety of interacting factors. First, naturally, is the mitochondrial mutation itself, which may have one or more direct consequences for the operation of the mitochondrial translational machinery. Second, other mtDNA sequence polymorphisms ('mitochondrial haplotype') might modify, mitigate or exacerbate the molecular effects of the primary pathological mutation. Third, nuclear genes whose products must interact with a mutant tRNA or rRNA could also affect the outcome, by virtue of their own structural polymorphisms, variable expression levels or else tissue-specific isoforms. Environmental factors and a variety of physiological or epigenetic responses could also act within the organism to alter the phenotypic expression of a mtDNA mutation, in much the same way that nuclear mutations said to be of variable penetrance can result in a variable spectrum of disease. Finally, the specific consequences of heteroplasmy need to be taken into account, since variation in the amount and tissue-patterns of representation of a mutant tRNA could result in drastically different outcomes.

Bearing in mind these potentially complicating factors, significant advances in our understanding of the pathological mechanisms of mitochondrial disease mutations have come from analyses of cybrid cell lines, in which patient-derived mtDNA carrying a defined mutation has been transferred into a control nuclear background,[27] via fusion to a ρ^0 cell line (i.e. an engineered cell line lacking its own mtDNA). Not only has this allowed nuclear genetic or developmental effects to be set aside: it has also allowed the molecular and physiological effects of different levels of heteroplasmy to be tested directly. Conversely, testing the same mutation in different cell backgrounds has revealed unexpected and potentially significant effects attributable to the nucleus. One methodological drawback of these model systems is that the cell types most commonly affected by mitochondrial disease are very different from the tumour-derived ρ^0 cell lines used to create cybrids. Cultured cell lines in general are also far less dependent on mitochondrial respiration than terminally differentiated cell types *in vivo*, such as skeletal muscle or neurons. Nevertheless, cybrid studies have given valuable clues to the molecular mechanisms by which mutations in genes for the mitochondrial translation machinery bring about cellular dysfunction. Additional information has come from studies of patient-derived (e.g. lymphoblastoid) cell lines or technically more difficult analyses carried out directly on biopsy material.

We now consider mechanistic findings in regard to each of the major mutations or mutation classes described in the previous section.

MERRF mutations in tRNA^{Lys}

Most cybrid studies on tRNA^{Lys} have focused on the A8344G mutation, but rather similar findings have emerged in regard to the mutation at np 8356,[29] and may be generalizable to other mutations in the tRNA^{Lys} gene associated with a MERRF-like clinical phenotype. In the case of this heteroplasmic mutation, there is a clear relationship between mutant load in the patient's tissues, especially muscle, and clinical phenotype.[6] Thus, relatives with <70 per cent A8344G mutant mtDNA in muscle are usually asymptomatic, although some may suffer from lipoma,[28,30] whereas patients with >90 per cent mutant mtDNA invariably have a severe disease including myoclonic seizues in almost all cases.[6] This correlation holds up also at the level of the individual muscle fibre, where mutant loads of >90 per cent are indicative of OXPHOS dysfunction.[31] The precise tissue distribution of mutant *versus* mtDNA molecules thus can also play a role in precise details of the clinical phenotype.

In both patient-derived myoblasts[32] and 143B osteosarcoma cell cybrids[28,33] the A8344G mutation shows a nice illustration of the threshold effect, also confirming the pathological nature of the mutation. Heteroplasmy levels of up to 85 per cent can apparently be tolerated without drastic effect, but as the proportion of mtDNA carrying the mutation rises above 90 per cent there is a sharp decline in respiratory capacity, with progressive loss of mitochondrial protein synthesis. The pattern of mitochondrial translation products can be conveniently visualized on SDS–PAGE gels by pulse-labelling with ^{35}S-methionine in the presence of low concentrations of emetine, which specifically suppresses cytosolic translation. Different translation products can be identified immunologically, and there appears to be a relationship between lysine content and the degree to which the synthesis of different translation products is affected by very high levels of the mutation.[34] This strongly suggests a simple loss of function mechanism, whereby the mutant tRNA is unable to decode lysine codons. At very high levels of the mutation, a reproducible set of truncated polypeptides is detected on SDS–PAGE, and these are believed to represent the products of ribosomes stalled at lysine codons and/or released products arising from frameshifts at such positions.[34]

It is not known how these translational abnormalities impact the respiratory chain enzymes, of which cytochrome *c* oxidase seems to be the most severely affected. The assembly of cytochrome *c* oxidase and other respiratory enzyme complexes may simply be starved of necessary subunits. Alternatively, truncated polypeptides synthesized at a lower level might interfere with assembly even in cells where full-length products are still being made in substantial amounts.

Aminoacylation of tRNA^{Lys} seems to be impaired in at least some 143B osteosarcoma cybrid cell lines that are almost homoplasmic for the mutation.[34] However, this may not always apply *in vivo*, since the mutant tRNA was judged to be efficiently aminoacylated in muscle biopsy samples from patients.[35] In HeLa cell cybrids,[36] there is loss of hypermodification of the wobble base U of the mutant tRNA (U34 in the conventional nomenclature) which is believed to be responsible for restricting its decoding capacity to codons ending in a purine. The implication is that the mutant tRNA might misread AAY asparagine codons, incorrectly inserting lysine into mitochondrial translation products at these positions. However, no such misreading can be detected *in vitro*:[37] instead, the mutant, unmodified tRNA seems simply to be incapable of reading cognate codons. It remains formally possible that misreading could occur in some cell types *in vivo*, or in some genetic backgrounds. A rather similar set of findings has been made in relation to the A3243G mutation, as discussed below, therefore it is tempting to suggest that different clinical phenotypes associated with specific tRNA mutations may result from the synthesis of specific, abnormal translation products in some tissues, which would be different in every case since a different set of codons would be misread. However, at this time there is no concrete evidence for codon misreading *in vivo* in MERRF or any other mitochondrial tRNA disorder.

Pathological mutations in tRNA$^{Leu(UUR)}$

Of the various pathological mutations in tRNA$^{Leu(UUR)}$, A3243G has been by far the most extensively analysed, although useful data on other mutations, particularly those at np 3260, 3271 and 3302 have been reported. *In vivo* there appears to be a lower threshold level of heteroplasmy required to produce disease for A3243G than for A8344G,[16,38] but in terms of biochemical effects in cybrid cells the opposite seems to apply, with a very high level (>98 per cent) of A3243G mutant mtDNA required to provoke a major defect in mitochondrial protein synthesis.[12,39–41] However, in at least some tissues, for example, brain, a clear metabolic defect is evident at much lower levels of heteroplasmy, and is even linearly related to heteroplasmy level.[42] The expression of the metabolic defect in different tissue appears to depend directly on energy demand.[43]

Cybrid studies have yielded a rather similar picture as for the A8344G mutation. However, there is less consistency, perhaps reflecting greater effects of mtDNA haplotype and/or nuclear background, which may in turn underlie clinical variability. The most general statement that can be made about A3243G from cybrid and also *in vitro* studies is that the mutation impairs, to some degree, or at least in some context, almost every aspect of tRNA$^{Leu(UUR)}$ function.[44] This probably reflects a destabilizing effect of the mutation on the tertiary structure of the tRNA, although detailed structural studies have, rather remarkably, not been reported. Abnormal folding probably affects tRNA processing, tRNA turnover, aminoacylation, base modification and perhaps even interaction with the ribosome.

In both 143B osteosarcoma[39–41] and A549 lung carcinoma cybrids,[12] the A3243G mutation manifests a clear threshold effect related to the heteroplasmy level, which is also modulated in individual cell lines by mtDNA copy number.[45] Below approximately 70 per cent mutant mtDNA there is little effect on mitochondrial function, but even up to 90 per cent mutant mtDNA only a mild deficiency of Complex I activity is evident.[40] Above the 90 per cent level oxygen consumption falls sharply, and there is a clear quantitative effect on mitochondrial protein synthesis, as well as reported abnormalities in the pattern of translation products, most clearly affecting one polypeptide,[40] provisionally identified as ND6. Finally, at mutant levels of 98 per cent or above, mitochondrial protein synthesis typically is severely impaired, and mitochondrial redox complexes containing mtDNA-encoded subunits are no longer assembled. However, some cybrid cell lines with very high levels of mutant mtDNA retain significant mitochondrial protein synthesis activity,[46] perhaps indicating the possibility that some compensatory mechanism may, in some instances, be inducible.

Shortly after its discovery, it was noticed that the A3243G mutation falls within the tridecamer sequence that serves as a binding site for the mitochondrial transcriptional terminator mTERF.[47] The precise physiological role of mTERF is not completely clear, but *in vitro* its binding serves to block onward transcription initiated at the upstream of the two mapped promoters of the heavy strand.[48] This seems to make sense as a mechanism for restricting the transcriptional event to just the rRNA genes (plus two tRNAs, phenylalanine and valine).

The rRNAs are needed in much larger quantities than the mRNAs and tRNAs encoded on the remainder of the heavy-strand transcription unit (see Chapter 2). Exactly how this functions *in vivo*, and how it relates to the use of the two alternate promoters of the heavy strand, remains unclear. However, *in vitro*, the A3243 mutation impairs transcriptional termination within the tRNA[Leu(UUR)] gene.[47] This has given rise to many speculations on the significance of this *in vivo*, although there is no evidence that the ratio of rRNAs to mRNAs in mitochondria of A3243G patients is abnormal in patients or even in cybrids.[41] Moreover, the pattern of protein binding around the transcription termination site appears to be completely unaffected by the mutation[49] in 143B osteosarcoma cybrids. Once again, the question arises of whether such findings in cybrids are generalizable to other cell types. Some other mutations in tRNA[Leu(UUR)] with a clinical phenotype that overlaps that of A3243G fall outside of the mTERF binding site, although it has been suggested that mTERF may require accessory factors for activity, and these other mutations may affect their interaction with the mtDNA.

The biosynthesis and/or stability of A3243G mutant tRNA[Leu(UUR)] are abnormal in a variety of cell backgrounds, as well as *in vivo*. The steady-state abundance of the mutant tRNA is up to four-fold depressed in A549 lung carcinoma cybrids,[12] and is also typically very low in 143B osteosarcoma,[49,50] though apparently not in HeLa cell[51] cybrids. *In vivo*, there is more variability,[35] although the effect is usually in the same direction. A proposed RNA processing intermediate, comprising tRNA[Leu(UUR)] still joined to the immediately upstream (16S rRNA) and downstream (ND1) transcripts, and designated 'RNA 19', accumulates in most cybrid cells containing A3243G mutant mtDNA.[12,52] This also applies to cybrids containing mtDNA with the mutations T3271C[39] or A3302G,[53] in the latter case accompanied by increased levels of other RNA processing intermediates in a tissue-specific fashion. Such findings raise the possibility that the mutation interferes with RNA maturation, although significant accumulation of RNA 19 is not obvious in all cases, therefore it could be a secondary effect, or potentially mitigated by a compensatory response. The accumulation of RNA 19 suggested a possible gain of function mechanism whereby the precursor-like transcript may compete with *bona fide* ND1 (or other) mRNA(s) for ribosomes and/or translation factors.[52] In support of this, Complex I activity and also the synthesis of specific ND subunits, including ND1, are affected at mutant levels that do not cause a complete loss of mitochondrial protein synthesis, yet nevertheless are well above the threshold for pathogenicity in patients.[40]

Similarly conflicting data have emerged from studies of tRNA[Leu(UUR)] aminoacylation in different cell backgrounds. In A549 lung carcinoma cybrids, almost no aminoacylated mutant tRNA can be detected,[54] whereas 143B cybrids with almost 100 per cent mutant mtDNA do contain at least some aminoacylated product.[49] In HeLa cell cybrids, aminoacylation, like the overall steady-state level of tRNA[Leu(UUR)] seem only slightly affected by the mutation.[51]

A straightforward loss of function hypothesis to account for the pathological effects of the A3243G mutation is strongly supported by the fact that in the A549 lung carcinoma background, heteroplasmy for an anticodon mutation in tRNA[Leu(CUN)], G12300A, predicted to create a novel suppressor tRNA capable of decoding the UUR codon group, restores mitochondrial protein synthesis and respiratory function to cells that are close to 100 per cent for A3243G mutant mtDNA. This restoration of phenotype can be serially passaged with mtDNA, by cybrid transfer into the same cell background. However, the situation appears less clear cut when the same mtDNA is passaged by cybridization into the 143B osteosarcoma cell background, which gives an intermediate respiratory phenotype (N Hance, SK Lehtinen,

HT Jacobs, and IJ Holt, unpublished data). Whilst this might be due to some defect in the maturation of the suppressor tRNA in the 143B cell background, the finding hints that the effects of the mutation on protein synthesis and respiratory function may not be purely attributable to loss of functional tRNA[Leu(UUR)], and could involve, for example, codon misreading by the low proportion of tRNA[Leu(UUR)] that is aminoacylated in this cell background.

A simple deficiency of UUR decoding capacity may not be the whole story even in A549 cybrids. In cybrid cells with 95 per cent mutant mtDNA, oxygen consumption is only approximately 25 per cent that in control cybrids, but the amount of mitochondrial translation products accumulated in a 60 min period of labelling with ^{35}S-methionine is almost the same as in control cells, with only very minor quantitative abnormalities. During shorter labelling times, there does, however, appear to be some decrease in the amount of label incorporated in mutant compared with control cells (El Meziane *et al.*, 1998*a* and M Lehtola, SK Lehtinen and HT Jacobs, unpublished data). One possibility is that the translation products made are structurally abnormal, that is, contain misincorporated amino acids, or that the assembly of functional redox complexes is in some way linked directly to the rate of translation. Support for the concept of structurally aberrant translation products comes from studies of patient-derived lymphoblastoid cells carrying 70 per cent A3243G mutant mtDNA, where the amount of incorporation of leucine was decreased compared with control cells.[55] This would imply that a deficiency of UUR decoding capacity could lead to the insertion of other amino acids at these codon positions.

Studies of tRNA base modification have suggested just the opposite, namely that, exactly as for the A8344G mutation, the A3243G mutation results in a failure of wobble-base U hypermodification,[51] which could potentially result in misreading of UUY phenylalanine codons as leucine. The same defect is apparent in A549 lung carcinoma cell cybrids (T Yasukawa, personal communication), but here would be arguably less damaging, since the mutant tRNA is only very poorly aminoacylated. In a similar study, the wobble-base defect was not detected in 143B osteosarcoma cybrids:[56] instead, a quantitative deficiency of methylation of a G residue in the D-arm of the tRNA, of unknown functional significance, was found.[56] Failure of wobble-base hypermodification in HeLa cell cybrids has also been found for the tRNA[Leu(UUR)] mutation T3271C.[51]

The tRNA[Ser(UCN)] mutations

Compared with the A3243G and A8344G mutations, those affecting tRNA[Ser(UCN)] are associated with mainly very mild clinical phenotypes, and commonly are homoplasmic. Their effects on cellular phenotype are correspondingly modest, perhaps not surprising in view of the fact that *in vivo* they mainly affect only the auditory system. The basis of this tissue specificity is not understood. In cultured cells, homoplasmy for either the A7445G or 7472insC mutations typically causes only a very slight growth impairment on selective media, with respiratory enzyme activities hardly different from control cells.[57–60] However, in some nuclear or mitochondrial genetic backgrounds, a more pronounced biochemical phenotype is evident.[61,62] As already noted in the case of the A3243G mutation, a relatively low mtDNA copy number can exacerbate the biochemical phenotype in osteosarcoma cybrids bearing the 7472insC mutation.[57]

At the molecular level, the A7445G mutation is probably the best understood. Because the mutation lies 1 bp 3′ to the tRNA coding sequence, it cannot directly or primarily affect the stability, aminoacylation capacity or translational properties of the tRNA itself. Instead, it seems to affect pre-tRNA processing.[59,61] resulting in a drop in the steady-state level of tRNA$^{Ser(UCN)}$ of approximately 60–65 per cent, and giving rise to a modest but variable translational defect. This variability seems to be correlated with clinical severity, being most pronounced in mutant cells derived from families having many severely affected members. This has been suggested to result from mtDNA haplotype (i.e. the spectrum of other sequence polymorphisms carried in mtDNA from the given family), although nuclear background could also play a role.[61] On the other strand, the mutation effects a silent change in the COXI stop codon, but there is no evidence for any effects on COXI mRNA or its translation. The tRNA processing defect also affects the steady-state level of ND6 mRNA which, like tRNA$^{Ser(UCN)}$, is encoded on the light-strand of mtDNA. It is believed that the two transcripts are generated via a common processing pathway with which the mutation somehow interferes. The clinical significance, if any, of this ND6 mRNA deficiency is unclear.

Another deafness-associated tRNA$^{Ser(UCN)}$ mutation, 7472insC, also entrains a 65 per cent drop in the steady-state level of the tRNA, but again this results in only a very modest, quantitative defect in protein synthesis, in this case with no significant effect on ND6 mRNA processing.[57] One suggested reason for the decrease in the level of tRNA$^{Ser(UCN)}$ in 7472insC mutant cells is that the mutation, which introduces an extra nucleotide into the T-arm of the tRNA, might alter its structure in a way that impairs its half-life.[57] However, more recent data indicate that a synthesis defect, rather than reduced half-life, underlies the decreased steady-state level of tRNA$^{Ser(UCN)}$ (M Toompuu and HT Jacobs, unpublished data)

Aminoacylation by serine is not drastically impaired,[57] although sensitive assays indicate that it is diminished by approximately 25 per cent (M Toompuu and HT Jacobs, unpublished data). Furthermore, no differences can be detected in the pattern of base modification of the mutant tRNA. One possibility is that the specific effect of A7445G on ND6 mRNA is somehow associated with the palmoplantar keratoderma that is apparently a unique feature of its clinical phenotype. Obviously, similar studies on other tRNA$^{Ser(UCN)}$ mutations will help clarify some of these issues.

The A1555G mutation in 12S rRNA

The clinical interaction of this mutation with aminoglycoside antibiotics is mirrored in lymphoblastoid cell lines derived from patients,[63] as well as in HeLa cell cybrids containing patient-derived mtDNA,[64] which are rendered hypersensitive to streptomycin. Although studies of mitochondrial protein synthesis in mutant cells have revealed no obvious abnormalities, a reasonable hypothesis is that the combination of the mutation and the drug impair the fidelity of mitochondrial translation, as is known to occur in bacteria, whose SSU rRNAs are structurally more similar to the mutant than to wild-type 12S rRNA. The reason why this leads to such a tissue-specific phenotype remains unknown.

There has been much speculation that individuals with the A1555G mutation who develop hearing loss without any known treatment with aminoglycosides may be susceptible because of their nuclear genotype.[24] Studies in 143B osteosarcoma cell cybrids strongly support this: mutant cybrids are growth impaired on galactose medium, which selects for respiratory competence, regardless of whether the mitochondrial donor cell line itself was susceptible.[65] In contrast, the degree to which donor cell lines are phenotypically affected appears to depend on whether the individual from whom they were derived was clinically affected.[63]

There are several candidate genes for such an effect, since the conserved accuracy centre of the ribosome includes not only the domain of SSU rRNA to which np 1555 maps, but also three relatively well conserved ribosomal proteins, designated S12, S4, and S5 in bacteria. These are relatively unusual amongst ribosomal proteins, in having rather clear orthologues in mitochondria. Most mitoribosomal proteins bear little or no structural resemblance to those of eubacteria,[66] see Chapter 2). In bacteria, mutations in S12 commonly result in amino-glycoside resistance associated with more stringent translation,[67] whereas mutations in S4 and S5 have the opposite effect, and promote enhanced ribosomal ambiguity.[68,69]

The human gene for mitoribosomal protein S12 (*RPMS*12) has been characterized[70,71] and its coding region analysed in 15 patients and unaffected relatives having the A1555G mutation. No differences were seen (V Migliosi, ZH Shah and HT Jacobs, unpublished data). Therefore, if *RPMS*12 is really involved in modifying the A1555G phenotype it must be via the unlikely route of a regulatory mutation that has yet to be identified. S4 and S5 remain candidates.

Concluding remarks

Mitochondrial DNA sequence diversity in the human population is considerable. Until recently, the prevailing view has been that this variation is selectively neutral, and that it only impinges on phenotype via rare but drastic mutations that cause a clear pathological state. However, more attention should be paid to possibly 'sub-clinical' phenotypic manifestations of mtDNA variation, that could affect virtually any tissue. Overt phenotypes may only manifest in combination with specific nutritional or other environmental factors, the A1555G mutation providing an obvious paradigm. Nuclear background could be another important determinant, the studies with the A3243G mutation being highly suggestive of this. Even without such precipitating factors, mtDNA variation could have a significant influence on development, since it is already clear that the amount and quality of mitochondrial protein synthesis can have important and complex effects on model organisms. Even if these effects are sometimes subtle, they may represent a pool of genetic variation whose importance in phenotypic outcome may be comparable with variation in the much larger nuclear genome.

Acknowledgements

I thank the members of my lab for permission to quote their unpublished findings, and for their many contributions to the ideas set out here. My research is supported by funding from the Academy of Finland, Tampere University Hospital Medical Research Fund, and the European Union.

References

1. Anderson S, Bankier AT, Barrell BG, de Bruijn MH, Coulson AR, Drouin J, Eperon IC, Nierlich DP, Roe BA, Sanger F, Schreier PH, Smith AJ, Staden R, and Young IG (1981). Sequence and organization of the human mitochondrial genome. *Nature* **290**: 457–465.
2. MITOMAP (2001). A Human Mitochondrial Genome Database. Center for Molecular Medicine, Emory University, Atlanta, GA, USA. http://www.gen.emory.edu/mitomap.html

3. Sternberg D, Chatzoglou E, Laforet P, Fayet G, Jardel C, Blondy P, Fardeau M, Amselem S, Eymard B, and Lombes A (2001). Mitochondrial DNA transfer RNA gene sequence variations in patients with mitochondrial disorders. *Brain* 124: 984–994.

4. Moraes CT, Ciacci F, Bonilla E, Jansen C, Hirano M, Rao N, Lovelace RE, Rowland LP, Schon EA, and DiMauro S (1993*a*). Two novel pathogenic mitochondrial DNA mutations affecting organelle number and protein synthesis. *J. Clin. Invest.* 92: 2906–2915.

5. Moraes CT, Ciacci F, Silvestri G, Shanske S, Sciacco M, Hirano M, Schon EA, Bonilla E, and DiMauro S (1993*b*). Atypical clinical presentations associated with the MELAS mutation at position 3243 of human mitochondrial DNA. *Neuromusc. Disord.* 3: 43–50.

6. Chinnery PF, Howell N, Lightowlers RN, and Turnbull DM (1998). MELAS and MERRF. The relationship between maternal mutation load and the frequency of clinically affected offspring. *Brain* 121: 1889–1894.

7. Shoffner JM, Lott MT, Lezza AM, Seibel P, Ballinger SW, and Wallace DC (1990). Myoclonic epilepsy and ragged-red fiber disease (MERRF) is associated with a mitochondrial DNA tRNA(Lys) mutation. *Cell.* 61: 931–937.

8. Silvestri G, Moraes CT, Shanske S, Oh SJ, and DiMauro S (1992). A new mtDNA mutation in the tRNA(Lys) gene associated with myoclonic epilepsy and ragged-red fibers (MERRF). *Am. J. Hum. Genet.* 51: 1213–1217.

9. Goto Y, Nonaka I, and Horai S (1990). A mutation in the tRNA(Leu)(UUR) gene associated with the MELAS subgroup of mitochondrial encephalomyopathies. *Nature.* 348: 651–653.

10. Majamaa K, Moilanen JS, Uimonen S, Remes AM, Salmela PI, Karppa M, Majamaa-Voltti KA, Rusanen H, Sorri M, Peuhkurinen KJ, and Hassinen IE (1998). Epidemiology of A3243G, the mutation for mitochondrial encephalomyopathy, lactic acidosis, and strokelike episodes: prevalence of the mutation in an adult population. *Am. J. Hum. Genet.* 63: 447–454.

11. van den Ouweland JM, Lemkes HH, Ruitenbeek W, Sandkuijl LA, de Vijlder MF, Struyvenberg PA, van de Kamp JJ, and Maassen JA (1992). Mutation in mitochondrial tRNA(Leu)(UUR) gene in a large pedigree with maternally transmitted type II diabetes mellitus and deafness. *Nat. Genet.* 1: 368–371.

12. El Meziane A, Lehtinen S, Hance N, Nijtmans LGJ, Dunbar D, Holt IJ, and Jacobs HT (1998*a*). A tRNA suppressor mutation in human mitochondria. *Nat. Genet.* 18: 350–353.

13. Dunbar DR, Moonie PA, Jacobs HT, and Holt IJ (1995). Different cellular backgrounds confer a marked advantage to either mutant or wild-type mitochondrial genomes. *Proc. Natl Acad. Sci. USA* 92: 6562–6566.

14. Silvestri G, Rana M, Odoardi F, Modoni A, Paris E, Papacci M, Tonali P, and Servidei S (2000). Single-fiber PCR in MELAS(3243) patients: correlations between intratissue distribution and phenotypic expression of the mtDNA(A3243G) genotype. *Am. J. Med. Genet.* 94: 201–206.

15. Ozawa M, Nonaka I, and Goto Y (1998). Single muscle fiber analysis in patients with 3243 mutation in mitochondrial DNA: comparison with the phenotype and the proportion of mutant genome. *J. Neurol. Sci.* 159: 170–175.

16. Chinnery PF, Howell N, Lightowlers RN, and Turnbull DM (1997). Molecular pathology of MELAS and MERRF. The relationship between mutation load and clinical phenotypes. *Brain* 120: 1713–1721.

17. Chinnery PF, Zwijnenburg PJ, Walker M, Howell N, Taylor RW, Lightowlers RN, Bindoff L, and Turnbull DM (1999). Nonrandom tissue distribution of mutant mtDNA. *Am. J. Med. Genet.* 85: 498–501.

18. Bakker A, Barthelemy C, Frachon P, Chateau D, Sternberg D, Mazat JP, and Lombes A (2000). Functional mitochondrial heterogeneity in heteroplasmic cells carrying the mitochondrial DNA mutation associated with the MELAS syndrome (mitochondrial encephalopathy, lactic acidosis, and strokelike episodes). *Pediatr. Res.* 48: 143–150.

19. Prezant TR, Agapian JV, Bohlman MC, Bu XD, Ötzas S, Qiu WQ, Arnos KS, Cortopassi GA, Jaber L, Rotter JI, Shohat M, and Fischel-Ghodsian N (1993). Mitochondrial ribosomal RNA

mutation associated with both antibiotic-induced and non-syndromic deafness. *Nat. Genet.* **4**: 289–294.

20. Casano RA, Johnson DF, Bykhovskaya Y, Torricelli F, Bigozzi M, and Fischel-Ghodsian N (1998). Inherited susceptibility to aminoglycoside ototoxicity: genetic heterogeneity and clinical implications. *Am. J. Otolaryngol.* **20**: 151–156.

21. Hutchin T, Haworth I, Higashi K, Fischel-Ghodsian N, Stoneking M, Saha N, Arnos C, and Cortopassi G (1993). A molecular basis for human hypersensitivity to aminoglycoside antibiotics. *Nucleic Acids Res.* **21**: 4174–4179.

22. Mathijs G, Claes S, Longo-Mbenza B, and Cassiman JJ (1996). Non-syndromic deafness associated with a mutation and a polymorphism in the mitochondrial 12S ribosomal RNA gene in a large Zairean pedigree. *Eur. J. Hum. Genet.* **4**: 46–51.

23. Estivill X, Govea N, Barcelo E, Badenas C, Romero E, Moral L, Scozzri R, D'Urbano L, Zeviani M, and Torroni A (1998). Familial progressive Sensorineural deafness is mainly due to the mtDNA A1555G mutation and is enhanced by treatment with aminoglycosides. *Am. J. Hum. Genet.* **62**: 27–35.

24. Bykhovskaya Y, Yang H, Taylor K, Hang T, Tun RY, Estivill X, Casano RA, Majamaa K, Shohat M, and Fischel-Ghodsian N (2001). Modifier locus for mitochondrial DNA disease: linkage and linkage disequilibrium mapping of a nuclear modifier gene for maternally inherited deafness. *Genet. Med.* **3**: 177–180.

25. Melberg A, Akerlund P, Raininko R, Silander HC, Wibom R, Khaled A, Nennesmo I, Lundberg PO, and Olsson Y (1996). Monozygotic twins with MELAS-like syndrome lacking ragged-red fibers and lactacidaemia. *Acta Neurol. Scand.* **94**: 233–241.

26. Van Camp G and Smith RJH (2001). Hereditary Hearing Loss Homepage. Department of Medical Genetics, University of Antwerp, Belgium. http://www.uia.ac.be/dnalab/hhh

27. King MP and Attardi G (1996). Mitochondria-mediated transformation of human rho(0) cells. *Methods Enzymol.* **264**: 313–334.

28. Holme E, Larsson NG, Oldfors A, Tulinius M, Sahlin P, and Stenman G (1993). Multiple symmetric lipomas with high levels of mtDNA with the tRNA(Lys) AG(8344) mutation as the only manifestation of disease in a carrier of myoclonus epilepsy and ragged-red fibers (MERRF) syndrome. *Am. J. Hum. Genet.* **52**: 551–556.

29. Masucci JP, Schon EA, and King MP (1997). Point mutations in the mitochondrial tRNA(Lys) gene: implications for pathogenesis and mechanism. *Mol. Cell. Biochem.* **174**: 215–219.

30. Gamez J, Playan A, Andreu AL, Bruno C, Navarro C, Cervera C, Arbos MA, Schwartz S, Enriquez JA, and Montoya (1998). Familial multiple symmetric lipomatosis associated with the A8344G mutation of mitochondrial DNA. *Neurology* **51**: 258–260.

31. Moslemi AR, Tulinius M, Holme E, and Oldfors A (1998). Threshold expression of the tRNA(Lys) A8344G mutation in single muscle fibres. *Neuromusc. Dis.* **8**: 345–349.

32. Hanna MG, Nelson IP, Morgan-Hughes JA, Harding AE (1995). Impaired mitochondrial translation in human myoblasts harbouring the mitochondrial DNA tRNA lysine 8344 A–>G (MERRF) mutation: relationship to proportion of mutant mitochondrial DNA. *J. Neurol. Sci.* **130**: 154–160.

33. Yoneda M, Miyatake T, and Attardi G (1994). Complementation of mutant and wild-type human mitochondrial DNAs coexisting since the mutation event and lack of complementation of DNAs introduced separately into a cell within distinct organelles. *Mol. Cell. Biol.* **14**: 2699–2712.

34. Enriquez JA, Chomyn A, and Attardi G (1995). MtDNA mutation in MERRF syndrome causes defective aminoacylation of tRNA(Lys) and premature translation termination. *Nat. Genet.* **10**: 47–55.

35. Börner GV, Zeviani M, Tiranti V, Carrara F, Hoffmann S, Gerbitz KD, Lochmuller H, Pongratz D, Klopstock T, Melberg A, Holme E, and Pääbo S (2000). Decreased aminoacylation of mutant tRNAs in MELAS but not in MERRF patients. *Hum. Mol. Genet.* **9**: 467–475.

36. Yasukawa T, Suzuki T, Ishii N, Ueda T, Ohta S, and Watanabe K (2000*a*). Defect in modification at the anticodon wobble nucleotide of mitochondrial tRNA(Lys) with the MERRF encephalomyopathy pathogenic mutation. *FEBS Lett.* **467**: 175–178.

37. Yasukawa T, Suzuki T, Ishii N, Ohta S, and Watanabe K (2001). Wobble modification defect in tRNA disturbs codon-anticodon interaction in a mitochondrial disease. *EMBO J.* **20**: 4794–4802.

38. Laforet P, Ziegler F, Sternberg D, Rouche A, Frachon P, Fardeau M, Eymard B, and Lombes A (2001). 'MELAS' (A3243G) mutation of mitochondrial DNA: a study of the relationships between the clinical phenotype in 19 patients and morphological and molecular data. *Rev. Neurol.* **156**: 1136–1147.

39. Koga Y, Davidson M, Schon EA, and King MP (1995). Analysis of cybrids harboring MELAS mutations in the mitochondrial tRNA(Leu(UUR)) gene. *Muscle Nerve.* **3**: S119–S123.

40. Dunbar DR, Moonie PA, Zeviani M, and Holt IJ (1996). Complex I deficiency is associated with 3243G:C mitochondrial DNA in osteosarcoma cell cybrids. *Hum Mol Genet.* **5**: 123–129.

41. Chomyn A, Martinuzzi A, Yoneda M, Daga A, Hurko O, Johns D, Lai ST, Nonaka I, Angelini C, and Attardi G (1992). MELAS mutation in mtDNA binding site for transcription termination factor causes defects in protein synthesis and in respiration but no change in levels of upstream and downstream mature transcripts. *Proc. Natl Acad. Sci. USA* **89**: 4221–4225.

42. Dubeau F, De Stefano N, Zifkin BG, Arnold DL, and Shoubridge EA (2000). Oxidative phosphorylation defect in the brains of carriers of the tRNAleu(UUR) A3243G mutation in a MELAS pedigree. *Ann. Neurol.* **47**: 179–185.

43. James AM, Sheard PW, Wei YH, and Murphy MP (1999). Decreased ATP synthesis is phenotypically expressed during increased energy demand in fibroblasts containing mitochondrial tRNA mutations. *Eur. J. Biochem*: **259**: 462–469.

44. Jacobs HT and Holt IJ (2000). The np 3243 MELAS mutation: damned if you aminoacylate, damned if you don't. *Hum. Mol. Genet.* **9**: 463–465.

45. Bentlage HA and Attardi G (1996). Relationship of genotype to phenotype in fibroblast-derived transmitochondrial cell lines carrying the 3243 mutation associated with the MELAS encephalomyopathy: shift towards mutant genotype and role of mtDNA copy number. *Hum. Mol. Genet.* **5**: 197–205.

46. Janssen GM, Maassen JA, and van Den Ouweland JM (1999). The diabetes-associated 3243 mutation in the mitochondrial tRNA(Leu(UUR)) gene causes severe mitochondrial dysfunction without a strong decrease in protein synthesis rate. *J. Biol. Chem.* **274**: 29744–29748.

47. Hess JF, Parisi MA, Bennett JL, and Clayton DA (1991). Impairment of mitochondrial transcription termination by a point mutation associated with the MELAS subgroup of mitochondrial encephalomyopathies. *Nature* **351**: 236–239.

48. Kruse B, Narasimhan N, and Attardi G (1989). Termination of transcription in human mitochondria: identification and purification of a DNA binding protein factor that promotes termination. *Cell* **58**: 391–397.

49. Chomyn A, Enriquez JA, Micol V, Fernandez-Silva P, and Attardi G (2000). The mitochondrial myopathy, encephalopathy, lactic acidosis, and stroke-like episode syndrome-associated human mitochondrial tRNALeu(UUR) mutation causes aminoacylation deficiency and concomitant reduced association of mRNA with ribosomes. *J. Biol. Chem.* **275**: 19198–19209.

50. Hayashi J, Ohta S, Takai D, Miyabayashi S, Sakuta R, Goto Y, and Nonaka I (1993). Accumulation of mtDNA with a mutation at position 3271 in tRNA(Leu)(UUR) gene introduced from a MELAS patient to HeLa cells lacking mtDNA results in progressive inhibition of mitochondrial respiratory function. *Biochem. Biophys. Res. Commun.* **197**: 1049–1055.

51. Yasukawa T, Suzuki T, Ueda T, Ohta S, and Watanabe K (2000b). Modification defect at anticodon wobble nucleotide of mitochondrial tRNAs(Leu)(UUR) with pathogenic mutations of mitochondrial myopathy, encephalopathy, lactic acidosis, and stroke-like episodes. *J. Biol. Chem.* **275**: 4251–4257.

52. Schon EA, Koga Y, Davidson M, Moraes CT, and King MP (1992). The mitochondrial tRNA(Leu(UUR)) mutation in MELAS: a model for pathogenesis. *Biochim. Biophys. Acta* **1101**: 206–209.

53. Bindoff LA, Howell N, Poulton J, McCullough DA, Morten KJ, Lightowlers RN, Turnbull DM, and Weber K (1993). Abnormal RNA processing associated with a novel tRNA mutation in mitochondrial DNA. A potential disease mechanism. *J. Biol. Chem.* **268**: 19559–19564.

54. El Meziane A, Lehtinen SK, Holt IJ, and Jacobs HT (1998*b*). Mitochondrial tRNALeu isoforms in lung carcinoma cybrid cells containing the np 3243 mtDNA mutation. *Hum. Mol. Genet.* **7**: 2141–2147.

55. Flierl A, Reichmann H, and Seibel P (1997). Pathophysiology of the MELAS 3243 transition mutation. *J. Biol. Chem.* **272**: 27189–27196.

56. Helm M, Florentz C, Chomyn A, and Attardi G (1999). Search for differences in post-transcriptional modification patterns of mitochondrial DNA-encoded wild-type and mutant human tRNALys and tRNALeu(UUR). *Nucleic Acids Res.* **27**: 756–763.

57. Toompuu M, Tiranti V, Zeviani M, and Jacobs HT (1999). Molecular phenotype of the np 7472 deafness-associated mitochondrial mutation in osteosarcoma cell cybrids. *Hum. Mol. Genet.* **8**: 2275–2283.

58. Tiranti V, Chariot P, Carella F, Toscano A, Soliveri P, Girlanda P, Carrara F, Fratta GM, Reid FM, Mariotti C, and Zeviani M (1995). Maternally inherited hearing loss, ataxia and myoclonus associated with a novel point mutation in mitochondrial tRNASer(UCN) gene. *Hum. Mol. Genet.* **4**: 1421–1427.

59. Reid FM, Rovio A, Holt IJ, and Jacobs HT (1997). Molecular phenotype of a human lymphoblastoid cell-line homoplasmic for the np 7445 deafness-associated mitochondrial mutation. *Hum. Mol. Genet.* **6**: 443–449.

60. Hyslop SJ, James AM, Maw M, Fischel-Ghodsian N, and Murphy MP (1997). The effect on mitochondrial function of the tRNA Ser(UCN)/COI A7445G mtDNA point mutation associated with maternally-inherited sensorineural deafness. *Biochem. Mol. Biol. Int.* **42**: 567–575.

61. Guan MX, Enriquez JA, Fischel-Ghodsian N, Puranam RS, Lin CP, Maw MA, and Attardi G (1998). The deafness-associated mitochondrial DNA mutation at position 7445, which affects tRNASer(UCN) precursor processing, has long-range effects on NADH dehydrogenase subunit ND6 gene expression. *Mol. Cell. Biol.* **18**: 5868–5879.

62. Jaksch M, Klopstock T, Kurlemann G, Dorner M, Hofmann S, Kleinle S, Hegemann S, Weissert M, Muller-Hocker J, Pongratz D, and Gerbitz KD (1998). Progressive myoclonus epilepsy and mitochondrial myopathy associated with mutations in the tRNA(Ser(UCN)) gene. *Ann. Neurol.* **44**: 635–640.

63. Guan MX, Fischel-Ghodsian N, and Attardi G (1996). Biochemical evidence for nuclear gene involvement in phenotype of non-syndromic deafness associated with mitochondrial 12S rRNA mutation. *Hum. Mol. Genet.* **5**: 963–971.

64. Inoue K, Takai D, Soejima A, Isobe K, Yamasoba T, Oka Y, Goto Y, and Hayashi J (1996). Mutant mtDNA at 1555 A to G in 12S rRNA gene and hypersusceptibility of mitochondrial translation to streptomycin can be co-transferred to rho⁰ HeLa cells. *Biochem. Biophys. Res. Commun.* **223**: 496–501.

65. Guan MX, Fischel-Ghodsian N, and Attardi G (2001). Nuclear background determines biochemical phenotype in the deafness-associated mitochondrial 12S rRNA mutation. *Hum Mol Genet.* **10**: 573–580.

66. O'Brien TW, Liu J, Sylvester JE, Mougey EB, Fischel-Ghodsian N, Thiede B, Wittmann-Liebold B, and Graack HR (2000). Mammalian mitochondrial ribosomal proteins (4). Amino acid sequencing, characterization, and identification of corresponding gene sequences. *J. Biol. Chem.* **275**: 18153–18159.

67. Timms AR and Bridges BA (1993). Double, independent mutational events in the rpsL gene of Escherichia coli: an example of hypermutability? *Mol. Microbiol.* **9**: 335–342.

68. Piepersberg W, Noseda V, and Bock A (1979). Bacterial ribosomes with two ambiguity mutations: effects of translational fidelity, on the response to aminoglycosides and on the rate of protein synthesis. *Mol. Gen. Genet.* **171**: 23–34.

69. Alksne LE, Anthony RA, Liebman SW, and Warner JR (1993). An accuracy center in the ribosome conserved over 2 billion years. *Proc. Natl Acad. Sci. USA* **90**: 9538–9541.

70. Shah ZH, O'Dell K, Miller SCM, An X, and Jacobs, HT (1997). Metazoan nuclear genes for mito-ribosmal protein S12. *Gene* **204**: 55–62.

71. Spirina O, Bykhovskaya Y, Kajava AV, O'Brien TW, Nierlich DP, Mougey EB, Sylvester JE, Graack HR, Wittmann-Liebold B, and Fischel-Ghodsian N (2000). Heart-specific splice-variant of a human mitochondrial ribosomal protein (mRNA processing; tissue specific splicing). *Gene* **261**: 229–234.

8 Pathogenic mitochondrial DNA mutations in genes that encode respiratory chain subunits

Neil Howell

Introduction

It has been 20 years since the publication of the sequence of the human mitochondrial genome[1] and more than 10 years since the 'dawn' of studies on mitochondrial genetic diseases. With regard to the topic of this review, pathogenic mtDNA mutations in protein-encoding genes, 'volume' has greatly exceeded 'space'. This is not a physical riddle, but the welcome reality of the current state of research. That is, the literature on such mtDNA mutations is now so large (and getting larger), that no single review of reasonable length can adequately summarize and critically evaluate the results. Therefore, this review must of necessity offer a somewhat skewed appraisal of this area. With that constraint in mind, the main topic of this review is Leber's hereditary optic neuropathy (LHON), the obvious choice for someone who has been investigating this mitochondrial disease for more than a decade. Beyond the advantage of familiarity, there are other reasons for this choice. LHON is probably the most prevalent mitochondrial disease (leaving aside the controversy over whether ageing is—to some extent—a mitochondrial disease). It is arguably the most diligently investigated, so that one has the advantage that there is a substantial body of published work available for summary and analysis.

Despite the high quality and quantity of LHON research, however, there remains much to be learned. One hears at scientific gatherings that LHON is so unusual that it is not a 'typical' mitochondrial disease. This is true in the sense that LHON has some features that are apparently unique, but it is not clear which mitochondrial disease could fulfill that role and each has features that defy easy explanation. Optimistically, those particular features of LHON may provide some insights into other mitochondrial diseases, and I have tried in this review to point out how LHON is relevant to other mitochondrial diseases. This may be one way of saying that everything looks like a nail when the only tool you have is a hammer, but I have endeavoured to keep a broad perspective on mitochondrial diseases. The field of mitochondrial disease research is established in terms of a substantial body of high-quality experimental data, and this knowledge is now being used to guide the next generation of experiments that are aimed at greater insight into molecular pathophysiology and potential therapeutic approaches.

Leber hereditary optic neuropathy (LHON): Mutations in Complex I genes

Clinical and genetic studies of LHON

LHON, as it is now termed, was first reported in detail by Theodor Leber in 1871. Typically, LHON is an acute or subacute loss of central vision, usually painless, that occurs predominantly in young males. Detailed reviews of the pathophysiology, epidemiology, and genetics of LHON are available,[2–6] and the following are some key summary points.

1. Beginning with the LHON pedigrees reported by Leber in 1871,[7] it can be seen that the risk of developing the optic neuropathy shows *maternal* transmission. It is now understood that the primary aetiological event or factor in LHON is a mutation in the maternally inherited mtDNA.

2. The optic neuropathy is due to loss of retinal ganglion cells and degeneration of the optic nerve. It is very likely that the ganglion cells die through a mitochondrial apoptotic pathway, rather than a necrotic one as discussed by Howell.[5] LHON has a very similar clinical presentation to the autosomally inherited optic neuropathies and to the toxic-nutritional amblyopias. LHON involves a preferential loss of P-ganglion cells (those with smaller cell diameters), particularly those that subserve central vision.[8] An optic neuropathy with a similar focal pathology to LHON is also caused, as a side effect, by systemic treatment of humans either with chloramphenicol, an antibacterial agent that also inhibits mitochondrial protein synthesis,[4] or with ethambutol, an antimycobacterial drug. Studies of the effects of ethambutol on rat retinal ganglion cells indicated that the drug acts through a glutamate excitotoxic pathway in which mitochondrial calcium levels are increased and in which there is evidence of decreased mitochondrial respiratory chain function.[9] The authors note that ethambutol causes retinal ganglion cells to be more sensitive to normal levels of glutamate, the principal neurotransmitter of these cells. Taken together, these results indicate that retinal ganglion cell function and/or viability is particularly sensitive to some *specific* pathway or activity of mitochondrial energy metabolism, and not to just any reduction of respiratory chain activity. This specificity is also attested by the observations that, in other mitochondrial diseases, it is the retinal pigmented epithelium that is most often affected.[10]

3. In the vast majority of LHON patients, the optic neuropathy is the sole *clinical* abnormality, although there are indications of elevated frequencies of other neurological deficits, most notably a multiple sclerosis (MS)-like syndrome, among LHON family members. Although one suspects that careful examination would reveal a substantial spectrum of subtle, sub- or preclinical abnormalities, the point remains that the pathology is impressively focal. In this regard, typical or classical LHON is different from other mitochondrial diseases where the types and severities of the abnormalities are broadly heterogeneous.[11] In contrast, there are a small proportion of LHON families in which there are severe abnormalities, such as dystonia or encephalopathy, that overshadow the optic neuropathy.

4. LHON has an incomplete penetrance and most family members remain clinically unaffected throughout life. This characteristic indicates that other aetiological factors—genetic and/or environmental—are involved secondarily to the LHON mtDNA mutation. The characteristic feature of sudden onset suggests that the primary mtDNA mutation causes a compromised energy metabolism in the retinal ganglion cells and optic nerve and that these secondary factors exacerbate metabolism beyond a crisis point where the optic nerve can no longer function and vision is lost. Finally, males are affected approximately 4–5 times more often than females. The obvious explanation for this disparity is an X-linked modifier locus, but the accumulating experimental data argue against this explanation.

Since the identification of the first LHON mutation,[12] hundreds of LHON patients and family members have been analysed to identify the underlying pathogenic mtDNA mutations.

The first point of interest is that LHON mutations occur in mitochondrial genes that encode subunits of Complex I (NADH – ubiquinone oxidoreductase). There may be some rare exceptions, but those results have not been convincing. There is broad agreement that approximately 95 per cent of classic LHON cases result from one of three mtDNA mutations:[13] (i) a G → A transition at nucleotide 3460 that results in the substitution of THR for ALA at amino acid position 52 of the ND1 gene; (ii) a G → A transition at nucleotide 11778 (ND4/ARG340 changed to HIS); and (iii) a T → C transition at nucleotide 14484 (ND6/MET64 changed to VAL). The 11778 LHON mutation is the most prevalent, and it occurs in ~65 per cent of all patients. The 14484 mutation occurs in 15–20 per cent of patients while the 3460 mutation occurs in 10–15 per cent. A number of other mtDNA mutations that cause LHON have been identified: these usually occur in single pedigrees and they also occur in mitochondrial genes that encode Complex I subunits.[14,15] In ~15 per cent of LHON patients, the mtDNA mutation is heteroplasmic (i.e. both wildtype and mutant alleles are present in an individual). As would be expected, the risk of developing the optic neuropathy is related to mutation load, and males with a load of the 11778 LHON mutation in blood of less than 60 per cent have a low risk of vision loss.[16] In this regard, LHON is atypical, because the pathogenic mutation in other mitochondrial diseases is almost invariably heteroplasmic.[11] There are subtle differences among these three LHON mutations in the features of the optic neuropathy, but there is a clear difference in terms of recovery of vision after the acute phase.[17] Recovery of vision is very rare in 11778 LHON patients (on the order of 4 per cent), but it is relatively frequent in 14484 LHON patients (~50 per cent if vision is lost before the age of 30 years). At least in 14484 LHON patients, therefore, there can be a prolonged period of time in which retinal ganglion cells lose function but do not commit to a cell death pathway.

The genetics of the 'LHON plus' families, with their wider array—and greater severity—of clinical abnormalities, has turned out to be more complex. Shoffner *et al.*[18] reported that a G → A mutation at nucleotide 14459 (ND6/ALA72 changed to VAL) caused LHON plus dystonia in three unrelated families. The pathological specificity of this mutation has been challenged by the occurrence of this mutation in two unrelated Australian families who are affected with Leigh syndrome (subacute necrotizing encephalomyopathy) but who have no history of optic neuropathy or dystonia.[19] De Vries *et al.*[20] reported that a large family in which LHON was associated with hereditary spastic dystonia carried a heteroplasmic mutation at nucleotide 11696 (ND4/VAL312 changed to ILE) and a homoplasmic mutation at nucleotide 14596 (ND6/MET26 changed to ILE). Either mutation, or both, may be the primary pathogenic event, but the maternal transmission of the abnormalities is unequivocal so that a mitochondrial genetic aetiology seems certain. The Australian neurologist David Wallace[21] described a family (now designated QLD1) in which the optic neuropathy is overwhelmed by a variety of maternally inherited severe neurological abnormalities, including a fatal infantile encephalopathy. It appears that the optic neuropathy is caused by the 14484 LHON mutation and that the neurological abnormalities are caused by a mutation at nucleotide 4160 (ND1/LEU285 changed to PRO).[22] Determination of the complete mtDNA sequence from the QLD1 LHON pedigree does not reveal any other mutations that are likely to contribute to the complex clinical presentation (N Howell and C Herrnstadt, unpublished data). Finally, mutations at nucleotides 13513 (ND5/ASP393 changed to ASN) and 13514 (ND5/ASP393 changed to GLY) are associated with what is described as a LHON/MELAS overlap syndrome.[23,24] These mutations have been identified in several unrelated individuals and they are usually—but not always—associated with an LHON-like optic neuropathy. The neurological abnormalities are lumped under the term 'MELAS', but they are quite heterogeneous and include bilateral hearing loss, pyramidal signs, memory loss, and muscle atrophy in addition to the characteristic stroke-like episodes.

It was noticed some years ago that certain mtDNA polymorphisms occurred at higher frequency in LHON patients than in normal controls.[25] A plausible explanation has been proposed, but discussion of this phenomenon first requires a few remarks about the evolution of the human mitochondrial genome. Analysis of mtDNAs from any of the three major ethnic groups (Caucasians or Europeans, Asians, and Africans) reveals that the sequences can be phylogenetically grouped according to the presence of a small number of distinctive polymorphisms. For example, there are nine such European *haplogroups* that are easily and unambiguously assigned according to the allele status at a relatively small number of sites (not surprisingly, there are multiple phylogenetic subgroups within each haplogroup that can be discerned with high resolution analysis). The mtDNAs from LHON patients who carry the 3460 mutation have the same distribution among the European haplogroups as do mtDNAs from the general population. In marked contrast, ~75 per cent of the mtDNAs from 14484 LHON pedigrees belong to haplogroup J, although only ~10 per cent of mtDNAs from the general European population belong to this haplogroup.[26,27] There appears to be a preferential association, or haplogroup clustering, of the 11778 LHON mutation with haplogroup J but the effect is quite weak. Phylogenetic analysis of LHON mtDNAs from different pedigrees indicates that a simple 'founder' effect can be ruled out, and the evidence indicates that the 14484 LHON mutation has arisen many times during human evolution (Howell *et al.*[28] N Howell and DA Mackey, unpublished observations). Alternatively, it has been proposed that LHON haplogroup clustering reflects a higher penetrance of the 14484 mutation when it is 'embedded' within a haplogroup J background. Because of the higher penetrance, therefore, there is a biased sampling of individuals who carry LHON mutations: families who carry a LHON mutation, but who lack affected members, will not come to the attention of geneticists. It is presumed that one or more polymorphisms within haplogroup J mtDNAs has a phenotype that increases penetrance of the 14484 LHON mutation (this point is discussed further in the next section). There is no current challenge to the haplogroup clustering of the 14484 LHON mutation, but the penetrance explanation is difficult to prove. Penetrance in LHON pedigrees is a complicated phenomenon and it appears to be influenced by a number of factors (see the discussion by Riordan-Eva *et al.*[12] and Howell[4,5]).

Thus far, it can be concluded that LHON involves the selective loss (or damage) of retinal ganglion cells, and particularly the smaller diameter cells that function in central vision. There are compelling arguments that this group of ganglion cells is highly dependent upon mitochondrial respiratory chain function[8] and that is—in turn—exquisitely vulnerable to conditions that impair function. For example, there is an energetic 'choke point' in the region where the unmyelinated axons sharply bend at the optic nerve head and transverse the lamina cribosa, and one might suppose that even a mild respiratory chain deficit would compromise the function of the optic nerve in this region.[4,5] It is interesting that it is also these ganglion cells that are more susceptible to NMDA-induced excitotoxicity than are the larger diameter ones (the opposite trend occurs for kainate-induced excitotoxicity), although there are no differences in the distribution of glutamate receptors among the retinal ganglion cells.[29] However, this rather simplistic view would predict that optic neuropathy would be the 'lowest common denominator' among mitochondrial diseases, and this is clearly not the case.[11] Instead, it appears that retinal ganglion cells are especially vulnerable to certain types of mitochondrial respiratory chain compromise or insult.

Biochemical studies, structure–function relationships, and LHON

Ten years of biochemical studies have not yet resolved all of the issues that surround the mitochondrial respiratory chain defects produced by LHON mutations (reviewed by Brown[30] and Howell).[5,6] The recent comprehensive analyses of Brown *et al.*[31] yielded results that are in accord with the bulk of earlier biochemical studies and that serve as a good starting point for further discussion. These investigators analysed both lymphoblastoid lines from LHON patients and transmitochondrial cybrid lines to which the mitochondrial LHON mutations had been transferred.[31] Their studies encompassed the three major LHON mutations (those at nucleotides 3460, 11778, and 14484) and they compared the results to those obtained for the 14459 mutation (for which LHON is associated with dystonia). The 14459 mutation caused no measurable defect in the rate of State III mitochondrial respiration; the 14484 mutation produced only a mild defect; and the 3460 and 11778 mutations produced slightly greater defects (~20 per cent in cybrid lines). In contrast, the 14459 and 3460 mutations produced marked reductions (60–70 per cent) in Complex I activity, whereas the 11778 and 14484 mutations caused little, if any, reduction. The 'disconnect' between State III respiration rates and Complex I activities is noteworthy, and it suggests that the latter—at least in these cells— is not rate-limiting for the former.

The mutation equivalent to the 3460 LHON mutation has been introduced into the ND1-encoding gene of *Paracoccus denitrificans*.[32] It was found that the V_{max} for short-chain quinone analogs was decreased ~20 per cent, whereas the K_m values were nearly doubled. Those results, as well as other studies, indicate that the ND1 subunit is involved in the quinone catalytic site of Complex I. Studies of both the 11778 and 14484 LHON mutations also suggest a possible role for these Complex I subunits in quinone/quinol binding and redox catalysis. For example, Carelli *et al.*[33] observed that Complex I activity was normal in 14484 LHON patients, but that the complex was more sensitive to quinol-like inhibitors.

Other studies, however, are not compatible with these findings. For example, Oostra *et al.*[34] found that the 14484 LHON mutation was associated with a 50 per cent reduction in mitochondrial Complex I activity. In order to avoid the problems with isolation and assay of mitochondria, we assayed the lactate : pyruvate ratio in fibroblast cell cultures from normals and from LHON patients (Howell, unpublished data). This ratio is a function of the mitochondrial NAD/NADH ratio and it is thus an indirect, but reliable, assay of mitochondrial respiratory chain function. In these experiments, it was observed that the 11778 LHON mutation was associated with a mild impairment of the respiratory chain, whereas the 14484 mutation was clearly associated with a more severe defect. This is the opposite trend to the biochemical studies, but one must be cautious not to rely too heavily on preliminary results from non-neural cell types. There seems a danger in extrapolating from these systems to the retinal ganglion cells, which—unfortunately—are largely inaccessible to biochemical analysis.

One would have a greater sense of comfort if the *in vitro* biochemical studies were in better agreement with the reports of *in situ* assays of mitochondrial respiratory chain activity (reviewed by Howell).[5] For example, Lodi *et al.*[35] used ^{31}P magnetic resonance spectroscopy to assess energy metabolism in skeletal muscle of LHON patients. In contrast to the biochemical studies of isolated mitochondria, these investigators observed that the maximal rate of ATP synthesis was ~30 per cent of normal during the exercise recovery phase in 11778 LHON patients.[36] Furthermore, the equivalent rate was ~50 per cent in patients who harboured the 14484 LHON mutation, a result that is more compatible with our assays of fibroblast mitochondrial energy metabolism but that differs from the biochemical studies.[31] The most striking result, however, was that the 3460 LHON mutation—despite the consistent finding of a marked Complex I deficiency *in vitro*—was associated with only a mild defect in muscle energy production. Those last results are complemented by the recent study of Cock *et al.*[37] that involve biochemical assays of mitochondrial function in fibroblasts from 3460 LHON patients. As with other studies (see previous discussion), these investigators measured a marked decrease (~60 per cent) in Complex I activity. Their key observation, however, was that there was no significant impairment in ATP production. In contrast, when the assays were repeated with fibroblasts from a patient with mitochondrial cardiomyopathy, there were defects in *both* Complex I activity and ATP production. In addition, it has been reported by Cock *et al.*,[38] on the basis of cybrid fusions to different nuclear genetic donor cells, that the Complex I defect in 3460 was phenotypically suppressed in one nuclear genetic background, but expressed in a different one. As discussed previously, it has been proposed that when the 14484 and—to a lesser extent—11778 LHON mutations occur within a haplogroup J mtDNA, the penetrance of the optic neuropathy is increased. Lodi *et al.*,[36] have recently shown the energetic dysfunction *in vivo* associated with the 11778 LHON mutation is not increased as a function of a haplogroup J background. One awaits similar analyses with the 14484 LHON mutation, which shows the greatest haplogroup clustering. All of these results underscore the fact that the pathophysiology of LHON involves more than a simple respiratory chain defect.

The results of Carelli *et al.*[38] add additional important details. These investigators studied an affected 14484 LHON patient in whom vision improved coincident with treatment with idebenone, a quinone analogue, and vitamin B_{12}. One interesting point is that this patient, before idebenone treatment and 6 months after its discontinuation, had elevated blood lactate after cycloergometer exercise, a result indicative of a defect in mitochondrial energy production. Histological examination of muscle tissue failed to reveal abnormal frequencies of ragged red fibres or cytochrome oxidase-deficient fibres, hallmarks of other mitochondrial diseases. Mitochondrial morphology was also normal, but the authors reported mitochondrial proliferation in this tissue. This last result is particularly intriguing in view of the report by Sadun *et al.*[40] that the ocular muscle of an 11778 LHON patient also showed marked mitochondrial proliferation. It appears that muscle, but not retinal ganglion cells, compensate—or at least attempt to—for the mitochondrial respiratory chain defect in LHON by producing more mitochondria.

It is irrefutable that mutations in at least 3 of the 7 mitochondrially encoded Complex I subunits cause LHON. In contrast to the ND1 and ND4 subunits, which may have only one LHON mutation each (3460 and 11778, respectively), there are multiple LHON mutations in the ND6 gene. In a recent study, Chinnery *et al.*[15] carried out secondary structure modelling of this subunit and they obtained some interesting and potentially important results. It was found that the LHON mutations localized to a specific region of the subunit that involved both a transmembrane hydrophobic cleft or pocket and residues in the adjacent extramembrane hydrophilic loops (Fig. 8.1). It may also be noted that the two mutations, I26M and A72V, for which the LHON is compounded with severe abnormalities putatively map to the hydrophilic loops, whereas the 'LHON only' mutations map to the hydrophobic pocket. This is the first evidence of a relationship between a mitochondrial disease and a specific region of a respiratory chain subunit. Now the question is, what is the function of this region and how does its alteration lead to LHON?

On the basis of the analysis of the ND6 LHON mutations, and of the various biochemical studies, it was suggested[15] that the 3460/ND1, the 11778/ND4, and the ND6 mutations all affect amino acid sequences that constitute a single large quinone redox site within Complex I.

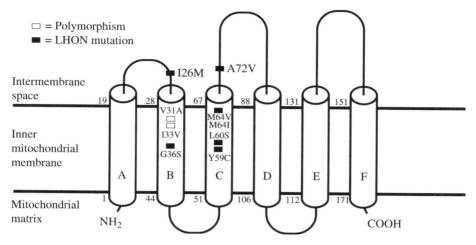

Fig. 8.1 Predicted transmembrane topology of the mitochondrial ND6 subunit of Complex I. The cylinders represent transmembrane helices as predicted with the *TMpred* program. The small filled boxes denote the putative locales of LHON mutations, whereas the two open boxes indicate the amino acid positions altered by polymorphisms occurring in clinically normal individuals (see Chinnery *et al.* for additional details, discussion, and references). [This figure was reprinted from Chinnery *et al.* (2001) with the permission of Oxford University Press.]

While this remains an attractive hypothesis, there are two problems with it. In the first place, it does not account for reports of LHON mutations that map to the ND2 and ND5 subunits.[14,41] The quinone binding region may be large, but it is difficult to imagine that there is a single functional domain that involves the structural interactions of 5 of the 7 mitochondrial subunits. The second concern is prompted by the emerging picture of Complex I structure and function (reviewed by Friedrich).[42] It is now proposed that Complex I is composed of three subcomplexes or modules that are distinct both functionally and structurally (they also appear to have different evolutionary origins that can be traced). The soluble extramembrane NADH dehydrogenase carries out the oxidation of NADH and then transfers the reducing equivalents to a small connecting fragment. The hydrophobic membrane-embedded subcomplex is proposed to have two functional domains, one of which carries out quinone redox reactions that are coupled to proton translocation and a second that carries out conformation-linked proton translocation (thus, there are two putative sites of transmembrane proton translocation in Complex I). The seven mitochondrial subunits localize to this hydrophobic membrane subcomplex. According to this model, the ND1 subunit—along with two nuclear-encoded subunits—is involved in quinone/quinol binding and the ND5 subunit is involved in the redox-linked proton translocation. The ND2 and ND4 subunits are proposed to function in the conformation-linked proton translocation step. Thus, the possibility that LHON mutations affect a single specific step in Complex I function seems to be waning, although the current model[42] will undoubtedly undergo further modification and refinement. It is interesting that it has not yet been possible to determine the structural or functional role of the ND6 subunit, which thus far has defied attempts at isolation with the subcomplexes.[43]

At this point, it is difficult to confidently espouse a simple unified model for the molecular pathophysiology of LHON. The common link among the different LHON mutations, most recently proposed by Brown et al.[14] and Sadun et al.,[8] is that LHON mutations alter Complex I activity in such a way as to increase ROS (reactive oxygen species) production through perturbation of the quinone redox reactions. The increased ROS production would thus lead to oxidative stress, triggering retinal ganglion cell dysfunction and—eventually—cell death. Wong and Cortopassi[44] showed that LHON cybrid cells were more sensitive to killing by ROS, suggesting that their anti-oxidant systems may have been 'overloaded' as a result of the mutations. Klivenyi et al.[45] have recently reported that the concentration of plasma α-tocopherol was reduced in 11778 LHON family members, irrespective of whether they were affected. They suggested that this result reflected increased oxidative stress as a result of the LHON mutation. Finally, an oxidative stress mechanism for LHON suggests an explanation for the predominance of affected males relative to females. It was noted previously that a specific X-linked modifier locus was unlikely. An alternative explanation is that females are less vulnerable to development of the optic neuropathy because of their higher oestrogen levels during the time window when risk is the highest. There is compelling evidence that oestrogen compounds are both neuroprotective and neurotrophic, but—moreover—there is evidence that oestrogens can act on mitochondria to relieve oxidative stress.[46] These results not only point the way to additional avenues of experimental investigation, but they also suggest possible preventive strategies for at-risk LHON family members. With regard to therapy, it is noteworthy that retinal ganglion cell death in glaucoma (the most prevalent eye disease that involves degeneration of the retinal ganglion cells and optic nerve) appears to occur through a mitochondrial apoptotic pathway. The potential of drugs that act on mitochondria and prevent the early steps in the apoptotic cascade for the treatment of glaucoma has been noted.[48]

ADOA and LHON

Autosomal dominant optic atrophy (ADOA) typically presents in childhood with slow bilateral vision loss, optic nerve pallor, colour vision abnormalities, and centrocecal defects in the visual fields.[49] A more recent study by Votruba et al.[50] extends those studies and makes the additional important point that the presentation of the ophthalmological abnormalities is highly variable (even among patients of the same age), a characteristic shared with LHON. The pathology of ADOA, therefore, is very similar to that of LHON, although the latter typically (but not invariantly) has an onset later in life and a vision loss that is asynchronous in a substantial number of cases. In fact, the two disorders can be difficult to distinguish.[51,52] It has recently been shown that a large number of ADOA cases are caused by mutations in the *OPA*1 gene.[52–55] The protein encoded by the *OPA*1 gene appears to be a widely-expressed member of the GTP-binding dynamin family that is particularly abundant in the retina. Most importantly, this protein is localized in the mitochondrion and it may be important for maintenance of structural and genetic integrity on the basis of its possible homology to the yeast *Mgm*1/*Msp*1 proteins.

As discussed above, previous studies have focussed on the nature of the mitochondrial respiratory chain defects caused by LHON mutations. Should the ADOA mutations suggest another avenue for investigation? There is preliminary evidence that the *OPA*1 mutations alter the structure of the mitochondrial reticulum in monocytes, and one would certainly like to know if similar abnormalities are present in the retinal ganglion cells. Thus far, no studies of respiratory chain function in ADOA patients have been carried out, and—conversely—no studies of the mitochondrial reticulum in LHON patients have been performed. It is difficult, at this point, to see any 'connection' between the structural defects of mitochondria in ADOA patients and the Complex I functional defects in LHON patients. The common pathology, however, suggests that such a connection may indeed exist, and should therefore be investigated.

Other mitochondrial diseases that involve respiratory chain subunits

Mutations in genes that encode subunits of cytochrome oxidase

A number of pathogenic mutations have been identified that map to one of the three mitochondrial genes that encode subunits of cytochrome oxidase (COX), and we have summarized the genetic and clinical results in Table 8.1. The most striking result is that, in contrast to LHON, the clinical abnormalities are very heterogeneous although muscle and CNS are most frequently involved. In this regard, these mutations are similar to those that cause other classical mitochondrial diseases, such as MELAS (mitochondrial encephalopathy with lactic acidosis and stroke-like episodes) and MERRF (myoclonic epilepsy with ragged red fibers). Secondly, most of the mutations appear to be somatic and thus they are not inherited. The

Table 8.1 Pathogenic mtDNA mutations in cytochrome *c* oxidase genes

Mutation	Clinical presentation	Reference
COX3/F251L	MELAS; blindess; hearing loss	80
COX3/del[a]	Myoglobinuria	81
COX1/M273T; COX1/I280T	Sideroblastic anaemia (two patients)	82
COX1/del[b]	Delayed onset; progressive spastic paraparesis; fatal motor neuron disease	83
COX3/W249term[c]	Encephalopathy; lactic acidosis; exercise intolerance; myalgia; myopathy and muscle weakness	84
COX1/G343term	Early onset; hearing loss; myoclonic epilepsy; cerebellar ataxia; cerebellar atrophy; muscle weakness; optic atrophy	56
COX/M1T	Ataxia; optic atrophy; pigmentary retinopathy; muscle wasting; encephalomyopathy	58
COX2/M29K	Muscle weakness; fatigue	57
COX1/W6term	Myglobinuria; exercise intolerance	85
COX2/W104term	Early onset; failure to thrive; microcephaly; hypotonia; pigmentary retinopathy; cardiomyopathy	86

[a] This mutation comprises a15 bp in-frame deletion starting at nucleotide 9497; 5 amino acids are removed starting with residue W95.
[b] This mutation comprises a 5pb out-of-frame deletion of one of two CGAGC repeats at nucleotides 6015–6024. The amino acid sequence is normal until residue ALA39, after which it is then frame-shifted. The fourth codon distal to the ALA39 residue, as a result of the frame-shift, is a termination codon.
[c] 'term' indicates a nonsense mutation.

mutations are always heteroplasmic, and—in multiple instances—they appear to be predominantly localized to one tissue or stem cell population. It is likely that high mutation loads in other tissues would be lethal, possibly even at the embryonic stage. The level of mutation varies markedly among individual muscle fibers, and some of the studies have shown a relationship between mutation load and the biochemical deficit in COX activity.[56] The mtDNA mutations tend to be severe and they usually lead to a marked deficiency of COX activity, but there is nothing to be gleaned beyond that at this point. Often there is evidence that assembly of the COX complex is altered, but this is to be expected when a crucial subunit is missing.[57] There is one mutation that deserves comment. Clark *et al.*[58] identified a mutation at nucleotide 7587 that changes the initiation MET codon of the COX2 gene to THR. These investigators concluded, on the basis of their results, that there was no translation of this subunit. This stringency does not extend to other mitochondrial initiation codons. For example, there is a polymorphism at nucleotide 3308 that also changes the ND1 initiation codon from MET to THR. This polymorphism occurs in a major subgroup of the African L1 haplogroup[59] and its prevalence within the population indicates that it is a phenotypically benign sequence change. It is not known if the mitochondrial translation machinery uses the next available MET codon in the ND1 mRNA (there is one at amino acid position iii), but the disparity between these two situations is interesting.

Mutations in the mitochondrial cytochrome b gene

The cytochrome *b* protein is the only subunit of Complex III (ubiquinol – cytochrome *c* oxidoreductase) that is encoded in the human mitochondrial genome. Beginning with the report of Dumoulin *et al.*,[60] a number of cytochrome *b* mutations have been identified in patients with an exercise intolerance that is often accompanied by proximal limb weakness (see especially publications by Andreu *et al.*[61] and Keightley *et al.*[62] for summaries of previous studies). In these patients, the mutation is heteroplasmic and it is limited to muscle tissue. The prevailing view is that these mutations are somatic in origin, rather than germ line, and probably limited to the affected tissue.[61] These cytochrome *b* mutations, similar to the pathogenic COX mutations, appear to affect amino acid residues that are close to the redox centres and that severely affect Complex III activity (see figure 3 of Andreu *et al.*).[61]

In addition to this group of somatic mutations with a relatively mild clinical presentation, there are a small group of other pathogenic cytochrome *b* mutations.

1. A mutation at nucleotide 15243 (GLY166 changed to GLU) was identified in a patient who died of severe hypertrophic cardiomyopathy at the age of 9 years. The mutation was not detected in the mother's leukocytes, so the mutation might have arisen *de novo* in the patient.[63]

2. De Coo *et al.*[64] have described a patient with a delayed-onset, progressive, and severe Parkinsonism/MELAS overlap syndrome. The presentation of an akinetic rigid syndrome as a teenager was followed by an encephalopathy that included seizures and stroke-like episodes. Biochemical analysis indicated a marked Complex III deficiency and genetic analysis identified a 4-bp deletion of mtDNA nucleotides 14787–14790. This deletion affects the amino acid sequence beginning with residue ILE14. The mutation was detected in multiple tissues from the patient, but in none of those from his mother, results that indicate a *de novo* origin. Subsequent cybrid analyses of this mutation showed absence of the

cytochrome *b* protein not only caused a Complex III deficiency but also to an increased production of ROS.[65]

3. Keightley *et al.*[62] have summarized their long-term studies of a patient who first developed exercise intolerance and lactic acidosis, who had a Complex III defect upon biochemical analysis, and who subsequently developed an encephalopathy. Sequence analysis of muscle mtDNA identified a heteroplasmic mutation at nucleotide 15242 that changes the GLY166 codon to a termination codon. This mutation was present in multiple tissues of the patient, but was absent from the mother. The wider tissue distribution, relative to that of patients with only exercise intolerance, provides a plausible explanation for the more severe clinical abnormalities.

4. Andreu *et al.*[66] have reported the follow-up analysis of an infant who died in 1984 of histiocytoid cardiomyopathy. Genetic analysis of postmortem liver and kidney tissue identified a mutation at nucleotide 15498 that changes the GLY2251 residue to ASP. The altered amino acid residue is in close proximity to one of the cytochrome *b* quinone/quinol redox centres and is likely to impair binding and electron transfer at this site. The authors point out that previous studies had shown that this rare condition is associated with aggregates of enlarged mitochondria with abnormal cristae, and they suggested that this disorder may have a mitochondrial aetiology.

Mutations in a mitochondrial ATP synthase gene

Mutations at nucleotide 8993 of the mitochondrial ATP6 gene, which encodes one of the sub-units of Complex V or the ATP synthase, cause a clinically heterogeneous disorder (reviewed by Howell.[5] Both a pathogenic T → G transversion in the mtDNA L-strand sequence and a T → C transition at nucleotide 8993 have been identified in NARP/MILS families with the latter mutation generally being clinically milder at equivalent loads.[67] These sequence changes result in substitution of ARG and PRO for the LEU at position 156 in the ATPase 6 subunit.

The predominant clinical abnormalities in families are neuropathy, ataxia, and retinitis pigmentosa, thus leading to the acronym NARP. However, other abnormalities occur, including sensorineural deafness, strokes, and hypocitrullinaemia.[68] These mutations are heteroplasmic in different family members, and severities of clinical abnormalities are related to mutation load,[67] and very high levels of the 8993 mutation cause maternally inherited Leigh syndrome, thus leading to the more complete acronym NARP/MILS. The ophthalmological abnormalities are more heterogeneous than just retinitis pigmentosa and defects in rod and cone function have been identified (see the recent studies of Chowers *et al.*[69] and Kerrison *et al.*).[70] It is worth re-emphasizing the differences in ophthalmological pathology between NARP/MILS and LHON, and how these differences refute mechanistically simple pathophysiologies.

The 8993 NARP mutation appears to have an unusual pattern of segregation and transmission. Thus, in many instances, the NARP mutation—in contrast to other pathogenic mtDNA mutations—appears to reach very high mutation loads in a relatively small number of generations (reviewed by Howell;[5] see also the recent studies of Ferlin *et al.*[70] and White *et al.*).[72] Vergani *et al.*[73] have carried out some experiments that complement the transmission analyses of pedigrees. These investigators analysed the segregation of the 8993 T → G mutation in two sets of cybrid lines (different nuclear donor lines were used), and they observed in both sets that there was an accumulation of mtDNA molecules that carry this pathogenic mutation. They concluded that this mutation segregates in these cybrid cells under positive selection, rather than by random genetic drift as is the case for other pathogenic mtDNA mutations.[74] Vergani *et al.*[73] note that the NARP mutation has relatively little effect on phenotype (there is, at most, a subtle respiratory chain defect) and therefore a basis for positive selection is difficult to identify. Furthermore, it was also observed that mtDNA was often completely lost in cybrid lines during passage, a finding that is also difficult to reconcile with positive selection for the NARP mutation. In other studies of cybrid lines, Manfredi *et al.*[75] obtained evidence that, under conditions where the cells have to rely more heavily on mitochondrial energy production, the 8993 mutation segregated under *negative* selection. Finally, careful longitudinal analysis of patients indicated that there was *no* change in mutation load over time and no significant tissue variation in mutation load, results that indicate a lack of selection.[72] These results underscore the sensitivity of mtDNA segregation and transmission to a complex array of factors, including cellular energy demands.

Biochemical studies suggest, not surprisingly, that the NARP mutations are associated with a defect in mitochondrial energy production (ATP synthesis), but the results also indicate that the phenotype may differ by tissue type or nuclear genetic background. Thus, Manfredi *et al.*[75] showed that fibroblast cultures from NARP patients divided at a normal rate under conditions that favoured glycolysis, but relatively slowly when the cells were grown under conditions that favoured mitochondrial oxidative phosphorylation. For reasons that are not yet clear, these cells were more sensitive to oligomycin, an inhibitor of oxidative phosphorylation. They also measured normal activities of the electron transfer complexes, but a decreased rate of ATP synthesis, in NARP cybrid lines. Geromel *et al.*[76] also used fibroblasts for their studies and showed that there was an increased level of apoptosis in these cultures that was paralleled by large increases in the levels of both the manganese-dependent SOD (superoxide dismutase) and the copper, zinc-dependent SOD. It appears, therefore, that the NARP mutation causes an increase in the generation of ROS, which—in turn—promotes cell death. Yet it is far from clear how two types of pathogenic mtDNA mutations, LHON and NARP, could both cause their very disparate clinical abnormalities through increased production of ROS in mitochondria.

Baracca *et al.*[77] isolated mitochondria from platelets collected from normal subjects and NARP patients. There was a marked impairment in mitochondrial ATP synthesis, although—and this was unexpected on the basis of previous results—ATP-driven proton transport appeared normal. In this regard, Nijtmans *et al.*[78] have obtained results that stand on its head the standard hypothesis of a pure 'catalytic' 8993 NARP mutation that causes faulty proton translocation through the ATP synthase complex. Instead, while they also measured decreased ATP synthesis by the assembled complex, their results also point towards a 'structural' effect of the mutation that perturbs assembly and stability of the complex. These investigators suggest that there may be tissue-specific differences in ATP synthase subunits that determine tissue-specific energetic crises in NARP patients. These are important results and one suspects that the implications are far-reaching and extend beyond NARP to other mitochondrial diseases.

Conclusions

What are we learning about mitochondrial genetic diseases? In the first place, we are discovering that these diseases are much more prevalent, and of greater impact on the health care system, than was apparent when the first pathogenic mtDNA mutations were first identified in the late 1980s. Second, we are learning that the pathogenesis and aetiology of the mitochondrial genetic diseases are very complex. The differences between different diseases are more obvious than their similarities. It is not unfounded optimism, however, to offer the view that there has been real progress in the areas of diagnosis and counselling, and that the studies of pathophysiology are pointing the way towards treatment, especially approaches that might slow or ameliorate the onset of the clinical abnormalities. While onset can be sudden and/or very early in life, many mitochondrial diseases have a later onset and there should be opportunities for medical intervention. Third, we are learning a lot about mitochondrial biogenesis, mitochondrial genetics, and the interaction of different organelles to maintain cell function and viability.

Another important area of inquiry—but one that is not without controversy—is the possible role of mitochondrial dysfunction in a much broader range of disorders. Many neurodegenerative disorders—including Alzheimer's disease and Parkinson's disease (see Chapter 12)—are associated with mitochondrial respiratory chain defects that are similar, at least in some ways, with those caused by pathogenic mtDNA mutations.[79] It is beyond the scope of this review to detail those studies, but it is not beyond the scope to note that what we are learning about LHON, NARP/MILS, and other recognized mitochondrial genetic diseases may be a crucial jumping-off point for investigating a much broader collection of diseases.

Acknowledgements

The support of my research on LHON by the Eierman Foundation is gratefully acknowledged. A list of those who have contributed to my thinking on the issues reviewed here would be very long indeed, but I would especially acknowledge the long and productive collaborations with Drs Doug Turnbull and Patrick Chinnery (University of Newcastle) and with Dr David Mackey (University of Tasmania). Finally, I thank Oxford University Press for permission to reprint Fig. 8.1 here from Chinnery *et al.* (2001).

References

1. Anderson S, Bankier AT, Barrell BG, de Bruijn MHL, Coulson AR, Drouin J, Eperon IC, Nierlich DP, Roe BA, Sanger F, Schreier PH, Smith AJH, Staden R, and Young IG (1981). Sequence and organization of the human mitochondrial genome. *Nature* **290**: 457–465.
2. Riordan-Eva P, Sanders MD, Govan GG, Sweeney MG, Da Costa J, and Harding AE (1995). The clinical features of Leber's hereditary optic neuropathy defined by the presence of a pathogenic mitochondrial DNA mutation. *Brain* **118**: 319–338.
3. Kleiner L and Sherman J (1996). Leber's hereditary optic neuropathy: historical and contemporary considerations. *Optom. Clin.* **5**: 77–112.
4. Howell N (1997*a*). Leber hereditary optic neuropathy: Mitochondrial mutations and degeneration of the optic nerve. *Vision Res.* **37**: 3495–3507.
5. Howell N (1999*a*). Human mitochondrial diseases: answering questions and questioning answers. *Intern. Rev. Cytol.* **186**: 49–116.
6. Howell N (1999*b*). Leber hereditary optic neuropathy: Potential opportunities/potential pitfalls for drug therapy of optic nerve degenerative disorders. *Drug Dev. Res.* **46**: 34–43.
7. Leber T (1871). Über hereditare und congenital-angelegte Sehnervenleiden. *Graefe's Arch. Ophthalmol.* **17** (Part 2): 249–291.

8. Sadun AA, Win PH, Ross-Cisneros FN, Walker SO, and Carelli V (2000). Leber's hereditary optic neuropathy differentially affects smaller axons in the optic nerve. *Trans. Am. Ophthalmol. Soc.* **98**: 223–235.

9. Heng JE, Vorwerk CK, Lessell E, Zurakowski D, Levin LA, and Dreyer EB (1999). Ethambutol is toxic to retinal ganglion cells via an excitotoxic pathway. *Invest. Ophthalmol. Vision Sci.* **40**: 190–196.

10. Isashiki Y, Nakagawa M, Ohba N, Kamimura K, Sakoda Y, Higuchi I, Izumo S, and Osame M (1998). Retinal manifestations in mitochondrial diseases associated with mitochondrial DNA mutation. *Acta Ophthalmol. Scand.* **76**: 6–13.

11. Chinnery PF, Howell N, Lightowlers RN, and Turnbull DM (1997). Molecular pathology of MELAS and MERRF. The relationship between mutation load and clinical phenotypes. *Brain* **120**: 1713–1721.

12. Wallace DC, Singh G, Lott MT, Hodge JA, Schurr TG, Lezza AMS, Elsas LJ, and Nikoskelainen E (1988). Mitochondrial DNA mutation associated with Leber's hereditary optic neuropathy. *Science* **242**: 1427–1430.

13. Mackey DA, Öostra R-J, Rosenberg T, Nikoskelainen E, Bronte-Stewart J, Poulton J, Harding AE, Govan G, Bolhuis PA, Norby S, Bleeker-Wagemakers EM, Savontaus M-L, Chan C, and Howell N (1996). Primary pathogenic mitochondrial DNA mutations in multigeneration pedigrees with Leber hereditary optic neuropathy. *Am. J. Hum. Genet.* **59**: 481–485.

14. Brown MD, Zhadanov S, Allen JC, Hosseini S, Newman NJ, Atamonov VV, Mikhailovskaya IE, Sukernik RI, and Wallace DC (2001). Novel mtDNA mutations and oxidative phosphorylation dysfunction in Russian LHON families. *Hum. Genet.* **109**: 33–39.

15. Chinnery PF, Brown DT, Andrews RM, Singh-Kler R, Riordan-Eva P, Lindley J, Appelgarth DA, Turnbull DM, and Howell N (2001*a*). The mitochondrial *ND6* gene is a hot spot for mutations that cause Leber's hereditary optic neuropathy. *Brain* **124**: 209–218.

16. Chinnery PF, Andrews RM, Turnbull DM, and Howell N (2001*b*). Leber hereditary optic neuropathy: Does heteroplasmy influence the inheritance and expression of the G11778A mitochondrial DNA mutation? *Am. J. Med. Genet.* **98**: 235–243.

17. Johns DR (1994). Genotype-specific phenotypes in Leber's hereditary optic neuropathy. *Clin. Neurosci.* **2**: 146–150.

18. Shoffner JM, Brown MD, Stugard C, Jun AS, Pollock S, Haas RH, Kaufman A, Koontz D, and Kim Y (1995). Leber's hereditary optic neuropathy plus dystonia is caused by a mitochondrial DNA point mutation. *Ann. Neurol.* **38**: 163–169.

19. Kirby DM, Kahler SG, Freckmann M-L, Reddihough D, and Thorburn DR (2000). Leigh disease caused by the mitochondrial DNA G14459A mutation in unrelated families. *Annal. Neurol.* **48**: 102–104.

20. De Vries DD, Went LN, Bruyn GW, Scholte HR, Hofstra RMW, Bolhuis PA, and van Oost BA (1996). Genetic and biochemical impairment of mitochondrial complex I activity in a family with Leber hereditary optic neuropathy and hereditary spastic dystonia. *Am. J. Hum. Genet.* **58**: 703–711.

21. Wallace DC (1970). A new manifestation of Leber's disease and a new explanation for the agency responsible for its unusual pattern of inheritance. *Brain* **93**: 121–132.

22. Howell N (1994). Primary LHON mutations: Trying to separate "fruyt" from "chaf". *Clin. Neurosci.* **2**: 130–137.

23. Pulkes T, Eunson L, Patterson V, Siddiqui A, Wood NW, Nelson IP, Morgan-Hughes JA, and Hanna MG (1999). The mitochondrial DNA G13513A transition in ND5 is associated with a LHON/MELAS overlap syndrome and may be a frequent cause of MELAS. *Ann. Neurol.* **46**: 916–919.

24. Corona P, Antozzi C, Carrara F, D'Incerti L, Lamantea E, Tiranti V, and Zeviani M (2001). A novel mtDNA mutation in the ND5 subunit of complex I in two MELAS patients. *Ann. Neurol.* **49**: 106–110.

25. Johns DR and Berman J (1991). Alternative simultaneous complex I mitochondrial DNA mutations in Leber's hereditary optic neuropathy. *Biochem. Biophys. Res. Commun.* **174**: 1324–1330.

26. Brown MD, Sun F, and Wallace DC (1997). Clustering of Caucasian Leber hereditary optic neuropathy patients containing the 11778 or 14484 mutations on an mtDNA lineage. *Am. J. Hum. Genet.* **60**: 381–387.

27. Torroni A, Petrozzi M, D'Urbano L, Sellitto D, Zeviani M, Carrara F, Carducci C, Leuzzi V, Carelli V, Barboni P, De Negri A, and Scozzari R (1997). Haplotype and phylogenetic analyses suggest that one European-specific mtDNA background plays a role in the expression of Leber hereditary optic neuropathy by increasing the penetrance of the primary mutations 11778 and 14484. *Am. J. Hum. Genet.* **60**: 1107–1121.

28. Howell N, Kubacka I, Halvorson S, Howell B, McCullough DA, and Mackey D (1995). Phyloegentic analysis of mitochondrial genomes from Leber hereditary optic neuropathy pedigrees. *Genetics* **140**: 285–302.

29. Vorwerk CK, Kreutz MR, Böckers TM, Brosz M, Dreyer EB, and Sabel BA (1999). Susceptibility of retinal ganglion cells to excitotoxicity depends on soma size and retinal eccentricity. *Curr. Eye Res.* **19**: 59–65.

30. Brown MD (1999). The enigmatic relationship between mitochondrial dysfunction and Leber's hereditary optic neuropathy. *J. Neurol. Sci.* **165**: 1–5.

31. Brown MD, Trounce IA, Jun AS, Allen JC, and Wallace DC (2000). Functional analysis of lymphoblast and cybrid mitochondria containing the 3460, 11778, or 14484 Leber's hereditary optic neuropathy mitochondrial DNA mutation. *J. Biol. Chem.* **275**: 39831–39836.

32. Zickermann V, Barquera B, Wikström M, and Finel M (1998). Analysis of pathogenic human mitochondrial mutation ND1/3460 and mutations of strictly conserved residues in its vicinity, using the bacterium *Paracoccus denitrificans. Biochemistry* **37**: 11792–11796.

33. Carelli V, Ghelli A, Bucchi L, Montagna P, De Negri A, Leuzzi V, Carducci C, Lenaz G, Lugaresi E, and Degli Esposti M (1999). Biochemical features of mtDNA 14484 (ND6/M64V) point mutation associated with Leber's hereditary optic neuropathy. *Ann. Neurol.* **45**: 320–328.

34. Oostra R-J, Van Galen MJM, Bolhuis PA, Bleeker-Wagemakers EM, and Van den Bogert C (1995) The mitochondrial DNA mutation ND6*14,484C associated with Leber hereditary optic neuropathy, leads to deficiency of complex I of the respiratory chain. *Biochem. Biophy. Res. Commun.* **215**: 1001–1005.

35. Lodi R, Taylor DJ, Tabrizi SJ, Kumar S, Sweeney M, Wood NW, Styles P, Radda GK, and Schapira AHV (1997). In vivo skeletal muscle mitochondrial function in Leber's hereditary optic neuropathy assessed by ^{31}P magnetic resonance spectroscopy. *Ann. Neurol.* **42**: 573–579.

36. Lodi R, Montagna P, Cortelli P, Iotti S, Cevoli S, Carelli V, and Barbiroli B (2000). "Secondary" 4216/ND1 and 13708/ND5 Leber's hereditary optic neuropathy mitochondrial DNA mutations do not further impair *in vivo* mitochondrial oxidative metabolism when associated with the 11778/ND4 mitochondrial DNA mutation. *Brain* **123**: 1896–1902.

37. Cock HR, Cooper JM, and Schapira AHV (1999). Functional consequences of the 3460-bp mitochondrial DNA mutation associated with Leber's hereditary optic neuropathy. *J. Neurol. Sci.* **165**: 10–17.

38. Cock HR, Tabrizi SJ, Cooper JM, and Schapira AHV (1998). The influence of nuclear background on the biochemical expression of 3460 Leber's hereditary optic neuropathy. *Ann. Neurol.* **44**: 187–193.

39. Carelli V, Barboni P, Zacchini A, Mancini R, Monari L, Cevoli S, Liguori R, Sense M, Lugaresi E, and Montagna P (1998) Leber's hereditary optic neuropathy (LHON) with 14484/ND6 mutation in a North African patient. *J. Neurol. Sci.* **160**: 183–188.

40. Sadun AA, Kashima Y, Wurdeman AE, Dao J, Heller K, and Sherman J (1994). Morphological findings in the visual system in a case of Leber's hereditary optic neuropathy. *Clin. Neurosci.* **2**: 165–172.

41. Howell N, Halvorson S, Burns J, McCullough DA, and Poulton J (1993). When does bilateral optic atrophy become Leber's hereditary optic neuropathy? *Am. J. Hum. Genet.* **53**: 959–963.

42. Friedrich T (2001). Complex I: a chimaera of a redox and conformation-driven proton pump? *J. Bioenerg. Biomembr.* **33**: 169–177.

43. Sazanov LA, Peak-Chew SY, Fearnley IM, and Walker JE (2000). Resolution of the membrane domain of bovine complex I into subcomplexes: implications for structural organization of the enzyme. *Biochemistry* **39**: 7229–7235.

44. Wong A and Cortopassi G (1997). mtDNA mutations confer cellular sensitivity to oxidant stress that is partially rescued by calcium depletion and cyclosporin A. *Biochem. Biophys. Res. Commun.* **234**: 511–515.

45. Klivenyi P, Karg E, Rozsa C, Horvath R, Komoly S, Nemeth I, Turi S, and Vecsei L. (2001). α-Tocopherol/lipid ratio in blood is decreased in patients with Lebers hereditary optic neuropathy and asymptomatic carriers of the 11778 mtDNA mutations. *J. Neurol. Neurosurg. Psychiatry* **70**: 359–362.

46. Wang J, Green PS, and Simpkins JW (2001). Estradiol protects against ATP depletion, mitochondrial membrane potential decline and the generation of reactive oxygen species induced by 3-nitropropionic acid in SK-N-SH human neuroblastoma cells. *J. Neurochem.* **77**: 804–811.

47. Tatton WG, Marchbank NJ, Mackey DA, Craig JE, Newbury-Ecob RA, Bennett CP, Vize CJ, Desai SP, Black GCM, Patel N, Teimory M, Markham AF, Inglehearn CF, and Churchill AJ (2001b). Spectrum, frequency and penetrance of *OPA1* mutations in dominant optic atrophy. *Hum. Mol. Genet.* **10**: 1369–1378.

48. Tatton WG, Chalmers-Redman RME, Sud A, Podos SM, and Mittag TW (2001a). Maintaining mitochondrial membrane impermeability: An opportunity for new therapy in glaucoma? *Survey Ophthalmol.* **45** (Suppl. 3): S277–S283.

49. Johnston PB, Gaster RN, Smith VC, and Tripathi RC (1979). A clinico-pathological study of autosomal dominant optic atrophy. *Am. J. Ophthalmol.* **88**: 868–875.

50. Votruba M, Fitzke FW, Holder GE, Carter A, Bhattacharya SS, and Moore AT (1998). Clinical features in affected individuals from 21 pedigrees with dominant optic atrophy. *Arch. Ophthalmol.* **116**: 351–358.

51. Jacobson DM and Stone EM (1991). Difficulty differentiating Leber's from dominant optic neuropathy in a patient with remote visual loss. *J. Clin. Neuroophthalmol.* **11**: 152–157.

52. Toomes C, Marchbank NJ, Mackey DA, Craig JE, Newbury-Ecob RA, Bennett CP, Vize CJ, Desai SP, Black GC, Patel N, Teimory M, Markham AF, Inglehearn CF, and Churchill AJ (2001). Spectrum, frequency and penetrance of *OPA1* mutations in dominant optic atrophy. *Hum. Mol. Genet.* **10**: 1369–1378.

53. Alexander C, Votruba M, Pesch UEA, Thiselton DL, Mayer S, Moore A, Rodriguez M, Kellner U, Leo-Kottler B, Auburger G, Bhattacharya SS, and Wissinger B (2000). *OPA1*, encoding a dynamin-related GTPase, is mutated in autosomal dominant optic atrophy linked to chromosome 3q28. *Nat. Genet.* **26**: 211–215.

54. Delettre C, Lenaers G, Griffoin J-M, Gigarel N., Lorenzo C, Belenguer P, Pelloquin L, Grosgeorge J, Turc-Carel C, Perret E, Astarie-Dequeker C, Lasquellec L, Arnaud B, Ducommun B, Kaplan J, and Hamel CP (2000). Nulcear gene *OPA1*, encoding a mitochondrial dynamin-related protein, is mutated in dominant optic atrophy. *Nat. Genet.* **26**: 207–210.

55. Pesch UEA, Leo-Kottler B, Mayer S, Jurklies B, Kellner U, Apfelstedt-Sylla E, Zrenner E, Alexander C, and Wissinger B (2001). *OPA1* mutations in patients with autosomal dominant optic atrophy and evidence for semi-dominant inheritance. *Hum. Mol. Genet.* **10**: 1359–1368.

56. Bruno C, Martinuzzi A, Tang Y, Andreu AL, Pallotti F, Bonilla E, Shanske S, Fu J, Sue CM, Angelini C, DiMauro S, and Manfredi G (1999). A stop-codon mutation in the human myDNA cytochrome *c* oxidase I gene disrupts the functional structure of Complex IV. *Am. J. Hum. Genet.* **65**: 611–620.

57. Rahman S., Taanman J-W, Cooper JM, Nelson I, Hargreaves I, Meunier B, Hanna MG, Garcia JJ, Capaldi RA, Lake BD, Leonard JV, and Schapira AHV (1999). A missense mutation of cytochrome oxidase subunit II causes defective assembly and myopathy. *Am. J. Hum. Genet.* **65**: 1030–1039.

58. Clark KM, Taylor RW, Johnson MA, Chinnery PF, Chrzanowska-Lightowlers ZMA, Andrews RM, Nelson IP, Wood NW, Lamont PJ, Hanna MG, Lightowlers RN, and Turnbull DM (1999). An mtDNA mutation in the initiation codon of the cytochrome c oxidase subunit II gene results in lower levels of the protein and a mitochondrial encephalomyopathy. *Am. J. Hum. Genet.* **64**: 1330–1339.

59. Rocha H, Flores C, Campos Y, Arenas J, Vilarinho L, Santorelli FM, and Torroni A (1999). About the 'pathological' role of the mtDNA T3308C mutation . . . *Am. J. Hum. Genet.* **65**: 1457–1459.

60. Dumoulin R, Sagnol I, Ferlin T, Bozon D, Stepien G, and Mousson B (1996). A novel gly290asp mitochondrial cytochrome *b* mutation linked to a complex III deficiency in progressive exercise intolerance. *Mol. Cell. Probes* **10**: 389–391.

61. Andreu A, Hanna MG, Reichmann H, Bruno C, Penn AS, Tanji K, Pallotti F, Iwata S, Bonilla E, Lach B, Morgan-Hughes J, and DiMauro S (1999). Exercise intolerance due to mutations in the cytochrome *b* gene of mitochondrial DNA. *N. Eng. J. Med.* **341**: 1037–1044.

62. Keightley JA, Anitori R, Burton MD, Quan F, Buist NRM, and Kennaway NG (2000). Mitochondrial encephalomyopathy and complex III deficiency associated with a stop-codon mutation in the cytochrome *b* gene. *Am. J. Hum. Genet.* **67**: 1400–1410.

63. Valnot I, Kassis J, Chretien D, de Lonlay P, Parfait B, Munnich A, Kachaner J, Rustin P, and Rötig A (1999). A mitochondrial cytochrome *b* mutation but no mutations of nuclearly encoded subunits in ubiquinol cytochrome *c* reductase (complex III) deficiency. *Hum. Genet.* **104**: 460–466.

64. De Coo IFM, Renier WO, Ruitenbeek W, Ter Laak HJ, Bakker M, Schägger H, Van Oost BA, and Smeets HJM (1999). A 4-base pair deletion in the mitochondrial cytochrome *b* gene associated with Parkinsonism/MELAS overlap syndrome. *Ann. Neurol.* **45**: 130–133.

65. Rana M, de Coo I, Diaz F, Smeets H, and Moraes CT (2000). An out-of-frame cytochrome *b* gene deletion from a patient with Parkinsonism is associated with impaired complex III assembly and an increase in free radical production. *Ann. Neurol.* **48**: 774–781.

66. Andreu AL, Checcarelli N, Iwata S, Shanske S, and DiMauro S (2000). A missense mutation in the mitochondrial cytochrome *b* gene in a revisited case with histiocytoid cardiomyopathy. *Pediat. Res.* **48**: 311–314.

67. White SL, Collins VR, Wolfe R, Cleary MA, Shanske S, DiMauro S, Dahl H-HM, and Thorburn DR (1999*a*). Genetic counseling and parental diagnosis for the mitochondrial DNA mutations at nucleotide 8993. *Am. J. Hum. Genet.* **65**: 474–482.

68. Parfait B, de Lonlay P, von Kleist-Retzow JC, Cormier-Daire V, Chretien D, Rötig A, Rabier D, Saudubray JM, Rustin P, and Munnich A (1999). The neurogenic weakness, ataxia and retnitis pigmentosa (NARP) syndrome mtDNA mutation (T8993G) triggers muscle ATPase deficiency and hypocitrullinaemia. *Eur. J. Pediatr.* **158**: 55–58.

69. Chowers T, Lerman-Sagie T, Elpeleg ON, Shaag A, and Merin S (1999). Cone and rod dysfunction in the NARP syndrome. *Br. J. Ophthalmol.* **83**: 190–193.

70. Kerrison JB, Biousse V, and Newman NJ (2000). Retinopathy of NARP syndrome. *Arch. Ophthalmol.* **118**: 298–299.

71. Ferlin T, Landrieu P, Rambaud C, Fernandez H, Duloulin R, Rustin P, and Mousson B (1997). Segregation of the G8993 mutant mitochondrial DNA through generations and embryonic tissues in a family at risk of Leigh syndrome. *J. Pediatr.* **131**: 447–449.

72. White SL, Shanske S, McGill JJ, Mountain H, Geraghty MT, Di Mauro S, Dahl H-HM, and Thorburn DR (1999*b*). Mitochondrial DNA mutations at nucleotide 8993 show a lack of tissue- or age-related variation. *J. Inherit. Metabolic Dis.* **22**: 899–914.

73. Vergani L, Rossi R, Brierley CH, Hanna M, and Holt IJ (1999). Introduction of heteroplasmic mitochondrial DNA (mtDNA) from a patient with NARP into two human_° cell lines is associated either with selection and maintence of NARP mutant mtDNA or failure to maintain mtDNA. *Hum. Mol. Genet.* **8**: 1751–1755.

74. Chinnery PF, Thorburn DR, Samuels DC, White SL, Dahl H-HM, Turnbull DM, Lightowlers RN, and Howell N (2000). The inheritance of mitochondrial DNA heteroplasmy: random drift, selection or both? *Trends Genet.* **16**: 500–505.

75. Manfredi G, Gupta N, Vazquez-Memije ME, Sadlock JE, Spinazzola A, De Vivo DC, and Schon EA (1999). Oligomycin induces a decrease in the cellular content of a pathogenic mutation in the human mitochondrial ATPase 6 gene. *J. Biol. Chem.* **274**: 9386–9391.

76. Geromel V, Kadhom N, Cebalos-Picot I, Ouari O, Polidori A, Munnich A, Rötig A, and Rustin P (2001). Superoxide-induced massive apoptosis in cultured skin fibroblasts harboring the neurogenic ataxia retinitis pigmentosa (NARP) mutation in the ATPase-6 gene of the mitochondrial DNA. *Hum. Mol. Genet.* **10**: 1221–1228.

77. Baracca A, Barogi S, Carelli V, Lenaz G, and Solaini G (2000). Catalytic activities of mitochondrial ATP synthase in patients with mitochondrial T8993G mutation in the Atpase 6 gene encoding subunit *a. J. Biol. Chem.* **275**: 4177–4182.

78. Nijtmans LGJ, Henderson NS, Attardi G, and Holt IJ (2001). Impaired ATP synthase assembly associated with a mutation in the human ATP synthase subunit 6 gene. *J. Biol. Chem.* **276**: 6755–6762.

79. Manfredi G and Beal MF (2000). The role of mitochondria in the pathogenesis of neurodegenerative diseases. *Brain Pathol* **10**: 462–472.

80. Manfredi G, Schon EA, Moraes CT, Bonilla E, Berry GT, Sladky JT, and DiMauro S (1995). A new mutation associated with MELAS is located in a mitochondrial DNA polypeptide-coding gene. *Neuromusc. Disord.* **5**: 391–398.

81. Keightley JA, Hoffbuhr KC, Burton MD, Salas VM, Johnston WSW, Penn AMW, Buist NRM, and Kennaway NG (1996). A microdeletion in cytochrome c oxidase (COX) subunit III associated with COX deficiency and recurrent myoglobinuria. *Nat. Genet.* **12**: 410–416.

82. Gattermann N, Retzlaff S, Wang Y-L, Hofhaus G, Heinisch J, Aul C, and Schneider W (1997). Heteroplasmic point mutations of mitochondrial DNA affecting subunit I of cytochrome c oxidase in two patients with acquired idiopathic sideroblastic anemia. *Blood* **90**: 4961–4972.

83. Comi GP, Bordoni A, Salani S, Franceschina L, Sciacco M, Prelle A, Fortunato F, Zeviani M, Napoli L, Bresolin N, Moggio M, Ausenda CD, Taanman J-W, and Scarlato G (1998). Cytochrome oxidase subunit I microdeletion in a patient with motor neuron disease. *Ann. Neurol.* **43**: 110–116.

83. Hanna MG, Nelson IP, Rahman S, Lane RJM, Land J, Heales S, Cooper MJ, Schapira AHV, Morgan-Hughes JA, and Wood NW (1998). Cytochrome c oxidase deficiency associated with the first-stop-codon point mutation in human mtDNA. *Am. J. Hum. Genet.* **63**: 29–36.

84. Karadimas CL, Greenstein P, Sue CM, Joseph JT, Tanji K, Haller RG, Taivassalo T, Davidson MM, Shanske S, Bonilla E, and DiMauro S (2000). Recurrent myoglobinuria due to a nonsense mutation in the COX I gene of mitochondrial DNA. *Neurology* **55**: 644–649.

85. Campos Y, Garcia-Redondo A, Fernandez-Moreno MA, Martinez-Pardo M, Goda G, Rubio JC, Martin MA, del Hoyo P, Cabello A, Bornstein B, Garesse R, and Arenas J (2001). Early-onset multisystem mitochondrial disorder caused by a nonsense mutation in the mitochondrial DNA *cytochrome c oxidase II* gene. *Ann. Neurol.* **50**: 409–413.

Section III   Nuclear genes and mitochondrial disease

9 Multiple mitochondrial DNA deletions and mitochondrial DNA depletion

Anu Suomalainen-Wartiovaara

Mitochondrial mtDNA maintenance is a complex process. In the yeast *Saccharomyces cerevisiae* over a hundred genes have been identified whose deletion causes loss or instability of mtDNA.[1] However, progress in elucidating the equivalent mechanisms in mammals lags behind that of yeast, and the factors regulating mtDNA stability in mammals are only now beginning to be unravelled. The progress made in yeast, as well as in bacteria and bacteriophages, can be of enormous benefit to understanding human pathologies as there is considerable conservation of mtDNA maintenance proteins. Comparison of the proteins of lower organisms with the human genome enables the identification of human homologues, and thereby accelerates elucidation of the disease mechanisms underlying mtDNA instability.

The major protein of human mtDNA replication is believed to be mtDNA polymerase γ(POLG).[2–4] Mitochondrial DNA replication can proceed by two different modes, either by an asynchronous or by a conventional replication mode (see Chapter 1 for details). Replication by either mode requires minimally the presence of single-stranded DNA binding protein (mtSSB), a DNA polymerase, a primase, DNA helicase, DNA ligase, and topoisomerases. These proteins, or at least activities, have been identified in vertebrate mitochondria.[5–13] The mammalian mitochondrial DNA processing proteins are not closely related to other eukaryotic DNA replication systems, but have their closest relatives in *Escherichia coli* and T-odd bacteriophages.[2]

Practically any defective protein involved in mtDNA replication, maintenance, segregation, or mtDNA organization within mitochondria, could precipitate loss or instability of mtDNA, although many such defects would be lethal at an early stage of development.

Diseases associated with mtDNA depletion

In humans, mtDNA depletion can be either spontaneous or induced. Iatrogenic mtDNA depletion can be a side effect of zidovudine or other nucleoside analog therapy of HIV-infected patients. Inhibition of POLG by these substances leads to decreased mtDNA copy number, which can lead to a secondary myopathy.[14] However, after drug withdrawal, normal mtDNA levels are restored. MPP$^+$, a drug that can cause a Parkinson's disease-like phenotype, has also been suggested to cause mtDNA depletion by destabilizing the D-loop region of mtDNA, releasing the nascent H-strands.[15]

Spontaneously occurring mtDNA depletion syndrome (MDS) is a severe infantile inherited disease, characterized by tissue-specific lack of mtDNA.[16] The mtDNA levels in affected tissues are typically less than 10 per cent of those of controls (Fig. 9.1). The MDS pedigrees display an autosomal recessive pattern of inheritance, since the parents are unaffected.

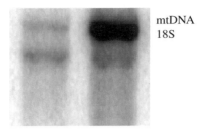

mtDNA
18S

Fig. 9.1 Depletion of mtDNA in Southern blot DNA analysis. Left lane: MDS patient's muscle DNA sample; right lane: control muscle DNA. The mtDNA signal in MDS patient's line is about 10% of the control's signal. A nuclear probe, detecting 18S rRNA gene (18S) controls equal loading of DNA on both lanes.

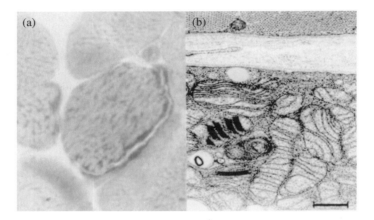

Fig. 9.2 (a) Ragged red fibres in the muscle sample of a patient with a mitochondrial myopathy. In the modified Gomori trichrome staining increased numbers of mitochondria are detected subsarcolemmally and within the fibre. (×800; courtesy of Prof Matti Haltia.) (b) Electron micrograph of a ragged red fibre. In the upper part of the figure, normal structure of a muscle fibre is seen. The muscle fibre in the lower part of the figure is filled with abnormal, large mitochondria, containing distorted cristae and 'parking lot' inclusions. (×22,600; courtesy of Dr Anders Paetau.) (See Plate 4.)

A single sibship may include patients with different affected tissues, which is typical for diseases with mtDNA mutations. The syndrome can be divided into myopathic and hepatopathic forms, which show somewhat different disease progression. The hepatopathic form usual presents neonatally, with severe liver failure leading to death before the age of 1 year.[16–21] Onset can occasionally be later in life.[22] Children with myopathic symptoms usually manifest the disease around 1 year of age and rapidly lose their motor skills.[23–29] Exceptionally, presentation may be as late as adulthood.[30] Symptoms may include retarded development, encephalopathy, or renal tubulopathy. Paradoxically, disease severity does not always correlate with the extent of mtDNA depletion.[26,27] Histological analyses of patients' muscle sometimes reveals ragged red fibres (RRFs, Fig. 9.2a), a classical feature of mitochondrial disease,[23,28] however, usually RRFs are absent.[26] Notwithstanding this, cytochrome *c* oxidase is always low in affected tissues, as are respiratory Complexes I and III.

Mechanisms of mtDNA depletion

Two nuclear genes underlying MDS were recently described, both associated with mtDNA synthesis. The myopathic form was ascribed to mutations in the gene-encoding thymidine kinase 2 (TK2),[31] whereas the hepatopathic form was ascribed to mutations in the gene-encoding deoxyguanosine kinase (dGK, or DGUOK).[32,33] However, the trait was proven to be genetically heterogeneous: screening of patient material from one neuro-muscular centre revealed that only 11 per cent of myopathic and 14 per cent of hepatopathic patients had TK2 or dGK mutations.[32,34] The clinical outcome of the TK2 mutations was shown to be variable, also including spinal muscular atrophy-type disease.[35] Since the primary findings are recent, it remains to be seen whether the outcomes are extended even further.

Thymidine kinase 2 and dGK are enzymes required for mitochondrial nucleoside, dNTP, synthesis. The building blocks of DNA, nucleosides dATP, dTTP, dGTP, and dCTP, are needed in balanced concentrations for accurate mtDNA synthesis. Either excess or deficiency of one or more dNTPs can cause error-prone DNA synthesis or cease it completely. Specific dNTP transporters in the inner mitochondrial membrane import dNTPs from the cytosol.[36,37] However, in non-replicating cells, such as neurons and muscle cells, the cytoplasmic dNTP synthesis is downregulated, but the mtDNA replication continues independent of cell cycle. In those conditions, the mitochondrial dNTP pools are dependent on salvage, recycling of the used dNTPs. The salvage pathway depends on the action of the two enzymes, dGK and TK2, which together allow the synthesis of all the four nucleosides needed for mtDNA replica-tion.[38,39] Previous studies showed that increased thymidine levels can cause mtDNA deple-tion and/or deletion formation in mitochondrial neurogastrointestinal encephalomyopathy, MNGIE.[40] The characterization of the defects of dGK and TK2, focuses the MDS research towards the regulation of the mitochondrial dNTP pools, and all the proteins involved are obvious candidates to cause the disease. Furthermore, the question, how TK2 and dGK defects result in highly tissue-specific phenotypes remains to be answered.

Since MDS is a genetically heterogeneous disease, alternative pathogenetic mechanisms may result in the same phenotype. The disease could result from a defect in any part of the mtDNA replication machinery: mutations in the mtDNA regulatory region, in mtDNA pro-cessing enzymes, or their regulatory proteins or substrates. Possible candidates, nuclear-encoded mtDNA maintenance proteins (mtSSB, endonuclease G, POLG, mtTFA, and NRF1), were excluded by haplotype analysis as causative in one MDS family.[41] Mitochondrial DNA replication is inactive from fertilization to the blastocyst stage. Defective control of mtDNA replication resumption after its arrest in early embryogenesis, could lead to low amounts of mtDNA in some stem cell populations.[16] Sequencing of mtDNA regulatory regions failed to reveal any MDS associated mutations in one material,[16] but another study found mtDNA point mutations that were putatively associated with disease pathogenesis.[42] When compar-ing the outcome of different studies it should be borne in mind that MDS is a heterogeneous disorder, therefore the falsification of a hypothesis to explain the disease in one family does not exclude it as a cause of MDS in other pedigrees.

Animal models of tissue-specific depletion have been created by inactivating the mouse gene for mitochondrial transcription factor A,[43–46] which encodes the protein necessary for replication priming and transcription initiation of mtDNA.[47] MDS patients have been shown to have low mtTFA levels in affected tissues.[48,49] However, this may be a secondary phenomenon since mtTFA levels are known to decrease in parallel with a decrease in mtDNA number.[50] Inactivation of nuclear respiratory factor 1 (NRF1) in mouse blastocysts also leads to mtDNA depletion, resulting in early embryonal lethality.[51] Since NRF1 regulates the levels of mtTFA, the depletion of mtDNA is likely to be a result of low mtTFA levels.

To conclude, MDS is genetically heterogeneous, and the data accumulated so far suggests that defects affecting intramitochondrial dNTP pools are in a key role in its pathogenesis.

Disorders with multiple mtDNA deletions

The second type of mtDNA instability in humans is multiple large-scale mtDNA deletions. Small amounts of mtDNA with large-scale rearrangements can be found in normal individuals,[52] as well as be generated by nonspecific disease processes such as inflammation in inclusion body myositis,[53] degeneration during ageing[54,55] or degenerative disease.[56,57] The nature of these mutations resembles closely those found in diseases associated with multiple mtDNA deletions.[52,58] However, since they account for only a very small proportion of mitochondrial DNA present in tissues, it remains to be determined whether or not such a low mutant mtDNA load has any pathological effect.

The disorders associated with multiple mtDNA deletions have variable clinical outcomes, the most common being chronic progressive external ophthalmoplegia and muscle weakness with exercise intolerance (Table 9.1). The primary causative genes are nuclear encoded, since the pedigrees reported all follow a Mendelian pattern of inheritance, either autosomal recessive[59,60] or dominant.[61] Four causative genes have recently been discovered: in autosomal dominant and recessive progressive external ophthalmoplegia (adPEO, arPEO) and in MNGIE. These discoveries bring new insights into the mechanisms of mtDNA maintenance in humans.

Mitochondrial neurogastrointestinal encephalomyopathy (MNGIE)

Autosomal recessively inherited MNGIE is characterized by PEO, severe gastrointestinal dysmotility, peripheral neuropathy, cachexia, and diffuse leukoencephalopathy on brain MRI.[59,62] The disease onset ranges from 5 months to 43 years of age.[62] Histological or biochemical analyses may indicate mitochondrial dysfunction. Southern analysis of the patients' muscle mtDNA often shows either multiple mtDNA deletions and/or depletion of mtDNA, but in some patients neither of these are seen.[59] The disease gene was mapped to chromosome 22q13.32-qter,[63] and subsequently the disease was shown to be caused by mutations in the thymidine phosphorylase (TP) gene.[40] Sixteen different mutations in ethnically diverse MNGIE pedigrees have been found,[64] indicating that mutations in TP gene are the major cause of the MNGIE disease. The mutations lead to a decrease in the enzyme activity to 5 per cent of controls,[40] which results in highly increased thymidine concentrations in the cells and plasma.[65]

Considerations of pathogenic mechanisms in MNGIE

TP mutations provided the first indication that disturbed dNTP pools promote mtDNA deletion formation and depletion. TP is a multifunctional enzyme involved in the regulation of

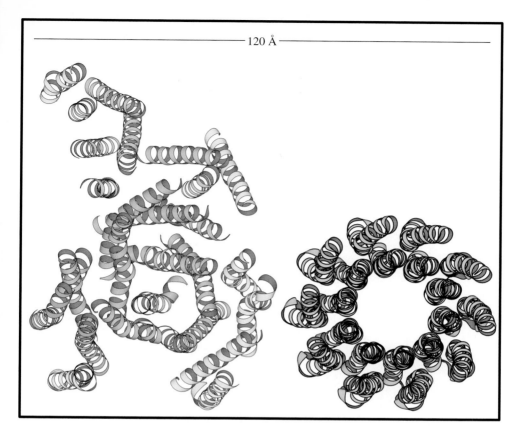

Plate 1. Packing density of Complex IV and H$^+$–ATP synthase in the inner mitochondrial membrane.

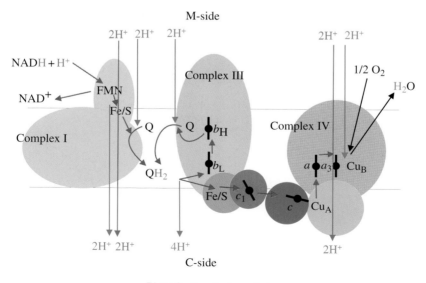

Plate 2. Respiratory chain.

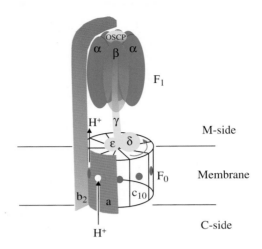

Plate 3. H$^+$–ATP synthase.

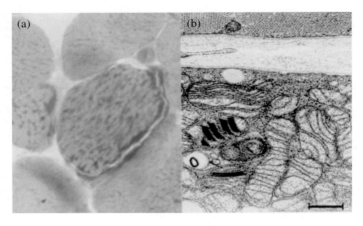

Plate 4. (a) Ragged red fibres in the muscle sample of a patient with a mitochondrial myopathy. (b) Electron micrograph of a ragged red fibre.

Table 9.1 Clinical symptoms associated with multiple mtDNA deletions

Classical symptoms	Additional features	Reference
PEO, muscle weakness	Vestibular areflexia, tremor	61, 70
PEO	Peripheral neuropathy	76
PEO, mitochondrial myopathy		78, 99, 100
	Ataxia, ketoacidotic coma	101
PEO, exercise intolerance	Dysphagia, cataracts, early death	71
	Recurrent myoglobinuria	102
PEO, exercise intolerance	Major depression	69
	Idiopathic dilated cardiomyopathy	103
PEO	Peripheral neuropathy, leukoencephalopathy, gastrointestinal symptoms and dysmotility (MNGIE)	59, 104, 105
	Periodic paralysis	106
	Flaccid tetraplegia, parkinsonism, hyperCPKemia	107
Muscle weakness	Sideroblastic anaemia, pancreatic insufficiency	108
	Multiple symmetrical lipomatosis	109
PEO		110
	Hypertrophic cardiomyopathy, muscle wasting	111
PEO, muscle wasting, weakness	Ataxia, hearing loss	112
	Neonatal hyperthermia	113
PEO, exercise intolerance	Hypogonadism, ataxia, neuropathy, cataracts, hypoacusia, parkinsonism, pes cavus, tremor, depression, rhabdomyolysis	72, 73, 114
PEO, proximal and facial muscle weakness	Cardiomyopathy	60
	Wolfram syndrome	115
PEO	Pigmentary retinopathy, ataxia, peripheral neuropathy	116
PEO	Sensory ataxic neuropathy, dysarthria	117, 118
PEO	Myoclonus epilepsy with ragged red fibres, sensory neuropathy	119
	Ataxia, dysphonia, optic atrophy, sensory neuropathy, multiple symmetrical lipomatosis	120
PEO, child onset	Cerebellar ataxia	121
Muscle weakness	Ataxia, dementia, bulbar syndrome	121

cellular dTTP levels for DNA synthesis, and in physiological and tumour-associated angiogenesis.[66] TP drives the thymidine salvage pathway: it catalyses the breakdown of thymidine to be reused for dTTP synthesis (reviewed by Brown and Bicknell).[66] TP produces 2-deoxyribose as a byproduct of dTTP synthesis, which is an endothelial cell chemo-attractant in angiogenesis induction. TP has also been shown to regulate glial cell proliferation and cortical neuron trophism,[67] which might explain the encephalopathy seen in MNGIE. The TP is widely expressed in tissues, although paradoxically it is not present in skeletal muscle, which is the major tissue showing mtDNA rearrangements. However, aberrant extracellular thymidine pools could affect the balance of intramitochondrial dNTP pools and lead to error-prone mtDNA synthesis and generation of mtDNA deletions and depletion. Previously, depletion of thymidine pools had been shown to result specifically in mtDNA mutagenesis in cultured human cells.[68]

The pathogenesis of MNGIE is closely related to MDS, but also connects depletion mechanisms and mtDNA deletion formation (below). Subtle differences in the increased thymidine levels may thus result in a complete block of mtDNA synthesis and depletion, or modification of the polymerase kinetics, resulting in mtDNA deletions.

Autosomal dominant progressive external ophthalmoplegia (adPEO)

Autosomal dominant progressive external ophthalmoplegia is a rare inherited disorder, with an incidence of 1 : 100,000 in the Finnish and Italian populations. It is clinically characterized with ophthalmoparesis, ptosis and exercise intolerance. Different families have variable additional symptoms, such as severe retarded depression, peripheral neuropathy, hypoacusis, hypogonadism, ataxia, tremor, cataracts, and rhabdomyolysis.[69–73] Disease-onset varies from 18 to 40 years of age.[70,74] Families with similar symptoms, yet autosomal recessive inheritance, have been found (unpublished data of the author).[75] Morphological analyses of patients' muscle show RRFs and cytochrome *c* oxidase negative fibers. The proportion of these may, however, be only 3–10 per cent of all muscle fibres.[74] Electron microscopy reveals abnormal mitochondria with distorted cristae and various inclusions (Fig. 9.2b). Biochemical analysis of the muscle respiratory chain activities often shows mild deficiency of respiratory chain Complexes I, III, and IV, which are the enzymes containing mtDNA-encoded components, or can even fall within the normal range.[74] Southern blot analysis of patient's muscle specimen confirms the diagnosis, showing multiple large-scale deletions of mtDNA (Fig. 9.3). The quality of Southern blotting is critical and multiple deletions are probably under-diagnosed for this reason. Autopsy studies showed that the highest proportion of mutant mtDNA was greater than 60 per cent of total mtDNA in the basal ganglia and cerebral cortex, followed by the skeletal and ocular muscles and the heart with over 40 per cent deleted mtDNA (Fig. 9.3).[74] Leukocytes do not contain mutant mtDNA, detectable by Southern blotting; hence analysis of blood DNA is uninformative for this disorder. The deletion breakpoints are sometimes,[61,76–78] but not always,[74,79] flanked by short repeated sequences, which might suggest recombination or slippage-mispairing of mtDNA strands during replication. The deletions probably arise as somatic mutations, and accumulate in non-dividing cell types, since they are not present in cultured PEO cells (Carrozo *et al.*[80] and unpublished results of the author).

Using linkage analysis, we demonstrated that adPEO was genetically heterogeneous. A locus on chromosome 10q24 was linked to the disease in a Finnish and a Pakistani family,[81,82] whereas chromosome 4q34–35 carries a disease locus for a set of Italian families.[83] We showed that chromosome 4-linked adPEO is caused by mutations in adenine nucleotide translocator 1 (ANT1), the heart and muscle-specific isoform of the ADP/ATP transporter.[84] Two different missense mutations, both affecting a conserved site in a local transmembrane α helix, were identified in six Italian families. Two new missense mutations were found in a Greek[85] and in a Japanese family.[86]

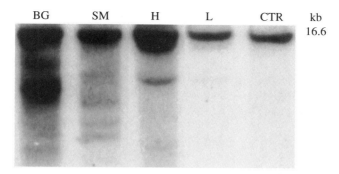

Fig. 9.3 Multiple mtDNA deletions in Southern blot analysis. Total DNA was extracted from various organs (BG, basal ganglia; SM, skeletal muscle; H, heart; L, leukocytes; CTR, control muscle), and probed with a cloned fragment of human mtDNA, containing the 16S and 12S rRNA genes. In the control sample, only one signal from the full-size mtDNA is seen (16.6 kb), whereas in the patient's tissue samples, several additional, faster migrating mtDNA populations are seen, representing mtDNA with deletions of different sizes. The highest proportion of mutant mtDNA is present in the basal ganglia and in different brain regions, whereas the leukocytes do not harbour mutant mtDNA.

The form of adPEO linked to chromosome 10 was found recently to be caused by mutations in a new mitochondrial protein, named Twinkle, with homology to the primase/helicase gene 4 of the T7 bacteriophage.[11] Twinkle is also a possible component of a mammalian mitochondrial nucleoid (see Chapter 2 for details). We described eleven different mutations in Twinkle gene in 12 families with different ethnic backgrounds; they include missense mutations and an in-frame duplication of a 39-bp sequence.[11] Two new mutations in Australian patients were recently described.[87]

The third protein underlying both dominant and recessive PEO is the mitochondrial DNA polymerase gamma (POLG).[75] Mutations in this gene result in a more variable phenotype, including PEO and myopathy, but often also ataxia, sensory neuropathy, extrapyramidal syndrome, and cataracts (Van Goethem *et al.* and Lamantea *et al.*:[75,88] the author, unpublished). POLG mutations seem to be the most frequent cause of familial PEO (Lamantea *et al.*;[88] the author, unpublished). In our material analysed to date, the POLG mutation Y955C[75] accounts for over 50 per cent of all dominant cases of PEO. This specific mutation should therefore be the primary diagnostic genetic test in adPEO families.

The grade of genetic heterogenity in familial PEO is remarkable: about 20 per cent of the families in our material do not have mutations in ANT1, Twinkle, or POLG.

Possible mechanism underlying mtDNA deletion formation

The knowledge about the genes underlying adPEO and MNGIE offers new insights into the mechanisms of mtDNA maintenance and stability in human cells. All these gene defects described so far seem to be involved directly with mtDNA replication and maintenance.

The POLG is believed to be the chief enzyme in DNA replication in the mitochondria. Indeed, it turns out to be the most frequent cause of familial PEO with multiple mtDNA deletions.[75]

Within the POLG protein, the aminoterminal part includes the conserved exonuclease domains, in charge of the proofreading DNA synthesis, whereas the carboxyterminal part includes the catalytic polymerase domains, which execute dNTP binding and DNA synthesis. The recessive PEO mutations cluster into the exonuclease region, whereas dominant mutations occur in the polymerase region (Lamantea *et al.*[88] and the author, unpublished). The most frequently described mutation, changing a cysteine for a highly conserved tyrosine at amino acid position 955, results in a clear increase in the POLG error-rate, and this is associated with decreased dNTP binding affinity.[89] In addition to multiple mtDNA deletions, POLG may also introduce point mutations, which would explain the more severe clinical phenotype of these patients when compared with those with Twinkle or ANT1 mutations. That is, in the case of POLG mutations, full genome length mtDNAs as well as partially deleted mtDNAs may be non-functional due to the point mutations, whereas the dysfunctional mtDNAs associated with Twinkle or ANT1 mutations are presumed to be only those that are partially deleted.

The primary function of ANT in the inner membrane is to transport ADP in and ATP out of mitochondria, making ANT the key supplier of ATP for cellular processes. The protein functions as a homodimer.[90] ANT dysfunction could cause a mitochondrial disease simply by impairing ADP/ATP transport, that is, by not providing enough ADP for the respiratory chain, and thus, ATP for myriad cellular functions. However, the mechanism by which defective ANT1 compromises mtDNA stability is as yet unknown. In yeast, expression of the translocator, engineered to carry a PEO-mutation, resulted in no acute changes in mtDNA integrity, but impaired respiratory growth capacity[84] and increased petite-colony formation.[84,91] Given the possible role of imbalanced dNTP pools in mtDNA deletion formation in MNGIE, it was tempting to suggest that ANT would affect dATP pools within mitochondria. However, the K_m of ANT for ADP is 10–15 times lower than its K_m for dADP, which does not support the idea that dADP is a physiological substrate for ANT.[90,92] Moreover, a probable human mitochondrial deoxynucleotide transporter was recently characterized that transports dADP efficiently *in vitro*, and could potentially supply dADPs for mtDNA synthesis.[36,93] The ANT1 is therefore unlikely to affect dATP transport. Nevertheless, being the regulator of mitochondrial and cytosolic adenine nucleotide levels, the defect in ADP/ATP transport could affect dNTP synthesis. dATP can be synthesized from ADP or dADP, and the enzymes needed for these reactions are present in mammalian mitochondria, as well as the cytosol.[94–96] Deficient ADP/ATP transport, especially upon increased demand in stress situations, could affect dNTP pools by limiting ADP for dATP synthesis, or ATP for dNTP phosphorylation. This, in turn, could affect POLG fidelity, or Twinkle-helicase function, leading to the formation of multiple mtDNA deletions. Over time the primary ADP/ATP transport defect may start to affect oxidative phosphorylation, enhancing the existing mitochondrial dysfunction caused by mtDNA deletions.

How then does a defect in a putative mitochondrial helicase, Twinkle, fit into the picture of mtDNA deletion predisposition? A dysfunctional replication helicase could cause increased replication pausing and thereby promote illegitimate recombination. This could be due to hetero-oligomerization of the mutant and wild-type proteins in the ring helicase; cells overexpressing mutant forms of Twinkle did not show defects in multimerization.[11] It is also possible to suggest a gain-of-function type of action for Twinkle. One of the Twinkle missense mutations occurred at a conserved site that had been described previously in the phage T7 gene4. The T7 mutation enhanced the dTTPase activity of the protein, in the absence of DNA template. Clearly, this would cause an imbalance of dNTPs. Accordingly, dNTP imbalance may account for multiple deletions as a result of Twinkle, ANT1 and MNGIE mutations. Both the mitochondrial helicase activity described previously,[8] and the increased helicase activity in Twinkle overexpressing lines are dATP or ATP specific. Therefore, ANT1 mutations might even cause mtDNA deletions by perturbing Twinkle function.

To conclude, multiple mtDNA deletions in familial PEO and MNGIE may arise either directly from mutations in POLG or indirectly due to disturbed dNTP pools, as they also reduce the fidelity of the polymerase. Alternatively, a dNTP imbalance may affect other mitochondrial DNA-processing enzymes, such as Twinkle, involved in mtDNA replication or repair. When generated, the partially deleted mtDNA molecules replicate faster than larger wild-type molecules,[97,98] and the mutant mtDNA may thus increase in proportion over time. When a critical, possibly tissue-specific, threshold in the level of mutant mtDNA is exceeded, respiratory chain deficiency, and disease ensue.

References

1. Contamine V and Picard M (2000). Maintenance and integrity of the mitochondrial genome: a plethora of nuclear genes in the budding yeast. *Microbiol. Mol. Biol. Rev.* **64**: 281–315.
2. Lecrenier N, Van Der Bruggen P, and Foury F (1997). Mitochondrial DNA polymerases from yeast to man: a new family of polymerases. *Gene* **185**: 147–152.
3. Ropp PA and Copeland WC (1996). Cloning and characterization of the human mitochondrial DNA polymerase, DNA polymerase gamma. *Genomics* **36**: 449–458.
4. Gray H and Wong TW (1992). Purification and identification of subunit structure of the human mitochondrial DNA polymerase. *J. Biol. Chem.* **267**: 5835–5841.
5. Mignotte B, Barat, M, and Mounolou, JC (1985). Characterization of a mitochondrial protein binding to single-stranded DNA. *Nucleic Acids Res.* **13**: 1703–1716.
6. Wong TW and Clayton DA (1985). In vitro replication of human mitochondrial DNA: accurate initiation at the origin of light-strand synthesis. *Cell* **42**: 951–958.
7. Wong TW and Clayton DA (1986). DNA primase of human mitochondria is associated with structural RNA that is essential for enzymatic activity. *Cell* **45**: 817–825.
8. Hehman GL and Hauswirth WW (1992). DNA helicase from mammalian mitochondria. *Proc. Natl Acad. Sci. USA* **89**: 8562–8566.
9. Bogenhagen DF and Pinz KG (1998). The action of DNA ligase at abasic sites in DNA. *J. Biol. Chem.* **273**: 7888–7893.
10. Lakshmipathy U and Campbell C (1999). The human DNA ligase III gene encodes nuclear and mitochondrial proteins. *Mol. Cell. Biol.* **19**: 3869–3876.
11. Spelbrink JN, Li F-y, Tiranti V, Nikali K, Yuan Q-P, Tariq M, Wanrooij S, Garrido N, Comi G, Morandi L, Santoro L, Toscano A, Fabrizi G-M, Somer H, Poulton J, Croxen R, Beeson D, Suomalainen A, Jacobs HT, Zeviani M, and Larsson C (2001). Human mitochondrial DNA instability caused by defective Twinkle, a phage T7 primase/helicase-like protein localized in mitochondrial nucleoids. *Nat. Genet.* **28**: 223–231.
12. Wang Y, Lyu YL, and Wang JC (2002). Dual localization of human DNA topoisomerase IIIalpha to mitochondria and nucleus. *Proc. Natl Acad. Sci. USA* **99**: 12114–12119.
13. Zhang H, Barcelo JM, Lee B, Kohlhagen G, Zimonjic DB, Popescu NC, and Pommier Y (2001). Human mitochondrial topoisomerase I. *Proc. Natl Acad. Sci. USA* **98**: 10608–10613.
14. Arnaudo E, Dalakas M, Shanske S, Moraes CT, DiMauro S, and Schon EA (1991). Depletion of muscle mitochondrial DNA in AIDS patients with zidovudine-induced myopathy. *Lancet* **337**: 508–510.
15. Umeda S, Muta T, Ohsato T, Takamatsu C, Hamasaki N, and Kang D (2000). The D-loop structure of human mtDNA is destabilized directly by 1-methyl-4-phenylpyridinium ion (MPP+), a parkinsonism-causing toxin. *Eur. J. Biochem.* **267**: 200–206.

16. Moraes CT, Shanske S, Tritschler HJ, Aprille JR, Andreetta F, Bonilla E, Schon EA, and DiMauro S (1991). mtDNA depletion with variable tissue expression: a novel genetic abnormality in mitochondrial diseases. *Am. J. Hum. Genet.* **48**: 492–501.

17. Mazziotta MR, Ricci E, Bertini E, Vici CD, Servidei S, Burlina AB, Sabetta G, Bartuli A, Manfredi G, Silvestri G, *et al.* (1992). Fatal infantile liver failure associated with mitochondrial DNA depletion. *J. Pediatr.* **121**: 896–901.

18. Maaswinkel-Mooij PD, Van den Bogert C, Scholte HR, Onkenhout W, Brederoo P, and Poorthuis BJ (1996). Depletion of mitochondrial DNA in the liver of a patient with lactic acidemia and hypoketotic hypoglycemia [see comments]. *J. Pediatr.* **128**: 679–683.

19. Bakker HD, Scholte HR, Dingemans KP, Spelbrink JN, Wijburg FA, and Van den Bogert C (1996). Depletion of mitochondrial deoxyribonucleic acid in a family with fatal neonatal liver disease [see comments]. *J. Pediatr.* **128**: 683–687.

20. Bakker HD, Van den Bogert C, Scholte HR, Zwart R, Wijburg FA, and Spelbrink JN (1996). Fatal neonatal liver failure and depletion of mitochondrial DNA in three children of one family. *J. Inherit. Metab. Dis.* **19**: 112–114.

21. Morris AA, Taanman JW, Blake J, Cooper JM, Lake BD, Malone M, Love S, Clayton PT, Leonard JV, and Schapira AH (1998). Liver failure associated with mitochondrial DNA depletion. *J. Hepatol.* **28**: 556–563.

22. Ducluzeau PH, Lachaux A, Bouvier R, Streichenberger N, Stepien G, and Mousson B (1999). Depletion of mitochondrial DNA associated with infantile cholestasis and progressive liver fibrosis. *J. Hepatol.* **30**: 149–155.

23. Tritschler HJ, Andreetta F, Moraes CT, Bonilla E, Arnaudo E, Danon MJ, Glass S, Zelaya BM, Vamos E, Telerman-Toppet N, *et al.* (1992). Mitochondrial myopathy of childhood associated with depletion of mitochondrial DNA. *Neurology* **42**: 209–217.

24. Telerman-Toppet N, Biarent D, Bouton JM, de Meirleir L, Elmer C, Noel S, Vamos E, and DiMauro S (1992). Fatal cytochrome c oxidase-deficient myopathy of infancy associated with mtDNA depletion. Differential involvement of skeletal muscle and cultured fibroblasts. *J. Inherit. Metab. Dis.* **15**: 323–326.

25. Figarella-Branger D, Pellissier JF, Scheiner C, Wernert F, and Desnuelle C (1992). Defects of the mitochondrial respiratory chain complexes in three pediatric cases with hypotonia and cardiac involvement. *J. Neurol. Sci.* **108**: 105–113.

26. Macmillan CJ and Shoubridge EA (1996). Mitochondrial DNA depletion: prevalence in a pediatric population referred for neurologic evaluation. *Pediatr. Neurol.* **14**: 203–210.

27. Campos Y, Martin MA, Garcia-Silva T, del Hoyo P, Rubio JC, Castro-Gago M, Garcia-Penas J, Casas J, Cabello A, Ricoy JR, and Arenas J (1998). Clinical heterogeneity associated with mitochondrial DNA depletion in muscle. *Neuromusc. Disord.* **8**: 568–573.

28. Vu TH, Sciacco M, Tanji K, Nichter C, Bonilla E, Chatkupt S, Maertens P, Shanske S, Mendell J, Koenigsberger MR, Sharer L, Schon EA, DiMauro S, and DeVivo DC (1998). Clinical manifestations of mitochondrial DNA depletion. *Neurology* **50**: 1783–1790.

29. Kirches EJ, Winkler K, Warich-Kirches M, Szibor R, Wien F, Kunz WS, von Bossanyi P, Bajaj PK, and Dietzmann K (1998). mtDNA depletion and impairment of mitochondrial function in a case of a multisystem disorder including severe myopathy. *J. Inherit. Metab. Dis.* **21**: 400–408.

30. Vu TH, Tanji K, Valsamis H, DiMauro S, and Bonilla E (1998). Mitochondrial DNA depletion in a patient with long survival. *Neurology* **51**: 1190–1193.

31. Saada A, Shaag A, Mandel H, Nevo Y, Eriksson S, and Elpeleg O (2001). Mutant mitochondrial thymidine kinase in mitochondrial DNA depletion myopathy. *Nat. Genet.* **29**: 342–344.

32. Mandel H, Szargel R, Labay V, Elpeleg O, Saada A, Shalata A, Anbinder Y, Berkowitz D, Hartman C, Barak M, Eriksson S, and Cohen N (2001). The deoxyguanosine kinase gene is mutated in individuals with depleted hepatocerebral mitochondrial DNA. *Nat. Genet.* **29**: 337–341.

33. Taanman JW, Kateeb I, Muntau AC, Jaksch M, Cohen N, and Mandel H (2002). A novel mutation in the deoxyguanosine kinase gene causing depletion of mitochondrial DNA. *Ann. Neurol.* **52**: 237–239.

34. Salviati L, Sacconi S, Mancuso M, Otaegui D, Camano P, Marina A, Rabinowitz S, Shiffman R, Thompson K, Wilson CM, Feigenbaum A, Naini AB, Hirano M, Bonilla E, DiMauro S, and Vu TH (2002). Mitochondrial DNA depletion and dGK gene mutations. *Ann. Neurol.* **52**: 311–317.

35. Mancuso M, Salviati L, Sacconi S, Otaegui D, Camano P, Marina A, Bacman S, Moraes CT, Carlo JR, Garcia M, Garcia-Alvarez M, Monzon L, Naini AB, Hirano M, Bonilla E, Taratuto AL, DiMauro S, and Vu TH (2002). Mitochondrial DNA depletion: mutations in thymidine kinase gene with myopathy and SMA. *Neurology* **59**: 1197–1202.

36. Dolce VV, Fiermonte G, Runswick MJ, Palmieri F, and Walker JE (2001). The human mitochondrial deoxynucleotide carrier and its role in the toxicity of nucleoside antivirals. *Proc. Natl Acad. Sci. USA* **98**: 2284–2288.

37. Bridges EG, Jiang Z, and Cheng YC (1999). Characterization of a dCTP transport activity reconstituted from human mitochondria. *J. Biol. Chem.* **274**: 4620–4625.

38. Johansson M, Bajalica-Lagercrantz S, Lagercrantz J, and Karlsson A (1996). Localization of the human deoxyguanosine kinase gene (DGUOK) to chromosome 2p13. *Genomics* **38**: 450–451.

39. Wang L, Munch-Petersen B, Herrstrom Sjoberg A, Hellman U, Bergman T, Jornvall H, and Eriksson S (1999). Human thymidine kinase 2: molecular cloning and characterisation of the enzyme activity with antiviral and cytostatic nucleoside substrates. *FEBS Lett.* **443**: 170–174.

40. Nishino I, Spinazzola A, and Hirano M (1999). Thymidine phosphorylase gene mutations in MNGIE, a human mitochondrial disorder. *Science* **283**: 689–692.

41. Spelbrink JN, Van Galen MJ, Zwart R, Bakker HD, Rovio A, Jacobs HT, and Van den Bogert C (1998). Familial mitochondrial DNA depletion in liver: haplotype analysis of candidate genes. *Hum. Genet.* **102**: 327–331.

42. Barthelemy C, de Baulny HO, and Lombes A (2002). D-loop mutations in mitochondrial DNA: link with mitochondrial DNA depletion? *Hum. Genet.* **110**: 479–487.

43. Larsson NG, Wang J, Wilhelmsson H, Oldfors A, Rustin P, Lewandoski M, Barsh GS, and Clayton DA (1998). Mitochondrial transcription factor A is necessary for mtDNA maintenance and embryogenesis in mice [see comments]. *Nat. Genet.* **18**: 231–236.

44. Wang J, Wilhelmsson H, Graff C, Li H, Oldfors A, Rustin P, Bruning JC, Kahn CR, Clayton DA, Barsh GS, Thoren P, and Larsson NG (1999). Dilated cardiomyopathy and atrioventricular conduction blocks induced by heart-specific inactivation of mitochondrial DNA gene expression. *Nat. Genet.* **21**: 133–137.

45. Silva JP, Kohler M, Graff C, Oldfors A, Magnuson MA, Berggren PO, and Larsson NG (2000). Impaired insulin secretion and beta-cell loss in tissue-specific knockout mice with mitochondrial diabetes [In Process Citation]. *Nat. Genet.* **26**: 336–340.

46. Sorensen L, Ekstrand M, Silva JP, Lindqvist E, Xu B, Rustin P, Olson L, and Larsson NG (2001). Late-onset corticohippocampal neurodepletion attributable to catastrophic failure of oxidative phosphorylation in MILON mice. *J. Neurosci.* **21**: 8082–8090.

47. Fisher RP, Lisowsky T, Parisi MA, and Clayton DA (1992). DNA wrapping and bending by a mitochondrial high mobility group-like transcriptional activator protein. *J. Biol. Chem.* **267**: 3358–3367.

48. Larsson NG, Oldfors A, Holme E, and Clayton DA (1994). Low levels of mitochondrial transcription factor A in mitochondrial DNA depletion. *Biochem. Biophy. Res. Commun.* **200**: 1374–1381.

49. Poulton J, Morten K, Freeman-Emmerson C, Potter C, Sewry C, Dubowitz V, Kidd H, Stephenson J, Whitehouse W, Hansen FJ, *et al.* (1994). Deficiency of the human mitochondrial transcription factor h-mtTFA in infantile mitochondrial myopathy is associated with mtDNA depletion. *Hum. Mol. Genet.* **3**: 1763–1769.

50. Davis AF, Ropp PA, Clayton DA, and Copeland WC (1996). Mitochondrial DNA polymerase gamma is expressed and translated in the absence of mitochondrial DNA maintenance and replication. *Nucleic Acids Res.* **24**: 2753–2759.

51. Huo L and Scarpulla RC (2001). Mitochondrial DNA instability and peri-implantation lethality associated with targeted disruption of nuclear respiratory factor 1 in mice. *Mol. Cell. Biol.* **21**: 644–654.

52. Kajander OA, Rovio AT, Majamaa K, Poulton J, Spelbrink JN, Holt IJ, Karhunen PJ, and Jacobs HT (2000). Human mtDNA sublimons resemble rearranged mitochondrial genoms found in pathological states. *Hum. Mol. Genet.* **9**: 2821–2835.

53. Oldfors A, Moslemi AR, Fyhr IM, Holme E, Larsson NG, and Lindberg C (1995). Mitochondrial DNA deletions in muscle fibers in inclusion body myositis. *J. Neuropathol. Experimental Neurol.* **54**: 581–587.

54. Cortopassi GA and Arnheim N (1990). Detection of a specific mitochondrial DNA deletion in tissues of older humans. *Nucleic Acids Res.* **18**: 6927–6933.

55. Corral-Debrinski M, Horton T, Lott MT, Shoffner JM, Beal MF, and Wallace DC (1992). Mitochondrial DNA deletions in human brain: regional variability and increase with advanced age. *Nat. Genet.* **2**: 324–329.

56. Yamamoto H, Tanaka M, Katayama M, Obayashi T, Nimura Y, and Ozawa T (1992). Significant existence of deleted mitochondrial DNA in cirrhotic liver surrounding hepatic tumor. *Biochem. Biophy. Res. Commun.* **182**: 913–920.

57. Mansouri A, Fromenty B, Berson A, Robin MA, Grimbert S, Beaugrand M, Erlinger S, and Pessayre D (1997). Multiple hepatic mitochondrial DNA deletions suggest premature oxidative aging in alcoholic patients. *J. Hepatol.* **27**: 96–102.

58. Moslemi AR, Lindberg C, and Oldfors A (1997). Analysis of multiple mitochondrial DNA deletions in inclusion body myositis. *Hum. Mutation* **10**: 381–386.

59. Hirano M, Silvestri G, Blake DM, Lombes A, Minetti C, Bonilla E, Hays AP, Lovelace RE, Butler I, Bertorini TE, *et al.* (1994). Mitochondrial neurogastrointestinal encephalomyopathy (MNGIE): clinical, biochemical, and genetic features of an autosomal recessive mitochondrial disorder. *Neurology* **44**: 721–727.

60. Bohlega S, Tanji K, Santorelli FM, Hirano M, al-Jishi A, and DiMauro S (1996). Multiple mitochondrial DNA deletions associated with autosomal recessive ophthalmoplegia and severe cardiomyopathy. *Neurology* **46**: 1329–1334.

61. Zeviani M, Servidei S, Gellera C, Bertini E, DiMauro S, and DiDonato S (1989). An autosomal dominant disorder with multiple deletions of mitochondrial DNA starting at the D-loop region. *Nature* **339**: 309–311.

62. Hirano M and Vu TH (2000). Defects of intergenomic communication: where do we stand? *Brain Pathol.* **10**: 451–461.

63. Hirano M, Garcia-de-Yebenes J, Jones AC, Nishino I, DiMauro S, Carlo JR, Bender AN, Hahn AF, Salberg LM, Weeks DE, and Nygaard TG (1998). Mitochondrial neurogastrointestinal encephalomyopathy syndrome maps to chromosome 22q13.32-qter. *Am. J. Hum. Genet.* **63**: 526–533.

64. Nishino I, Spinazzola A, Papadimitriou A, Hammans S, Steiner I, Hahn CD, Connolly AM, Verloes A, Guimaraes J, Maillard I, Hamano H, Donati MA, Semrad CE, Russell JA, Andreu AL, Hadjigeorgiou GM, Vu TH, Tadesse S, Nygaard TG, Nonaka I, Hirano I, Bonilla E, Rowland LP, DiMauro S, and Hirano M (2000). Mitochondrial neurogastrointestinal encephalomyopathy: an autosomal recessive disorder due to thymidine phosphorylase mutations. *Ann. Neurol.* **47**: 792–800.

65. Spinazzola A, Marti R, Nishino I, Andreu AL, Naini A, Tadesse S, Pela I, Zammarchi E, Donati MA, Oliver JA, and Hirano M (2002). Altered thymidine metabolism due to defects of thymidine phosphorylase. *J. Biol. Chem.* **277**: 4128–4133.

66. Brown NS and Bicknell R (1998). Thymidine phosphorylase, 2-deoxy-D-ribose and angiogenesis. *Biochem. J.* **334**: 1–8.

67. Asai K, Nakanishi K, Isobe I, Eksioglu YZ, Hirano A, Hama K, Miyamoto T, and Kato T (1992). Neurotrophic action of gliostatin on cortical neurons. Identity of gliostatin and platelet-derived endothelial cell growth factor. *J. Biol. Chem.* **267**: 20311–20316.

68. Hoar DI and Dimnik LS (1985). Induction of mitochondrial mutations in human cells by methotrexate. *Basic Life Sci.* **31**: 265–282.

69. Suomalainen A, Majander A, Haltia M, Somer H, Lonnqvist J, Savontaus ML, and Peltonen L (1992). Multiple deletions of mitochondrial DNA in several tissues of a patient with severe retarded depression and familial progressive external ophthalmoplegia. *J. Clin. Invest.* **90**: 61–66.

70. Zeviani M, Bresolin N, Gellera C, Bordoni A, Pannacci M, Amati P, Moggio M, Servidei S, Scarlato G, and DiDonato S (1990). Nucleus-driven multiple large-scale deletions of the human mitochondrial genome: a new autosomal dominant disease. *Am. J. Hum. Genet.* **47**: 904–914.

71. Servidei S, Zeviani M, Manfredi G, Ricci E, Silvestri G, Bertini E, Gellera C, Di Mauro S, Di Donato S, and Tonali P (1991). Dominantly inherited mitochondrial myopathy with multiple deletions of mitochondrial DNA: clinical, morphologic, and biochemical studies. *Neurology* **41**: 1053–1059.

72. Melberg A, Arnell H, Dahl N, Stalberg E, Raininko R, Oldfors A, Bakall B, Lundberg PO, and Holme E (1996). Anticipation of autosomal dominant progressive external ophthalmoplegia with hypogonadism. *Muscle Nerve* **19**: 1561–1569.

73. Melberg A, Holme E, Oldfors A, and Lundberg PO (1998). Rhabdomyolysis in autosomal dominant progressive external ophthalmoplegia. *Neurology* **50**: 299–300.

74. Suomalainen A, Majander A, Wallin M, Setala K, Kontula K, Leinonen H, Salmi T, Paetau A, Haltia M, Valanne L, Lonnqvist J, Peltonen L, and Somer H (1997). Autosomal dominant progressive external ophthalmoplegia with multiple deletions of mtDNA: clinical, biochemical, and molecular genetic features of the 10q-linked disease. *Neurology* **48**: 1244–1253.

75. Van Goethem G, Dermaut B, Lofgren A, Martin JJ, and Van Broeckhoven C (2001). Mutation of POLG is associated with progressive external ophthalmoplegia characterized by mtDNA deletions. *Nat. Genet.* **28**: 211–212.

76. Yuzaki M, Ohkoshi N, Kanazawa I, Kagawa Y, and Ohta S (1989). Multiple deletions in mitochondrial DNA at direct repeats of non-D-loop regions in cases of familial mitochondrial myopathy. *Biochem. Biophy. Res. Commun.* **164**: 1352–1357.

77. Ohno K, Tanaka M, Ino H, Suzuki H, Tashiro M, Ibi T, Sahashi K, Takahashi A, and Ozawa T (1991). Direct DNA sequencing from colony: analysis of multiple deletions of mitochondrial genome. *Biochim. Biophys. Acta* **1090**: 9–16.

78. Kawashima S, Ohta S, Kagawa Y, Yoshida M, and Nishizawa M (1994). Widespread tissue distribution of multiple mitochondrial DNA deletions in familial mitochondrial myopathy. *Muscle Nerve* **17**: 741–746.

79. Moslemi AR, Melberg A, Holme E, and Oldfors A (1996). Clonal expansion of mitochondrial DNA with multiple deletions in autosomal dominant progressive external ophthalmoplegia [see comments]. *Ann. Neurol.* **40**: 707–713.

80. Carrozzo R, Davidson MM, Walker WF, Hirano M, and Miranda AF (1999). Cellular and molecular studies in muscle and cultures from patients with multiple mitochondrial DNA deletions. *J. Neurol. Sci.* **170**: 24–31.

81. Suomalainen A, Kaukonen J, Amati P, Timonen R, Haltia M, Weissenbach J, Zeviani M, Somer H, and Peltonen L (1995). An autosomal locus predisposing to deletions of mitochondrial DNA. *Nat. Genet.* **9**: 146–151.

82. Li FY, Tariq M, Croxen R, Morten K, Squier W, Newsom-Davis J, Beeson D, and Larsson C (1999). Mapping of autosomal dominant progressive external ophthalmoplegia to a 7-cM critical region on 10q24. *Neurology* **53**: 1265–1271.

83. Kaukonen J, Zeviani M, Comi GP, Piscaglia MG, Peltonen L, and Suomalainen A (1999). A third locus predisposing to multiple deletions of mtDNA in autosomal dominant progressive external ophthalmoplegia [letter]. *Am. J. Hum. Genet.* **65**: 256–261.

84. Kaukonen J, Juselius JK, Tiranti V, Kyttala A, Zeviani M, Comi GP, Keranen S, Peltonen L, and Suomalainen A (2000). Role of adenine nucleotide translocator 1 in mtDNA maintenance. *Science* **289**: 782–785.

85. Napoli L, Bordoni A, Zeviani M, Hadjigeorgiou GM, Sciacco M, Tiranti V, Terentiou A, Moggio M, Papadimitriou A, Scarlato G, and Comi GP (2001). A novel missense adenine nucleotide translocator-1 gene mutation in a Greek adPEO family. *Neurology* **57**: 2295–2298.

86. Komaki H, Fukazawa T, Houzen H, Yoshida K, Nonaka I, and Goto Y (2002). A novel D104G mutation in the adenine nucleotide translocator 1 gene in autosomal dominant progressive external ophthalmoplegia patients with mitochondrial DNA with multiple deletions. *Ann. Neurol.* **51**: 645–648.

87. Lewis S, Hutchison W, Thyagarajan D, and Dahl HH (2002). Clinical and molecular features of adPEO due to mutations in the Twinkle gene. *J. Neurol. Sci.* **201**: 39–44.

88. Lamantea E, Tiranti V, Bordoni A, Toscano A, Bono F, Servidei S, Papadimitriou A, Spelbrink H, Silvestri L, Casari G, Comi GP, and Zeviani M (2002). Mutations of mitochondrial DNA polymerase gammaA are a frequent cause of autosomal dominant or recessive progressive external ophthalmoplegia. *Ann. Neurol.* **52**: 211–219.

89. Ponamarev MV, Longley MJ, Nguyen D, Kunkel TA, and Copeland WC (2002). Active site mutation in DNA polymerase gamma associated with progressive external ophthalmoplegia causes error-prone DNA synthesis. *J. Biol. Chemistry* **277**: 15225–15228.

90. Klingenberg M (1976). In: *The Enzymes of Biological Membranes: Membrane Transport* (ed AN Martonosi), New York: Plenum Publishing Corp., pp. 383–483.

91. Chen XJ (2002). Induction of an unregulated channel by mutations in adenine nucleotide translocase suggests an explanation for human ophthalmoplegia. *Hum. Mol. Genet.* **11**: 1835–1843.

92. Halestrap AP, Woodfield KY, and Connern CP (1997). Oxidative stress, thiol reagents, and membrane potential modulate the mitochondrial permeability transition by affecting nucleotide binding to the adenine nucleotide translocase. *J. Biol. Chem.* **272**: 3346–3354.

93. Rosenberg MJ, Agarwala R, Bouffard G, Davis J, Fiermonte G, Hilliard MS, Koch T, Kalikin LM, Makalowska I, Morton DH, Petty EM, Weber JL, Palmieri F, Kelley RI, Schaffer AA, and Biesecker LG (2002). Mutant deoxynucleotide carrier is associated with congenital microcephaly. *Nat. Genet.* **32**: 175–179.

94. Bodenstein-Lang J, Buch A, and Follmann H (1989). Animal and plant mitochondria contain specific thioredoxins. *FEBS Lett.* **258**: 22–226.

95. Young P, Leeds JM, Slabaugh MB, and Mathews CK (1994). Ribonucleotide reductase: evidence for specific association with HeLa cell mitochondria. *Biochem. Biophys. Res. Commun.* **203**: 46–52.

96. Milon L, Meyer P, Chiadmi M, Munier A, Johansson M, Karlsson A, Lascu I, Capeau J, Janin J, and Lacombe ML (2000). The human nm23-H4 gene product is a mitochondrial nucleoside diphosphate kinase. *J. Biol. Chem.* **275**: 14264–14272.

97. Moraes CT, Kenyon L, and Hao H (1999). Mechanisms of human mitochondrial DNA maintenance: the determining role of primary sequence and length over function. *Mol. Biol. Cell* **10**: 3345–3356.

98. Diaz F, Bayona-Bafaluy MP, Rana M, Mora M, Hao H, and Moraes CT (2002). Human mitochondrial DNA with large deletions repopulates organelles faster than full-length genomes under relaxed copy number control. *Nucleic Acids Res.* **30**: 4626–4633.

99. Otsuka M, Niijima K, Mizuno Y, Yoshida M, Kagawa Y, and Ohta S (1990). Marked decrease of mitochondrial DNA with multiple deletions in a patient with familial mitochondrial myopathy. *Biochem. Biophys. Res. Commun.* **167**: 680–685.

100. Kiyomoto BH, Tengan CH, Moraes CT, Oliveira AS, and Gabbai AA (1997). Mitochondrial DNA defects in Brazilian patients with chronic progressive external ophthalmoplegia. *J. Neurol. Sci.* **152**: 160–165.

101. Cormier V, Rotig A, Tardieu M, Colonna M, Saudubray JM, and Munnich A (1991). Autosomal dominant deletions of the mitochondrial genome in a case of progressive encephalomyopathy. *Am. J. Hum. Genet.* **48**: 643–648.

102. Ohno K, Tanaka M, Sahashi K, Ibi T, Sato W, Yamamoto T, Takahashi A, and Ozawa T (1991). Mitochondrial DNA deletions in inherited recurrent myoglobinuria. *Ann. Neurol.* **29**: 364–369.

103. Suomalainen A, Paetau A, Leinonen H, Majander A, Peltonen L, and Somer H (1992). Inherited idiopathic dilated cardiomyopathy with multiple deletions of mitochondrial DNA. *Lancet* **340**: 1319–1320.

104. Johns DR, Threlkeld AB, Miller NR, and Hurko O (1993). Multiple mitochondrial DNA deletions in myo-neuro-gastrointestinal encephalopathy syndrome [letter]. *Am. J. Ophthalmol.* **115**: 108–109.

105. Uncini A, Servidei S, Silvestri G, Manfredi G, Sabatelli M, Di Muzio A, Ricci E, Mirabella M, Di Mauro S, and Tonali P (1994). Ophthalmoplegia, demyelinating neuropathy, leukoencephalopathy, myopathy, and gastrointestinal dysfunction with multiple deletions of mitochondrial DNA: a mitochondrial multisystem disorder in search of a name. *Muscle Nerve* **17**: 667–674.

106. Prelle A, Moggio M, Checcarelli N, Comi G, Bresolin N, Battistel A, Bordoni A, and Scarlato G (1993). Multiple deletions of mitochondrial DNA in a patient with periodic attacks of paralysis. *J. Neurol. Sci.* **117**: 24–27.

107. Checcarelli N, Prelle A, Moggio M, Comi G, Bresolin N, Papadimitriou A, Fagiolari G, Bordoni A, and Scarlato G (1994). Multiple deletions of mitochondrial DNA in sporadic and atypical cases of encephalomyopathy. *J. Neurol. Sci.* **123**: 74–79.

108. Casademont J, Barrientos A, Cardellach F, Rotig A, Grau JM, Montoya J, Beltran B, Cervantes F, Rozman C, Estivill X, *et al.* (1994). Multiple deletions of mtDNA in two brothers with sideroblastic anemia and mitochondrial myopathy and in their asymptomatic mother. *Hum. Mol. Genet.* **3**: 1945–1949.

109. Klopstock T, Naumann M, Schalke B, Bischof F, Seibel P, Kottlors M, Eckert P, Reiners K, Toyka KV, and Reichmann H (1994). Multiple symmetric lipomatosis: abnormalities in complex IV and multiple deletions in mitochondrial DNA. *Neurology* **44**: 862–866.

110. Ville-Ferlin T, Dumoulin R, Stepien G, Matha V, Bady B, Flocard F, Carrier H, Mathieu M, and Mousson B (1995). Fine mapping of randomly distributed multiple deletions of mitochondrial DNA in a case of chronic progressive external ophthalmoplegia. *Mol. Cell. Probes* **9**: 207–214.

111. Takei Y, Ikeda S, Yanagisawa N, Takahashi W, Sekiguchi M, and Hayashi T (1995). Multiple mitochondrial DNA deletions in a patient with mitochondrial myopathy and cardiomyopathy but no ophthalmoplegia. *Muscle Nerve* **18**: 1321–1325.

112. Kawai H, Akaike M, Yokoi K, Nishida Y, Kunishige M, Mine H, and Saito S (1995). Mitochondrial encephalomyopathy with autosomal dominant inheritance: a clinical and genetic entity of mitochondrial diseases. *Muscle Nerve* **18**: 753–760.

113. Melegh B, Bock I, Gati I, and Mehes K (1996). Multiple mitochondrial DNA deletions and persistent hyperthermia in a patient with Brachmann-de Lange phenotype. *Am. J. Med. Genet.* **65**: 82–88.

114. Cottrell DA, Ince PG, Blakely EL, Johnson MA, Chinnery PF, Hanna M, and Turnbull DM (2000). Neuropathological and histochemical changes in a multiple mitochondrial DNA deletion disorder. *J. Neuropathol. Experi. Neurol.* **59**: 621–627.

115. Barrientos A, Volpini V, Casademont J, Genis D, Manzanares JM, Ferrer I, Corral J, Cardellach F, Urbano-Marquez A, Estivill X, and Nunes V (1996). A nuclear defect in the 4p16 region predisposes to multiple mitochondrial DNA deletions in families with Wolfram syndrome. *J. Clin. Invest.* **97**: 1570–1576.

116. Chalmers RM, Brockington M, Howard RS, Lecky BR, Morgan-Hughes JA, and Harding AE (1996). Mitochondrial encephalopathy with multiple mitochondrial DNA deletions: a report of two families and two sporadic cases with unusual clinical and neuropathological features. *J. Neurol. Sci.* **143**: 41–45.

117. van Domburg PH, Gabreels-Festen AA, Gabreels FJ, de Coo R, Ruitenbeek W, Wesseling P, and ter Laak H (1996). Mitochondrial cytopathy presenting as hereditary sensory neuropathy with progressive external ophthalmoplegia, ataxia and fatal myoclonic epileptic status. *Brain* **119** (Pt 3): 997–1010.

118. Fadic R, Russell JA, Vedanarayanan VV, Lehar M, Kuncl RW, and Johns DR (1997). Sensory ataxic neuropathy as the presenting feature of a novel mitochondrial disease. *Neurology* **49**: 239–245.

119. Blumenthal DT, Shanske S, Schochet SS, Santorelli FM, DiMauro S, Jaynesm M, and Bodensteiner J (1998). Myoclonus epilepsy with ragged red fibers and multiple mtDNA deletions. *Neurology* **50**: 524–525.

120. Mancuso M, Bianchi MC, Santorelli FM, Tessa A, Casali C, Murri L, and Siciliano G (1999). Encephalomyopathy with multiple mitochondrial DNA deletions and multiple symmetric lipomatosis: further evidence of a possible association [letter]. *J. Neurol.* **246**: 1197–1198.

121. Paul R, Desnuelle C, Pouget J, Pellissier JF, Richelme C, Monfort MF, Butori C, Saunieres A, and Paquis-Flucklinger V (2000). Importance of searching for associated mitochondrial DNA alterations in patients with multiple deletions. *European J. Hum. Genet.* **8**: 331–338.

10 Nuclear gene mutations in mitochondrial disorders

Massimo Zeviani and Massimo Pandolfo

Introduction

Neurological syndromes are the most common clinical presentations of mitochondrial disorders, a group of human diseases characterized by defects of mitochondrial energy production.[1] Mitochondrial energy metabolism is composed of several pathways. However, the term 'mitochondrial disorders' is to a large extent restricted to clinical syndromes associated with abnormalities of the final pathway, oxidative phosphorylation (OXPHOS).[2] The OXPHOS takes place in the inner mitochondrial membrane where it is mediated by the respiratory chain and ATP synthase. From a genetic standpoint, the respiratory chain is unique, as it is formed through the complementation of two genetic systems, nuclear and mitochondrial DNA (mtDNA). Because of this dual genetic control, OXPHOS disorders can result from mutations in mitochondrial or nuclear genes, encoding either structural components of the five enzymes, or factors controlling their expression, assembly, function and turnover.

The most relevant contribution to the elucidation of the molecular basis of mitochondrial disorders has come from the discovery of an impressive and ever expanding number of pathogenic mutations of mtDNA.[3] Some mutations are rather frequent and account for most of the cases with a known genetic aetiology. Other mutations are rare and have been found only in one or a few families. However, mutations of mtDNA account only for 40 per cent of adult mitochondrial cases.[4,5] This figure is substantially smaller for mitochondrial disorders of infants, where known mtDNA mutations account for less than 10 per cent of cases.[6] Many yet-to-be-discovered mutations of mtDNA will doubtless turn out to be responsible for a substantial proportion of mitochondrial syndromes. Notwithstanding this observation, it is now clear that many neuro-paediatric syndromes are due to abnormalities in OXPHOS-related nuclear genes. Nuclear gene products account for more than 90 per cent of the mitochondrial proteins related to OXPHOS. However, currently the number of defined mitochondrial disorders caused by defects of nuclear genes is still small. Most of the cases in which a mtDNA mutation cannot be found are classified as mitochondrial on the basis of a biochemical defect, or the observation of typical morphological clues, or a combination of the two.

Clinical considerations

The clinical presentation of defects of the respiratory chain is heterogeneous, with onset ranging from neonatal to adult life. The clinical features include fatal infantile multisystem syndromes, encephalomyopathy, or isolated myopathy sometimes associated with cardiomyopathy.

In paediatric patients the most frequent clinical features are severe psychomotor delay, generalized hypotonia, lactic acidosis, and signs of cardio-respiratory failure.

Patients with later onset usually show signs of myopathy associated with variable involvement of the CNS (ataxia, hearing loss, seizures, polyneuropathy, pigmentary retinopathy, and, more rarely, movement disorders). Other patients complain only of muscle weakness or wasting with exercise intolerance. However, it has become more and more frequent to observe syndromes dominated by abnormalities in specific neurological systems or functions, such as ataxia, dystonia, or spastic paraparesis. Moreover, the absence of typical biochemical or morphological clues of mitochondrial abnormalities does not exclude a mitochondrial origin of clinical syndromes previously classified with the generic term of 'neurodegenerative disease'. Typical examples of this new category of 'mitochondrial' disorder are Friedreich's ataxia and other clinical entities associated with malfunctioning of mitochondrial iron metabolism.

Leigh syndrome

In infants and children, the most common clinical and neuropathological presentation is that of Leigh syndrome.[7] Affected infants show severe psychomotor delay, cerebellar, and pyramidal signs, dystonia, respiratory abnormalities, uncoordinated eye movements, and recurrent vomiting. Ragged red fibres are absent. The MRI picture reflects the typical neuropathological findings that define this condition (Fig. 10.1). Symmetric lesions usually involve the medulla, the pontine tegmentum and the periaqueductal region, and, in the cerebellum, the

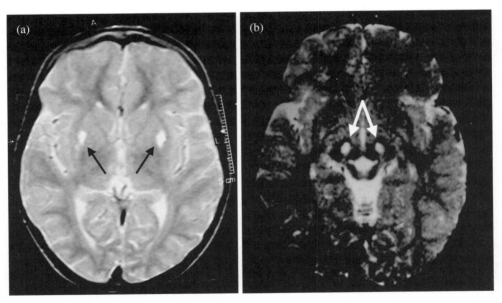

Fig. 10.1 Neuropathological findings in Leigh syndrome. (a) Axial T2-weighted brain NMR image of a Leigh syndrome patient with a mutation in COX subunit III. Note the symmetrical hyperintense areas in the posterior basal ganglia (arrows) and in the heads of caudate nuclei. (b) Axial T2-weighted brain NMR image of a Leigh syndrome patient with a mutation in SURF1 gene. Note the symmetrical hyperintense areas in the subthalamic nuclei (arrows) and periaqueductal area.

dentate nuclei and the deep white matter surrounding these nuclei. Basal ganglia and posterior fossa structures may be involved simultaneously. Rarely, however, one group of structures or nuclei may improve while another becomes involved. Occasionally, the signal changes may spare completely the brainstem and cerebellum, being confined to basal ganglia, particularly the putamina and subthalamic nuclei.

LS is clearly a genetically heterogeneous entity.[8,9] In some cases it is attributable to mtDNA mutations, as in the case of NARP/MILS, in others the defect is X-linked or sporadic, as in the case of the defect of the E1a subunit of pyruvate dehydrogenase (PDH). In still other cases it is attributable to an autosomal recessive defect of a nuclear gene. Defects of Complexes I and IV, or, more rarely, Complex II, have been reported in autosomal recessive LS. However, the attribution of these disorders to nuclear-gene defects has for long remained speculative, since it was based on biochemical findings only. Two recent discoveries have contributed to a rapid advance in our understanding of LS.[10] One was the identification of mutations in genes encoding different subunits of Complex II and Complex I in LS associated with biochemical defects of these complexes. The molecular dissection of the structural components of Complex I in LS is still ongoing, and is likely to contribute further to the elucidation of the genetic basis of Complex I deficiency in LS. The second important contribution has been the discovery of SURF-1, a gene already well known in humans, as the gene responsible for most of the cases of LS due to a defect of Complex IV (cytochrome *c* oxidase, COX). Interestingly, the product of SURF-1 is not a subunit of COX, but, like its yeast homologue, is an integral component of the mitochondrial inner membrane, probably involved in enzyme assembly.

In any case, all defects described to date in patients with LS affect terminal oxidative metabolism and are likely to impair energy production. The typical neuropathological findings of LS are therefore the expression of the damage produced by faulty oxidative metabolism on the developing brain, irrespective of the specific biochemical or genetic causes.[8]

Genetically defined defects of OXPHOS-related nuclear genes

Nuclear genes encode hundreds of proteins related to mitochondrial metabolism and OXPHOS.[11–13] Nevertheless, the identification of nuclear genes responsible for OXPHOS-related disorders has proceeded at a much slower pace, compared to the discovery and characterization of mtDNA mutations. The reasons for such a gap are numerous, including the rarity of the syndromes, their genetic heterogeneity, and our ignorance of the nuclear gene OXPHOS repertoire in humans. Thus, until recently, the attribution of mitochondrial syndromes to nuclear gene defects was entirely circumstantial. In most cases it was based on the observation of familial syndromes with Mendelian inheritance and severe isolated defects of the respiratory-chain complexes, not associated with mtDNA lesions. However, the situation is changing, rapidly thanks to the discovery of several OXPHOS-related genes in humans,[10] and to the identification in some of them of mutations responsible for different clinical syndromes. These achievements make it possible to propose four groups of nuclear gene defects related to mitochondrial disorders.

1. Defects of nuclear genes encoding structural components of respiratory chain complexes.
2. Defects of genes encoding factors involved in the assembly of the respiratory chain complexes.

3. Defects of genes encoding factors involved in metabolic pathways influencing the bio-genesis of mitochondria, including OXPHOS.

4. Defects of genes altering the stability of mtDNA.

We shall describe here the current knowledge on the first three groups of disorders, while the last group is discussed in the preceding chapter.

In the first two groups are defects that are clearly associated with a specific biochemical impairment of one of the respiratory chain complexes. The third group includes protein products that play a role in different mitochondrial metabolic pathways, which are indirectly associated with the mitochondrial energy pathway. In these cases the pathogenesis cannot be attributed to a specific OXPHOS defect, although abnormalities of the respiratory chain can contribute to the development of organ impairment and clinical phenotype. Table 10.1 lists the general classification of genetically-defined defects of OXPHOS-related nuclear genes.

Defects of nuclear genes encoding structural components of respiratory chain complexes

Defects of Complex I subunits
In mammalian mitochondria Complex I catalyses the oxidation of NADH by ubiquinone. It consists of 42–43 subunits with a total molecular mass of 10,000 kDa. Seven subunits (ND1–ND6, and ND4L) are encoded by mtDNA, the others by nuclear genes.[14] The cDNAs

Table 10.1 Classification of mitochondrial disorders due to nuclear gene defects

Protein	Function	Phenotype
Structural components of respiratory chain		
NDUFS1	Complex I	Encephalopathy
NDUFS2	Complex I	Encephalocardiomyopathy
NDUFS4	Complex I	Leigh syndrome
NDUFS8	Complex I	Leigh syndrome
NDUFS7	Complex I	Leigh syndrome
NDUVV1	Complex I	Leukodystrophy, myoclonus
Flavoprotein	Complex II	Leigh syndrome
SDHD, SDHC	Complex II	Inherited paragangliomas
CoQ10 deficiency	Complex I–III, II–III	Ataxia, myopathy
Respiratory chain assemblers		
SURF-1	COX assembler	Leigh syndrome
SCO1	Copper incorporation	Encephalo-epatopatia neonatale
SCO2	Copper incorporation	Deficit di COX
COX 10	Haeme a synthesis	Deficit di COX
Mitoproteins indirectly related to OXPHOS		
Paraplegin	Metalloprotease	Hereditary spastic paraparesis
DDP1	Mitotransporter	X-linked dystonia deafness syndrome
OPA1	Dynamin	Autosomals dominant optic atrophy
ABC7	Iron exporter	Sideroblastic anaemia/ataxia (X-linked)
Frataxin	Iron storage	Friedreich's ataxia
Proteins controlling mtDNA metabolism		
Thymidine phosphatase	Nucleoside pool	MNGIE
ANT1	ADP/ATP translocator	adPEO
Locus on 10q	?	adPEO

of 35 of the human nuclear genes coding for Complex I subunits have been sequenced, but for many of them the function is unknown. In *B. taurus*, Complex I is organized in an L-shaped structure, with a peripheral arm protruding into the mitochondrial matrix.[15] Most of the electron carriers of Complex I, such as flavin mononucleotides (FMNs) and iron-sulfur clusters, are localized in the peripheral arm.

Isolated Complex I deficiency is relatively frequent among mitochondrial disorders.[16] The primary underlying genetic defect may either be at the mtDNA or at the nuclear DNA level. Given the complexity of the enzyme, its dual genetic origin, and the lack of information about the factors involved in its assembly, turnover and regulation, it is not surprising that the vast majority of Complex I defects have been defined on the basis of biochemical findings alone.[17] Isolated Complex I deficiency is rare in early childhood, or at least rarely diagnosed. The clinical presentation is a progressive neurological disorder, often Leigh syndrome, occasionally complicated by cardiomyopathy, or multisystem involvement. In most patients, lactic acidemia with increased lactate : pyruvate ratios is observed, and the outcome is usually fatal. Unfortunately, the defect may be absent in amniocytes or trophoblast cells, making prenatal enzymatic diagnosis of the defect impossible.[18]

It has only been in the last three years that several disease-associated mutations in nuclear-encoded subunits of Complex I have been discovered. No major mutation hotspot has been identified to date, although the NDUFS4 18 kDa subunit is affected more frequently than other subunits. The first case was that of a patient affected by Leigh syndrome carrying two compound heterozygous transitions in the nuclear-encoded NDUFS8 (TYKY) subunit of Complex I.[19] The first mutation was a C236T (P79L), and the second mutation was a G305A (R102H). Both mutations were absent in 70 control alleles and co-segregated within the family. The NDUFS8 is a highly conserved, polypeptide of 210 amino acids, containing two 4Fe4S ferrodoxin consensus patterns, which have long been thought to provide the binding site for the iron–sulphur cluster N2. Leigh syndrome was again the clinical and neuropathological presentation in 2 siblings carrying the first missense mutation within another nuclear encoded Complex I subunit, NDUFS7.[20] Mutations in the 18 kDa NDUFS4 subunit has been reported in four patients.[21–23] All of them suffered of Leigh syndrome, although different, all the mutations were either frameshift or stop mutations predicting the early truncation of the protein. Abolition of cAMP-dependent phosphorylation of the NDUFS4 18 kDa subunit, and lack of activation of the complex, have been demonstrated in one case,[24] while absence of fully-assembled Complex I has been shown in a second.[23] Mutant NDUFV1 subunit of mitochondrial Complex I has been reported in two cases, in association with leukodystrophy and myoclonic epilepsy.[25] Screening of the NDUFS2 cDNA revealed three missense mutations resulting in the substitution of conserved amino acids in three families of patients affected by cardiomyopathy and encephalomyopathy.[26] All had severe Complex I deficiency in muscle homogenate and, in several cases, cultured fibroblasts. Interestingly, combined defects of Complex I and Complex III activities were observed in association with a 5-bp deletion in the NDUFS4 gene, suggesting that disruption of Complex I can perturb other respiratory chain enzymes.[22] Very recently,[27] in 3/36 patients with isolated Complex I deficiency, five new point mutations and one large deletion have been identified in the NDUFS1 gene (del222, D252G, M707V, R241W, and R557X). Six novel NDUFV1 mutations were found in three other patients (Y204C, C206G, E214K, IVS 8+41, A432P, and del nt 989–990). The six unrelated patients presented with hypotonia, ataxia, psychomotor retardation, or Leigh syndrome. Some patients failed to show Complex I deficiency in isolated fibroblasts. Thus screening for

Complex I nuclear gene mutations is necessary in patients with Complex I deficiency, even when normal respiratory enzyme activities in cultured fibroblasts are observed.

Defects of Complex II subunits

Complex II (succinate : ubiquinone oxidoreductase; EC 1.3.5.1) is composed of four sub-units.[28] It catalyses the oxidation of succinate to fumarate and feeds electrons to ubiquinone (see Chapter 4). A soluble functional heterodimer, succinate dehydrogenase (SDH), consists of a 70 kDa flavoprotein subunit (Fp) containing the active site, and a covalently bound FAD and a 30 kDa iron–sulphur protein subunit (Ip) carrying three distinct iron–sulphur clusters. The corresponding genes or cDNAs of the four subunits have been identified.[29–34] A nuclear psuedogene of the Fp subunit is present in the human genome which means that genetic screening has to be carried out via reverse-transcribed cDNA. The SDH complex is anchored to the matrix-face of the inner mitochondrial membrane by two smaller subunits (SDHC, 15 kDa, and SDHD, 12 kDa) carrying cytochrome b558 and the ubiquinone-binding sites. All four subunits are nuclear-encoded. Mitochondrial disease involving Complex II is rare, representing 2 per cent cases of respiratory chain deficiency.[35] Clinically, Leigh syndrome is the most common presentation, but myopathy, encephalopathy, and isolated cardiomyopathy have also been reported.

Only three families with mutations of Complex II have so far been identified. A mutation in the nuclear-encoded flavoprotein (Fp) subunit gene of SDH was found in two siblings with Complex II deficiency presenting as Leigh syndrome.[36] Both patients were homozygous for an R554W substitution in the Fp subunit. The deleterious effect of the Arg to Trp substitution on the catalytic activity of SDH was observed in a SDH-deficient yeast strain transformed with mutant Fp cDNA. Another case of LS and SDH deficiency resulted from two hetero-zygous missense mutations in the Fp gene; a heterozygous C → T transition, changing an Ala to a Val in one allele, and an A–C substitution changing the Met translation initiation codon to a Leu in the second allele.[37] The latter mutant transcript represented only 10 per cent of total Fp transcripts suggesting that the loss of the start codon leads to transcript instability. A third, interesting pedigree composed of two affected sisters has more recently been reported.[38] Both patients presented with late-onset neurodegenerative disease including optic atrophy, ataxia, and a proximal myopathy. The syndrome was associated with a partial deficiency of Complex II (approximately 50 per cent of control values) in muscle and platelets. The defect was not expressed in cultured skin fibroblasts or immortalized lymphocytes. The affected family members were shown to carry a C → T transition in one allele of the nuclear gene encoding the flavoprotein subunit of Complex II. Mutation of the equivalent base in *Escherichia coli* (*E. Coli*) generates an inactive enzyme unable to bind flavin adenine dinuc-leotide covalently. Compatible with these findings, the patients have an approximate 50 per cent decrease in Complex II activity. These results suggest that genetic defects of nuclear-encoded subunits of the mitochondrial respiratory chain can behave as co-dominant traits, and result in late-onset neurodegenerative disease.

Complex II mutations in paragangliomas

An interesting discovery concerning defects of Complex II has recently been obtained from studies on paragangliomas, usually benign tumours of neuroectodermal origin affecting the parasympathic ganglia. In 10–50 per cent of the cases, paraganglioma are inherited in an auto-somal dominant fashion with incomplete penetrance. Three loci, PGL1, PGL2, and PGL3 have been linked to inherited paragangliomas in different families. Mutations of SDHD, the gene encoding the smallest subunit of Complex II, which anchors SDH to the inner mito-chondrial membrane, are responsible for the PGL1 type, which includes a peculiar form of paraganglioma, affecting the carotid body.[39] Mutations of the SDHC subunit, which also acts as an anchoring structure of Complex II, is responsible for the PGL3 type.[40] In both cases, the tumor seems to be caused by a loss-of-heterozygosity (LOH) mechanism, due to somatic deletions in the responsible locus, occurring in the affected tissue of individuals carrying an inherited mutation in one allele of the genes. More recently, mutations of the SDHD gene or of LOH markers flanking the gene, have been identified in a high percentage of non-familiar phaechromocytomas,[41] another type of tumour derived from the neuroectoderm, which affects the medullary tissue of the adrenal glands and is associated with severe arterial hyper-tension. The pathogenesis of paraganglioma induced by LOH of different genes of Complex II remains to be explained. As far as the tumour of the carotid body is concerned, it is interest-ing to note that the main role of this organ is to act as a 'chemosensor' of the concentration of oxygen supplied by the cerebral arteries to the brain. An intrinsic defect of cellular respi-ration could stimulate the compensatory proliferation of the parangliar cells, triggering a cascade ultimately leading to neoplastic transformation of the tissue.

Coenzyme Q$_{10}$ deficiency

Coenzyme Q$_{10}$ (CoQ$_{10}$), or ubiquinone, is a lipophilic component of the electron-transport chain, which transfers electrons from Complexes I or II, and from the oxidation of fatty acids and branched-chain amino acids via flavin-linked dehydrogenases to Complex III (ubiquinone–cytochrome *c* reductase).[42] The CoQ$_{10}$ also plays a role as an antioxidant and as a membrane stabilizer.[43] In 1989 Ogashara *et al.*[44] described a syndrome associated with CoQ$_{10}$ deficiency in muscle, which was probably the first example of a Mendelian defect in the respir-atory chain. That syndrome, which was characterized by the triad of recurrent myoglobinuria, brain involvement (seizures, ataxia, and mental retardation) and ragged red fibres (RRF)/lipid storage in muscle, was confirmed in an additional case.[45] A later report described a child with ataxia, cerebellar atrophy, and generalized seizures, whose muscle biopsy showed Complex III deficiency and severe CoQ$_{10}$ deficiency.[46] More recently, six patients with cerebellar ataxia, pyramidal signs, and seizures, but with only unspecific myopathic change and no myoglobinuria, have been found to have very low levels of CoQ$_{10}$ in muscle (26–35 per cent of normal).[47] Crucially, all six patients appeared to respond to CoQ$_{10}$ supplementation: strength increased, ataxia improved, and seizures became less frequent. Thus, although the biochemical and molecular bases remain undefined, primary CoQ$_{10}$ deficiency is a potentially important cause of familial myoglobinuria, or ataxia, or both, and should be considered in the differential diagnosis of these conditions as CoQ$_{10}$ administration seems to improve the clinical picture.

*Defects of genes encoding factors involved in the assembly of
the respiratory chain complexes*

This group comprises so far only defects of genes encoding assembly factors of cytochrome *c* oxidase (COX, Complex IV) and one factor involved in the assembly of Complex III.

COX (EC 1.9.3.1), the terminal component of the mitochondrial respiratory chain, is a mul-tiheteromeric enzyme embedded in the mitochondrial inner membrane, consisting of a pro-tein backbone bound to two copper-containing prosthetic groups; cytochromes *a* and *a$_3$*.[48] COX transfers electrons from reduced cytochrome *c* to molecular oxygen, contributing, like Complex I and Complex III, to the formation of a transmembrane proton gradient which fuels the conversion of ADP to ATP, by the ATP synthetase. Like Complex I, COX comprises products of both nuclear and mitochondrial DNA.[49] Human COX is composed of 13 subunits: I, II, III, IV, Va, Vb, VIa, VIb, VIc, VIIa, VIIb, VIIc, and VIII, only the three largest (I–III) are encoded by mtDNA.[50] Two of the nuclear-encoded subunits VIa and VIIa are present in two tissue-specific isoforms: one isoform is expressed ubiquitously, while the other is restricted to heart and skeletal muscle.[51,52] All of the human COX genes have been completely sequenced.[55,56]

COX deficiency is possibly the most frequent biochemical abnormality in mitochondrial disease.[57] In infancy, the most frequent manifestation of isolated, profound COX deficiency is Leigh syndrome, although other phenotypes, including severe cardiomyopathy, or complex encephalocardiomyopathies have also been reported.[58] The COX defects are associated with mutations of mitochondrial tRNA genes, and also a few mutations in mtDNA genes encoding COX subunits.[59–62] No mutation in any nuclear-encoded COX subunit has yet been reported, while all of the nuclear-gene defects of COX so far identified are due to mutations in enzyme assembly factors. The 13 subunits of COX are inserted in the inner mitochondrial membrane, and assembled together into the nascent complex in an ordered fashion. Four COX assembly intermediates can be detected.[63] It has been proposed that these subcomplexes represent major steps in the COX assembly process, as illustrated in Fig. 10.2. In the first step (S1) subunit I is inserted in the inner mitochondrial membrane, followed by the binding of haeme a and haeme a_3 and a first copper atom (CuB). In the second step (S2) subunit IV is added to the nascent complex. A third step (S3) in the assembly process is believed to start with the binding of subunit II, which carries a copper pair (CuA), and subunit III, followed by subunits

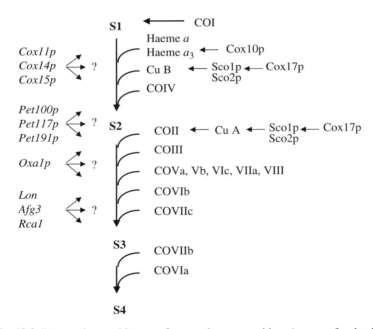

Fig. 10.2 Proposed assembly steps for cytochrome *c* oxidase (see text for details).

Va, Vb, VIc, VIIa, VIII, VIb, and VIIc. In the final step (S4) a fully assembled holoenzyme is obtained by insertion of subunits VIIb and VIa. From studies on yeast, several factors have been implicated in the assembly process of COX, and some human homologues have been identified.[64] These include four nuclear-encoded proteins, which have been implicated in severe COX deficiency, namely Surf-1, Sco-1, Sco-2, and COX-10. Other factors, such as COX11, COX15, and COX17 are candidates for COX deficiency of unknown cause.

Surf-1 mutations

In 1998 a disease locus for LS^{COX} was mapped to chromosome 9q34, and analysis of SURF-1, a candidate gene in the region, revealed deleterious mutations in most of the LS^{COX} patients investigated.[65,66] Subsequent studies have shown that SURF-1 mutations are the most common cause of LS^{COX}, and that the association between LS and SURF-1 mutations is highly specific, since no SURF-1 mutation has been detected in a COX-deficient patient without LS.[67–69] Nevertheless, the condition is genetically heterogeneous as mutational analysis and complementation assays in cell culture indicate that a minority of LS^{COX} cases is not associated with a SURF-1 mutation.

Although the precise function of SURF-1 remains to be elucidated, studies on the yeast homologue SHY-1 suggest that SURF-1 is involved in the maintenance of COX activity and mitochondrial respiration.[72] To understand better the role of the product of SURF-1 (Surf-1p) and the pathogenesis of LS^{COX}, the expression, mitochondrial targeting and possible interactions of Surf-1p with other components of the mitochondrial inner compartment have been investigated in normal and disease conditions.[73,74] Mature Surf-1 protein (Surf-1p) is a 30 kDa hydrophobic polypeptide that is imported into mitochondria as a larger precursor, which is processed to the mature product by cleaving of an amino-terminal leader polypeptide. Like SHY-1,[72] Surf-1p is tightly bound to the mitochondrial inner membrane.[73,74] The same studies revealed that the protein is absent from cell lines carrying SURF-1 loss-of-function mutations, regardless of their type and position. Moreover, RNA analysis indicated the virtual absence of SURF-1 transcripts in these cell lines suggesting that a number of SURF-1 mutations lead to severe instability of Surf-1 mRNA. Artificial constructs of truncated or partially deleted SURF-1 cDNAs failed to restore COX activity when expressed in SURF-1 null mutant cells, suggesting that many regions of the protein are essential for function.[73,74] No protein was detected also in the few missense mutations found in SURF-1 gene in association with LS.[75] To test the hypothesis that Surf-1p plays a role in COX assembly, the accumulation of COX assembly intermediates was investigated by using Blue Native-2D gel electrophoresis.[73] The results indicate that the absence of Surf-1p causes the accumulation of early intermediates S1 (COXI alone) and S2 (COXI + COXIV), suggesting that Surf-1p is indeed a COX assembler, involved in the formation of subcomplex S3. It is likely that this involves the incorporation of subunit II into the COXI + IV intermediate, a crucial step which is believed to produce the rapid, 'cascade-like' assembly of the other COX subunits. Moreover, detection of residual amounts of fully assembled complex suggests a certain degree of redundancy of the COX assembly function of Surf-1p. It is interesting to notice that the 2D-gel patterns obtained from different Surf-1 mutant cell lines are virtually identical to each other. However, they clearly differ from the patterns obtained in both normal controls, and COX-deficient cell lines not associated with SURF-1 mutations. The consistency of these results is in agreement with the observation that the clinical and biochemical features of Surf-1 mutant LS^{COX} patients are fairly homogeneous. In particular, the defect of COX activity appears to be the only OXPHOS abnormality in these patients, it is widespread to all tissues of the body, including skin fibroblasts, and it is quite severe, although a residual activity ranging from 5 to 20 per cent can usually be found.

SURF-1 is the first nuclear gene to be consistently mutated in a major category of respiratory chain defects. DNA and protein analysis can now be used to accurately diagnose LS^{COX}, a common subtype of Leigh syndrome.

Sco-1, Sco-2, and COX-10 mutations

In yeast, two related COX assembly genes, SCO1 and SCO2 (for synthesis of cytochrome c oxidase), enable subunits I and II to be incorporated into the holoenzyme.[76,77] The precise functions of these proteins are unclear; however, both SCO1 and SCO2 are believed to be involved in the incorporation of copper atoms in the catalytic sites of the nascent complex.[78] This incorporation, which also requires COX17,[79] is carried out in the initial phase of COX assembly, and is believed to be necessary to promote incorporation of the first protein subunits of the complex, including subunits I and II and stabilize the assembly. Mutations in the human homologue of SCO2, mapped on chromosome 22, were linked to a newly recognized fatal cardioencephalomyopathy, with COX deficiency.[80] To date, five mutations in SCO2 have been reported, one nonsense mutation (Q53X) and four missense mutations (E140K, L151P, R171W, and S225F) in seven unrelated families.[80–82] Interestingly, all patients to date have been compound heterozygotes, and even more remarkably, the E140K mutation was common to all affected individuals. SCO-1 mutations have been found in a single, large family with multiple cases of neonatal ketoacidotic comas and isolated COX deficiency.[83] Mutation screening revealed compound heterozygosity for SCO1 gene mutations in the patients. One mutant allele harboured a 2-bp frameshift deletion (ΔGA; nt 363–364) resulting in a premature stop codon and a highly unstable mRNA; the other mutation (C520T) changed a highly conserved proline to leucine (P174L). This proline, adjacent to the CxxxC copper-binding domain of SCO1, is likely to play a crucial role in the three-dimensional structure of the domain. Curiously, the clinical presentations of SCO1- and SCO2-deficient patients differ markedly from that of patients harbouring mutations in other COX assembly and/or maturation genes, such as Leigh syndrome, caused by mutations in SURF1.[82] The COX-10 gene product is a haemeA : farnesyltransferase,[84] which catalyses the first step in the conversion of protoheme to the haeme A prosthetic groups of the enzyme, a crucial step of COX maturation. A homozygous missense mutation in the COX10 gene was found in the affected members of a consanguineous family with an isolated COX defect leading to an early onset leukoencephalopathy.[85]

BCS-1 mutations in Complex III deficiency

BCS1L is an assembly factor for Complex III in yeast, and its homologue has been identified in human. BCS1L mutations have been reported in six patients with severe Complex III deficiency, from four unrelated families and presenting neonatal proximal tubulopathy, hepatic involvement, and encephalopathy.[86]

Perturbation of mitochondrial metabolic pathways that indirectly affect OXPHOS

Some neurodegenerative disorders that do not feature overt OXPHOS deficiency have been attributed to mutations in mitochondrial proteins indirectly related to respiration and energy production. This observation further broadens the concept of mitochondrial disease and extends the possible involvement of mitochondrial energy metabolism to a previously unsuspected large number of clinical phenotypes.

Mutations of paraplegin, a mitochondrial metalloprotease, in
hereditary spastic paraplegia

Hereditary spastic paraplegia (HSP) is characterized by progressive weakness and spasticity of the lower limbs due to degeneration of corticospinal axons.[87] HSPs are a genetically heterogeneous group of neurodegenerative disorders affecting approximately 1 in 10,000 individuals.[88,89] In 1999, patients from a chromosome 16q24.3-linked HSP family[90] were found to carry a homozygous 9.5 kb deletion involving a gene encoding a novel protein, named paraplegin.[91] Two additional paraplegin mutations, both frameshifts, were found in a complicated and in a standard form of HSP. The function of paraplegin remains to be elucidated. Immunofluorescence analysis and import experiments showed that paraplegin localizes to mitochondria. This molecule is highly homologous to a mitochondrial subclass of yeast ATPases. Members of this subclass are the ATP-dependent metallopeptidases AFG3, RCA1, and YME1 (also known as Yta10p, Yta12p, and Yta11p, respectively), originally identified by genomic sequencing and complementation studies in yeast.[92] In yeast, AFG3 and RCA1 form a membrane-embedded complex which has both a protease activity, needed for ATP-dependent degradation of mitochondrial translation products, and a chaperon-like function, mediating assembly of membrane-associated ATP synthase.[93] Correct folding and assembly of these proteins is needed for functional respiratory chain processes. Yeast strains carrying mutations in AFG3, RCA, or YME1 genes are deficient in assembled respiratory and ATPase complexes.[94] The ATP-binding, GPPGCGKT, and HEXXH motifs, typical of zinc-dependent binding domains, are completely conserved between paraplegin, AFG3, RCA1, and YME1. Furthermore, the homology is not limited to these domains but spans almost the entire protein. Paraplegin represented the first vertebrate homologue of this class of protein. Subsequently, other members of the same protein family have been identified in humans, but no mutations in any of these genes has been found so far, in association with HSP or other diseases.

Analysis of muscle biopsies from two patients of the original family carrying the homozygous Paraplegin deletion showed typical signs of mitochondrial pathology, namely ragged red and COX-deficient fibres.[91] An additional family with a paraplegin mutation has more recently been reported in the northeast of England.[95] Interestingly, this paraplegin mutation co-segregates with an HSP phenotype in an apparent dominant manner. The phenotype of this paraplegin-related HSP family described had several striking features including amyotrophy, raised creatine kinase, sensorimotor peripheral neuropathy, and OXPHOS defect on muscle biopsy. In other cases, 'mitochondrial clues' failed to be found in muscle biopsies of paraplegin-related HSP patients. It is difficult to explain why a defect in an apparently ubiquitous protein required for mitochondrial function affects primarily specific axonal populations, such as the corticospinal tracts and the dorsal columns. These are the longest axons in the human body and may be more sensitive to an impairment of the mitochondrial protein degradation machinery. However, taking into account that muscle is not the primary tissue involved in HSP, the presence of, albeit inconsistent, signs of a mitochondrial myopathy in patients with paraplegin mutations is highly suggestive of an involvement of the mitochondrial energy metabolism in this form of HSP.

In yeast, many of the factors involved in the biogenesis of mitochondrial respiratory chain are known to cooperate. For instance, inactivation of either *AFG3* or *RCA1* can be complemented by overexpression of the *LON* gene.[96] In the case of HSP, it is possible that other mitochondrial factors with a similar function can compensate paraplegin defects, at least in part, thus reducing the severity of symptoms. As in yeast, defects in paraplegin may cause an accumulation of incompletely synthesized mitochondrial translation products and unassembled subunits of ATP-synthase or respiratory chain complexes, leading to axonal degeneration. The decline in OXPHOS and the increase of mitochondrial DNA mutations with age may contribute to the progressive nature of HSP phenotype.

Mutations of Tim8/9, a mitochondrial transporter, in X-linked deafness dystonia syndrome

The human deafness dystonia syndrome (Mohr–Tranebjaerg syndrome, MTS/DFN-1, OMIM 304700) is a recessive, X-linked neurodegenerative disorder characterized by progressive sensorineural deafness, cortical blindness, dystonia, dysphagia, and paranoia.[97,98] It is usually caused by truncation or deletion of an 11-kDa protein (referred to as DDP-1)[99] whose gene is located on Xq21.3-Xq22, although a *de novo* missense mutation of DDP-1 has recently been found in a singleton DFN-1 case.[100] DDP1 is closely related to the ORF YJR135w-a in *Saccharomyces cerevisiae.*[101] DDP-1 and YGR135w-a (referred to as Tim8p) are similar to Tim9p, Tim10p, and Tim12p, which mediate the import of mitochondrial carrier proteins. DDP-1, Tim8p, and Tim13p are localized to the mitochondrial intermembrane space, and the yeast homologue of DDP-1, Tim8p, interacts with the import system for multispanning inner membrane proteins. The DDP-1 transcript is ubiquitously expressed in human tissues, indicating that DDP-1 is important for basic cellular processes. Loss of DDP-1 may manifest itself selectively in different tissue types because the energy requirements of tissues may differ, particularly during development. DDP-1 may be important for import of a subset of metabolite carriers that can have a crucial role in neural development of mammals. Although this question remains open, the present results show clearly that the human deafness dystonia syndrome is a novel type of mitochondrial disease that most likely reflects a defect in mitochondrial protein import. The demonstration that the DDP-1 protein is probably involved in the import of the mitochondrial proteins implies that the underlying defect of the Mohr–Tranebjaerg syndrome is a defect in mitochondrial OXPHOS, specifically due to deficiencies in carrier proteins like ANT. This hypothesis is bolstered by the observation that the phenotypes associated with systemic OXPHOS defects resulting from mutations in the mtDNA give an array of clinical symptoms that nicely overlap with those of the Mohr–Tranebjaerg syndrome. Hence, deafness and dystonia associated with basal ganglia degeneration can now be linked to mitochondrial defects resulting from nDNA as well as mtDNA mutations, like the ND6 mutation associated with Leber's-dystonia syndrome.[102]

Mutations of OPA1, a gene encoding a mitochondrial dynamin-like protein, in autosomal dominant optic atrophy

Dominant optic atrophy 1 (OPA1, OMIM 165500) is a hereditary optic neuropathy causing decreased visual acuity, colour vision deficits, a centrocecal scotoma, and optic nerve pallor.[103] It is characterized by an insidious onset of optic atrophy in early childhood with moderate to severe decrease of visual acuity, blue–yellow dyschromatopsia, and centrocecal scotoma of varying density. Many affected members of the families may be unaware of having the disease or of its hereditary aspects. Visual acuity in affected subjects is highly variable. A mild degree of temporal or diffuse pallor of the optic disc and minimal colour vision defects, in the context of the family with dominant optic atrophy, are highly suggestive of an individual being affected, even if visual acuity is normal. Morphologically, there is evidence of degeneration of the ganglion cell layer, predominantly from central retina. Alexander *et al.*[104] and Delettre *et al.*[105] independently identified a gene (OPA1) in the optic atrophy-1 candidate region that encodes a polypeptide with homology to dynamin-related GTPases. Both groups identified mutations in this gene causing autosomal dominant optic atrophy. The presence of numerous loss-of-function heterozygous mutations in affected individuals suggests that haploinsufficiency of OPA1 may be the pathogenetic mechanism in this condition.

OPA1 is a 960-amino acid polypeptide, weakly similar to Msp1 and Mgm1, two dynamin-related protein identified in *Schizosaccharomyces pombe* and *Saccharomyces cerevisiae*, respectively.[106,107] Both proteins have a GTPase domain, a central dynamin domain conserved among all dynamins, and an amino-terminal domain required for mitochondrial localization. Likewise, OPA1 is targeted to mitochondria; Msp1 and Mgm1 are essential for the maintenance and inheritance of mitochondria, possibly controlling their proliferation and cellular distribution.[108]

Interestingly, the pathophysiology and clinical symptoms observed in autosomal dominant optic atrophy overlap with those in LHON (see Chapter 8). LHON is caused by mutations in mtDNA-encoded genes for subunits of Complex I of the respiratory chain. These mutations are believed to lead to insufficient energy supply in the highly energy-demanding neurons of the optic nerve (notably the papillomacular bundle) and to cause blindness by a compromise of axonal transport in retinal ganglion cells. It is possible that mutations in OPA1 affect mitochondrial integrity, resulting in impairment of energy supply. In the long term, this may affect normal metabolic processes in retinal ganglion cells and consequently their survival.

Defects of mitochondrial metabolism of iron (I): mutations of ABC7 in X-linked sideroblastic anaemia with ataxia syndrome (XLSA/A)

In XLSA/A (OMIM 300135), affected males have a moderate hypochromic microcytic anaemia with ring sideroblasts on bone marrow examination as in typical X-linked sideroblastic anaemia due to defects of delta-aminolevulinate synthase. However, XLSA/A patients have increased, rather than normal or low, free erythrocyte protoporphyrin levels, no excessive parenchymal iron storage in adulthood, and lack of correction by pyridoxine supplementation.[109] The ataxia can be evident by age 1 year, is usually nonprogressive, and is accompanied by long motor tract signs (hyperactive deep tendon reflexes, positive Babinski sign, clonus). These features distinguish it from the more common X-linked sideroblastic anaemia (XLSA; OMIM 301300), which does not have a neurologic component, is typically at least partially pyridoxine-responsive, and is caused by mutations in the erythroid-specific 5-aminolevulinate synthase (ALAS2) gene at Xp11. A missense mutation, Ile400 to Met in ABC7, a gene mapping to Xq13, was found in a family with 5 affected males with ASAT.[110] The gene contains 16 exons, and the protein comprises 750 amino acids. A second missense mutation was later found in exon 10 of the *ABC7* gene in 2 affected brothers with XLSA/A.[111] The mutation was a G–A transition at nucleotide 1305 of the full-length cDNA, resulting in a charge inversion caused by the substitution of Lys for Glu at residue 433 C-terminal to the putative sixth transmembrane domain of ABC7.

The human protein ABC7 belongs to the adenosine triphosphate-binding cassette transporter superfamily,[112–114] and its yeast orthologue, Atm1p,[115] plays a central role in the maturation of cytosolic iron–sulphur (Fe/S) cluster-containing proteins.[116] Expression of normal ABC7 complemented the defect in the maturation of cytosolic Fe/S proteins in a yeast strain in which the *ATM1* gene had been deleted (atm1 cells). In contrast, the expression of mutated ABC7 (E433K) or Atm1p (D398K) proteins in atm1 cells led to a low efficiency of cytosolic Fe/S protein maturation. These data demonstrate that both the molecular defect in XLSA/A and the impaired maturation of a cytosolic Fe/S protein result from an ABC7 mutation in the reported family.[117]

A role of the yeast ABC transporter protein, Atm1p, in the generation of cytosolic Fe/S proteins has recently been identified. It was proposed that Atm1p was involved in the export of a component required for cytosolic Fe/S protein assembly. Consistent with this idea, Atm1p was required for maturation of the cytosolic Fe/S cluster-containing protein, isopropyl malate isomerase (Leu1p), but not for the assembly of mitochondrial Fe/S proteins.

The connections between the ABC7 defect, the mitochondrial iron overloading evidenced by the presence of ringed sideroblasts, and the XLSA/A disease phenotype remains to be elucidated. The relationship between ABC7-dependent Fe/S protein maturation in the cytosol and haeme synthesis is also far from understood. The combined haematologic evidence for functional iron deficiency in the proband (microcytic, hypochromic anaemia with low serum iron, low transferrin saturation, and elevated sTfR) suggests that the iron imported into the mitochondria is unavailable for ferrochelatase-catalysed insertion into protoporphyrin IX. It is possible that some cytosolic Fe/S protein is critical to this process or that oxidative stress induced by iron overload might interfere with haeme biosynthesis or stability. The anaemia caused by decreased haeme concentration could promote aberrant erythropoiesis, leading to increased gastrointestinal iron absorption. Reticuloendothelial iron loading with increased serum ferritin, as seen in the probands, would result from the scavenging of ineffective red cell precursors. The presence of cerebellar ataxia in XLSA/A indicates that, as evidenced in Friedreich's ataxia, iron plays an important role in cerebellar cells. Delineation of the underlying mechanisms requires further investigations of the molecular pathology of the XLSA/A erythroblast and neural cells.

Defects of mitochondrial metabolism of iron (II): mutations of
frataxin in Friedreich's ataxia
Friedreich ataxia (FA) is an inherited recessive disorder characterized by progressive neurological disability and heart abnormalities that may be fatal. The disease, which currently has no treatment, affects roughly 1 in 50,000 people. The first symptoms usually appear in childhood, but age of onset varies from infancy to adulthood. Atrophy of sensory and cerebellar pathways causes ataxia, dysarthria, fixation instability, deep sensory loss and loss of tendon reflexes. Corticospinal degeneration leads to muscle weakness and extensor plantar responses. A hypertrophic cardiomyopathy may contribute to disability and cause premature death. Other common problems include kyphoscoliosis, pes cavus, and, in 10 per cent of patients, diabetes mellitus. Typically, patients lose the ability to walk 15 years after the onset of symptoms and have a reduced life expectancy, although mild cases have been observed.

The FA gene (FRDA) encodes a protein of 210 amino acids, called frataxin. The gene is expressed in all cells, but at variable levels in different tissues and during development. Frataxin expression is generally higher in mitochondria-rich cells, such as cardiomyocytes and neurons. FA is the result of Frataxin deficiency, which in most cases stems from a triplet expansion in the FRDA gene.[118–120] The majority of patients are homozygous for a GAA triplet repeat sequence expansion (TRS) in the first intron of the gene, 5 per cent are heterozygous for a GAA expansion and a point mutation in the frataxin coding sequence. Repeats in normal chromosomes contain up to ~40 triplets, whereas 90 to >1000 triplets are seen in chromosomes of affected patients. Expanded alleles show meiotic and mitotic instability. The severity and age of onset of the disease are in part determined by the size of the expanded triplet, in particular of the smaller allele. However, differences in GAA expansions account for only about 50 per cent of the variability in age of onset, indicating that other factors influence phenotype. These may include somatic mosaicism for expansion size, modifier genes and environmental factors.

Frataxin does not resemble any protein of known function. It is highly conserved during evolution,[121] with homologues in mammals, invertebrates, yeast, and plants. The protein is targeted to mitochondria,[121–123] and localized in the mitochondrial matrix.[123] Gene disruption (knock out) of the yeast frataxin homologue gene (YFH1) leads to accumulation of iron in mitochondria.[124] Most YFH1 knock-out strains, called ΔYFH1, have defects in, or lose mtDNA, they are consequently OXPHOS deficient and cannot grow on non-fermentable substrates.[125] Loss of respiratory competence occurs only when iron is included in the culture medium suggesting that mitochondrial damage is the consequence of iron toxicity. Iron in mitochondria can react with reactive oxygen species (ROS) that form in these organelles. Even in normal mitochondria, some electrons from the respiratory chain are lost, mostly from reduced ubiquinone (probably its semiquinone form), and directly reduce molecular oxygen to superoxide (O_2^-). Mitochondrial Mn-dependent superoxide dismutase (SOD2) generates hydrogen peroxide (H_2O_2) from $O_2^{\cdot-}$, then glutathione peroxidase oxidizes glutathione to convert H_2O_2 to H_2O. Iron may intervene in this process and generate the hydroxyl radical ($OH^\cdot$) through the Fenton reaction (Fe(II) + H_2O_2 → Fe(III) + $OH^\cdot$+ OH^-); $OH^\cdot$ is highly toxic and causes lipid peroxidation, protein and nucleic acid damage. Occurrence of the Fenton reaction in ΔYFH1 yeast cells is suggested by their greatly enhanced sensitivity to H_2O_2.[126] Disruption of frataxin causes a general disturbance of iron metabolism in yeast. Because iron is trapped in mitochondria, a deficit in cytosolic iron results, causing a marked induction (ten–fifty-fold) of the high-affinity iron transport system of the cell membrane.[126] As a consequence, iron crosses the plasma membrane in large amounts and accumulates further in mitochondria. Normal human frataxin is able to complement the defect in ΔYFH1 cells, while human frataxin carrying a point mutation found in FA patients is unable to do so, strongly suggesting that the function of yfh1p is conserved in human frataxin.

Experiments involving induction of frataxin expression from a plasmid transformed into ΔYFH1 yeast cells indicate that the protein stimulates a flux of non-haeme iron out of mitochondria,[126] but the mechanism and transporter remain obscure. Haeme synthesis is normal in ΔYFH1 yeast, suggesting that ferrochelatase function and transport of haeme out of mitochondria are unaffected by frataxin deficiency.

The current experimental data may be interpreted in different ways, therefore it is not yet possible to state whether mitochondrial damage is the consequence of increased free radical production, or is in part a direct consequence of the primary function of frataxin. Several mitochondrial enzymes are known to be impaired in ΔYFH1 yeast cells, as well as cardiac tissue from FA patients, particularly respiratory chain Complexes I, II, and III, and aconitase.[127] These enzymes all contain iron–sulphur (Fe–S) clusters in their active sites. Fe–S clusters are remarkably sensitive to free radicals, so a deficit can be reasonably ascribed to oxidative damage. However, a specific synthetic pathway has been recently discovered for Fe–S clusters in yeast mitochondria.[128] Remarkably, defects in several enzymes in the pathway lead to mitochondrial iron accumulation, similar to those observed in ΔYFH1. This has prompted some researchers to suggest that yeast frataxin may itself be involved in Fe–S cluster synthesis.[128]

The structure of frataxin is the object of intensive analysis.[129,130] Frataxin does not have any feature resembling a known iron-binding site. Studies on its crystal structure study demonstrated that iron binds the frataxin monomer nonspecifically. Hopefully, a more extensive correlation between structural data and biochemical findings will soon be available, which will clarify the issue of iron binding.

Several observations in humans and human cell lines reinforce the hypothesis that altered iron metabolism, free radical damage, and mitochondrial dysfunction all occur in FA. Involvement of iron was suggested twenty years ago as deposits are found in myocardial cells from FA patients.[131] Iron accumulation has been demonstrated by magnetic resonance imaging (MRI) in the dentate nucleus, a component of the central nervous system that is severely affected in FA.[132] The observation of a moderate, but significant increase in iron concentration in the mitochondrial fraction from FA fibroblasts has been reported.[133] Oxidative stress is suggested by the observation that FA patients have an increased lipid peroxidation product,[134] as well as increased 8-hydroxy-2'-deoxyguanosine (8OH2'dG), a marker of oxidative DNA damage, in urine.[135] In addition, fibroblasts of patients with FA are sensitive to low doses of H_2O_2.[136] Another hint of a possible role of free radicals is the observation that vitamin E deficiency produces a phenotype resembling FA.[137] Vitamin E localizes in mitochondrial membranes where it acts as a free radical scavenger.

Mitochondrial dysfunction has been demonstrated *in vivo* in FA. Magnetic resonance spectroscopy analysis of skeletal muscle shows a reduced rate of ATP synthesis after exercise, which is inversely correlated to GAA expansion sizes.[138] Rötig *et al.*[127] also demonstrated the same multiple enzyme deficiencies found in $\Delta YFH1$ yeast (deficit of respiratory Complexes I, II and III, and of aconitase) in endomyocardial biopsies of two FA patients.

The generation of a frataxin knock-out mouse.[139] has revealed that homozygous knock-out mice die as early as embryonic day 7 (E7). While total absence of frataxin leads to cell death in the early embryo, a reduced level of the protein, as observed in patients, may only affect some cells that are dependent on a normal level of frataxin to survive through some critical step in their development, for example, sensory neurons of the dorsal root ganglia. These cells are lost very early in FA, the loss seems to be non-progressive, and may therefore be developmental. Two viable mouse models have been generated using a conditional gene targeting approach. One was a heart and striated muscle frataxin-deficient line, the other had a more generalized deficiency.[140] The mice reproduced important progressive pathophysiological and biochemical features of the human disease. These were cardiac hypertrophy associated with progressive intramitochondrial iron accumulation in the former case, and large sensory neuron dysfunction in the more generalized frataxin-deficient line. Both FA knock-out strains displayed Complex I–III and aconitase deficiency. These animals provide an important resource for pathophysiological studies and for testing new treatments. However, they do not mimic perfectly the situation in humans because conditional gene targeting leads to complete loss of frataxin in some cells at a specific time in development, while FA is characterized by partial frataxin deficiency in all cells, throughout life. Therefore, there is still a need to develop new animal models of the disease.

Prospects for therapy in FA

Based on the hypothesis that iron-mediated oxidative damage plays a major role in the pathogenesis of Friedreich ataxia, removal of excess mitochondrial iron and/or antioxidant treatment may in principle be attempted. However, removal of excess mitochondrial iron is problematic with the currently available drugs. Desferioxamine (DFO) is effective in chelating iron in the extracellular fluid and cytosol, but not in mitochondria. Furthermore, DFO toxicity may be higher when there is no overall iron overload. Thus, chelation therapy has a number of unknowns: it is probably best that it is tested in trials involving a small number of closely monitored patients. Iron depletion by phlebotomy, though less risky, presents the same uncertainties concerning possible efficacy. As far as antioxidants are concerned, these include a long list of molecules with specific mechanisms of action and pharmacokinetic properties. To have the potential to be effective in FA, an antioxidant must protect against damage caused by free radicals, act in the mitochondrial compartment and be able to cross the blood–brain barrier. At this time, coenzyme Q derivatives appear plausible therapeutic agents and are currently under trial.[141] However, new information on frataxin function and pathogenesis is needed to progress towards effective treatment of the disease.

Acknowledgements

We are indebted to Ms B Geehan for revising the manuscript. We thank Drs Mario Savoiardo, and Laura Farina, for the NMR images. Supported by Fondazione Telethon-Italy (Grant No. 1180 to M.Z.), Fondazione Pierfranco e Luisa Mariani (Ricerca 2000 grant to M.Z.), Ricerca Finalizzata Min. San. ICS 030.3/RF98.37, and EU Human Capital and Mobility network grant on 'Mitochondrial Biogenesis in Development and Disease'.

References

1. Zeviani M and Taroni F (1994). Mitochondrial diseases. *Baillieres Clin. Neurol.* **2**: 315–334.
2. Zeviani M and Antozzi C (1997). Mitochondrial disorders. *Mol. Hum. Reprod.* **3**: 133–148.
3. MITOMAP (2000). A Human Mitochondrial Genome Database. Center for Molecular Medicine, Emory University, Atlanta, GA, USA. http://www.gen.emory.edu/mitomap.html.
4. Chinnery PF, Johnson MA, Wardell TM, Singh-Kler R, Hayes C, Brown DT, Taylor RW, Bindoff LA, and Turnbull DM (2000). The epidemiology of pathogenic mitochondrial DNA mutations. *Ann Neurol.* **48**: 188–193.
5. Chinnery PF and Turnbull DM (2000). Mitochondrial DNA mutations in the pathogenesis of human disease. *Mol. Med. Today* **6**: 425–432.
6. Zeviani M, Tiranti V, and Piantadosi C (1998). Mitochondrial disorders. *Medicine* **77**: 59–72.
7. Leigh D (1951). Subacute necrotizing encephalomyelopathy in an infant. *J. Neurol. Neurosurg. Psychiatry* **14**: 216–221.
8. DiMauro S and De Vivo DC (1996). Genetic heterogeneity in Leigh Syndrome. *Ann. Neurol.* **40**: 5–7.
9. Rahman S, Blok RB, Dahl H-H, Danks DM, Kirby DM, Chow CW, Christodoulou J, and Thorburn DR (1996). Leigh syndrome: clinical features and biochemical and DNA abnormalities. *Ann. Neurol.* **39**: 343–351.
10. Sue CM and Schon EA (2000). Mitochondrial respiratory chain diseases and mutations in nuclear DNA: a promising start? *Brain Pathol.* **10**: 441–450.
11. Attardi G and Schatz G (1988). Biogenesis of mitochondria. *Annu. Rev. Cell. Biol.* **4**: 289–333.
12. Poyton RO and JE McEwen (1996). Crosstalk between nuclear and mitochondrial genomes. *Annu. Rev. Biochem.* **65**: 563–607.
13. Tzagoloff A and Dieckmann CL (1990). PET genes of *Saccharomyces cerevisiae. Microbiol. Rev.* **54**: 211–225.

14. Smeitink J and van den Heuvel L (1999). Human mitochondrial complex I in health and disease. *Am. J. Hum. Genet.* **64**: 1505–1510.

15. Grigorieff N (1998). Three-dimensional structure of bovine NADH : ubiquinone oxidoreductase (complex I) at 22 Å in ice. *J. Mol. Biol.* **277**: 1033–1046.

16. Morris AAM, Leonard JV, Brown GK, Bidouki SK, Bindoff LA, Woodward CE, Harding AE, Lake BD, Harding BN, Farrell MA, Bell, JE, Mirakhur M, and Turnbull D (1996). Deficiency in respiratory chain complex I is a common cause of Leigh disease. *Ann. Neurol.* **40**: 25–30.

17. Robinson BH (1998). Human complex I deficiency: clinical spectrum and involvement of oxygen free radicals in the pathogenicity of the defect. *Biochim. Biophys. Acta* **1364**: 271–286.

18. Faivre L, Cormier-Daire V, Chretien D, Christoph von Kleist-Retzow J, Amiel J, Dommergues M, Saudubray JM, Dumez Y, Rotig A, Rustin P, and Munnich A (2000). Determination of enzyme activities for prenatal diagnosis of respiratory chain deficiency. *Prenat. Diagn.* **20**: 732–737.

19. Loeffen J, Smeitink J, Triepels R, Smeets R, Schuelke M, Sengers R, Trijbels F, Hamel B, Mullaart R, and van den Heuvel, L (1998). The first nuclear-encoded complex I mutation in a patient with Leigh syndrome. *Am. J. Hum. Genet.* **63**: 1598–1608.

20. Triepels RH, van den Heuvel LP, Loeffen JLCM, Buskens CAF, Smeets RJP, Gozalbo MFR, Budde SMS, Mariman EC, Wijburg FA, Barth PG, Trijbels JMF, and Smeitink JAM (1999). Leigh syndrome associated with a mutation in the NDUFS7 (PSST) nuclear encoded subunit of complex I. *Ann. Neurol.* **45**: 787–790.

21. van den Heuvel L, Ruitenbeek W, Smeets R, Gelman-Kohan Z, Elpeleg O, Loeffen J, Trijbels F, Mariman E, de Bruijn D, and Smeitink J (1998). Demonstration of a new pathogenic mutation in human complex I deficiency: a 5-bp duplication in the nuclear gene encoding the 18-kD (AQDQ) subunit. *Am. J. Hum. Genet.* **62**: 262–268.

22. Budde SM, van den Heuvel LP, Janssen AJ, Smeets RJ, Buskens CA, DeMeirleir L, Van Coster R, Baethmann M, Voit T, Trijbels JM, and Smeitink JA (2000). Combined enzymatic complex I and III deficiency associated with mutations in the nuclear encoded NDUFS4 gene. *Biochem. Biophys. Res. Commun.* **275**: 63–68.

23. Petruzzella V, Vergari R, Puzziferri I, Boffoli D, Lamantea E, Zeviani M, and Papa S (2001). A nonsense mutation in the NDUFS4 gene encoding the 18 kDa (AQDQ) subunit of complex I abolishes assembly and activity of the complex in a patient with Leigh-like syndrome. *Hum. Mol. Genet.* **10**: 529–535.

24. Papa S, Scacco S, Sardanelli AM, Vergari R, Papa F, Budde S, van den Heuvel L, and Smeitink J (2001). Mutation in the NDUFS4 gene of complex I abolishes cAMP-dependent activation of the complex in a child with fatal neurological syndrome. *FEBS Lett.* **489**: 259–262.

25. Schuelke M, Smeitink J, Mariman E, Loeffen J, Plecko B, Trijbels F, Stockler-Ipsiroglu S, and van den Heuvel L (1999). Mutant NDUFV1 subunit of mitochondrial complex I causes leukodystrophy and myoclonic epilepsy. *Nat. Genet.* **21**: 260–261.

26. Loeffen J, Elpeleg O, Smeitink J, Smeets R, Stockler-Ipsiroglu S, Mandel H, Sengers R, Trijbels F, and van den Heuvel L (2001). Mutations in the complex I NDUFS2 gene of patients with cardiomyopathy and encephalomyopathy. *Ann. Neurol.* **49**: 195–201.

27. Benit P, Chretien D, Kadham N, de Lonlay-Debeney P, Cormier-Daire V, Cabral A, Peudenier S, Rustin P, Munnich A, and Rötig A (2001). Large-scale deletion and point mutations of the nuclear NDUFV1 and NDUFS1 genes in mitochondrial complex I deficiency *Am. J. Hum. Genet.* **68**: 1344–1354.

28. Ackrell BAC, Johnson MK, Gunsalus RP, and Cecchini G (1990). Structure and function of succinate dehydrogenase and fumarate reductase. In: *Chemistry and Biochemistry of Flavoproteins 3* (ed. F Muller). Boca Raton, Florida: CRC Press, pp. 229–297.

29. Kita K, Oya H, Gennis RB, Ackrell BA, and Kasahara MN (1990). Human complex II (succinate-ubiquinone oxidoreductase): cDNA cloning of iron sulfur (Ip) subunit of liver mitochondria. *Biochem. Biophys. Res. Commun.* **166**: 101–108.

30. Hirawake H, Wang H, Kuramochi T, Kojima S, and Kita K (1994). Human complex II (succinate-ubiquinone oxidoreductase): a cDNA cloning of the flavoprotein (Fp) subunit of liver mitochondria. *J. Biochem.* **116**: 211–217.

31. Hirawake H, Taniwaki M, Tamura A, Amino H, Tomitsuka E, and Kita K (1999). Characterization of the human SDHD gene encoding the small subunit of cytochrome b (cybS) in mitochondrial succinate-ubiquinone oxidoreductase. *Biochim. Biophys. Acta* **1412**: 295–300.

32. Hirawake H, Taniwaki M, Tamura A, Kojima S, and Kita K (1997). Cytochrome b in human complex II (succinate-ubiquinone oxidoreductase): cDNA cloning of the components in liver mito-chondria and chromosome assignment of the genes for the large (SDHC) and small (SDHD) sub-units to 1q21 and 11q23. *Cytogenet. Cell. Genet.* **79**: 132–138.

33. Morris AAM, Farnsworth L, Ackrell BAC, Turnbull DM, and Birch-Machin MA (1994). The cDNA sequence of the flavoprotein subunit of human heart succinate dehydrogenase. *Biochim. Biophys. Acta* **1185**: 125–128.

34. Au HC, Ream-Robinson D, Bellew LA, Broomfield PLE, Saghbini M, and Scheffler IE (1995). Structural organization of the gene encoding the human iron-sulfur subunit of the succinate dehydrogenase. *Gene* **159**: 249–253.

35. Rustin P, Bourgeron T, Parfait B, Chretien D, Munnich A, and Rötig A (1997). Inborn errors of the Krebs cycle: a group of unusual mitochondrial diseases in human. *Biochim. Biophys. Acta* **1361**: 185–197.

36. Bourgeron T, Rustin P, Chretien D, Birch-Machin M, Bourgeois M, Viegas-Pequignot E, Munnich A, and Rotig A (1995). Mutation of a nuclear succinate dehydrogenase gene results in mitochondrial respiratory chain deficiency. *Nat. Genet.* **11**: 144–149.

37. Parfait B, Chretien D, Rötig A, Marsac C, Munnich A, and Rustin P (2000). Compound hetero-zygous mutations in the flavoprotein gene of the respiratory chain complex II in a patient with Leigh syndrome. *Hum. Genet.* **106**: 236–243.

38. Birch-Machin MA, Taylor RW, Cochran B, Ackrell BA, and Turnbull DM (2000). Late-onset optic atrophy, ataxia, and myopathy associated with a mutation of a complex II gene. *Ann. Neurol.* **48**: 330–335.

39. Baysal BE, Ferrell RE, Willett-Brozick JE, Lawrence EC, Myssiorek D, Bosch A, van der Mey A, Taschner PE, Rubinstein WS, Myers EN, Richard CW, Cornelisse CJ, Devilee P, and Devlin B (2000). Mutations in SDHD, a mitochondrial complex II gene, in hereditary paraganglioma. *Science* **287**: 848–851.

40. Niemann S and Muller U (2000). Mutations in SDHC cause autosomal dominant paraganglioma, type 3. *Nat. Genet.* **26**: 268–270.

41. Gimm O, Armanios M, Dziema H, Neumann HP, and Eng C (2000). Somatic and occult germ-line mutations in SDHD, a mitochondrial complex II gene, in nonfamilial pheochromocytoma. *Cancer Res.* **60**: 6822–6825.

42. Olson RE and Rudney H (1983). Biosynthesis of ubiquinone. *Vitam. Horm.* **40**: 1–43§.

43. Lenaz G, Fato R, Castelluccio C, Genova ML, Bovina C, Estornell E, Valls V, Pallotti F, and Parenti-Castelli G (1993). The function of coenzyme Q10 in mitochondria. *J. Clin. Invest.* **71**: S66–S70.

44. Ogasahara S, Engel AG, Frens D, and Mack D (1989). Muscle coenzyme Q deficiency in familial mitochondrial encephalomyopathy. *Proc. Natl Acad. Sci. USA* **86**: 2379–2382.

45. Sobreira C, Hirano M, Shanske S, Keller RK, Haller RG, Davidson E, Santorelli FM, Miranda AF, Bonilla E, Mojon DS, Barreira AA, King MP, and DiMauro S (1997). Mitochondrial encephalomyo-pathy with coenzyme Q10 deficiency. *Neurology* **48**: 1238–1243.

46. Boitier E, Degoul F, Desguerre I, Charpentier C, Francois D, Ponsot G, Diry M, Rustin P, and Marsac C (1998). A case of mitochondrial encephalomyopathy associated with a muscle coenzyme Q10 deficiency. *J. Neurol. Sci.* **156**: 41–46.

47. Musumeci O, Naini A, Slonim AE, Skavin N, Hadjigeorgiou GL, Krawiecki N, Weissman BM, Tsao C-Y, Mendell JR, Shanske S, DeVivo DC, Hirano M, and DiMauro S (2001). Familial cere-bellar ataxia with muscle coenzyme Q10 deficiency. *Neurology* **56**: 849–855.

48. Babcock GT and Wikström M (1992). Oxygen activation and the conservation of energy in cell respiration. *Nature* **356**: 301–309.
49. Saraste M (1990). Structural features of cytochrome oxidase. *Q. Rev. Biophys.* **23**: 331–366.
50. Taanman JW (1997). Human cytochrome c oxidase: structure, function, and deficiency. *J. Bioenerg. Biomembr.* **29**: 151–163.
51. Fabrizi GM, Sadlock J, Hirano M, Mita S, Koga Y, Rizzuto R, Zeviani M, and Schon EA (1992). Differential expression of genes specifying two isoforms of subunit VIa of human cytochrome c oxidase. *Gene* **119**: 307–312.
52. Arnaudo E, Hirano M, Seelan RS, Milatovich A, Hsieh CL, Fabrizi GM, Grossman LI, Francke U, and Schon EA (1992). Tissue-specific expression and chromosome assignment of genes specifying two isoforms of subunit VIIa of human cytochrome c oxidase. *Gene* **119**: 299–305.
53. Iwata S, Ostermeier C, Ludwig B, and Michel H (1995). Structure at 2.8 A resolution of cytochrome c oxidase from Paracoccus denitrificans. *Nature* **376**: 660–669.
54. Tsukihara T, Aoyama H, Yamashita E, Tomizaki T, Yamaguchi H, Shinzawa-Itoh K, Nakashima R, Yaono R, and Yoshikawa S (1996). The whole structure of the 13-subunit oxidized cytochrome c oxidase at 2.8 A. *Science* **272**: 1136–1144.
55. Grossman LI and Lomax MI (1997). Nuclear genes for cytochrome c oxidase. *Biochim. Biophys. Acta* **1352**: 174–192.
56. Anderson S, Bankier AT, Barrell BG, de Bruijn MHL, Coulson AR, Drouin J, Eperon IC, Nierlich DP, Roe BA, Sanger F, Schreier PH, Smith AJH, Staden R, and Young IG (1981). Sequence and organization of the human mitochondrial genome. *Nature* **290**: 457–465.
57. DiMauro S, Hirano M, Bonilla E, Moraes CT, and Schon EA (1994). Cytochrome c oxidase deficiency: progress and problems. In: *Mitochondrial Disorders in Neurology* (eds AVH Schapira and DiMauro), Oxford: Butterworth-Heinemann, pp. 91–115.
58. DiMauro S and Bonilla E (1997). Mitochondrial Encephalomyopathies. In: *The Molecular and Genetic Basis of Neurological Disease* (eds RN Rosenberg, SB Prusiner, S DiMauro, and RL Barchi), Boston: Butterworth-Heinemann, pp. 201–235.
59. Comi GP, Bordoni A, Salani S, Franceschina L, Sciacco M, Prelle A, Fortunato F, Zeviani M, Napoli L, Bresolin N, Moggio M, Ausenda CD, Taanman JW, and Scarlato G (1998). Cytochrome c oxidase subunit I microdeletion in a patient with motor neuron disease. *Ann. Neurol.* **43**: 110–116.
60. Bruno C, Martinuzzi A, Tang Y, Andreu AL, Pallotti F, Bonilla E, Shanske S, Fu J, Sue CM, Angelini C, DiMauro S, and Manfredi G (1999). A stop-codon mutation in the human mtDNA cytochrome c oxidase I gene disrupts the functional structure of complex IV. *Am. J. Hum. Genet.* **65**: 1245–1249.
61. Hoffbuhr KC, Davidson E, Filiano BA, Davidson M, Kennaway NG, and King MP (2000). A pathogenic 15-base pair deletion in mitochondrial DNA-encoded cytochrome c oxidase subunit III results in the absence of functional cytochrome c oxidase. *J. Biol. Chem.* **275**: 13994–14003.
62. Tiranti V, Corona P, Greco M, Taanman JW, Carrara F, Lamantea E, Nijtmans L, Uziel G, and Zeviani M (2000). A novel frameshift mutation of the mtDNA COIII gene leads to impaired assembly of cytochrome c oxidase in a patient affected by Leigh-like syndrome. *Hum. Mol. Genet.* **9**: 2733–2742.
63. Nijtmans LGJ, Taanman JW, Muijsers AO, Speijer D, and Van den Bogert C (1998). Assembly of cytochrome c oxidase in cultured human cells. *Eur. J. Biochem.* **254**: 389–394.
64. Petruzzella V, Tiranti V, Fernandez P, Ianna P, Carrozzo R, and Zeviani M (1998). Identification and characterization of human cDNAs specific to BCS1, PET112, SCO1, COX15, and COX11, five genes involved in the formation and function of the mitochondrial respiratory chain. *Genomics* **54**: 494–504.
65. Tiranti V, Hoertnagel K, Carrozzo R, Galimberti C, Munaro M, Granatiero M, Zelante L, Gasparini P, Marzella R, Rocchi M, Bayona-Bafaluy MP, Enriquez A, Uziel G, Bertini E, Dionisi-Vici C, Franco B, Meitinger T, and Zeviani M (1998). Mutations of SURF-1 in Leigh Disease associated with cytochrome c oxidase deficiency. *Am. J. Hum. Genet.* **63**: 1609–1621.

66. Zhu Z, Yao J, Johns T, Fu K, de Bie I, Macmillan C, Cuthbert AP, Newbold RF, Wang J-C, Chevrette M, Brown GK, Brown RM, and Shoubridge E (1998). Surf1, a factor involved in the biogenesis of cytochrome c oxidase, is mutated in Leigh Syndrome. *Nat. Genet.* **20**: 337–343.

67. Tiranti V, Jaksch M, Hofmann S, Galimberti C, Bezold R, Lulli L, Freisinger P, Bindoff L, Comi G-P, Uziel G, Zeviani M, and Meitinger T (1999). Loss-of-function mutations of SURF-1 are specifically associated with Leigh Syndrome with Cytochrome c oxidase deficiency. *Ann. Neurol.* **46**: 161–166.

68. Teraoka M, Yokoyama Y, Ninomiya S, Inoue C, Yamashita S, and Seino Y (1999). Two novel mutations of SURF-1 in Leigh syndrome with cytochrome c oxidase deficiency. *Hum. Genet.* **105**: 560–563.

69. Pequignot MO, Desguerre I, Dey R, Tartari M, Zeviani M, Agostino A, Benelli C, Fouque F, Prip-Buus C, Marchant D, Abitbol M, and Marsac C (2001). New splicing-site mutations in the SURF1 gene in Leigh syndrome patients. *J. Biol. Chem.* Feb 6; [epub ahead of print]

70. Munaro M, Tiranti V, Sandona D, Lamantea E, Uziel G, Bisson R, and Zeviani M (1997). A single cell complementation class is common to several cases of cytochrome c oxidase-defective Leigh's syndrome. *Hum. Mol. Genet.* **6**: 221–228.

71. Brown RM and Brown GK (1996). Complementation analysis of systemic cytochrome oxidase deficiency presenting as Leigh syndrome. *J. Inherit. Metab. Dis.* **19**: 752–760.

72. Mashkevich G, Repetto B, Glerum DM, Jin C, and Tzagoloff A (1997). SHY1, the yeast homolog of the mammalian SURF-1 gene, encodes a mitochondrial protein required for respiration. *J. Biol. Chem.* **272**: 14356–14364.

73. Tiranti V, Galimberti C, Nijtmans L, Bovolenta S, Perini MP, and Zeviani M (1999). Characterization of SURF-1 expression and Surf-1p function in normal and disease conditions. *Hum. Mol. Genet.* **8**: 2533–2540.

74. Yao J and Shoubridge EA (1999). Expression and functional analysis of SURF1 in Leigh syndrome patients with cytochrome c oxidase deficiency. *Hum. Mol. Genet.* **8**: 2541–2549.

75. Poyau A, Buchet K, Bouzidi MF, Zabot MT, Echenne B, Yao J, Shoubridge EA, and Godinot C (2000). Missense mutations in SURF1 associated with deficient cytochrome c oxidase assembly in Leigh syndrome patients. *Hum. Genet.* **106**: 194–205.

76. Buchwald P, Krummeck G, and Rodel G (1991). Immunological identification of yeast *SCO1* protein as a component of the inner mitochondrial membrane. *Mol. Gen. Genet.* **229**: 413–420.

77. Schulze M and Rodel G (1988). *SCO1*, a yeast nuclear gene essential for accumulation of mitochondrial cytochrome *c* oxidase subunit II. *Mol. Gen. Genet.* **211**: 492–498.

78. Glerum DM, Shtanko A, and Tzagoloff A (1996). SCO1 and SCO2 act as high copy suppressors of a mitochondrial copper recruitment defect in *Saccharomyces cerevisiae*. *J. Biol. Chem.* **271**: 20531–20535.

79. Glerum DM, Shtanko A, and Tzagoloff A (1996). Characterization of COX17, a yeast gene involved in copper metabolism and assembly of cytochrome oxidase. *J. Biol. Chem.* **271**: 14504–14509.

80. Papadopoulou LC, Sue CM, Davidson. MM, Tanji K, Nishino I, Sadlock JE, Krishna S, Walker W, Selby J, Glerum DM, Van Coster R, Lyon G, Scalais E, Lebel R, Kaplan P, Shanske S, DeVivo DC, Bonilla E, Hirano M, DiMauro S, and Schon EA (1999). Fatal infantile cardioencephalomyopathy with COX deficiency and mutations in SCO2, a COX assembly gene. *Nat. Genet.* **23**: 333–337.

81. Jaksch M, Ogilvie I, Yao J, Kortenhaus G, Bresser HG, Gerbitz KD, and Shoubridge EA (2000). Mutations in SCO2 are associated with a distinct form of hypertrophic cardiomyopathy and cytochrome c oxidase deficiency. *Hum. Mol. Genet.* **9**: 795–801.

82. Sue CM, Karadimas C, Checcarelli N, Tanji K, Papadopoulou LC, Pallotti F, Guo FL, Shanske S, Hirano M, De Vivo DC, Van Coster R, Kaplan P, Bonilla E, and DiMauro S (2000). Differential features of patients with mutations in two COX assembly genes, SURF-1 and SCO2. *Ann. Neurol.* **47**: 589–595.

83. Valnot I, Osmond S, Gigarel N, Mehaye B, Amiel J, Cormier-Daire V, Munnich A, Bonnefont JP, Rustin P, and Rotig A (2000). Mutations of the SCO1 gene in mitochondrial cytochrome c oxidase deficiency with neonatal-onset hepatic failure and encephalopathy. *Am. J. Hum. Genet.* **67**: 1104–1109.

84. Glerum DM and Tzagoloff A (1997). Isolation of a human cDNA for haeme A : farnesyltransferase by functional complementation of a yeast cox10 mutant. *Hum. Genet.* **101**: 247–250.

85. Valnot I, von Kleist-Retzow JC, Barrientos A, Gorbatyuk M, Taanman JW, Mehaye B, Rustin P, Tzagoloff A, Munnich A, and Rotig A (2000). A mutation in the human haeme A:farnesyltransferase gene (COX10) causes cytochrome c oxidase deficiency. *Hum. Mol. Genet.* **9**: 1245–1249.

86. de Lonlay P, Valnot I, Barrientos A, Gorbatyuk M, Tzagoloff A, Taanman JW, Benayoun E, Chretien D, Kadhom N, Lombes A, de Baulny HO, Niaudet P, Munnich A, Rustin P, and Rotig A (2001). A mutant mitochondrial respiratory chain assembly protein causes complex III deficiency in patients with tubulopathy, encephalopathy and liver failure. *Nat. Genet.* **29**: 57–60.

87. Harding AE (1981). Genetic aspects of autosomal dominant late onset cerebellar ataxia. *J. Med. Genet.* **18**: 436–441.

88. Fink JK (1997). Advances in hereditary spastic praplegia. *Curr. Opin. Neurol.* **10**: 313–318.

89. Filla A, De Michele G, Marconi R, Bucci L, Carillo C, Castellano AE, Iorio L, Kniahynicki C, Rossi F, and Campanella G (1992). Prevalence of hereditary ataxias and spastic paraplegias in Molise, a region of Italy. *J. Neurol.* **239**: 351–353.

90. De Michele G, De Fusco M, Cavalcanti F, Filla A, Marconi R, Volpe G, Monticelli A, Ballabio A, Casari G, and Cocozza S (1998). A new locus for autosomal recessive hereditary spastic paraplegia maps to chromosome 16q24.3. *Am. J. Hum. Genet.* **63**: 135–139.

91. Casari G, De Fusco M, Ciarmatori S, Zeviani M, Mora M, Fernandez P, De Michele G, Filla A, Cocozza S, Marconi R, Durr A, Fontaine B, and Ballabio A (1998). Spastic paraplegia and OXPHOS impairment caused by mutations in paraplegin, a nuclear-encoded mitochondrial metalloprotease. *Cell* **93**: 973–983.

92. Tzagoloff A, Yue J, Jang J, and Paul MF (1994). A new member of a family of ATPases is essential for assembly of mitochondrial respiratory chain and ATP synthetase complexes in *Saccharomyces cerevisiae*. *J. Biol. Chem.* **269**: 26144–26151.

93. Arlt H, Tauer R, Feldmann H, Neupert W, and Langer T n(1996). The YTA10-12 complex, an AAA protease with chaperone-like activity in the inner membrane of mitochondria. *Cell* **85**: 875–885.

94. Paul M-F and Tzagoloff A (1995). Mutations in RCA1 and AFG3 inhibit F1-ATPase assembly in *Saccharomyces cerevisiae*. *FEBS Lett.* **373**: 66–70.

95. McDermott CJ, Dayaratne RK, Tomkins J, Lusher ME, Lindsey JC, Johnson MA, Casari G, Turnbull DM, Bushby K, and Shaw PJ (2001). Paraplegin gene analysis in hereditary spastic paraparesis (HSP) pedigrees in northeast England. *Neurology* **56**: 467–471.

96. Rep M, Maarten van Dijf J, Suda K, Schatz G, Grivell LA, and Suzuki CK (1996). Promotion of mitochondrial membrane complex assembly by a proteolytically inactive yeast Lon. *Science* **274**: 103–106.

97. Mohr J and Mageroy K (1960). Sex-linked deafness of a possibly new type. *Acta Genet. Statist. Med.* **10**: 54–62.

98. Tranebjaerg L, Schwartz C, Eriksen H, Andreasson S, Ponjavic V, Dahl A, Stevenson RE, May M, Arena F, Barker D, Elverland HH, and Lubs H (1995). A new X linked recessive deafness syndrome with blindness, dystonia, fractures, and mental deficiency is linked to Xq22. *J. Med. Genet.* **32**: 257–263.

99. Jin H, May M, Tranebjaerg L, Kendall E, Fontan G, Jackson J, Subramony SH, Arena F, Lubs H, Smith S, Stevenson R, Schwartz C, and Vetrie D (1996). A novel X-linked gene, DDP, shows mutations in families with deafness (DFN-1), dystonia, mental deficiency and blindness. *Nat. Genet.* **14**: 177–180.

100. Tranebjaerg L, Hamel BCJ, Gabreels FJM, Renier WO, and Van Ghelue M (2000). A de novo missense mutation in a critical domain of the X-linked DDP gene causes the typical deafness-dystonia-optic atrophy syndrome. *Europ. J. Hum. Genet.* **8**: 464–467.

101. Koehler CM, Leuenberger D, Merchant S, Renold A, Junne T, and Schatz G (1999). Human deafness dystonia syndrome is a mitochondrial disease. *Proc. Natl Acad. Sci. USA* **96**: 2141–2146.

102. Wallace DC and Murdock DG (1999). Mitochondria and dystonia: the movement disorder connection? *Proc. Natl Acad. Sci. USA* **96**: 1817–1819.

103. Johnston RL, Seller MJ, Behnam JT, Burdon MA, and Spalton DJ (1999). Dominant optic atrophy: refining the clinical diagnostic criteria in light of genetic linkage studies. *Ophthalmology* **106**: 123–128.

104. Alexander C, Votruba M, Pesch UEA, Thiselton DL, Mayer S, Moore A, Rodriguez M, Kellner U, Leo-Kottler B, Auburger G, Bhattacharya SS, and Wissinger B (2000). OPA1, encoding a dynamin-related GTPase, is mutated in autosomal dominant optic atrophy linked to chromosome 3q28. *Nat. Genet.* **26**: 211–215.

105. Delettre C, Lenaers G, Griffoin, JM, Gigarel N, Lorenzo C, Belenguer P, Pelloquin L, Grosgeorge J, Turc-Carel C, Perret E, Astarie-Dequeker C, Lasquellec L, Arnaud B, Ducommun B, Kaplan J, and Hamel CP (2000). Nuclear gene OPA1, encoding a mitochondrial dynamin-related protein, is mutated in dominant optic atrophy. *Nat. Genet.* **26**: 207–210.

106. Pelloquin L, Belenguer P, Menon Y, and Ducommun B (1998). Identification of a fission yeast dynamin-related protein involved in mitochondrial DNA maintenance. *Biochem. Biophys. Res. Commun.* **251**: 720–726.

107. Jones BA and Fangman WL (1992). Mitochondrial DNA maintenance in yeast requires a protein containing a region related to the GTP-binding domain of dynamin. *Genes Dev.* **6**: 380–389.

108. Wong ED, Wagner JA, Gorsich SW, McCaffery JM, Shaw JM, and Nunnari J (2000). The dynamin-related GTPase, Mgm1p, is an intermembrane space protein required for maintenance of fusion competent mitochondria. *J. Cell. Biol.* **151**: 341–345.

109. Pagon RA, Bird TD, Detter JC, and Pierce I (1985). Hereditary sideroblastic anaemia and ataxia: an X linked recessive disorder. *J. Med. Genet.* **22**: 267–273.

110. Allikmets R, Raskind WH, Hutchinson A, Schueck ND, Dean M, and Koeller DM (1999). Mutation of a putative mitochondrial iron transporter gene (ABC7) in X-linked sideroblastic anaemia and ataxia (XLSA/A). *Hum. Molec. Genet.* **8**: 743–749.

111. Bekri S, Kispal G, Lange H, Fitzsimons E, Tolmie J, Lill R, and Bishop DF (2000). Human ABC7 transporter: gene structure and mutation causing X-linked sideroblastic anaemia with ataxia with disruption of cytosolic iron-sulfur protein maturation. *Blood* **96**: 3256–3264.

112. Savary S, Allikmets R, Denizot F, Luciani MF, Mattei MG, Dean M, and Chimini G (1997). Isolation and chromosomal mapping of a novel ATP-binding cassette transporter conserved in mouse and human. *Genomics* **41**: 275–278.

113. Shimada Y, Okuno S, Kawai A, Shinomiya H, Saito A, Suzuki M, Omori Y, Nishino N, Kanemoto N, Fujiwara T, Horie M, and Takahashi E (1998). Cloning and chromosomal mapping of a novel ABC transporter gene (hABC7), a candidate for X-linked sideroblastic anaemia with spinocerebellar ataxia. *J. Hum. Genet.* **43**: 115–122.

114. Csere P, Lill R, and Kispal G (1998). Identification of a human mitochondrial ABC transporter, the functional orthologue of yeast Atm1p. *FEBS Lett.* **441**: 266–270.

115. Leighton J and Schatz G (1995). An ABC transporter in the mitochondrial inner membrane is required for normal growth of yeast. *EMBO J.* **14**: 188–195.

116. Kispal G, Csere P, Guiard B, and Lill R (1997). The ABC transporter Atm1p is required for iron homeostasis. *FEBS Lett.* **418**: 346–357.

117. Bekri S, Kispal G, Lange H, Fitzsimons E, Tolmie J, Lill R, and Bishop DF (2000). Human ABC7 transporter: gene structure and mutation causing X-linked sideroblastic anaemia with ataxia with disruption of cytosolic iron-sulfur protein maturation. *Blood* **96**: 3256–3264.

118. Campuzano V, Montermini L, Moltó MD, Pianese L, Cossée M, Cavalcanti F, *et al.* (1996). Friedreich ataxia: autosomal recessive disease caused by an intronic GAA triplet repeat expansion. *Science* **271**: 1423–1427.

119. Bidichandani SI, Ashizawa T, and Patel PI (1997). Atypical Friedreich ataxia caused by compound heterozygosity for a novel missense mutation and the GAA triplet-repeat expansion. *Am. J. Hum. Genet.* **60**: 251–1256.

120. Cossee M, Durr A, Schmitt M, Dahl N, Trouillas P, Allinson P, Kostrzewa M, Nivelon-Chevallier A, Gustavson KH, Kohlschutter A, Muller U, Mandel JL, Brice A, Koenig M, Cavalcanti F, Tammaro A, De Michele G, Filla A, Cocozza S, Labuda M, Montermini L, Poirier J, and Pandolfo M (1999). Frataxin point mutations and clinical presentation of compound heterozygous Friedreich ataxia patients. *Ann. Neurol.* **45**: 200–206.

121. Koutnikova H, Campuzano V, Foury F, Dollé P, Cazzalini O, and Koenig M (1997). Studies of human, mouse and yeast homologues indicate a mitochondrial function for frataxin. *Nat. Genet.* **16**: 345–

122. Branda SS, Cavadini P, Adamec J, Kalousek F, Taroni F, and Isaya G (1999). Yeast and human frataxin are processed to mature form in two sequential steps by the mitochondrial processing peptidase. *J. Biol. Chem.* **274**: 22763–22769.

123. Priller J, Scherzer CR, Faber PW, MacDonald ME, and Young AB (1997). Frataxin gene of Friedreich's ataxia is targeted to mitochondria. *Ann. Neurol.* **42**: 265–269.

124. Babcock M, de Silva D, Oaks R, Davis-Kaplan S, Jiralerspong S, Montermini L, Pandolfo M, and Kaplan J (1997). Regulation of mitochondrial iron accumulation by Yfh1, a putative homolog of frataxin. *Science* **276**: 1709–1712.

125. Wilson RB and Roof DM (1997). Respiratory deficiency due to loss of mitochondrial DNA in yeast lacking the frataxin homologue. *Nat. Genet.* **16**: 352–357.

126. Radisky DC, Babcock MC, and Kaplan J (1999). The yeast frataxin homologue mediates mitochondrial iron efflux. Evidence for a mitochondrial iron cycle. *J. Biol. Chem.* **274**: 4497–4499.

127. Rötig A, deLonlay P, Chretien D, *et al.* (1997). Frataxin gene expansion causes aconitase and mitochondrial iron-sulfur protein deficiency in Friedreich ataxia. *Nat. Genet.* **17**: 215–217.

128. Lill R, Diekert K, Kaut A, *et al.* (1999). The essential role of mitochondria in the biogenesis of cellular iron-sulfur proteins. *Biol. Chem.* **380**: 1157–1166.

129. Dhe-Paganon S, Shigeta R, Chi YI, Ristow M, and Shoelson SE (2000). Crystal structure of human frataxin. *J. Biol. Chem.* **275**: 30753–30756.

130. Cho SJ, Lee MG, Yang JK, Lee JY, Song HK, and Suh SW (2000). Crystal structure of Escherichia coli CyaY protein reveals a previously unidentified fold for the evolutionarily conserved frataxin family. *Proc. Natl Acad. Sci. USA* **97**: 8932–8937.

131. Lamarche JB, Côté M, and Lemieux B (1980). The cardiomyopathy of Friedreich ataxia morphological observations in 3 cases. *Can. J. Neurol. Sci.* **7**: 389–396.

132. Waldvogel D, van Gelderen P, and Hallett M (1999). Increased iron in the dentate nucleus of patients with Friedreich ataxia. *Ann. Neurol.* **46**: 123–125.

133. Delatycki MB, Camakaris J, Brooks H, Evans-Whipp T, Thorburn DR, Williamson R, and Forrest SM (1999). Direct evidence that mitochondrial iron accumulation occurs in Friedreich ataxia. *Ann. Neurol.* **45**: 673–675.

134. Emond M, Lepage G, Vanasse M, and Pandolfo M (2000). Increased levels of plasma malondialdehyde in Friedreich ataxia. *Neurology* **55**: 1752–1753.

135. Schulz JB, Dehmer T, Schöls L, Mende H, Hardt C, Vorgerd M, Bürk K, Matson W, Dichgans J, Beal MF, and Bogdanov MB (2000). Oxidative stress in patients with Friedreich ataxia. *Neurology* **55**: 1719–1721.

136. Wong A, Yang J, Cavadini P, Gellera C, Lonnerdal B, Taroni F, and Cortopassi G (1999). The Friedreich ataxia mutation confers cellular sensitivity to oxidant stress which is rescued by chelators of iron and calcium and inhibitors of apoptosis. *Hum. Mol. Genet.* **8**: 425–430.

137. Ben Hamida M, Belal S, Sirugo G, Ben Hamida C, Panayides K, Ionannou P, Beckmann J, Mandel JL, Hentati F, Koenig M, *et al.* (1993). Friedreich ataxia phenotype not linked to chromosome 9 and associated with selective autosomal recessive vitamin E deficiency in two inbred Tunisian families. *Neurology* **43**: 2179–2183.

138. Lodi R, Cooper JM, Bradley JL, Manners D, Styles P, Taylor DJ, and Schapira AH (1999). Deficit of in vivo mitochondrial ATP production in patients with Friedreich ataxia. *Proc. Natl Acad. Sci. USA* **96**: 11492–11495.

139. Cossée M, Puccio H, Gansmuller A, *et al.* (2000). Inactivation of the Friedreich ataxia mouse gene leads to early embryonic lethality without iron accumulation. *Hum. Mol. Genet.* **9**: 1219–1226.

140. Puccio H, Simon D, Cossee M, Criqui-Filipe P, Tiziano F, Melki J, Hindelang C, Matyas R, Rustin P, and Koenig M (2001). Mouse models for Friedreich ataxia exhibit cardiomyopathy, sensory nerve defect and Fe-S enzyme deficiency followed by intramitochondrial iron deposits. *Nat. Genet.* **27**: 181–186.

141. Rustin P, von Kleist-Retzow JC, Chantrel-Groussard K, Sidi D, Munnich A, and Rotig A (1999). Effect of idebenone on cardiomyopathy in Friedreich's ataxia: a preliminary study. *Lancet* **354**: 477–479.

Section IV Cell function, neurodegenerative disorders, and ageing

11 The effects of mitochondrial DNA mutations on cell function

Andrew M James and Michael P Murphy

The pathophysiology of mitochondrial DNA (mtDNA) diseases is caused by increased cell death and dysfunction due to the accumulation of mutations to mtDNA. While disruption to oxidative phosphorylation is central to mtDNA diseases, many other factors such as Ca^{2+} dyshomeostasis, increased oxidative stress, and defective turnover of mitochondrial proteins may also contribute. The relative importance of these processes in causing cell dysfunction and death is uncertain. It is also unclear whether these damaging processes lead to the disease phenotype through affecting cell function, increasing cell death or a combination of the two. These uncertainties limit our understanding of mtDNA disease pathophysiology and our ability to develop rational therapies. Here, we outline how the accumulation of mtDNA mutations can lead to cell dysfunction by altering oxidative phosphorylation, Ca^{2+} homeostasis, oxidative stress, and protein turnover and discuss how these processes affect cell function and susceptibility to cell death. Better understanding these processes will eventually clarify why particular mtDNA mutations cause defined syndromes in some cases but not in others, and why the same mutation can lead to different phenotypes.

Introduction

There are broad similarities in the pathophysiology of all mtDNA diseases in that they chiefly affect post-mitotic and energy-demanding tissues such as nerve, muscle, or pancreatic cells. Furthermore, nuclear mutations that disrupt oxidative phosphorylation in all cells have similar phenotypes and affect the same tissues as mtDNA diseases,[1] indicating that oxidative phosphorylation defects are particularly damaging to specific cell and tissue types. Nevertheless, there are many puzzling features to the pathophysiology of mtDNA mutations, such as how a single mutation can lead to quite different syndromes,[2,3] how similar phenotypes can be caused by different mutations,[4,5] and why some specific mutations are associated with distinct phenotypes such as deafness,[5] diabetes,[3] or blindness.[6] As these aspects can only be partially explained by the selective propagation of particular mtDNA mutations,[7,8] different mtDNA mutations must have distinct effects on mitochondrial function. Greater understanding of the common and unique effects that different mtDNA mutations have on mitochondrial function coupled with knowledge of how they propagate, should provide a rational basis for understanding how each particular mtDNA mutation impacts upon different cell types. Coupled with knowledge of the nuclear background, life history, ageing, and environmental factors, the idiosyncrasies of mtDNA disease phenotype should become explainable. It may then become clear why some tRNA mutations lead to selective loss of cochlear function[5] while mutations to particular Complex I polypeptides lead to optic nerve death.[9]

Many of the consequences of mitochondrial diseases such as muscle weakness, fatigue, and lactic acidosis, are clearly related to defective oxidative phosphorylation. However, it is less clear why mitochondrial defects lead to symptoms such as the stroke-like episodes in MELAS[10] or the proliferation of keratinocytes in palmoplantar keratinocytosis.[11] In explaining these phenotypes it is important to determine whether mtDNA mutations act by promoting cell death and consequent cell loss, by affecting the function of still living cells, or both. In many mtDNA diseases there is evidence of cell death to post-mitotic cells that cannot be replaced by further cell division. This leads to muscle atrophy[12] and fibrosis in the heart,[13] as well as retinopathy,[14] gliosis,[15] demyelination,[16] and necrosis[17] in the brain. While there is evidence for increased apoptosis in mtDNA diseases,[18] the correlation between cell death and mitochondrial dysfunction is sometimes limited.[19] Furthermore, some symptoms of mtDNA diseases can arise before there is clear evidence of cell death,[20] suggesting that defective function of existing cells may be sufficient to cause the pathology.

Here, we review how mtDNA mutations affect aspects of mitochondrial function, including oxidative phosphorylation, Ca^{2+} homeostasis, oxidative stress, and protein turnover. We also discuss the consequences of these changes for the cell and how they might lead to cell dysfunction and death.

Oxidative phosphorylation defects caused by mtDNA mutation

An important aspect of mtDNA diseases is the threshold effect, whereby pathogenic mtDNA mutations disrupt oxidative phosphorylation when they are present above a certain level. The mutant load required to disrupt oxidative phosphorylation varies with cell and tissue type for poorly understood reasons and is also dependent on the nature of the mtDNA mutation.[21–25]

Mitochondrial DNA encodes 13 polypeptide components of Complexes I, III, IV, and V along with the ribosomal and transfer RNAs required for their translation and transcription.[26] Defects in the activity of individual complexes due to specific mutations in protein coding genes are known for all four complexes with mtDNA-encoded components.[27] In addition, a general defect in mitochondrial protein synthesis is caused by deletions that remove one or more tRNA genes[28] or point mutations within a tRNA gene.[29,30] They affect the four oxidative phosphorylation complexes with mtDNA-encoded polypeptides (Fig. 11.1) and the degree of disruption usually correlates with the number of mitochondrially encoded subunits. The effects on mitochondrial function of disrupting all four oxidative phosphorylation complexes are often quite distinct from the specific disruption of a single complex.

The respiratory chain transfers electrons from reduced substrates to oxygen and uses the difference in redox potential to pump protons across the inner membrane to establish a proton electrochemical potential gradient which is then used to drive ATP synthesis by Complex V, the ATP synthase (Fig. 11.1). This proton electrochemical potential gradient has both a membrane potential and a pH gradient component. In considering the pathophysiology of mtDNA diseases it is useful to differentiate between mutations that affect the respiratory chain and those that affect Complex V. Defects in Complexes I, III, or IV disrupt respiration, decrease the mitochondrial proton electrochemical potential gradient, and prevent mitochondrial ATP synthesis even when ATP synthase itself is unaffected. Defects due to large mtDNA

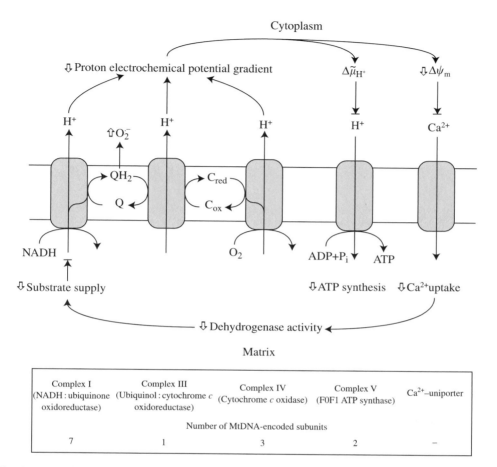

Fig. 11.1 Effects of mtDNA mutations on oxidative phosphorylation and calcium uptake. The figure shows how mitochondria use electrons supplied by dehydrogenases to pump protons across the mitochondrial inner membrane. The proton gradient is then used to generate ATP and sequester Ca^{2+} from the cytoplasm. Superoxide is produced as a byproduct of oxidative phosphorylation. The open arrows show an increase (⇑) or a decrease (⇓) in function due to mtDNA mutations. $O_2^{\cdot-}$, superoxide; Q, ubiquinone; QH_2, ubiquinol; C_{ox}, ferricytochrome *c*; C_{red}, ferrocytochrome *c*; $\Delta\mu_H^+$, proton motive force; $\Delta\psi_m$, mitochondrial membrane potential.

deletions or tRNA mutations will disrupt both the ability to form a proton electrochemical potential gradient as well as the capacity to synthesize ATP. In contrast, mutations in ATP synthase genes will not affect the ability of the mitochondrial respiratory chain to establish a proton electrochemical potential gradient but will diminish ATP synthesis (Fig. 11.1). While the endpoint of defective ATP synthesis is similar in all these situations, there are important differences that may be relevant to the pathology. For example, the presence of a membrane potential in the absence of ATP synthesis, will still allow mitochondrial Ca^{2+} accumulation, while an active ATP synthase in the absence of a functioning respiratory chain can still form a membrane potential by acting as a proton pump that consumes glycolytically generated ATP. Finally, the point at which electron transport is blocked in the respiratory chain will have significant consequences for the redox state of electron carriers, such as ubiquinone and cytochrome *c*. Inhibition of electron flow at Complex I or III would oxidize the electron carriers further down the respiratory chain, whereas blockage at Complexes III, IV, or V would reduce the transfer components upstream (Fig. 11.1). The effect of this on the redox state of the ubiquinone pool may have important implications for radical production, while the accumulation of NADH from inhibition of the respiratory chain will affect cell redox balance.

Consider first the effects of defective mitochondrial ATP synthesis on cell function. Any oxidative phosphorylation defect that completely blocked mitochondrial ATP synthesis would be fatal *in utero*, as evidenced by the embryonic lethality of knocking out mitochondrial transcription factor A (Tfam) in mice.[31] Hence in mtDNA diseases mitochondrial oxidative phosphorylation must be at least partially effective during the lifetime of the patient. This suggests a model of cell dysfunction and death in response to ATP synthesis defects, by which cells with the highest ATP demands will be most affected. While there is some truth in this model it is overly simplistic because many highly oxidative tissues such as the liver and kidney are not generally affected by mtDNA mutations to the same extent as neuronal and muscle tissue.[32]

The effects of defective mitochondrial ATP synthesis on cell function can be better understood by considering the example of fibroblasts that contain the MELAS or MERRF mutations. Digitonin-permeabilized cells have defective mitochondrial ATP synthesis when supplied with an excess of ADP, yet the ATP/ADP ratio was normal in the intact cells.[33] Superficially, these experiments appear contradictory, yet closer analysis revealed otherwise. In digitonin-permeabilized cells oxidative phosphorylation approximates State 3 conditions of high ATP turnover, while in intact cells in glucose-enriched culture medium it is closer to State 4, as turnover of ATP is low and glycolysis contributes to ATP generation. This suggests that the mitochondrial ATP synthesis deficiency observed in digitonin-permeabilized fibroblasts only becomes evident when ATP demand is high. To investigate this, ATP turnover was gradually increased with the Na^+/K^+-ionophore gramicidin to generate an ion flux across the plasma membrane and thus stimulate ATP turnover by the plasma membrane Na^+/K^+-ATPase. Wild-type cells were able to maintain their ATP/ADP ratio with a three-fold higher level of ATP turnover than cells containing the MELAS and MERRF mutations.[33] Thus, a plausible model *in vivo* is that tissues with variable ATP demands are most susceptible to the presence of mtDNA mutations. This is because cells that were continually incapable of meeting their ATP demands would die, compromising the viability of the organism *in utero*. In contrast, cells with variable ATP demands could survive in most situations but would express a defective phenotype when ATP demand was stimulated above basal levels. This would apply particularly to muscle and neuronal cells, which have uneven ATP demands resulting from variable ion fluxes across their membranes in response to external stimulation. Similarly, this might explain the susceptibility of pancreatic β-cells to mitochondrial dysfunction, as elevation of the cytosolic ATP/ADP ratio in response to increased plasma glucose levels is required to induce insulin secretion. Thus, we would predict that many cell types in mtDNA patients, should function relatively normally until there is increased ATP demand, at which point cells containing mtDNA mutations would be more likely to undergo a profound decrease in the cytoplasmic ATP/ADP ratio.

This loss of cytoplasmic ATP for extended periods during ATP demand will not only disrupt the primary functions of these cells, such as muscle contraction, nerve signal conduction, insulin secretion or transduction of sound, but will also increase the likelihood that the cell will undergo apoptotic or necrotic cell death. This may help explain why particular types of neuronal cells, such as optic nerve and cochlear hair cells, are lost as they experience variable stimulation in response to rapidly changing environmental stimuli. There may also be chronic effects of defective ATP synthesis, such as lowered protein synthesis and degradation, and less-effective DNA repair, which will also have consequences for long-term viability and render the cell susceptible to cell death. Therefore, defective mitochondrial ATP synthesis will have a number of quite subtle effects on cell function and is also likely to influence the probability of cell death, and the mechanisms by which this may occur are considered in the following sections.

Calcium dyshomeostasis caused by mtDNA mutations

The cytosolic free Ca^{2+} concentration is closely controlled and changes in the range of 0.1–1 μM are important signals in a range of pathways, including apoptotic, neuronal and hormonal signalling, and in the secretion of insulin.[34] Mitochondria affect cytoplasmic Ca^{2+} metabolism in two ways: indirectly via mitochondrially produced ATP that is used by Ca^{2+}-dependent ATPases to pump Ca^{2+} out of the cell or into intracellular stores (Fig. 11.2), such as the sarcoplasmic and endoplasmic reticula; and directly through the mitochondrial membrane potential which drives the uptake of Ca^{2+} into mitochondria through a Ca^{2+}-uniporter (Fig. 11.1). As Ca^{2+} has two positive charges the Nernst equation predicts that Ca^{2+}-uptake through the mitochondrial uniporter would lead to a million-fold uptake relative to the cytoplasm. However, this does not occur because of mitochondrial Ca^{2+}-export systems that exchange matrix Ca^{2+} for cytoplasmic Na^+ or H^+.[35] The combined action of the mitochondrial Ca^{2+}-uptake and extrusion system is that the matrix free Ca^{2+} concentration responds to changes in the cytoplasmic free Ca^{2+} concentration and thus alters the activity of matrix Ca^{2+}-dependent dehydrogenases and of mitochondrial ATP synthesis.[36] In addition, the uptake of Ca^{2+} by mitochondria both buffers and modulates intracellular calcium signals, and may also act as a sink for excess cytoplasmic Ca^{2+}, protecting the cell from calcium overload. As Ca^{2+}-uptake is independent of membrane potential above ~110 mV in isolated mitochondria,[37] the magnitude of the drop in mitochondrial membrane potential caused by mtDNA mutations may be insufficient to disrupt Ca^{2+} homeostasis.[25] Targeting the Ca^{2+} reporter protein aequorin, to the mitochondria of MERRF cybrids showed decreased mitochondrial Ca^{2+}-uptake after inositol-3-phosphate (IP$_3$) agonists stimulated Ca^{2+}-release from the endoplasmic reticulum. This defect in mitochondrial Ca^{2+}-uptake prevented Ca^{2+}-dependent stimulation of ATP production through activation of matrix dehydrogenases.[38] In contrast, the mitochondria of neuropathy, ataxia, and retinitis pigmentosa (NARP) cybrids, whose defect lies in ATP synthase, accumulated Ca^{2+} as well as wild-type cells.[38] Therefore, disruption of the mitochondrial membrane potential due to mtDNA mutations does interfere with mitochondrial Ca^{2+}-uptake.

Ca^{2+}-ATPases are continually pumping excess Ca^{2+} from the cytoplasm to the extracellular environment, or to intracellular Ca^{2+} depots, where the free Ca^{2+} concentration is in the millimolar range.[34] Mitochondria are indirectly involved in this aspect of Ca^{2+} metabolism because they generate the ATP used to drive these Ca^{2+}-pumps and disrupting the ATP supply will thus increase cytoplasmic free Ca^{2+} (Fig. 11.2). After a K^+-induced depolarization led to

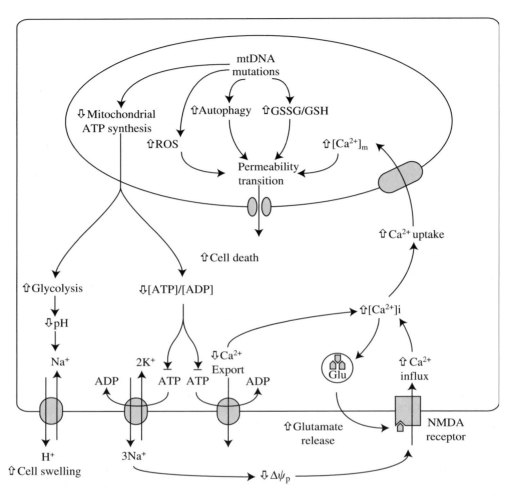

Fig. 11.2 How mtDNA mutations could promote cell death. This figure shows potential mechanisms by which mtDNA mutations could cause apoptotic or necrotic cell death. Decreased mitochondrial ATP synthesis increases reliance on glycolysis, which may in some situations lead to swelling and necrosis. In other situations (e.g. excitotoxicity) mtDNA mutations may cause cellular changes that open the mitochondrial permeability transition and trigger apoptosis. The open arrows show an increase (⇧) or a decrease (⇩) in function due to mtDNA mutations. $[Ca^{2+}]_m$, matrix calcium concentration; $[Ca^{2+}]_i$, cytoplasmic calcium concentration; GSSG/GSH, glutathione redox couple; ROS, reactive oxygen species; glu, glutamate; $\Delta\psi_p$, plasma membrane potential.

Ca^{2+}-influx from the extracellular environment, the cytoplasmic Ca^{2+} concentration in MELAS fibroblasts remained elevated for longer periods than wild-type cells, and often failed to return to basal levels.[23] Although ATP levels were similar in both MELAS and wild-type fibroblasts,[23,33] the ATP/ADP ratio was not measured during Ca^{2+}-influx and this will be the thermodynamic driving force for ATP hydrolysis by Ca^{2+}-ATPases.[33] Thus it remains possible that a decrease in the ATP/ADP ratio due to defective mitochondrial ATP synthesis caused the persistent increase in cytoplasmic Ca^{2+} following plasma membrane depolarization.[23] Interestingly, IP_3-stimulation of Ca^{2+} release from endoplasmic reticulum stores did not cause a similar persistent increase in cytoplasmic Ca^{2+}.[38] Thus the size of the Ca^{2+} reservoir (i.e. extracellular vs intracellular) and the period over which Ca^{2+} can flow to the cytoplasm may be important in determining whether mitochondrial dysfunction leads to Ca^{2+} overload.

Persistently elevated cytoplasmic Ca^{2+} not only disrupts Ca^{2+} signalling pathways, but also greatly increases the probability of cell death.[39,40] One situation where pathological increases in cytoplasmic Ca^{2+} are likely to occur is during glutamate excitotoxicity (Fig. 11.2). *In vivo*, plasma membrane depolarization following neuronal stimulation releases glutamate into the synaptic cleft. In most situations the plasma membrane is rapidly repolarised by the Na^+/K^+-ATPase, however ATP depletion of cultured neurons with cyanide, hypoxia, or hypoglycaemia makes glutamate stimulation neurotoxic.[41] This is because physiological concentrations of extracellular Mg^{2+} prevent activation of a glutamate-gated ion channel, the *N*-methyl-*D*-aspartate (NMDA) receptor, in a voltage dependent manner.[42] When oxidative phosphorylation does not generate sufficient ATP to repolarize the plasma membrane after glutamate stimulation this Mg^{2+} block on the NDMA receptor lifts, allowing activation of NMDA receptors by glutamate. Once activated the NMDA receptor allows fluxes of Ca^{2+}, Na^+, and K^+ across the plasma membrane causing further depolarization, glutamate release and Ca^{2+} overload.[41,43,44] A 'weak excitotoxic hypothesis' has been suggested to explain neuronal cell death in mtDNA disease.[45,46] In this, defective oxidative phosphorylation results in an ATP deficiency that makes nerves susceptible to failure of the Na^+/K^+-ATPase and subsequent plasma membrane depolarization. The plausibility of this hypothesis is supported by the finding in fibroblasts with mtDNA mutations, that stimulation of ATP turnover using a plasma membrane ionophore, resulted in plasma membrane depolarization at lower ion fluxes than in wild-type cells.[33] Something similar may also be occurring *in vivo*, as mice in which Tfam was selectively inactivated in neurons were more sensitive to the effects of seizures than control animals.[47] Even though the strength of seizures was similar in response to the glutamate agonist, kainic acid, post-seizure there was a marked increase in apoptosis in the brains of respiratory deficient mice when compared with controls.[47] This increased cell death is probably due to the prolonged duration of a Ca^{2+} transient leading to Ca^{2+} overload, thus mitochondrial dysfunction may change a metabolic signal to a pathological one. Similar increases in the duration of Ca^{2+} transients due to ATP depletion are also likely to promote cell death in other cell types harbouring mtDNA mutations.

The contribution of oxidative stress to mtDNA diseases

The role of the mitochondrial respiratory chain in radical production is well established with a significant proportion of the electrons that pass from reduced substrates to oxygen 'leaking' to form superoxide[48–50] (Fig. 11.3). Although relatively unreactive itself, superoxide is the parent of a number of other damaging reactive oxygen species (ROS).[51,52] Whether a cell experiences oxidative stress depends on the level of production of each oxidative species relative to its removal, and the effect of damage repair pathways. When these are out of balance, damage to mitochondrial respiratory complexes and mtDNA can arise leading to further mitochondrial dysfunction. While ROS are often considered as a single entity, each individual

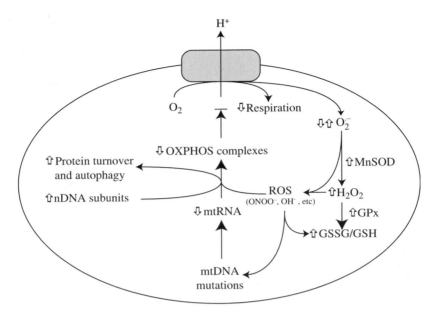

Fig. 11.3 How mtDNA mutations could increase protein turnover and oxidative stress. The figure shows mtDNA mutations could lead to an increase in the turnover of surplus, truncated, or ROS-damaged subunits. Those not turned over may form partial or defective complexes that produce greater amounts of superoxide and other damaging ROS. Increased ROS production may lead to a further decline in mitochondrial function through damage to mitochondrial lipid, protein and DNA. The open arrows show an increase ($\Uparrow$) or a decrease ($\Downarrow$) in function due to mtDNA mutations. $O_2^{\bullet-}$, superoxide; H_2O_2, hydrogen peroxide; MnSOD, manganese superoxide dismutase; GPx, glutathione peroxidase; ROS, reactive oxygen species; ONOO$^-$, peroxynitrite; OH$^\bullet$, hydroxyl radical; GSSG/GSH, glutathione redox couple.

ROS has its own mechanism of production and detoxification, and each has its own reaction profile with biological targets, consequently the pathological effects vary with the ROS involved. For example, superoxide itself is thought to be generated by semiquinone radicals in or near Complexes I and III, is scavenged by cytochrome *c* and superoxide dismutases in the matrix (MnSOD) and cytoplasm (Cu/Zn SOD), and directly damages iron–sulphur clusters in enzymes such as aconitase.[50] In contrast, hydrogen peroxide is produced by spontaneous and SOD-catalysed dismutation of superoxide, is removed by glutathione peroxidase, and causes hydroxyl radical formation and consequent damage to lipid, protein and DNA in the presence of ferrous iron.[51]

While mitochondrial radical production seems to be a consequence of normal mitochondrial function, the changes that occur to mitochondrial activity in mtDNA diseases may significantly increase ROS production and thereby contribute to the pathophysiology of these diseases. An increase in ROS could arise by a number of mechanisms. Firstly, inhibition of the respiratory chain can lead to a reduction of its electron carrying components and a consequent increase in ROS production (Fig. 11.1). Inhibition of ATP synthesis can also lead to reduction of respiratory carriers and an increase in mitochondrial membrane potential which also favours radical production.[53] MtDNA mutations that lead to incorrectly assembled complexes could increase superoxide formation by allowing greater interaction between oxygen and redox active respiratory chain components, such as the semiquinone radical. Finally, as Complexes I and III contain iron in iron–sulphur clusters, incorrectly assembled complexes might release iron and thereby increase mitochondrial production of hydroxyl radical through Fenton chemistry.

There are a number of reports of an induction of MnSOD as a consequence of mitochondrial dysfunction and this may have been due to an increase in ROS production[54,55] however in most cases it was not possible to measure an increase in ROS production directly. As mitochondrial dysfunction leads to the induction of a large number of nuclear-encoded mitochondrial genes,[56] MnSOD induction could often reflect increased mitochondrial biogenesis in response to mitochondrial dysfunction.[54] In one case where ROS was measured directly some, but not all, Complex I defects led to an increased steady state concentration of superoxide as measured by lucigenin chemiluminescence.[54,57] However, the implications of increased superoxide production in mtDNA disease pathogenesis are less clear as the patients with the poorest prognosis had an ~three-fold induction of MnSOD and lower steady-state concentrations of superoxide than controls.[54] One possible explanation is that MnSOD induction led to an increase in hydroxyl radical production and lipid peroxidation, through increased dismutation of superoxide to hydrogen peroxide.[58] However, this seems unlikely as mouse studies showed that MnSOD overexpression protected against lipid peroxidation and ischaemia-reperfusion damage to both neural and heart tissue.[59–61]

Decreased activity of the distal oxidative phosphorylation Complexes, III, IV, and V, increases the half-lives of partially reduced forms of upstream redox active components, such as ubiquinone, thus increasing endogenous radical production.[53] An increase in MnSOD and Cu/ZnSOD activity was observed when Complex V was damaged and this induction could be blocked by antioxidant spin traps.[55] The presence of a membrane potential may be important, as there was no induction of SOD caused by deficiencies in Complexes III or IV, even though mutations in these complexes would reduce the ubiquinone pool and other upstream redox carriers.[55]

A further mechanism for increased oxidative stress in mtDNA diseases is through decreased antioxidant protection. This can occur by a number of pathways: a decrease in mitochondrial NADPH concentration, which is partially dependent on the membrane potential-dependent transhydrogenase,[62] could lead to oxidation of the mitochondrial glutathione pool. This is supported by the finding that MELAS, MERRF, and LHON cybrids were sensitive to hydrogen peroxide-induced cell death, possibly because their peroxide-scavenging mitochondrial glutathione pool was oxidized:[63] Ferricytochrome *c* can accept electrons from superoxide converting it back to molecular oxygen[64] and mutations to Complexes IV and V could decrease the ability of the cytochrome *c* pool to scavenge superoxide: Ubiquinol is an important antioxidant that can protect against lipid peroxidation in the mitochondrial inner membrane,[65] and mutations to Complex I could oxidize the ubiquinone pool, decreasing the ubiquinol concentration.

An increase in oxidative stress is an attractive hypothesis to explain the progressive degenerative pathology of mtDNA diseases. A number of plausible mechanisms exist to link increased oxidative stress to mtDNA mutations, but in most cases concrete data is still lacking and the mechanisms remain unclear.

Alterations to mitochondrial turnover in mtDNA diseases

In mtDNA diseases truncated or incorrect mitochondrial polypeptides are produced, and these may be incorporated into oxidative phosphorylation complexes. This will lead to defective oxidative phosphorylation complexes that may accumulate if they are not rapidly turned over (Fig. 11.3). In addition, the inability to assemble correctly functioning mitochondria may lead to an upregulation of production of many mitochondrial polypeptides, or increase the biogenesis of the whole organelle, in an attempt to compensate for an energy deficit. For example, ragged red fibres (RRFs) are thought to arise as a consequence of an accumulation of mitochondria in the sarcoplasm of skeletal muscle[66] due to an induction of mitochondrial biogenesis in response to a metabolic deficiency. This response is a general one and involves increased replication of mtDNA[67,68] as well as induction of both mtDNA and nDNA-encoded genes.[56,69] Although mitochondrial biogenesis is stimulated in RRFs it commonly fails to correct the metabolic defect as Complex IV activity is often not detected with histochemical stains.[67,70] Although RRFs are a hallmark of mitochondrial diseases it is still unclear whether the accumulation of defective mitochondria in the sarcoplasm contributes to the pathophysiology or is simply a response to dysfunction. Even so, the production of defective mitochondria and mitochondrial proteins is likely to increase mitochondrial protein turnover.

The importance of correct protein degradation for mitochondrial function is illustrated by hereditary spastic paraplegia which is caused by mutations in paraplegin, a nuclear-encoded mitochondrial inner membrane metalloprotease that is thought to be involved in the turnover of mitochondrial oxidative phosphorylation complexes.[71] The yeast homologues of paraplegin are responsible for the degradation of incomplete, membrane-bound mitochondrial polypeptides[72] and are essential for assembly of inner membrane complexes and growth on respiratory substrates.[73,74] Interestingly, paraplegin mutations also lead to a disease phenotype that is similar to those of mtDNA diseases.[71] Therefore, it is possible that the accumulation of nuclear-encoded subunits or truncated mtDNA-encoded polypeptides in mtDNA diseases might disrupt mitochondrial function in a similar way. In addition to turnover through the activity of internal proteases, mitochondria are also turned over by autophagy whereby part of a mitochondrion is engulfed and fused with a lysosome for degradation.[75] Theoretically complete digestion of the material inside the resultant secondary lysosomes should leave no residual products. However, in practice incomplete digestion causes the remaining material to accumulate and form a family of morphologically diverse residual bodies, called lipofuscin or ceroid.[76] The accumulation of such partially degraded material correlates with cellular ageing in post-mitotic cells such as neurons,[77] and is accelerated in certain degenerative neurological conditions such as Alzheimer's,[78] Batten's,[79] and Huntington's diseases.[80] The hydrophobicity of the mtDNA-encoded subunits is likely to make them a difficult substrate for degradation by proteases as they may accumulate in insoluble bodies, as is the case for subunit c of the F_0F_1-ATPase.[81,82] While the nature of the undigested material in most residual bodies is uncertain it is often thought to include oxidatively damaged material that cannot be digested by enzymes.[77] Deletions, truncations, and point mutations in mtDNA protein encoding genes will directly produce abnormal peptides, and tRNA gene point mutations may have a similar effect, as incomplete base modification or inefficient tRNA aminoacylation in MERRF causes stalling of mitochondrial translation at lysine codons and the subsequent generation of truncated peptides.[83,84] The subsequent saturation of endogenous protein turnover pathways and the accumulation of undigested material is likely to be detrimental to the cell as a number of lysosomal storage diseases are caused by mutations in degradative enzymes.[85] However, the mechanism of cell damage due to the accumulation of ceroid and lipofuscin in these diseases is uncertain. In some cells with mtDNA mutations there are increases in secondary lysosomes and lipofuscin-like accumulations that may indicate increased autophagy of mitochondria.[25] Interestingly, ceroid accumulation is observed in a number of progressive myoclonic epilepsies of which MERRF is a member.[86]

How do mtDNA mutations lead to cell death?

In the last decade, mitochondria have been shown to play a central role in activating apoptotic cell death in response to cellular dysfunction. *In vitro*, under conditions of high Ca^{2+}, oxidative stress, and low ATP—a mitochondrial permeability transition pore (PTP) opens allowing diffusion of low molecular weight solutes across the mitochondrial inner membrane.[39] This leads to mitochondrial swelling which can rupture the outer mitochondrial membrane leading to the release of intermembrane space proteins, such as cytochrome *c*, SMAC/Diablo, apoptosis inducing factor (AIF), and endonuclease G into the cytoplasm, where they activate downstream pathways of cell death.[87] The protein components of the PTP are uncertain so it is still unclear how the PTP recognizes apoptotic signals and triggers release of proapoptotic proteins. However, the pore complex probably involves both inner membrane and outer membrane proteins and its susceptibility to induction seems to be regulated by both pro- and anti-apoptotic members of the Bcl-2 family.[88,89] The existence of mtDNA mutations is unlikely to prevent apoptotic cell death, as cells lacking a functional respiratory chain, due to complete elimination of mtDNA (ρ^0 cells), can still undergo cytochrome *c* release, caspase 3 activation, and apoptosis.[90–94] However, as mitochondria play a central role in integrating many of the signalling pathways that sense cellular dysfunction and decide whether to commit the cell to apoptosis, it is tempting to speculate that mitochondrial dysfunction caused by mtDNA mutations would promote cell death. Supporting this, progressive degeneration and loss of neural tissue is a common feature of mtDNA diseases, but it is unclear whether the mode of cell loss is necrotic or apoptotic, and the degree of cell loss varies considerably with brain region.[46] The influence of mtDNA mutations on cell death in other tissues is less clear as some studies of muscle biopsies from mtDNA patients have found increased caspase activity and DNA laddering,[18,95,96] while other investigators failed to detect these markers of apoptosis.[20] A further issue is that in muscle tissue an increase in apoptotic markers may not indicate cell death, as one study reported a high level of nuclear DNA fragmentation, without an associated loss of myofibres. One possibility is that nuclear redundancy in multinucleate myofibres may prevent cell loss in muscle tissue in spite of increases in apoptotic nuclei.[95] While cell loss is likely to be important in some mtDNA diseases, the extent to which it is due to apoptosis or necrosis is unclear and in those where cell death does occur it may not be pathologically significant in all tissues.

Cell death may be triggered by a range of quite distinct mechanisms, including increases in ROS, oxidation of the mitochondrial glutathione pool, chronic elevation of free Ca^{2+}, ATP depletion, or changes in intracellular pH, all of which can be affected by mtDNA mutations that cause mitochondrial dysfunction. ROS are an important proapoptotic signal in a range of biological systems in response to cell damage and in some cases may even be induced to signal cell death.[97] Even so, the direct evidence for an increase in oxidative stress as a result of mtDNA disease is inconclusive, although some mtDNA mutations do increase the expression of ROS detoxifying enzymes SOD, and glutathione peroxidase in cultured cells and in muscle biopsies from mtDNA patients.[54,55,96] One way in which ROS signals may affect the susceptibility of cells to apoptosis is through changes in the potential of the of the GSSG/2GSH couple which often correlates with the status of the cell. A reduced GSH pool (E_H ~-240 mV) signalling cell proliferation and a relatively oxidized GSH pool (E_H ~-170 mV) signalling apoptosis.[98] Excess production of peroxides oxidizes the glutathione pool and may also allow formation of critical protein dithiols on the PTP, which triggers pore opening and apoptosis in conjunction with Ca^{2+}-loading.[99] Oxidation of the glutathione pool may be exacerbated by a lower mitochondrial membrane potential decreasing the activity of the tran-shydrogenase, and hence the supply of NADPH for glutathione reduction. Interestingly, ρ^0 cells displayed little of the change in glutathione redox potential that was observed in parental wild-type cells during apoptosis because their pool of glutathione was already heavily oxidized.[93] In addition, MELAS, MERRF, and LHON cybrids were more susceptible to cell death on exposure to hydrogen peroxide than controls, and that this cell death was blocked by inhibitors of the PTP or of Ca^{2+}-depletion.[63] This suggests that proapoptotic pathways which require an oxidized glutathione pool would be enhanced in cells with defective mitochondria and that elevated Ca^{2+} would further favour the induction of apoptosis as it activates the PTP in conjunction with ROS.[100] It is likely that cells with defective mitochondria will be prone to Ca^{2+} overload as their capacity to pump Ca^{2+} out of the cytoplasm is reduced by a lower mito-chondrial membrane potential and decreased ATP synthesis.[23,33,38] Thus, vulnerability to Ca^{2+} overload leading to increased PTP induction, may also be a factor in the increased susceptibility to hydrogen peroxide induced cell death in MELAS, MERRF, and LHON cybrids.[63]

While ATP is important for maintaining ion gradients across membranes and is consumed by most energy requiring pathways in the cell it also inhibits the PTP.[39] During periods of ischaemia there is a progressive loss of adenine nucleotides as ATP and ADP are degraded to nucleosides, bases and phosphate. Both ATP and ADP, but not AMP, inhibit PTP opening in isolated mitochondria, while phosphate in conjunction with matrix Ca^{2+} promotes it.[39] This phenomenon may be important in mtDNA diseases as in resting ρ^0 cells there was a four-fold decrease in the concentration of ATP and ADP relative to wild-type cells and a similar downward trend in nucleotide concentration was observed in cybrids with mtDNA deletions.[101] A depleted adenine nucleotide pool may facilitate opening of the PTP during periods of ischaemia, as depletion of nucleotide levels below the threshold required for PTP induction would be easier to achieve. MtDNA defects also increase the reliance on glycolytic ATP production,[25,102] thus increasing the production of lactate that in extreme cases would harm the cell by lowering the intracellular pH. Attempts to rectify this using a plasma membrane Na^+/H^+-antiporter that is not osmotically neutral,[103] could lead to swelling and in extreme cases necrotic cell death. In support of this, blocking mitochondrial respiration with cyanide in the presence of glucose causes severe swelling and disruption in neurological tissue that can be prevented with inhibitors of glycolysis.[104]

A further mechanism by which mtDNA mutations may contribute to cell death is suggested by the link between mitochondrial autophagy and cell death pathways. Cyclosporin A, an inhibitor of the mitochondrial permeability transition and subsequent apoptosis, blocks autophagy in hepatocytes,[105] Beclin 1, a mammalian homologue of a yeast autophagy gene, interacts with the antiapoptotic gene Bcl-2[106] and apoptotic stimuli in neurons resulted a thirty-fold increase in autophagy.[107] In cells a link between mitochondrial turnover by autophagy and opening of PTP in response to mitochondrial dysfunction would provide a mechanism to selectively eliminate damaged mitochondria from within a healthy population. If mitochondrial dysfunction caused by mtDNA mutations triggered PTP opening and autophagy on a large scale in an attempt to eliminate defective mitochondria, the increased turnover of mitochondria could contribute to apoptotic cell death.

The role of mitochondrial dysfunction and increased cell death in mtDNA disease pathology

Understanding how and why cells die in response to mitochondrial dysfunction is critical for understanding the pathophysiology of mtDNA diseases and for developing therapies. In addition it is important for understanding what role mitochondrial dysfunction plays in ageing and in other degenerative diseases. A central concept in considering mitochondrial pathology is that of a 'threshold', or the point at which the capacity of a cell or tissue system is exceeded. It has generally been used in mtDNA diseases to define the proportion of a specific mtDNA mutation required to affect basal respiration or protein synthesis, but it can be used more extensively as there are likely to be multiple thresholds for different phenomena within a single cell. For example, the proportion of mutant mtDNA required to disrupt insulin secretion will differ from that required to cause cell death. Similar thresholds will occur for oxidative damage or lipofuscin/ceroid accumulation, as increases in ROS or defective protein synthesis will be countered by the action of antioxidants, proteases and lysosomes. A further aspect of this concept is 'stress', or the variable environmental signals that cause a threshold to be exceeded. For example, a mtDNA mutation that causes a decrease in the maximal rate of mitochondrial ATP synthesis will only express itself when environmental stimuli cause ATP turnover to exceed a combination of mitochondrial and glycolytic ATP generation.

The importance of the differing thresholds of pathways and the impact of environmental stress are nicely illustrated in a series of mice in which Tfam was selectively eliminated from certain cell types. Tfam is required for mtDNA transcription, and when initially healthy cells in specific tissues had Tfam deleted through activation of *cre-loxP* recombination there was a gradual decline in mtDNA transcription and mitochondrial function over time.[47,108–111] In a pancreatic Tfam-knockout mouse, a decline in Tfam led to decreased insulin secretion in response to glucose stimulation, a situation that mimics mitochondrial diabetes. Although blood glucose levels were significantly elevated in these mice at one month of age it still took several months before pancreatic β-islet area declined.[110] Neuronal Tfam-knockout mice were asymptomatic for 5 months, before dying within 2 weeks of the onset of symptoms from massive neurodegeneration.[47] When 4-month-old presymptomatic mice were challenged with the glutamate agonist kainic acid, a substantial increase in apoptosis was observed in neural tissue when compared with the wild-type.[47] These mouse models illustrate nicely how variably pathways within cells and tissues within the body depend on mitochondrial function and also demonstrate that cell death is the extreme consequence of progressive mitochondrial dysfunction.

Conclusion: what are the implications for mtDNA diseases?

Mitochondrial dysfunction leads to cells that are functionally compromised in a number of important ways. The most obvious metabolic defect caused by mitochondrial dysfunction is a deficiency in mitochondrial ATP synthesis. Although no mtDNA mutation will cause a complete cessation of mitochondrial ATP synthesis *in vivo*, under conditions where ATP turnover is increased, for example by ion influx, or ATP generation is decreased, for example by ageing, some cells will experience difficulty in meeting their energy requirements. Mitochondrial dysfunction thus creates a situation where ATP supply is generally sufficient to allow cell survival, but under certain conditions it will have pathological consequences. For example, if ATP demand exceeds the ability of the cell to deliver it aerobically the cell will start to generate it glycolytically and accumulate NADH, lactate and acid equivalents. A deficiency in oxidative metabolism will cause a cell to resort to glycolytic ATP production earlier during a period of high ATP hydrolysis than would a wild-type cell. In addition, turnover of NADH will be inhibited by a defective respiratory chain, preventing the cell from reconverting lactate to pyruvate after a period of ATP hydrolysis. The net effect is that mitochondrial dysfunction results in the cell being exposed to pH insults of greater severity, frequency, and duration.

A similar argument for an increase in severity and duration of intracellular Ca^{2+} dyshomeostasis in response to ATP depletion can be made, as defects in mitochondrial ATP synthesis will prolong increases in cytoplasmic Ca^{2+} by slowing extrusion of Ca^{2+} by the plasma membrane Ca^{2+}-ATPase. The spatiotemporal complexity of Ca^{2+} signalling and the large differences in Ca^{2+} channel expression between cell types,[34] mean that the occurrence of Ca^{2+} overload and dyshomeostasis will be tissue specific. These changes will be of pathological importance because of the cytotoxicity associated with chronically elevated cytoplasmic Ca^{2+} and one situation where mtDNA mutations might be particularly important in causing pathological increases in cytoplasmic Ca^{2+} is during glutamate excitotoxicity.

Events such as ATP depletion, pH changes, and Ca^{2+} overload are likely to occur in most mtDNA diseases so are unlikely to explain the differences caused by various mtDNA mutations. Two potential candidates for explaining the pathological heterogeneity of mtDNA diseases due to different mutations are oxidative stress and lipofuscin/ceroid accumulation.[77] Oxidative stress will not be present to the same extent in all mtDNA diseases and the damage caused will depend on the ROS species involved and on the patient's antioxidant status. Synthesis of abnormal polypeptides may be a common factor in mtDNA diseases, but whether they impact on pathology is likely to vary, as each mtDNA mutation will lead to a different pattern of abnormal or truncated polypeptides and iron. Some types of defective or oxidatively damaged protein may be resistant to degradation, leading to the accumulation of undigested protein that impairs mitochondrial function. This will be most relevant in postmitotic cells that cannot dilute out accumulated material by cell division, but could also occur because of spatial constraints. For example, substantial distances separate the synapses and cell bodies of neurons and increases in the biogenesis and degradation of mitochondria may strain axonal transport, particularly in the presence of defective ATP synthesis.

In conclusion, most mtDNA mutations will result in a cell prone to ATP depletion and in extreme cases calcium overload and cell death. The presence of increased oxidative stress and ceroid accumulation may further promote cell death in some mtDNA disease and possibly explain the wide clinical heterogeneity of mtDNA diseases. However, in most cases the details of the pathogenic mechanism remain unclear. The implications for therapy are that until effective gene therapies are available, there is potential to treat patients with agents designed to ameliorate oxidative damage, Ca^{2+} overload, or partially repair respiratory function.[112] However, many of the therapies are likely to be specific for a particular mutation, rather than generally applicable to all mtDNA diseases.

References

1. Zeviani M, Corona P, Nijtmans L, and Tiranti V (1999). Nuclear gene defects in mitochondrial disorders. *Ital. J. Neurol. Sci.* **20**: 401–408.
2. Goto Y, Nonaka I, and Horai S (1990). A mutation in the tRNA^Leu(UUR) gene associated with the MELAS subgroup of mitochondrial encephalomyopathies. *Nature* **348**: 651–653.
3. van den Ouweland JM, Lemkes HH, Ruitenbeek W, Sandkuijl LA, de Vijlder MF, Struyvenberg PA, van de Kamp JJ, and Maassen JA (1992). Mutation in mitochondrial tRNA(Leu)(UUR) gene in a large pedigree with maternally transmitted type II diabetes mellitus and deafness. *Nat. Genet.* **1**: 368–371.
4. Prezant TR, Agapian JV, Bohlman MC, Bu X, Oztas S, Qiu WQ, Arnos KS, Cortopassi GA, Jaber L, Rotter JI, *et al.* (1993). Mitochondrial ribosomal RNA mutation associated with both antibiotic-induced and non-syndromic deafness. *Nat. Genet.* **4**: 289–294.
5. Reid FM, Vernham GA, and Jacobs HT (1994). A novel mitochondrial point mutation in a maternal pedigree with sensorineural deafness. *Hum. Mutat.* **3**: 243–247.
6. Wallace DC, Singh G, Lott MT, Hodge JA, Schurr TG, Leeza AMS, Elsas II LJ, and Nikoskelainen EK (1988). Mitochondrial DNA mutation associated with Leber's hereditary optic neuropathy. *Science* **242**: 1427–1430.
7. Chinnery PF, Thorburn DR, Samuels DC, White SL, Dahl HM, Turnbull DM, Lightowlers RN, and Howell N (2000). The inheritance of mitochondrial DNA heteroplasmy: random drift, selection or both? *Trends Genet.* **16**: 500–505.
8. Goto Y (2001). Clinical and molecular studies of mitochondrial disease. *J. Inherit. Metab. Dis.* **24**: 181–188.
9. Chalmers RM and Schapira AH (1999). Clinical, biochemical and molecular genetic features of Leber's hereditary optic neuropathy. *Biochim. Biophys. Acta* **1410**: 147–158.
10. Pavlakis SG, Phillips PC, DiMauro S, De Vivo DC, and Rowland LP (1984). Mitochondrial myopathy, encephalopathy, lactic acidosis, and strokelike episodes: a distinctive clinical syndrome. *Ann. Neurol.* **16**: 481–488.
11. Sevior KB, Hatamochi A, Stewart IA, Bykhovskaya Y, Allen-Powell DR, Fischel-Ghodsian N, and Maw MA (1998). Mitochondrial A7445G mutation in two pedigrees with palmoplantar keratoderma and deafness. *Am. J. Med. Genet.* **75**: 179–185.
12. Kawai H, Akaike M, Yokoi K, Nishida Y, Kunishige M, Mine H, and Saito S (1995). Mitochondrial encephalomyopathy with autosomal dominant inheritance: a clinical and genetic entity of mitochondrial diseases. *Muscle Nerve* **18**: 753–760.
13. Ishikawa Y, Asuwa N, Ishii T, Masuda S, Kiguchi H, Hirai S, Akashi N, Yonenami K, and Fujisawa Y (1995). Severe mitochondrial cardiomyopathy and extra-neuromuscular abnormalities in mitochondrial encephalomyopathy, lactic acidosis, and stroke-like episode (MELAS). *Pathol. Res. Pract.* **191**: 64–75.
14. Kerrison JB, Howell N, Miller NR, Hirst L, and Green WR (1995). Leber hereditary optic neuropathy. Electron microscopy and molecular genetic analysis of a case. *Ophthalmology* **102**: 1509–1516.
15. Lombes A, Mendell JR, Nakase H, Barohn RJ, Bonilla E, Zeviani M, Yates AJ, Omerza J, Gales TL, Nakahara K, *et al.* (1989). Myoclonic epilepsy and ragged-red fibers with cytochrome oxidase deficiency: neuropathology, biochemistry, and molecular genetics. *Ann. Neurol.* **26**: 20–33.
16. Kalman B, Lublin FD, and Alder H (1997). Impairment of central and peripheral myelin in mitochondrial diseases. *Mult. Scler.* **2**: 267–278.
17. Terauchi A, Tamagawa K, Morimatsu Y, Kobayashi M, Sano T, and Yoda S (1996). An autopsy case of mitochondrial encephalomyopathy, lactic acidosis and stroke-like episodes (MELAS) with a point mutation of mitochondrial DNA. *Brain Dev.* **18**: 224–229.
18. Mirabella M, Di Giovanni S, Silvestri G, Tonali P, and Servidei S (2000). Apoptosis in mitochondrial encephalomyopathies with mitochondrial DNA mutations: a potential pathogenic mechanism. *Brain* **123**: 93–104.

19. Cottrell DA, Ince PG, Blakely EL, Johnson MA, Chinnery PF, Hanna M, and Turnbull DM (2000). Neuropathological and histochemical changes in a multiple mitochondrial DNA deletion disorder. *J. Neuropathol. Exp. Neurol.* **59**: 621–627.

20. Sciacco M, Fagiolari G, Lamperti C, Messina S, Bazzi P, Napoli L, Chiveri L, Prelle A, Comi GP, Bresolin N, *et al.* (2001). Lack of apoptosis in mitochondrial encephalomyopathies. *Neurology* **56**: 1070–1074.

21. Boulet L, Karpati G, and Shoubridge EA (1992). Distribution and threshold expression of the tRNA(Lys) mutation in skeletal muscle of patients with myoclonic epilepsy and ragged-red fibers (MERRF). *Am. J. Hum. Genet.* **51**: 1187–1200.

22. Larsson NG, Tulinius MH, Holme E, Oldfors A, Andersen O, Wahlstrom J, and Aasly J (1992). Segregation and manifestations of the mtDNA tRNA(Lys) A–>G(8344) mutation of myoclonus epilepsy and ragged-red fibers (MERRF) syndrome. *Am. J. Hum. Genet.* **51**: 1201–1212.

23. Moudy AM, Handran SD, Goldberg MP, Ruffin N, Karl I, Kranz-Eble P, DeVivo DC, and Rothman SM (1995). Abnormal calcium homeostasis and mitochondrial polarization in a human encephalomyopathy. *Proc. Natl Acad. Sci. USA* **92**: 729–733.

24. Dunbar DR, Moonie PA, Zeviani M, and Holt IJ (1996). Complex I deficiency is associated with 3243G:C mitochondrial DNA in osteosarcoma cell cybrids. *Hum. Mol. Genet.* **5**: 123–129.

25. James AM, Wei Y-H, Pang C-Y, and Murphy MP (1996). Altered mitochondrial function in fibroblasts containing MELAS or MERRF mitochondrial DNA mutations. *Biochem. J.* **318**: 401–407.

26. Chomyn A, Cleeter MWJ, Ragan CI, Riley M, Doolittle RF, and Attardi G (1986). URF6, last unidentified reading frame of human mtDNA, codes for an NADH dehydrogenase subunit. *Science* **234**: 614–618.

27. DiMauro S and Schon EA (2001). Mitochondrial DNA mutations in human disease. *Am. J. Med. Genet.* **106**: 18–26.

28. Hayashi J, Ohta S, Kikuchi A, Takemitsu M, Goto Y, and Nonaka I (1991). Introduction of disease-related mitochondrial DNA deletions into HeLa cells lacking mitochondrial DNA results in mitochondrial dysfunction. *Proc. Natl Acad. Sci. USA* **88**: 10614–10618.

29. Seibel P, Degoul F, Bonne G, Romero N, Francois D, Paturneau-Jouas M, Ziegler F, Eymard B, Fardeau M, Marsac C, *et al.* (1991). Genetic biochemical and pathophysiological characterization of a familial mitochondrial encephalomyopathy (MERRF). *J. Neurol. Sci.* **105**: 217–224.

30. King MP, Koga Y, Davidson M, and Schon EA (1992). Defects in mitochondrial protein synthesis and respiratory chain activity segregate with the tRNA[Leu(UUR)] mutation associated with mitochondrial myopathy, encephalopathy, lactic acidosis, and strokelike episodes. *Mol. Cell. Biol.* **12**: 480–490.

31. Larsson NG, Wang J, Wilhelmsson H, Oldfors A, Rustin P, Lewandoski M, Barsh GS, and Clayton DA (1998). Mitochondrial transcription factor A is necessary for mtDNA maintenance and embryogenesis in mice. *Nat. Genet.* **18**: 231–236.

32. Inoue K, Nakada K, Ogura A, Isobe K, Goto Y, Nonaka I, and Hayashi JI (2000). Generation of mice with mitochondrial dysfunction by introducing mouse mtDNA carrying a deletion into zygotes. *Nat. Genet.* **26**: 176–181.

33. James AJ, Sheard PW, Wei Y-H, and Murphy MP (1999). Decreased ATP synthesis is phenotypically expressed during increased energy demand in fibroblasts containing mitochondrial tRNA mutations: Implications for neurodegenerative and mitochondrial DNA diseases. *Eur. J. Biochem.* **259**: 462–469.

34. Berridge MJ, Lipp P, and Bootman MD (2000). The versatility and universality of calcium signalling. *Nat. Rev. Mol. Cell. Biol.* **1**: 11–21.

35. Gunter TE, Buntinas L, Sparagna G, Eliseev R, and Gunter K (2000). Mitochondrial calcium transport: mechanisms and functions. *Cell Calcium* **28**: 285–296.

36. Hansford RG and Zorov D (1998). Role of mitochondrial calcium transport in the control of substrate oxidation. *Mol. Cell. Biochem.* **184**: 359–369.

37. Goldstone TP, Roos I, and Crompton M (1987). Effects of adrenergic agonists and mitochondrial energy state on the Ca^{2+} transport systems of mitochondria. *Biochemistry* **26**: 246–254.
38. Brini M, Pinton P, King MP, Davidson M, Schon EA, and Rizzuto R (1999). A calcium signaling defect in the pathogenesis of a mitochondrial DNA inherited oxidative phosphorylation deficiency. *Nat. Med.* **5**: 951–954.
39. Crompton M (1999). The mitochondrial permeability transition pore and its role in cell death. *Biochem. J.* **341**: 233–249.
40. Duchen MR (2000). Mitochondria and calcium: from cell signalling to cell death. *J. Physiol.* **529**: 57–68.
41. Henneberry RL, Novelli A, and Lysko PG (1989). Neurotoxicity at the N-methyl-D-aspartate receptor in energy-comprimised neurons. An hypothesis for cell death in aging and disease. *Ann. NY Acad. Sci.* **568**: 225–233.
42. Mayer ML, Westbrook GL, and Guthrie PB (1984). Voltage-dependent block by Mg^{2+} of NMDA responses in spinal cord neurones. *Nature* **309**: 261–263.
43. Miller RJ, Murphy SN, and Glàum SR (1989). Neuronal Ca^{2+} channels and their regulation by excitatory amino acids. *Ann. NY Acad. Sci.* **568**: 149–158.
44. Siesjö BK Bengtsson F, Grampp W, and Theander S (1989). Calcium, excitotoxins, and neuronal death in the brain. *Ann. NY Acad. Sci.* **568**: 234–251.
45. Albin RL and Greenamyre JT (1992). Alternative excitotoxic hypotheses. *Neurology* **42**: 733–738.
46. Sparaco M, Bonilla E, DiMauro S, and Powers JM (1993). Neuropathology of mitochondrial encephalomyopathies due to mitochondrial DNA defects. *J. Neuropathol. Exp. Neurol.* **52**: 1–10.
47. Sorensen L, Ekstrand M, Silva JP, Lindqvist E, Xu B, Rustin P, Olson L, and Larsson NG (2001). Late-onset corticohippocampal neurodepletion attributable to catastrophic failure of oxidative phosphorylation in MILON mice. *J. Neurosci.* **21**: 8082–8090.
48. Chance B, Sies H, and Boveris A (1979). Hydroperoxide metabolism in mammalian organs. *Physiol. Rev.* **59**: 527–605.
49. Gutteridge JM and Halliwell B (2000). Free radicals and antioxidants in the year 2000. A historical look to the future. *Ann. NY Acad. Sci.* **899**: 136–147.
50. Raha S and Robinson BH (2000). Mitochondria, oxygen free radicals, disease and ageing. *Trends Biochem. Sci.* **25**: 502–508.
51. Beckman JS and Koppenol WH (1996). Nitric oxide, superoxide, and peroxynitrite: the good the bad and the ugly. *Am. J. Physiol.* **271**: C1424–C1437.
52. Murphy MP, Packer MA, Scarlett JL, and Martin SW (1998). Peroxynitrite: a biologically significant oxidant. *Gen. Pharmacol.* **31**: 179–186.
53. Korshunov SS, Skulachev VP, and Starkov AA (1997). High protonic potential actuates a mechanism of production of reactive oxygen species in mitochondria. *FEBS Lett.* **416**: 15–18.
54. Pitkänen S and Robinson BH (1996). Mitochondrial complex I deficiency leads to increased production of superoxide radicals and induction of superoxide dismutase. *J. Clin. Invest.* **98**: 345–351.
55. Geromel V, Kadhom N, Cebalos-Picot I, Ouari O, Polidori A, Munnich A, Rotig A, and Rustin P (2001). Superoxide-induced massive apoptosis in cultured skin fibroblasts harboring the neurogenic ataxia retinitis pigmentosa (NARP) mutation in the ATPase-6 gene of the mitochondrial DNA. *Hum. Mol. Genet.* **10**: 1221–1228.
56. Heddi A, Stepien G, Benke PJ, and Wallace DC (1999). Coordinate induction of energy gene expression in tissues of mitochondrial disease patients. *J. Biol. Chem.* **274**: 22968–22976.
57. Williams AJ and Cole PJ (1981). In vitro stimulation of alveolar macrophage metabolic activity by polystyrene in the absence of phagocytosis. *Br. J. Exp. Pathol.* **62**: 1–7.
58. Luo XP, Pitkänen S, Kassovskabratinova S, Robinson BH, and Lehotay DC (1997). Excessive formation of hydroxyl radicals and aldehydic lipid peroxidation products in cultured skin fibroblasts from patients with Complex I deficiency. *J. Clin. Invest.* **99**: 2877–2882.

59. Chen Z, Siu B, Ho YS, Vincent R, Chua CC, Hamdy RC, and Chua BH (1998). Overexpression of MnSOD protects against myocardial ischemia/reperfusion injury in transgenic mice. *J. Mol. Cell. Cardiol.* **30**: 2281–2289.

60. Keller JN, Kindy MS, Holtsberg FW, St Clair DK, Yen HC, Germeyer A, Steiner SM, Bruce-Keller AJ, Hutchins JB, and Mattson MP (1998). Mitochondrial manganese superoxide dismutase prevents neural apoptosis and reduces ischemic brain injury: suppression of peroxynitrite production, lipid peroxidation, and mitochondrial dysfunction. *J. Neurosci.* **18**: 687–697.

61. Macmillan-Crow LA, and Cruthirds DL (2001). Invited review: manganese superoxide dismutase in disease. *Free Radic. Res.* **34**: 325–336.

62. Drachev LA, Kondrashin AA, Semenov AY, and Skulachev VP (1980). Reconstitution of biological molecular generators of electric current. Transhydrogenase. *Eur. J. Biochem.* **113**: 213–217.

63. Wong A and Cortopassi G (1997). mtDNA mutations confer cellular sensitivity to oxidant stress that is partially rescued by calcium depletion and cyclosporin A. *Biochem. Biophys. Res. Commun.* **239**: 139–145.

64. Azzi A, Montecucco C, and Richter C (1975). The use of acetylated ferricytochrome c for the detection of superoxide radicals produced in biological membranes. *Biochem. Biophys. Res. Commun.* **65**: 597–603.

65. Forsmark P, Aberg F, Norling B, Nordenbrand K, Dallner G, and Ernster L (1991). Inhibition of lipid peroxidation by ubiquinol in submitochondrial particles in the absence of vitamin E. *FEBS Lett.* **285**: 39–43.

66. Scelsi R (1992). Morphometric analysis of skeletal muscle fibres and capillaries in mitochondrial myopathies. *Pathol. Res. Pract.* **188**: 607–611.

67. Mita S, Tokunaga M, Kumamoto T, Uchino M, Nonaka I, and Ando M (1995). Mitochondrial DNA mutation and muscle pathology in mitochondrial myopathy, encephalopathy, lactic acidosis, and strokelike episodes. *Muscle Nerve* Suppl. **3**: S113–S118.

68. Mita S, Tokunaga M, Uyama E, Kumamoto T, Uekawa K, and Uchino M (1998). Single muscle fiber analysis of myoclonus epilepsy with ragged-red fibers. *Muscle Nerve* **21**: 490–497.

69. Heddi A, Lestienne P, Wallace DC, and Stepien G (1993). Mitochondrial DNA expression in mitochondrial myopathies and coordinated expression of nuclear genes involved in ATP production. *J. Biol. Chem.* **268**: 12156–12163.

70. Reichmann H (1992). Enzyme activity analyses along ragged-red and normal single muscle fibres. *Histochemistry* **98**: 131–134.

71. Casari G, De Fusco M, Ciarmatori S, Zeviani M, Mora M, Fernandez P, De Michele G, Filla A, Cocozza S, Marconi R, *et al.* (1998). Spastic paraplegia and OXPHOS impairment caused by mutations in paraplegin, a nuclear-encoded mitochondrial metalloprotease. *Cell* **93**: 973–983.

72. Pajic A, Tauer R, Feldmann H, Neupert W, and Langer T (1994). Yta10p is required for the ATP-dependent degradation of polypeptides in the inner membrane of mitochondria. *FEBS Lett.* **353**: 201–206.

73. Tauer R, Mannhaupt G, Schnall R, Pajic A, Langer T, and Feldmann H (1994). Yta10p, a member of a novel ATPase family in yeast, is essential for mitochondrial function. *FEBS Lett.* **353**: 197–200.

74. Paul M-F and Tzagoloff A (1995). Mutations in *RCA1* and *AFG3* inhibit F_1-ATPase assembly in *Saccharomyces cerevisiae*. *FEBS Lett.* **373**: 66–70.

75. Klionsky DJ and Emr SD (2000). Autophagy as a regulated pathway of cellular degradation. *Science* **290**: 1717–1721.

76. Holtzman E (1989). *Lysosomes*. 1 ed. Plenum Press, New York.

77. Terman A (2001). Garbage catastrophe theory of aging: imperfect removal of oxidative damage? *Redox. Rep.* **6**: 15–26.

78. Nixon RA, Cataldo AM, and Mathews PM (2000). The endosomal–lysosomal system of neurons in Alzheimer's disease pathogenesis: a review. *Neurochem. Res.* **25**: 1161–1172.

79. Dawson G and Cho S (2000). Batten's disease: clues to neuronal protein catabolism in lysosomes. *J. Neurosci. Res.* **60**: 133–140.
80. Kegel KB, Kim M, Sapp E, McIntyre C, Castano JG, Aronin N, and DiFiglia M (2000). Huntingtin expression stimulates endosomal–lysosomal activity, endosome tubulation, and autophagy. *J. Neurosci.* **20**: 7268–7278.
81. Ezaki J, Wolfe LS, Higuti T, Ishidoh K, and Eiki K (1995). Specific delay of degradation of mito-chondrial ATP synthase subunit c in late infantile neuronal ceroid lipofuscinosis (Batten disease). *J. Neurochem.* **64**: 733–741.
82. Palmer DN, Bayliss SL, and Westlake VJ (1995). Batten disease and the ATP synthase subunit C turnover pathway. *Am. J. Med. Genetics* **57**: 260–265.
83. Enriquez JA, Chomyn A, and Attardi G (1995). MtDNA mutation in MERRF syndrome causes defect-ive aminoacylation of tRNA(Lys) and premature translation termination. *Nat. Genet.* **10**: 47–55.
84. Yasukawa T, Suzuki T, Ishii N, Ohta S, and Watanabe K (2001). Wobble modification defect in tRNA disturbs codon–anticodon interaction in a mitochondrial disease. *Embo. J.* **20**: 4794–4802.
85. Tomkinson B (1999). Tripeptidyl peptidases: enzymes that count. *Trends Biochem. Sci.* **24**: 355–359.
86. Delgado-Escueta AV, Ganesh S, and Yamakawa K (2001). Advances in the genetics of progressive myoclonus epilepsy. *Am. J. Med. Genet.* **106**: 129–138.
87. Bernardi P, Petronilli V, Di Lisa F, and Forte M (2001). A mitochondrial perspective on cell death. *Trends Biochem. Sci.* **26**: 112–117.
88. Harris MH and Thompson CB (2000). The role of the Bcl-2 family in the regulation of outer mito-chondrial membrane permeability. *Cell Death Differ.* **7**: 1182–1191.
89. Adams JM and Cory S (2001). Life-or-death decisions by the Bcl-2 protein family. *Trends Biochem. Sci.* **26**: 61–66.
90. Jacobson MD, and al e (1993). Bcl-2 blocks apoptosis in cells lacking mitochondrial DNA. *Nature* **361**: 365–369.
91. Asoh S, Mori T, Hayashi J, and Ohta S (1996). Expression of the apoptosis-mediator Fas is enhanced by dysfunctional mitochondria. *J. Biochem. (Tokyo)* **120**: 600–607.
92. Higuchi M, Aggarwal BB, and Yeh ET (1997). Activation of CPP32-like protease in tumor necrosis factor-induced apoptosis is dependent on mitochondrial function. *J. Clin. Invest.* **99**: 1751–1758.
93. Jiang S, Cai J, Wallace DC, and Jones DP (1999). Cytochrome c-mediated apoptosis in cells lack-ing mitochondrial DNA. Signaling pathway involving release and caspase 3 activation is conserved. *J. Biol. Chem.* **274**: 29905–29911.
94. Dey R and Moraes CT (2000). Lack of oxidative phosphorylation and low mitochondrial membrane potential decrease susceptibility to apoptosis and do not modulate the protective effect of Bcl-x(L) in osteosarcoma cells. *J. Biol. Chem.* **275**: 7087–7094.
95. Monici MC, Toscano A, Girlanda P, Aguennouz M, Musumeci O, and Vita G (1998). Apoptosis in metabolic myopathies. *Neuroreport* **9**: 2431–2435.
96. Di Giovanni S, Mirabella M, Papacci M, Odoardi F, Silvestri G, and Servidei S (2001). Apoptosis and ROS detoxification enzymes correlate with cytochrome c oxidase deficiency in mitochondrial encephalomyopathies. *Mol. Cell. Neurosci.* **17**: 696–705.
97. Hwang PM, Bunz F, Yu J, Rago C, Chan TA, Murphy MP, Kelso GF, Smith RA, Kinzler KW, and Vogelstein B (2001). Ferredoxin reductase affects p53-dependent, 5-fluorouracil-induced apoptosis in colorectal cancer cells. *Nat. Med.* **7**: 1111–1117.
98. Schafer FQ and Buettner GR (2001). Redox environment of the cell as viewed through the redox state of the glutathione disulfide/glutathione couple. *Free Radic. Biol. Med.* **30**: 1191–1212.
99. Chernyak BV and Bernardi P (1996). The mitochondrial permeability transition pore is modulated by oxidative agents through both pyridine nucleotides and glutathione at two separate sites. *Eur. J. Biochem.* **238**: 623–630.

100. Zoratti M and Zabo I (1995). The mitochondrial permeability transition. *Biocim. Biophys. Acta* **1241**: 139–176.
101. Porteous WK, James AM, Sheard PW, Porteous CM, Packer MA, Hyslop SJ, Melton JV, Pang CY, Wei YH, and Murphy MP (1998). Bioenergetic consequences of accumulating the common 4977-bp mitochondrial DNA deletion. *Eur. J. Biochem.* **257**: 192–201.
102. Baker SK, Tarnopolsky MA, and Bonen A (2001). Expression of MCT1 and MCT4 in a patient with mitochondrial myopathy. *Muscle Nerve* **24**: 394–398.
103. Demaurex N and Grinstein S (1994). Na^+/H^+ antiport: Modulation by ATP and role in cell volume regulation. *J. Exp. Biol.* **196**: 389–404.
104. Plum F (1983). What causes infarction in ischemic brain? The Robert Wartenberg lecture. *Neurology* **33**: 222–233.
105. Elmore SP, Qian T, Grissom SF, and Lemasters JJ (2001). The mitochondrial permeability transition initiates autophagy in rat hepatocytes. *Faseb. J.* **17**: 17.
106. Liang XH, Jackson S, Seaman M, Brown K, Kempkes B, Hibshoosh H, and Levine B (1999). Induction of autophagy and inhibition of tumorigenesis by beclin 1. *Nature* **402**: 672–676.
107. Xue L, Fletcher GC, and Tolkovsky AM (1999). Autophagy is activated by apoptotic signalling in sympathetic neurons: an alternative mechanism of death execution. *Mol. Cell. Neurosci.* **14**: 180–198.
108. Wang J, Wilhelmsson H, Graff C, Li H, Oldfors A, Rustin P, Bruning JC, Kahn CR, Clayton DA, Barsh GS, *et al.* (1999). Dilated cardiomyopathy and atrioventricular conduction blocks induced by heart-specific inactivation of mitochondrial DNA gene expression. *Nat. Genet.* **21**: 133–137.
109. Li H, Wang J, Wilhelmsson H, Hansson A, Thoren P, Duffy J, Rustin P, and Larsson NG (2000). Genetic modification of survival in tissue-specific knockout mice with mitochondrial cardiomyopathy. *Proc. Natl Acad. Sci. USA* **97**: 3467–3472.
110. Silva JP, Kohler M, Graff C, Oldfors A, Magnuson MA, Berggren PO, and Larsson NG (2000). Impaired insulin secretion and beta-cell loss in tissue-specific knockout mice with mitochondrial diabetes. *Nat. Genet.* **26**: 336–340.
111. Wang J, Silva JP, Gustafsson CM, Rustin P, and Larsson NG (2001). Increased in vivo apoptosis in cells lacking mitochondrial DNA gene expression. *Proc. Natl. Acad. Sci. USA* **98**: 4038–4043.
112. Murphy MP (2001). Development of lipophilic cations as therapies for disorders due to mitochondrial dysfunction. *Expert Opin. Biol. Ther.* **1**: 753–764.

12 Mitochondrial dysfunction in neurodegenerative disease

JM Cooper

Mitochondria are recognized for their key role in supplying ATP for normal cell function, which is particularly important for high-energy requiring cells such as neurones. However, the generation of free radicals by the respiratory chain and the involvement of the mitochondrion in cellular calcium buffering and regulation of apoptosis may also contribute to the involvement of mitochondrial dysfunction in disease. The first section of the chapter focuses on various factors that may influence mitochondrial function, and their relationship to pathogenesis. The second section reviews common neurodegenerative diseases (Parkinson's disease, Alzheimer's disease, and Huntington's disease) where mitochondrial respiratory chain dysfunction has been implicated in the disease mechanism. Those diseases with a specific and well-defined mitochondrial aetiology are covered elsewhere (e.g. mitochondrial encephalopathies (Chapter 5) and Friedreich's ataxia (Chapter 10)).

Role of mitochondrial dysfunction in disease pathogenesis

Decreased ATP supply

The primary role of the mitochondrial oxidative phosphorylation system (OPS) is the efficient supply of the high-energy phosphate compound ATP. Different cells in the body have different requirements for ATP and in general it is organs with the highest energy demand that are most vulnerable to OPS defects, namely the central nervous system (CNS), heart, skeletal muscle, retina, liver, and kidneys. While it is possible for cells without mitochondrial DNA (mtDNA; ρ^0 cells) to survive and grow in culture without a functional OPS, relying solely upon glycolysis for ATP production,[1] this cannot be translated to the whole organism.[2] The relationship between OPS dysfunction and decreased ATP synthesis is open to debate. Although *in vitro* evidence suggests that Complex I abnormalities of up to 70 per cent may be required before ATP synthesis is affected,[3] diseases manifest at lower thresholds,[4,5] implying a discrepancy between the *in vitro* and *in vivo* situations.

Neurones are very sensitive to ATP supply for normal cell function. The brain has very low stores of carbohydrate and therefore cannot maintain ATP synthesis via glycolysis alone for long periods accordingly it is highly dependent upon oxidative phosphorylation for efficient ATP synthesis. This dependence of the brain upon oxidative phosphorylation explains at least in part the sensitivity of the brain to a variety of toxins, even though they may be systemically administered. The basal ganglia are particularly sensitive to mitochondrial toxins. While the specificity of MPTP toxicity to the substantia nigra (see section on Parkinson's disease) may be in part dictated by the selective conversion and uptake characteristics of the toxin, this does not appear to be the case for 3-nitroproprionic acid, rotenone, carbon monoxide, or cyanide.[6–8]

Oxidative stress

A by-product of normal electron transfer catalysed by the oxidative phosphorylation enzyme complexes is the release of single electrons, which contribute significantly to the generation of cellular superoxide.[9,10] Inhibition of the mitochondrial respiratory chain (MRC) by a variety of toxins, including MPP$^+$, rotenone, and antimycin A, markedly increased the rate of superoxide formation[11,12] suggesting that oxidative stress may be induced by conditions that lead to mitochondrial inhibition. Indeed there is evidence that free radicals generated by inhibition of Complex I can lead to further inhibition of the complex leading to a vicious cycle.[13] The vulnerability of MRC components to oxidative damage suggests that MRC dysfunction could be secondary to increased free radical generation. While Complex I was the most vulnerable to oxidative damage when analysed using *in vitro* systems,[14,15] Complexes I and IV were equally vulnerable using *in vivo* models of oxidative damage.[16,17] However, the site of damage may also depend upon the free radical species involved as Complexes II and III were most vulnerable in SOD2 (mitochondrial MnSOD) knockout mice[18] and also to irreversible nitric oxide induced damage.[19] Consequently, when decreased mitochondrial respiratory chain function and oxidative stress co-exist it may not be apparent which is the primary event, or whether they may be secondary to other factors.

The CNS has several features that are thought to make it particular sensitive to free radical damage. It has a relatively high rate of oxidative phosphorylation and oxygen utilization, and therefore increased superoxide generation as a byproduct. Several neurotransmitters including dopamine and noradrenalin, autoxidize to give reactive quinones, in addition dopaminergic regions of the brain will also generate H_2O_2 via monoamine oxidase *b* (MAOb) metabolism of dopamine. Calcium movements within neurones are vital for normal function. Any perturbation in calcium export from cells can result in increased oxidative stress either via increased nitric oxide synthase (NOS) activity or decreased MRC function. Iron levels are relatively high in the brain but iron binding capacity in the cerebrospinal fluid (CSF) is relatively low. Consequently, the release of iron following CNS damage may contribute to an increase in the iron-catalysed degradation of H_2O_2 and oxidative damage. Catalase activities are relatively low in the brain, placing more emphasis on glutathione (GSH) and glutathione peroxidase activities for the removal of H_2O_2. The substrate for lipid peroxidation, polyunsaturated fatty acids (PUFA), are relatively abundant in the brain making it more vulnerable to lipid peroxidation

A modification of the free radical theory of ageing, places the mitochondion at the focal point of free radical damage which may accumulate with increasing age giving rise to mitochondrial dysfunction which contributes to cellular dysfunction.[20] MRC function has been reported to decline with increasing age[21,22] and therefore MRC dysfunction may be a prominent feature in post-mitotic cells of older individuals.

Calcium buffering, excitotoxicity, and apoptosis

The observation that mitochondria can accumulate calcium is well established. However, the physiological significance of this calcium transport, the extent to which pathological states may influence calcium transport into mitochondria or how abnormal mitochondrial calcium movements may influence mitochondrial function is beginning to be studied.

Mitochondria have a low resting calcium concentration maintained by a Na^+–Ca^{2+} exchanger, with the Na^+ balance maintained by the Na^+–H^+ exchange. Calcium import is via a uniporter and is dependant upon the mitochondrial membrane potential (MMP) and calcium concentration. Among the enzymes regulated by calcium concentration are the dehydrogenases (pyruvate dehydrogenase) associated with the tricarboxylic acid cycle, consequently, the rate of carbohydrate oxidation will be influenced by intra mitochondrial calcium concentrations, leading to up regulation of mitochondrial respiration and ATP synthesis.[23] Mitochondrial calcium uptake seems to occur only at high cytosolic calcium concentration, although these may be local to the mitochondria themselves if they are situated close to the sites of calcium entry to the cell.

In neurones cytosolic calcium increases rapidly after depolarization and opening of the voltage-gated calcium channels. Mitochondrial calcium uptake subsequently produces a rapid fall in cytosolic calcium and then slowly releases calcium back to the cytosol through the Na^+–Ca^{2+} antiport. Consequently, mitochondria may play a role in calcium signalling.

Although calcium uptake into mitochondria plays important physiological roles, it can also have deleterious effects. Conditions that change the MMP will influence calcium uptake with a collapse of the MMP preventing mitochondrial calcium uptake. Failure of mitochondrial calcium entry may lead to decreased carbohydrate oxidation and oxidative phosphorylation which will in turn lead to decreased MMP and ATP synthesis. Moreover increased mitochondrial calcium uptake may be particularly important in excitotoxicty and apoptosis.

Excitotoxicity describes the neurotoxic effects of increased postsynaptic stimulation by excitatory neurotransmitters such as glutamate and aspartate. When cortical cultures were treated with increasing concentrations of glutamate there was a dose-dependent loss of neurones with preservation of glial cells.[24] The mechanism of excitotoxic cell death is mediated via the activation of the *N*-methyl-*D*-aspartate (NMDA) ionotropic glutamate receptor. Glutamate activation of the NMDA receptor in addition to a drop in the membrane potential allows release of the magnesium block of the NMDA receptor and entry of calcium/sodium into the cell. This depolarization leads to the opening of voltage-gated calcium channels and further increases in intracellular calcium concentration. Under normal situations the release of glutamate into the extracellular space is transient with reuptake into the presynaptic neurone and surrounding glia sufficient to terminate NMDA stimulation. However, it is possible to have prolonged activation of NMDA receptors under circumstances where there is prolonged release of glutamate or similar NMDA agonist (quinolinic acid, homocysteine), or impaired re-uptake of glutamate. In fact there is evidence that impaired mitochondrial respiratory chain function leads to impaired Na/K ATPase activity and partial depolarization which relieves the voltage dependant Mg^{2+} block of the NMDA receptor channel enabling the channel to open even at relatively low glutamate concentrations[25] thus potentiating excitotoxicity.

The NMDA activation results in increased intracellular calcium, which is closely linked to the ensuing cell death.[26] The targets of impaired neuronal calcium homeostasis caused by excitotoxicity may involve kinases, phosphatases, proteases, phospholipases, neuronal nitric oxide synthase (nNOS), and mitochondria. Elevated intracellular calcium concentrations, lead to a decrease in MMP leading to cell death. It is not clear whether the decreased MMP is caused by opening of the MPT pore, involved in apoptosis, or due to decreased MRC function caused by NO inhibition of Complexes II and IV. The cell death is calcium and NOS dependant and can be prevented by depolarising the mitochondria[27] or by using NO scavengers, NOS inhibitors or neurones from neuronal NOS knockout mice.[28,29] It is possible that impaired MRC function and decreased MMP may influence calcium uptake into mitochondria thus affecting calcium-dependant activation of ATP synthesis[30] and also apoptosis. There is evidence that NMDA receptor activation results in increased free radical generation and oxidative stress,[31] which seem to predominantly involve mitochondrial ROS generation.[32] NO can be acting at several levels including regulation of cellular signalling, blood flow, guanylate cyclase activity, and the activity of other proteins by *S*-nitrosylation (reviewed by Kroncke *et al.* 1997).[33] However, inhibition of the mitochondrial respiratory chain at Complexes II, III, and IV are important targets of NO leading to cell dysfunction and death.

Mitochondria appear to play a key role regulating many apoptotic stimuli. Anti-apoptotic (i.e. bcl2) proteins are localised to the mitochondrial membranes and the pro-apoptotic cytochrome *c* and AIF (apoptosis-inducing factors) are located within the mitochondria and released after mitochondrial swelling.

Apoptosis is associated with a sequence of events leading to a fall in MMP, opening of the MPT pore and release of AIF into the cytoplasm. This precedes DNA fragmentation and chromatin condensation. Decreased MMP and increased intramitochondrial calcium have been correlated with a decrease in MMP, which may be influenced by decreased MRC function and free radical generation.[34] Opening of the pore dissipates the proton gradient and therefore MMP and the movement of solutes and small proteins between the matrix and cytosol leading to swelling and rupture of the mitochondrial outer membrane, release of cytochrome *c* from inter-membrane space. BCL-2 prevents MPT pore opening and therefore AIF release.

There is evidence that dysfunction of the MRC can lead to either cell death via apoptosis or necrosis depending upon the degree of inhibition. With severe inhibition of the MRC, ATP synthesis is severely impaired leading to a crisis in the cell function and a more rapid necrotic death, while mild inhibition of the MRC may affect cell death through other mechanisms possibly involving free radical generation, MMP or calcium uptake leading to apoptosis.[35] This may be the case with excitotoxicity with low concentrations of excitotoxins eliciting apoptosis and high concentrations necrosis.[36] The role of mitochondrial function seems important to the outcome following excitotoxic insult, with cells that can maintain mitochondrial function and ATP production may die by apoptosis and those that cannot maintain ATP supplies die by necrosis.[37] This can be seen in models of stroke where necrosis dominates in the ischaemic core while apoptosis is seen in the border region of the insult.[38]

Decreased MRC function in a variety of diseases including neurodegenerative diseases may decrease MMP thus making the cells more vulnerable to opening of the MPT pore and apoptosis. Apoptosis has been described in a variety of neurodegenerative diseases including; PD, HD, and AD, but this is not universally accepted.[39]

Mitochondrial dysfunction in neurodegenerative diseases

Over the last decade molecular genetics has made great strides in helping to identify the underlying cause of many neurodegenerative diseases. Patients with Huntington's disease (HD), Friedreich's ataxia (FRDA), and Wilson's disease (WD) have mutations in a single gene and therefore each disease has a common mechanism. In Alzheimer's disease (AD), Parkinson's disease (PD), hereditary spastic paraplegia (HSP), and amyotrophic lateral sclerosis (ALS) however, a genetic abnormality has been identified in only a fraction of patients and these are spread across several different genes. Consequently in the latter group each disease is likely to be linked to a variety of primary causes, involving genetic and environmental factors, possibly leading to a common pathway of cell dysfunction and disease.

The MRC dysfunction is apparent in many neurodegenerative diseases. However, the cause of the MRC defect and the role it plays in pathogenesis is different for each disease. In this respect it is possible to categorize these diseases into three groups; those that involve a genetic mutation directly affecting MRC components (Chapters 6–8 and 10); those involving a genetic defect of a mitochondrial protein not directly involved with the MRC (Chapter 10) and a third group where the MRC defect is more complex and likely to be secondary to other processes occurring as part of the disease mechanism. The evidence for mitochondrial respiratory chain dysfunction in the last group will be reviewed in the section following and their relationship to the primary causes or secondary factors associated with the diseases will be discussed.

Alzheimer's disease

Alzheimer's disease is the most common neurodegenerative disease with an incidence of up to 15 per cent of the population over 65 years.[40] Clinically, AD is characterized by a progressive loss of memory, disorientation in time and place and increased anxiety. A correct diagnosis requires positive neuropathological findings including loss of cortical cholinergic neurones, intraneural neurofibrillary tangles consisting of hyperphosphorylated tau, and abundant extracellular amyloid plaques composed of β-amyloid. The majority of patients present sporadically, however up to 20 per cent of patients show a familial pattern of inheritance. These patients invariably have an earlier onset, before 55 years, and a more aggressive course. Mutations of the amyloid precursor protein (APP),[41] and more commonly of the presenilin 1 and 2 genes[42,43] have been identified in this group of patients and may cause the disease by promoting the generation of β-amyloid.[44] In addition the presence of the APOE4 allele is also a risk factor for AD[45] which may promote β-amyloid aggregation or tau phosphorylation.

Decreased energy metabolism is well recognized in AD. Positron emission tomography (PET) studies have indicated that glucose metabolism is decreased in various cortical regions of AD brains.[46] Decreased cytochrome oxidase activity has been reported in a variety of AD brain regions[47] and platelets[48] and confirmed histochemically.[49] The underlying cause of this dysfunction is not known however, there is evidence that APP fragments inhibit cytochrome oxidase activity.[50] Although an increase in the incidence of several base changes in mitochondrial DNA has been reported in AD, including a A4336G change in the tRNA^{Gln} gene,[51,52] which may contribute to pathogenesis in some patients, no common mtDNA abnormality has yet been associated with AD.

There is extensive evidence of oxidative stress in AD affecting lipids, proteins, and DNA (reviewed by Butterfield *et al.*),[53] which may result directly from β-amyloid accumulation, or indirectly from free radical generation due to MRC dysfunction. Nitrotyrosine levels have been reported to be raised in AD hippocampus and corticol regions[54] although it is not known whether this is NO generated from an inflammatory response (iNOS) or via upregulation of nNOS following excitotoxicity. Mitochondrial morphological changes have been observed in normal myoblasts expressing APP cDNA similar to that seen in inclusion body myositis which shares the PHF and β-amyloid features with AD but in muscle.[55] This suggests that mitochondrial dysfunction may well be secondary to the β-amyloid and PHF pathology, that is, a consequence of increased oxidative stress.

Parkinson's disease

Parkinson's disease (PD) is the second most common neurodegenerative disease with a prevalence of approximately 1 in 400. It is characterized clinically by bradykinesia, akinaesia and tremor and pathologically by the loss of dopaminergic neurones in the pars compacta of the substantia nigra (SN), the substantia innominata and locus coeruleus. The presence of Lewy bodies in remaining neurones is a characteristic hallmark although these may be seen in other diseases and may be missing in patients with Parkinson's-like clinical features.[56] Onset of the clinical symptoms can be between the fourth and seventh decades with increasing age and family history the most consistent risk factors.

The PD is caused by heterogeneous primary abnormalities. Genetic factors are known to be important in at least a proportion of patients with known mutations exhibiting both autosomal dominant and recessive traits. Five families have been described with 2 different dominant point mutations in the α synuclein gene,[57,58] a mutation of the UCH L1 gene in one family[59] and a range of recessive mutations in a growing number of patients in the Parkin gene.[60] These patients tend to have an earlier onset than idiopathic PD and Lewy bodies are generally absent from patients with the Parkin mutations suggesting they are not classical PD patients. While the function of α synuclein is unclear it is known to be a major component of Lewy bodies in both the genetic and sporadic patients suggesting it plays a key role in pathogenesis of PD.[61] The UCHl1 and parkin are involved with the ubiquitination of damaged proteins and may result in the accumulation of such proteins in patients with mutations of these genes.[62]

The possible involvement of mitochondrial dysfunction in PD is supported by the selective dopaminergic cell loss and parkinsonism in primates (including humans) and/or rodents following exposure to various toxins that inhibit the MRC including MPTP, tetrahydroisoquinolines, iron, manganese, cyanide, rotenone, and carbon monoxide (reviewed by Cooper and Schapira).[63] This suggests that the SN is particularly sensitive to systemic perturbations of energy metabolism.

The mechanism of MPTP induced parkinsonism is relatively well understood.[64] Briefly MPTP crosses the blood brain barrier where it is converted to MPP^+ by the action of monoamine oxidase *b*. The MPP^+ is then selectively concentrated in the dopaminergic neurones by the dopamine transporter. MPP^+ is further concentrated in mitochondria where it inhibits Complex I of the respiratory chain thereby inducing ATP depletion. Transgenic mice over expressing SOD1[65] and neuronal NOS knockout mice[66] were both resistant to MPTP toxicity suggesting a role for NO and oxidative stress in addition to decreased ATP synthesis in MPTP toxicity.

Tetrahydroisoquinolines and isoquinolines can be produced in the brain from the condensation of dopamine with aldehydes. There is evidence that these compounds are inhibitors of Complex I. The injection of chemicals from these groups (1-benzyl-1,2,3,4-tetrahydroisoquinoline, *N*-methyl-salsolinol) into rats or mice have resulted in various pathological or clinical signs similar to those seen in PD including reduced striatal dopamine and selective loss of dopaminergic neurones (reviewed by Cooper and Schapira).[63] More recently, the chronic intravenous exposure of rats to the insecticide rotenone for 1–5 weeks resulted in a

Parkinsonian model involving the loss of nigrastriatal dopaminergic neurones, the presence of Lewy body-like inclusions and clinical signs of nigral degeneration.[7] This indicates that systemic exposure of toxins found in the environment could give clinical and pathological features very close to that seen in PD.

Decreased Complex I activity has been identified in the substantia nigra of a large group of patients with PD[67] and confirmed in an independent study.[68] While this defect could be secondary to degeneration or *L*-dopa therapy, Complex I activity was normal in other PD brain regions and in multiple system atrophy, a disease involving degeneration of the SN, which is treated using *L*-dopa.[69] This suggested the decrease in Complex I was disease-specific, and not secondary to *L*-dopa therapy or degeneration of the SN. Mitochondrial analyses of tissues outside the CNS are somewhat varied with a small but consistent Complex I defect in PD platelets[70,71] but less consistent results in skeletal muscle[72,73] and lymphoblasts.[74,75]

The analyses of ρ^0 cybrids generated from the transfer of PD platelet mitochondria from patients with decreased Complex I activity into A549 ρ^0 or SHSY5Y ρ^0 cells suggested the Complex I defect was transferred to the resulting cybrids.[76,77] The abnormalities of mtDNA responsible for the defect have not yet been identified. A number of studies of unselected PD patients have reported sequencing either the complete mitochondrial genome or the mitochondrial Complex I and transfer RNA genes of a variety of patients with PD.[78–80] A variety of polymorphisms have been identified that either have no predicted effect at the protein level or have uncertain significance. These data are difficult to explain unless the involvement of mtDNA in PD is restricted to a subgroup of patients, or the Complex I dysfunction is associated with a particular mtDNA haplotype. The presence of the common deletion (4977 bp) has been analysed in PD brains but levels were found to be similar to age matched individuals.[72]

The relationship between Lewy bodies and disease pathogenesis is not understood. However the connection between PD patients with mutations of the α synuclein gene and the presence of α synuclein in Lewy bodies of both these patients and sporadic patients places the formation of Lewy bodies right at the centre of the disease pathway. There are no data on mitochondrial function or oxidative stress in patients with PD of known cause. However, studies on cultured cells revealed no effect on mitochondrial function from overexpression of mutant or wild type α synuclein (unpublished experiments of the author). In addition to this the normal mitochondrial function in patients with diffuse Lewy body disease[81] suggests that mitochondrial dysfunction is not linked to α synuclein aggregation or Lewy body formation.

As α synuclein aggregation appears to play a central role in PD pathogenesis it is interesting to note that α synuclein positive inclusions were seen in rats chronically treated with rotenone or paraquat,[7,82] and in cell culture systems following MRC inhibition.[83] This raises the possibility that MRC inhibition or free radical generation may be important factors in PD pathogenesis leading to Lewy body formation, ATP depletion and oxidative damage.

A range of markers of oxidative stress and damage have been measured in PD brain samples and have indicated that free radical damage may play a key role in pathogenesis. Included in this are increased levels of lipid peroxidation, protein carbonyls, and DNA oxidation.[84,85] In addition there is an increase in nitrotyrosine residues on a protein component of Lewy bodies, α synuclein,[86] implying peroxynitrite damage is also a feature of PD pathology. Increased iron levels in PD SN have been reported by several groups,[87,88] and although this may be a nonspecific feature of neurodegeneration, iron can add to oxidative stress by catalysing the decomposition of H_2O_2 to the reactive hydroxyl radical. Changes in antioxidant defences are also indicative of oxidative stress, and with low levels of catalase in the brain GSH is particularly important for the oxidation of peroxides including H_2O_2. In PD, several groups have reported decreased levels of GSH in the SN which correlated with disease severity.[89,90] It is thought that the synthesis of GSH is unaffected in PD and that GSH levels are depleted due to increased oxidative stress, however the underlying cause of the increased oxidative stress is not known.

PD is almost certainly caused by heterogeneous factors. While it is possible that the underlying cause of the Complex I defect in PD is the primary cause of the disease in some patients, in others it may merely play a role in the pathway leading to α synuclein aggregation and dopaminergic cell loss. In the absence of an explicit mtDNA mutation in PD, the underlying cause of Complex I dysfunction may relate to specific mtDNA haplotype(s). The effect may be direct in particular neuronal cell types or stem from increased susceptibility to a toxin, which might be exogenous (MPTP, rotenone) or endogenous (free radicals, isoquinolines). The role of nuclear genes encoding Complex I subunits has yet to be investigated.

Huntington's disease

Huntington's disease (HD) is an autosomal dominant disorder with an incidence of approximately 1 in 20,000. It is characterized clinically by behavioural disturbance, chorea, dementia and ataxia with onset in the third to fifth decades of life. The classical pathological findings include the loss of neurones in the caudate and putamen in particular the medium spiny neurones,[91] and the more recently recognized neuronal intranuclear inclusions (NII).[92] The mutation responsible for HD is an expansion of the CAG repeat in exon 1 of the huntingtin gene on chromosome 4.[93] The repeat is expanded to greater than 36 CAG repeats in affected patients resulting in an expanded glutamine tract within the 350-kDa protein known as huntingtin. The age of onset and speed of disease progression is affected by the size of the CAG repeat with a younger onset and more rapid progression being associated with longer repeat lengths. The role of huntingtin is not known. It appears to be distributed within the cytosol and is widely expressed in neuronal and other tissues[94] with no clear correlation between the level of expression and site of neuropathological abnormality[95] suggesting cell-specific interactions may be important. Huntingtin is a highly conserved protein and expression is required for normal development.[96] Heterozygous knockout of the HD gene does not show a phenotype indicating the CAG mutation in HD is likely to produce a toxic gain of function.[97]

A transgenic model of HD (R6/2) generated using the N terminus of the protein with between 130–150 CAG repeats shows a movement disorder after 8 weeks of age, and death after 12–16 weeks.[98] Although the brains are smaller than normal and NII are present there is no significant degeneration. The role of NII in disease pathogenesis is not clear. They have been observed in HD brains and also the R6/2 mice and consist of ubiquitinated N-terminal portions of huntingtin which contain the expanded polyglutamine tract.[99] It is still debateable what role NII play in pathogenesis, rather than having a toxic role they have been proposed to be protective.[100]

Evidence for impaired energy metabolism in HD comes from a variety of different observations. The analyses of HD brain using PET identified decreased glucose metabolism in the striatum and cortex,[101] and increased lactate levels in the cortex and basal ganglia using proton magnetic resonance spectroscopy (MRS)[102] were confirmed with elevated lactate pyruvate ratios in the (CSF)[103] Analysis of MRC activities in HD brain identified a severe defect of Complexes II and III and a mild defect in Complex IV in the caudate nucleus and to a milder degree in the putamen which paralleled the severity of the pathology.[104–106] Although Complexes II and III were most severely affected in brain there was also an underlying Complex IV defect. This is of interest given the increased sensitivity of HD lymphoblasts to mitochondrial depolarization and apoptosis induced by the Complex IV inhibitor cyanide.[107] In addition, there is evidence that the androgen receptor involved in another CAG repeat disease, spinobulbar muscular atrophy (SBMA), interacts with subunit Vb of cytochrome oxidase[108] and may contribute to mitochondrial dysfunction in SBMA. However, to date there is no evidence that this is a common feature with CAG repeat diseases

In muscle ^{31}P MRS analysis revealed decreased mitochondrial ATP synthesis in both symptomatic and presymptomatic patients which correlated with the severity of the genetic mutation.[109] While a Complex I defect reported in HD skeletal muscle[110] is consistent with this it is not clear what relationship it has to the defect observed in the brain.

Models that induce HD pathology also suggest a mitochondrial role in disease pathogenesis. Ingestion of the Complex II inhibitor 3-nitroproprionic acid (3-NP),[111,112] or intrastriatal injections of malonate produced selective loss of medium spiny neurones in the rat.[113] This indicates that these cells are particularly sensitive to mitochondrial inhibition and in particular Complex II inhibition matching the biochemical defect in the striatum.

In the R6/2 mice at 12 weeks, there was a defect of Complex IV activity in the striatum, and cortex. Consistent with a bioenergetic deficit in this model creatine treatment improved survival and delayed clinical progression.[114]

Several observations have suggested that excitotoxicity may be involved in HD pathogenesis. First the NMDA agonist quinolinic acid induced striatal lesions in the rat similar to those seen in HD resulting in motor hyperactivity, learning deficits, and decreased glucose metabolism.[115,116] R6/2 mice have a decreased level of mGluR2 receptors that regulate glutamate release and therefore may impair feedback control of glutamate release thus predisposing the cells to excitotoxicity.[117] Toxicity due to intrastriatal injections of malonate and 3-NP in cultured cells was decreased by the NMDA antagonist MK 801.[113,118] The role of excitotoxicity in HD has been supported by increased striatal glutamate levels in HD caudate[119] and decreased numbers of NMDA receptors in HD striatum suggesting cells high in NMDA receptors are more vulnerable.[120] However, other factors must be important because HD pathology does not relate to areas high in NMDA receptors.[121]

Evidence of oxidative stress and damage in HD is limited. Increased 8 hydroxy-2-deoxyguanosine levels have been seen in HD caudate.[106] Aconitase activity is very sensitive to inactivation by free radicals and can be used to assess oxidative damage. Decreased aconitase activity has been detected in HD brain with the greatest inhibition in the caudate followed by the putamen and the cortex, mimicking the severity of pathology.[105] The decreased aconitase activity in the striatum and increased nitrotyrosine staining In R6/2 mouse brain is also indicative of oxidative damage.[19]

It is likely that mitochondrial dysfunction in HD is caused by excitotoxicity and the consequent generation of NO and free radicals, with inhibition of Complexes II/III and aconitase by NO and ONOO. This would account for the severity of the defect reflecting the pathological involvement in HD. In the R6/2 model Complexes II and III were not affected while aconitase was decreased in the striatum, consistent with a mild excitotoxic insult and very little cell death. It is not yet known how mutant huntingtin increases susceptibility to excitotoxicity but it could involve abnormal glutamate homeostasis.

Amyotrophic lateral sclerosis

Amyotrophic lateral sclerosis has a prevalence of approximately 1 in 20,000, it is characterized clinically by progressive muscular weakness and wasting with onset in the fifth decade and an average disease duration of between 3 and 5 years. Pathologically there is selective loss of motor neurones. Approximately 10 per cent of patients exhibit autosomal dominant inheritance (familial ALS, FALS) with approximately a quarter of these with one of more than 90 different mutations of the Cu/Zn superoxide dismutase gene (cytosolic form of the enzyme) on chromosome 21.[122] The SOD activity was decreased in FALS motor neurones but not sporadic patients.[123] Consistent with an impaired antioxidant capacity patient tissue from familial and sporadic ALS patients showed evidence of increased oxidative damage to proteins, lipid and DNA[124,125] and evidence of NO induced damage,[126] although changes were not consistently observed for all oxidative markers and all tissues.

Transgenic mice expressing mutant SOD1 but normal SOD activity developed an ALS-like disease[127,128] and had evidence of oxidative damage.[129] However, the observation that Cu/Zn SOD knockout mice developed normally suggests that loss of this activity does not lead to ALS *per se* although it did leave motor neurones more vulnerable to axon injury.[130] This suggested the SOD1 mutations probably produce a toxic gain of function, rather than a negative loss of function.

Mitochondria have been reported to be morphologically abnormal in ALS motor neurones[123,131] and mutant SOD1 transgenic mice.[132] The targeting of mitochondria by mutant SOD1 may be related to the recent observation that transgenic SOD1 can also be found in mitochondria[133] which is in agreement with the localization of the enzyme to the mitochondrial intermembrane space in yeast.[134] MRC dysfunction has been reported in ALS patients affecting either Complex I activity in skeletal muscle[135] or Complex IV activity in spinal cord motor neurones.[136] Decreased Complex IV activity has been association with a microdeletion of subunit I of Complex IV[137] adding further weight to the involvement of primary mtDNA abnormalities in at least a subset of patients with ALS and the importance of mitochondrial dysfunction in disease pathogenesis. A more general mitochondrial functional abnormality in ALS was reported in a recent study of spinal cord from ALS patients. In these patients there was an increase in mutant mtDNA and a general decrease in mitochondrial activities consistent with a loss of mitochondrial mass[138] which may reflect increased oxidative damage to mitochondria. The involvement of mitochondrial dysfunction is supported further by the use of creatine treatment to compensate for any bioenergetic defect in SOD1 mutant transgenic mice, which significantly delayed the loss of motor neurones and prolonged survival.[139]

There is indirect evidence of glutamate excitotoxicity in ALS.[140] The selective loss of motor neurones may be explained by the fact that motor neurones are more sensitive than inter-neurones in the dorsal horn to inhibition of the MRC,[141] with increased oxidative stress and MRC dysfunction making the cells more vulnerable to an excitotoxic insult resulting in elevated intracellular calcium concentrations, increased free radical generation and further MRC dysfunction leading to cell death.

Conclusion

There is substantial evidence that the mitochondrial respiratory chain and OPS is impaired in many neurodegenerative diseases, however, the underlying causes of this dysfunction and the role it plays in disease pathogenesis may vary considerably in different diseases. Mitochondrial dysfunction caused by mutations of mtDNA or nuclear genes encoding MRC subunits are clearly a primary cause of disease in the patients with classical mitochondrial encephalopathy (Chapter 5). This also appears to be the case in some patients with PD, AD, and ALS, however, there is no evidence that they are important in the majority of patients with these diseases. Endogenous and exogenous mitochondrial toxins may be involved in some diseases (PD). Alternatively, increased excitotoxicity (HD, ALS), altered mitochondrial bio- genesis (HSP, FRDA, see also Chapter 10) and increased oxidative stress and damage (ALS, PD, WD, FRDA) may account for the changes in MRC function found in neurodegenerative disease (Fig. 12.1). The causes of oxidative stress and their relationship with the known genetic abnormalities are beginning to be understood in several diseases including increased mitochondrial iron (FRDA) and copper (WD) levels and altered antioxidant defences (ALS).

With the observation that mitochondria can play a pivotal role in apoptosis and necrosis, the MRC changes observed in many of these diseases may play an important role in neuronal loss and may be a useful target for neuroprotective strategies.

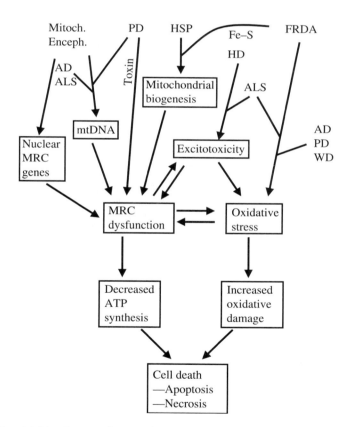

Fig. 12.1 Mitochondrial involvement in neurodegenerative diseases. Summary of the possible mecha- nisms leading to MRC dysfunction in: Parkinson's disease (PD), Huntington's disease (HD), Amyotrophic lateral sclerosis (ALS), Friedreich's ataxia (FRDA), Wilson's disease (WD), Hereditary spastic paraplegia (HSP), Alzheimer's disease (AD), and mitochondrial encephalopathies (mitoch. enceph.).

References

1. King MP and Attardi G (1989). Human cells lacking mtDNA: repopulation with exogenous mitochondria by complementation. *Science* **246**: 500–503.
2. Larsson NG, Wang J, Wilhelmsson H, Oldfors A, Rustin P, Lewardoski M, Barsh GS, and Clayton DA (1998). Mitochondrial transcription factor A is necessary for mtDNA maintenance and embryogenesis in mice. *Nat. Genet.* **18**: 231–236.
3. Davey GP and Clark JB (1996). Threshold effects and control of oxidative phosphorylation in non-synaptic rat brain mitochondria. *J. Neurochem.* **66**: 1617–1624.
4. Holt IJ, Harding AE, Cooper JM, *et al.* (1989). Mitochondrial myopathies: clinical and biochemical features of 30 patients with major deletions of muscle mitochondrial DNA. *Ann. Neurol.* **26**: 699–708.
5. Trounce I, Byrne E, Marzuki S, *et al.* (1991). Functional respiratory chain studies in subjects with CPEO and large heteroplasmic mitochondrial DNA deletions. *J. Neurol. Sci.* **102**: 92–99.
6. Gould DH and Gustine DL (1982). Basal ganglia degeneration, myelin alterations, and enzyme inhibition induced in mice by the plant toxin 3-nitropropanoic acid. *Neuropathol. Appl. Neurobiol.* **8**: 377–393.
7. Betarbet R, Sherer TB, MacKenzie G, Garcia-Osuna M, Panov AV, and Greenamyre JT (2000). Chronic systemic pesticude exposure reproduces features of Parkinson's disease. *Nat. Neurosci.* **3**: 1301–1306.
8. Uitti RJ, Rajput AH, Ashenhurst EM, and Rozdilsky B (1985). Cyanide induced parkinsonism: A clinicopathologic report. *Neurology* **35**: 921–925.
9. Boveris A and Chance B (1973). The mitochondrial generation of hydrogen peroxide. *Biochem. J.* **13**: 707–716.
10. Raha S and Robinson BH (2000). Mitochondria, oxygen free radicals, disease and ageing. *TIBS* **25**: 502–508.
11. Takeshige K and Minakami S (1979). NADH- and NADPH-dependent formation of superoxide anions by bovine heart submitochondrial particles. *Biochem. J.* **180**: 129–135.
12. Hasegawa E, Takeshige K, Oishi T, Murai Y, and Minikami S (1990). 1-methyl-4-phenylpyridinium (MPP$^+$) induces NADH dependent superoxide formation, and enhances NADH-dependent lipid peroxidation in bovine heart submitochondrial particles. *Biochem. Biophys. Res. Commun.* **170**: 1049–1055.
13. Cleeter MJW, Cooper JM, and Schapira AHV (1992). Irreversible inhibition of mitochondrial complex I by 1-methyl-4-phenylpyridinium: evidence for free radical involvement. *J. Neurochem.* **58**: 786–789.
14. Narabayashu M, Takeshige K, and Minikami S (1982). Alteration of inner-membrane components and damage to electron-transfer activities of bovine heart submitochondrial particles induced by NADPH-dependent lipid peroxidation. *Biochem. J.* **202**: 97–105.
15. Hillered L and Ernster L (1983). Respiratory activity of isolated rat brain mitochondria following in vitro exposure to oxygen radicals. *J. Cer. Blood Flow Metab.* **3**: 207–214.
16. Thomas PK, Cooper JM, King RHM, *et al.* (1993). Myopathy in vitamin E deficient rats: muscle fibre necrosis associated with disturbances of mitochondrial function. *J. Anat.* **183**: 451–461.
17. Hartley A, Cooper JM, and Schapira AHV (1993). Iron induced oxidative stress and mitochondrial dysfunction: relevance to Parkinson's disease. *Brain Res.* **627**: 349–353.
18. Melov S, Coskun P, Patel M, *et al.* (1999). Mitochondrial disease in superoxide dismutase 2 mutant mice. *Proc. Natl Acad. Sci. USA* **96**: 846–851.
19. Tabrizi, SJ, Workman J, Hart P, *et al.* (2000). Mitochondrial dysfunction and free radical damage in the huntington R6/2 transgenic mouse. *Ann. Neurol.* **47**: 80–86.
20. Miquel J (1991). An update on the mitochondrial-DNA mutation hypothesis of cell aging. *Mutat. Res.* **275**: 209–216.

21. Trounce I, Byrne E, and Marzuki S (1989). Decline in skeletal muscle mitochondrial respiratory chain function, possible factor in ageing. *Lancet* **1**: 637–639.
22. Cooper JM, Mann VM, and Schapira AHV (1992). Analyses of mitochondrial respiratory chain function and mitochondrial DNA deletion in human skeletal muscle: effect of ageing. *J. Neurol. Sci.* **113**: 91–98.
23. Rizzuto R, Bastianutto C, Brini M, Murgia M, and Pozzan T (1994). Mitochondrial calcium homeostasis in intact cells. *J. Cell Biol.* **126**: 1183–1194.
24. Choi DW, Maulucci-Gedde M, and Guthrie PB (1987). Glutamate toxicity in corticol cell culture. *J. Neurosci.* **7**: 357–368.
25. Novelli A, Reilly JA, Lysko PG, and Henneberry RC (1988). Glutamate becomes neurotoxic via the n-methyl-d-aspartate receptor when intracellular energy levels are reduced. *Brain Res.* **451**: 205–212.
26. Hyrc K, Handran SD, Rothman SM, and Goldberg MP (1997). Ionized intracellular calcium concentration predicts excitotoxic neuronal death: observations with low-affinity fluorescent calcium indicators. *J. Neurosci.* **17**: 6669–6677.
27. Stout AK, Raphael HM, Kanterewicz BI, Klann E, and Reynolds IJ (1998). Glutamate-induced neuron death requires mitochondrial calcium uptake. *Nat. Neurosci.* **1**: 366–373.
28. Dawson VL, Kizushi VM, Huang PL, *et al.* (1996). Resistance to neurotoxicity in corticol cultures from neuronal nitric oxidase deficient mice. *J. Neurosci.* **16**: 2463–2478.
29. Dawson V, Dawson TM, London ED, Bredt DS, and Snyder SH (1991). Nitric oxide mediates glutamate neurotoxicity in primary cortical cultures. *Proc. Natl Acad. Sci. USA* **88**: 6368–6371.
30. Brini M, Printon P, King MP, *et al.* (1999). A Calcium signalling defect in the pathogenesis of a mitochondrial DNA inherited oxidative phosphorylation defect. *Nat. Med.* **5**: 951–954.
31. Lafon-Cazal M, Pietri S, Culcasi M, and Bockaert J (1993). NMDA dependent superoxide production and neurotoxicity. *Nature* **364**: 535–537.
32. Dugan LL, Sensi SL, Canzoniero LM, *et al.* (1995). Mitochondrial production of reactive oxygen species I cultured forebrain neurons following NMDA receptor activiation. *J. Neurosci.* **15**: 6377–6388.
33. Kroncke K, Fehsel K, and Kolb-Bachofen V (1997). Nitric Oxide: Cytotoxicity versus cytoprotection-How, Why, When and Where? *Nitric Oxide Biol. Chem.* **1**: 107–120.
34. Richter C (1993). Pro-oxidants and mitochondrial calcium: their relationship to apoptosis and oncognesis. *FEBS Lett.* **325**: 104–107.
35. Hartley A, Stone JM, Heron C, Cooper JM, and Schapira AHV (1994). Complex I inhibitors induce dose dependent apoptosis in PC12 cells: relevance to Parkinson's disease. *J. Neurochem.* **63**: 1987–1990.
36. Bonfoco E, Krainc D, Ankarcrona M, Nicotera P, and Lipton SA (1995). Apoptosis and necrosis: two distinct events induced, respectively, by mild and intense insults with N-methyl-D-aspartate or nitric oxide/superoxide in cortical cell cultures. *Proc. Natl Acad. Sci. USA* **92**: 72162–72166.
37. Ankarcrona M, Dypbukt JM, Bonfoco E, *et al.* (1995). Glutamate-induced neuronal death: a succession of necrosis or apoptosis depending on mitochondrial function. *Neuron* **15**: 961–973.
38. Charriaut-Marlangue C, Margaill I, Borrega F, Plotkine M, and Ben-Ari Y (1996). NG-nitro-L-arginine methyl ester reduces necrotic but not apoptotic cell death induced by reversible focal ischemia in rat. *Eur. J. Pharmacol.* **310**: 137–140.
39. Tatton WG, Chalmers-Redman RM, Ju WY, Wadia J, and Tatton NA (1997). Apoptosis in neurodegenerative disorders: potential for therapy by modifying gene transcription *J. Neurol. Transm.* **49**: 245–268.
40. Katzman R (1986). Alzheimer's disease. *N. Engl. J. Med.* **314**: 964–973.
41. Goate A, Chartier-Harlin MC, Mullan M, *et al.* (1991). Segregation of a missense mutation in the amyloid precursor protein gene with familial Alzheimer's disease. *Nature* **21**: 349, 704–706.
42. Sherrington R, Rogaev EL, Liang Y, *et al.* (1995). Cloning of a gene bearing missense mutations in early-onset familial Alzheimer's disease. *Nature* **375**: 754–760.

43. Alzheimer's disease collaborative group (1995). The structure of the presenilin 1 (S182) gene and identification of six novel mutations in early onset AD families. *Nat. Genet.* **11**: 219–222.

44. Sinha S and Lieberburg I (1999). Cellular mechanisms of beta-amyloid production and secretion. *Proc. Natl Acad. Sci. USA* **96**: 11049–11053.

45. Corder EH, Saunders AM, Strittmatter WJ, *et al.* (1993). Gene dose of apolipoprotein E type 4 allele and the risk of Alzheimer's disease in late onset families. *Science* **261**: 828–829; 921–923.

46. McGeer EG, Peppard RP, McGeer PL, *et al.* (1990). [18]Fluorodeoxyglucose positron emission tomography studies in presumed Alzheimer's cases, including 13 serial scans. *Can. J. Neurol. Sci.* **171**: 1–11.

47. Kish SJ, Bergeron C, Rajput A, *et al.* (1992). Brain cytochrome oxidase in Alzheimer's disease. *J. Neurochem.* **59**: 776–779.

48. Parker WD, Mahr NJ, Filley CM, *et al.* (1994). Reduced platelet cytochrome c oxidase activity in Alzheimer's disease. *Neurology* **44**: 1086–1090.

49. Simonian N and Hyman BT (1993). Functional alterations in Alzheimer's disease: diminution of cytochrome oxidase in the hippocampal formation. *J. Neuropathol. Exp. Neurol.* **52**: 580–585.

50. Canevari L, Clark JB, and Bates TE (1999). β-amyloid fragment 25–35 selectively decreases complex IV activity in isolated mitochondria. *FEBS Lett.* **457**: 131–134.

51. Shoffner JM, Brown MD, Torrino A, *et al.* (1993). Mitochondrial DNA variants observed in Alzheimer's disease and Parkinson's disease patients. *Genomics* **17**: 171–184.

52. Egensperger R, Kosel S, Schnopp NM, Mehraein P, and Graeber MB (1997). Association of the mitochondrial tRNA(A4336G) mutation with Alzheimer's and Parkinson's diseases. *Neuropathol. Appl. Neurobiol.* **23**: 315–321.

53. Butterfield DA, Drake J, Pocernich C, and Castegna A (2001). Evidence of oxiative damage in Alzheimer's disease brain: central role for β-amyloid. *Trends Mol. Med.* **7**: 548–554.

54. Hensley K, Maidt ML, Yu Z, Sang H, Markesbery WR, and Floyd RA (1998). Electrochemical analysis of protein nitrotyrosine and dityrosine in the Alzheimer brain indicates region-specific accumulation. *J. Neurosci.* **18**: 8126–8132.

55. Askanas V, McFerrin J, Baqué S, Alvarez RB, Sarkazi E, and Engel WK (1996). Transfer of ß-amyloid precursor protein gene using adenovirus vector causes mitochondrial abnormalities in cultured normal human muscle. *Proc. Natl Acad. Sci. USA* **93**: 1314–1319.

56. Mori H, Kondo T, Yokochi M, *et al.* (1998). Pathologic and biochemical studies of juvenile parkinsonism linked to chromosome 6q. *Neurology* **51**: 890–892.

57. Polymeropoulos MH, Lavedan C, Leroy E, *et al.* (1997). Mutation in the a-synuclein gene identified in families with Parkinson's disease. *Science* **276**: 2045–2047.

58. Krüger R, Kuhn W, Muller T, *et al.* (1998). Ala30Pro mutation in the gene a-synuclein in Parkinson's disease. *Nat. Genet.* **18**: 106–108.

59. Leroy E, Boyer R, Auburger G, *et al.* (1998). The ubiquitin pathway in Parkinson's disease. *Nature* **395**: 451–452.

60. Kitada T, Asakawa S, Hattori N, *et al.* (1998). Mutations in the parkin gene cause autosomal recessive juvenile parkinsonism. *Nature* **392**: 605–608.

61. Spillantini MG, Schmidt ML, Lee VM, Trojanowski JQ, Jakes R, and Goedert M (1997). Alpha-synuclein in Lewy bodies. *Nature* **388**: 839–840.

62. Shimura H, Hattori N, Kubo S, *et al.* (2000). Familial Parkinson disease gene product, parkin, is a ubiquitin-protein ligase. *Nat. Genet.* **25**: 302–305.

63. Cooper JM and Schapira AHV (1997). Mitochondrial dysfunction in neurodegeneration. *J. Bioenerg. Biomembr.* **29**: 175–183.

64. Tipton KF and Singer TP (1993). Advances in our understanding of the mechanisms of the neurotoxicity of MPTP and related compounds. *J. Neurochem.* **61**: 1191–1206.

65. Przedborski S, Kostic V, Jackson-Lewis V, *et al.* (1992). Transgenic mice with increased Cu/Zn-superoxide dismutase activity are resistant to N-methyl-4-phenyl 1,2,3,6-tetrahydropyridine-induced neurotoxicity. *J. Neurosci.* **12**: 1658–1667.

66. Przedborski S, Donaldson D, Murphy PI, *et al.* (1996). Role of neuronal nitric oxide in 1-methyl-4-phenyl 1,2,3,6 tetrahydropyridine (MPTP)-induced dopaminergic neurotoxicity. *Proc. Natl. Acad. Sci. USA* **93**: 4565–4571.

67. Schapira AHV, Cooper JM, Dexter D, Clark JB, Jenner P, and Marsden CD (1990). Mitochondrial complex I deficiency in Parkinson's disease. *J. Neurochem.* **54**: 823–827.

68. Janetzky B, Hauck S, Youdim MBH, *et al.* (1994). Unaltered aconitase activity but decreased complex I activity in substantia nigra pars compacta of patients with Parkinson's disease. *Neurosci. Lett.* **169**: 126–128.

69. Gu M, Gash MT, Cooper JM, *et al.* (1997). Mitochondrial respiratory chain function in multiple system atrophy. *Mov. Disord.* **12**: 418–422.

70. Parker WD, Boyson SJ, and Parks JK (1989). Abnormalities of the electron transport chain in idiopathic Parkinson's disease. *Ann. Neurol.* **26**: 719–723.

71. Krige D, Carroll MT, Cooper JM, Marsden CD, and Schapira AHV (1992). Platelet mitochondrial function in Parkinson's disease. *Ann. Neurol.* **32**: 782–788.

72. Mann VM, Cooper JM, Krige D, Daniel SE, Schapira AHV, and Marsden CD (1992). Brain, skeletal muscle and platelet homogenate mitochondrial function in Parkinson's disease. *Brain* **115**: 333–342.

73. Anderson JJ, Bravi D, Ferrari R, *et al.* (1993). No evidence for altered muscle mitochondrial function in Parkinson's disease. *J. Neurol. Neurosurg. Psychiatry* **56**: 477–480.

74. Barroso N, Campos Y, Huertas R, *et al.* (1993). Respiratory chain enzyme activities in lymphocytes from untreated patients with Parkinson disease. *Clin. Chem.* **34**: 667–669.

75. Yoshino H, Nakagawa-Hattori Y, Kondo T, and Mizuno Y (1992). Mitochondrial complex I and II activities of lymphocytes and platelets in Parkinson's disease. *J. Neurol. Transmis.* **4**: 27–34.

76. Gu M, Cooper JM, Taanman JW, and Schapira AHV (1998*b*). Mitochondrial DNA transmission of the mitochondrial defect in Parkinson's disease. *Ann. Neurol.* **44**: 177–186.

77. Swerdlow RH, Parks JK, Miller SW, *et al.* (1996). Origin and functional consequences of the complex I defect in Parkinson's disease. *Ann. Neurol.* **40**: 663–671.

78. Kösel S, Grasbon-Frodl EM, Mautsch U, *et al.* (1998). Novel mutations of mitochondrial complex I in pathologically proven Parkinson disease. *Neurogenetics* **1**: 197–204.

79. Mayr-Wohlfart U, Rodel G, and Henneberg A (1997). Mitochondrial tRNA(Gln) and tRNA(Thr) gene variants in Parkinson's disease. *Eur. J. Med. Res.* **2**: 111–113.

80. Simon DK, Mayeux R, Marder K, Kowall NW, Beal MF, and Johns DR (2000). Mitochondrial DNA mutations in complex I and tRNA genes in Parkinson's disease. *Neurology* **54**: 703–709.

81. Gu M, Owen AD, Toffa SEK, *et al.* (1998*a*). Mitochondrial function, GSH and iron in neurodegeneration and Lewy body diseases. *J. Neurol. Sci.* **158**: 24–29.

82. Manning-Bog AB, McCormack AL, Li J, Uversky VN, Fink AL, and Di Monte DA (2002). The herbicide paraquat causes up-regulation and aggregation of alpha-synuclein in mice: paraquat and alpha-synuclein *J. Biol. Chem.* **277**: 1641–1644.

83. Lee H, Shin SY, Choi C, Lee YH, and Lee S (2002). Formation and removal of α-synuclein aggregates in cells exposed to mitochondrial inhibitors. *J. Biol. Chem.* **277**: 5411–5417.

84. Dexter DT, Holley AE, Flitter WD, *et al.* (1994). Increased levels of lipid hydroperoxides in the Parkinsonian substantia nigra: an HPLC and ESR study. *Mov. Disord.* **9**: 92–97.

85. Alam ZI, Daniel SE, Lees AJ, *et al.* (1997). A generalised increase in protein carbonyls in the brain in Parkinson's but not incidental Lewy body disease *J. Neurochem.* **69**: 1326–1329.

86. Giasson BI, Duda JE, Murray IVJ, *et al.* (2000). Oxidative damage linked to neurodegeneration by selective α-synuclein nitration in synucleinopathy lesions. *Science* **290**: 985–989.

87. Dexter DT, Wells FR, Lees AJ, *et al.* (1989). Increased nigral iron content and alterations in other metal ions occurring in brain in Parkinson's disease. *J. Neurochem.* **52**: 1830–1836.

88. Hirsch EC, Brandel J-P, Galle P, Javoy-Agid F, and Agid Y (1991). Iron and aluminium increase in the substantia nigra of patients with Parkinson's disease: an X-ray microanalysis. *J. Neurochem.* **56**: 446–451.

89. Sian J, Dexter DT, Lees AJ, *et al.* (1994). Alterations in glutathione levels in Parkinson's disease and other neurodegenerative disorders affecting basal ganglia. *Ann. Neurol.* **36**: 348–355.

90. Sofic E, Lange KW, Jellinger K, and Riederer P (1992). Reduced and oxidised glutathione in the substantia nigra of patients with Parkinson's disease. *Neurosci. Lett.* **142**: 128–130.

91. Ferrante RJ, Beal MF, Kowall NW, Richardson EP, and Martin JB (1987). Sparing of acetylcholinesterase-containing striatal neurons in Huntington's disease. *Brain Res.* **41**: 162–166.

92. Difiglia M, Sapp E, Chase KO, *et al.* (1997). Aggregation of huntingtin in neuronal intranuclear inclusions and dystrophic neurites in brain. *Science* **277**: 1990–1993.

93. Huntington's Disease Collaborative Research Group (1993). A novel gene containing a tri-nucleotide repeat that is expanded and unstable on Huntington's disease chromosomes. *Cell* **72**: 971–983.

94. Strong TV, Tagle DA, and Valdes JM, *et al.* (1993). Widespread expression of the human and rat Huntington's disease gene in brain and nonneural tissues. *Nat. Genet.* **5**: 259–265.

95. Trottier Y, Devys D, Imbert G, *et al.* (1995). Cellular localization of the Huntington's disease protein and discrimination of the normal and mutated form. *Nat. Genet.* **10**: 104–110.

96. Nasir J, Floresco SB, O'Kusky JR, *et al.* (1995). Targeted disruption of the Huntington's disease gene results in embryonic lethality and behavioral and morphological changes in heterozygotes. *Cell* **81**: 811–823.

97. Duyao MP, Auerbach AB, Ryan A, *et al.* (1995). Inactivation of the mouse Huntington's disease gene homolog Hdh. *Science.* **269**: 407–410.

98. Mangiarini L, Sathasivam K, Seller M, *et al.* (1996). Exon 1 of the HD gene with an expanded CAG repeat is sufficient to cause a progressive neurological phenotype in transgenic mice. *Cell* **87**: 493–506.

99. Davies SW, Turmaine M, Cozens BA, *et al.* (1997). Formation of neuronal intranuclear inclusions underlies the neurological dysfunction in mice transgenic for the HD mutation. *Cell* **90**: 537–548.

100. Saudou F, Finkbeiner S, Devys D, and Greenberg ME (1998). Huntingtin acts in the nucleus to induce apoptosis but death does not correlate with the formation of intranuclear inclusions. *Cell* **95**: 55–66.

101. Kuwert T, Lange HW, Langer K-J, Herzog H, Aulich A, and Feinendegen LE (1990). Cortical and subcortical glucose consumption measured by PET in patients with Huntington's disease. *Brain* **113**: 1405–1423.

102. Jenkins BG, Koroshetz WJ, Beal FM, and Rosen BR (1993). Evidence for impairment of energy metabolism in vivo in Huntington's disease using localize ^{1}H NMR spectroscopy. *Neurology* **43**: 2689–2695.

103. Koroshetz WJ, Jenkins BG, Rosen BR, and Beal MF (1997). Energy metabolism defects in Huntington's disease and effects of coenzyme Q_{10}. *Ann. Neurol.* **41**: 160–165.

104. Gu M, Cooper JM, Gash M, Mann VM, Javoy-Agid F, and Schapira AHV (1996). Mitochondrial defect in Huntington's disease caudate nucleus. *Ann. Neurol.* **39**: 385–389.

105. Tabrizi SJ, Cleeter M, Xuereb J, Taanman JW, Cooper JM, and Schapira AHV (1999). Biochemical abnormalities and excitotoxicity in Huntington's disease brain. *Ann. Neurol.* **45**: 25–32.

106. Browne SE Bowling AC, *et al.* (1997). Oxidative damage and metabolic dysfunction in Huntington's disease: selective vulnerability of the basal ganglia. *Ann. Neurol.* **41**: 646–653.

107. Sawa A, Wiegand GW, Cooper J, *et al.* (1999). Increased apoptosis of Huntington disease lymphoblasts associated with repeat-length dependent mitochondrial depolarization. *Nat. Med.* **5**: 1194–1198.

108. Beauchemin AMJ, Gottlieb B, Beitel LK, *et al.* (2001). Cytochrome c oxidase subunit Vb interacts with human androgen receptor: A potential mechanism for neurotoxicity in spinobulbar muscular atrophy. *Brain Res. Bull.* **56**: 285–297.

109. Lodi R, Schapira AH, Manners D, *et al*. (2000). Abnormal in vivo skeletal muscle energy metabolism in Huntington's disease and dentatorubropallidoluysian atrophy. *Ann. Neurol.* **48**: 72–76.
110. Arenas J, Campos Y, Ribacoba R, *et al*. (1998). Complex I defect in muscle from patients with Huntington's disease. *Ann. Neurol.* **43**: 397–400.
111. Ludolph AC, He F, Spencer PS, Hammerstad J, and Sabri M (1991). 3-nitropropionic acid: exogenous animal neurotoxin and possible human striatal toxin. *Can. J. Neurol. Sci.* **18**: 492–498.
112. Brouillet E, Hantraye P, Ferrante RJ, *et al*. (1995). Chronic mitochondrial energy impairment produces selective striatal degeneration and abnormal choreiform movements in primates. *Proc. Natl Acad. Sci. USA* **9**: 7105–7109.
113. Greene JG, Porter RHP, Eller RV, and Greenamyre JT (1993). Inhibition of succinate dehydrogenase by malonic acid produces an 'excitotoxic' lesion in rat striatum. *J. Neurochem.* **61**: 1151–1154.
114. Ferrante RJ, Andreassen OA, Jenkins BG, *et al*. (2000). Neuroprotective effects of creatine in a transgenic mouse model of Huntington's disease. *J. Neurosci.* **20**: 4389–4397.
115. Beal MF, Kowell NW, Ferrante RJ, and Cippolloni PB (1989). Quinolinic acid striatal lesions in primates as a model of Huntington's disease. *Ann. Neurol.* **26**: 137.
116. Sanberg PR, Calderon SF SF, Guordana M, Tew JM, and Norman AB (1989). The quinolenic acid model of Huntington's disease: locomotor abnormalities. *Exp. Neurol.* **105**: 45–53.
117. Cha JHJ, Kosinski CM, Kerner JA, *et al*. (1998). Altered brain neurotransmitter receptors in transgenic mice expressing a portion of an abnormal human Huntington disease gene. *Proc. Natl Acad. Sci. USA* **95**: 6480–6485.
118. Weller M and Paul SM (1993). 3-nitroprionic acid is an indirect excitotoxin in cultured cerebellar granule neurons. *Eur. J. Pharmacol.* **248**: 223–228.
119. Taylor-Robinson SD, Weeks RA, Bryant DJ, *et al*. (1996). Proton magnetic resonance spectroscopy in Huntington's disease: evidence in favour of the glutamate excitotoxic theory. *Mov. Disord.* **11**: 167–173.
120. Young AB, Greenmayre JT, Hollingsworth Z, *et al*. (1988). NMDA receptor losses in putamen from patietns with Huntington's disease. *Science* **241**: 981–983.
121. Wagster MV, Hedreen JC, Peyser CE, *et al*. (1994). Selective loss of kainic acid and AMPA binding in layer VI of frontal cortex in Huntington's disease. *Exp. Neurol.* **127**: 70–75.
122. Shaw CE, Enayat ZE, Chioza BA, *et al*. (1998). Mutations in all five exons of SOD-1 may cause ALS. *Ann. Neurol.* **43**: 390–393.
123. Sasaki S, Maruyama S, Yamane K, Sakuma H, and Takeishi M (1990). Ultrastructure of swollen proximal axons of anterior horn neurons in motor neuron disease *J. Neurol. Sci.* **97**: 233–240.
124. Ferrante RJ, Browne SE, Shinobu LA, *et al*. (1997*a*). Evidence of increased oxidative damage in both sporadic and familial amyotropgic lateral sclerosis. *J. Neurochem.* **69**: 2064–2074.
125. Bogdanov M, Brown RH, Matson W, *et al*. (2000). Increased oxidative damage to DNA in ALS patients. *Free Rad. Bio. Med.* **29**: 652–658.
126. Beal MF, Ferrante RJ, Browne SE, *et al*. (1997). Increased 3-nitrotyrosine in both sporadic and familial amyotrophic lateral sclerosis. *Ann. Neurol.* **42**: 644–654.
127. Gurney ME, Pu H, Chiu AY, *et al*. (1994). Motor neuron degeneration in mice that express a human CuZn superoxide dismutase mutation. *Science* **264**: 1772–1775.
128. Wong PC, Pardo CA, Borchelt DR, *et al*. (1995). An adverse property of a familial ALS-linked SOD1 mutation causes motor neuron disease characterized by vacuolar degeneration of mitochondria. *Neuron.* **14**: 1105–1116.
129. Ferrante RJ, Shinobu LA, and Schulz JB, *et al*. (1997*b*). Increased 3-nitrotyrosine and oxidative damage in mice with a human copper/zinc superoxide dismutase mutation. *Ann. Neurol.* **42**: 326–334.
130. Reaume AG, Elliott JL, Hoffman EK, *et al*. (1996). Motor neurons in Cu/Zn superoxide dismutase-deficient mice develop normally but exhibit enhanced cell death after axonal injury. *Nat. Genet.* **13**: 43–47.

131. Bowling AC, Schulz JB, Brown RH, *et al.* (1993). Superoxide dismutase activity, oxidative damage amd mitochondrial energy metabolism in familial and sporadic amyotrophic lateral sclerosis. *J. Neurochem.* **61**: 2322–2325.

132. Kong J and Xu Z (1998). Massive mitochondrial degeneration in motor neurons triggers the onset of amyotrophic lateral sclerosis in mice expressing a mutant SOD1. *J. Neurosci.* **18**: 3241–3250.

133. Higgins CMJ, Jung C, Ding H, and Xu Z (2002). Mutant Cu, Zn SOD that causes Motorneuron degeneration is present in mitochondria in the CNS. *J. Neurosci.* **22**:

134. Sturtz LA, Diekert K, Jensen LT, Lill R, and Culotta VC (2001). A fraction of yeast Cu,Zn-superoxide dismutase and its metallochaperone, CCS, localize to the intermembrane space of mitochondria. A physiological role for SOD1 in guarding against mitochondrial oxidative damage. *J. Biol. Chem.* **276**: 38084–38089.

135. Wiedemann FR, Winkler K, Kuznetsov AV, *et al.* (1998). Impairment of mitochondrial function in skeletal muscle of patients with amyotrophic lateral sclerosis. *J. Neurol. Sci.* **156**: 65–72.

136. Borthwick GM; Johnson MA, and Ince PG, *et al.* (1999). Mitochondrial enzyme activity in amyotrophic lateral sclerosis: Implications for the role of mitochondria in neuronal cell death. *Ann. Neurol.* **46**: 787–90.

137. Comi CP, Bordoni A, Salani S, *et al.* (1998). Cytochrome c oxidase subunit I microdeletion in a patient with motor neuron disease. *Ann. Neurol.* **43**: 110–116.

138. Wiedemann FR, Manfredi G, Mawrin C, Beal MF, and Schon EA (2002). Mitochondrial DNA and respiratory chain function in spinal cords of ALS patients. *J. Neurochem.* **80**: 616–625.

139. Klivenyi P, Ferrante RJ, Matthews RT, *et al.* (1999). Neuroprotective effects of creatine in a transgenic animal model of amylotrophic lateral sclerosis. *Nat. Med.* **5**: 347–350.

140. Shaw PJ and Ince PG (1997). Glutamate, excitotoxicity and amyotrophic lateral sclerosis. *J. Neurol.* **244**: S3–S14.

141. Kaal EC, Vlug AS, Versleijen MW, *et al.* (2000). Chronic mitochondrial inhibition induces selective motoneuron death in vitro: a new model for amyotrophic lateral sclerosis. *J. Neurochem.* **74**: 1158–1165.

13 Mechanisms underlying the age-related accumulation of mutant mitochondrial DNA

Aubrey DNJ de Grey

Introduction

The role of oxygen radical-mediated oxidative damage in ageing, first proposed by Harman in 1956,[1] has for many years been indisputable. For me, the most compelling evidence for it is the consistent finding that shorter-lived animals generate more superoxide as a percentage of their oxygen consumption, both across species and when calorically restricted and *ad libitum-*fed animals are compared. This and the many other less direct pieces of evidence in favour of the free radical theory of ageing have been expertly reviewed elsewhere[2–6] and will not be discussed here; however, towards the end of this review I will describe the potentially pivotal recent work of Zassenhaus's laboratory.[7]

The pervasiveness of the free radical theory in contemporary biogerontology is perhaps most clearly demonstrated by the frequency with which other, superficially unrelated, proposed mechanisms of ageing are now embellished to intertwine them with the free radical theory. Two prominent examples are the acceleration of both telomere shortening[8] and non-enzymatic glycosylation[9] by oxidative stress. But the first such elaboration of the free radical theory (for that is, in some senses, what such ideas are) was the simplest: that oxidative damage induces mutations, whose accumulation makes us progressively less viable, including (but not limited to) initiating cancer. This idea was explicitly set out by Harman in his original article,[1] along with the suggestion that oxidative damage would also affect components of the extracellular medium.

In that first paper, Harman further noted that the substances most likely to suffer damage from free radicals would be those closest to the free radicals' principal site(s) of production. It would be another decade before we acquired the crucial item of information that brings this point into conjunction with the proposed importance of DNA oxidation to ageing. That item was, of course, the discovery[10,11] that mitochondria possess their own DNA, encoding proteins essential to the process of oxidative phosphorylation.

Once we knew that mitochondria have their own DNA and are also probably the main site of production of toxic oxygen radicals, it was but a small leap of induction to propose that the mitochondrial DNA (mtDNA) was the likeliest site of accumulating mutations leading to ageing. Indeed, in 1972 exactly this was suggested—again by Harman:[12]

Free radicals 'escaping' from the respiratory chain . . . would be expected to produce deleterious effects mainly in the mitochondria . . . Are these effects mediated in part through alteration of mitochondrial DNA functions?

It is worth noting here that there is an unfortunate tendency nowadays to attribute this insight to an article published fully 17 years later[13] that failed to cite Harman's work. It is to be hoped that this amnesia will cease.

Comfort's (insufficiently) discomfiting objection

When a cell divides, the average number of mitochondria per cell in the two daughter cells is obviously half of what it was in the parent. This number must thus be doubled, on average, before those daughter cells are ready to divide again.

In a post-mitotic cell such as a neuron or a muscle fibre, however, no such requirement exists. In theory, mitochondria of such cells could exist indefinitely in a non-dividing state for the lifetime of their host cell, even if that were the lifetime of the organism. They would inevitably suffer degenerative (including oxidative) damage, but this could in theory be repaired by 'piecemeal' mechanisms analogous to those that keep the nucleus and its contents functioning.

In the 1960s, however, it was discovered that this is not what mitochondria of post-mitotic cell in fact do. Fletcher and Sanadi reported[14] that many constituents of mitochondria could be shown, by radiolabelling, to be recycled quite frequently—on the order of once a week to once a month. The classic studies in this area[15,16] established that this turnover rate was not a property of the individual constituent, but was uniform for almost all the material of the mitochondrial inner membrane or matrix—DNA or protein—though certain components of the outer membrane seemed to be recycled more rapidly. This indicated that mitochondrial maintenance is not a piecemeal, damage-targeted process as in the nucleus, but is instead performed at the level of the entire organelle: that is, some organelles are simply destroyed wholesale and presumably replaced by division of others. Electron microscopic evidence for this destruction was in fact already available:[17] it is termed autophagy or autophagocytosis. (In 1996, preliminary data belatedly emerged[18] on the rate of turnover in human tissues; analysis of mass spectroscopy of muscle needle biopsies implies a half-life of 2–3 months if most mitochondrial protein degradation is by autophagy. More measurements of human mitochondrial turnover rates are urgently needed.)

Enter Alex Comfort, just becoming better known in a more recreational context[19] but at that time also the prominent and hugely respected editor of *Experimental Gerontology*. In 1974 he published a wide-ranging review of the state of the nation as regards the biology of ageing, in which he touched briefly on Harman's then 2-year-old idea.[20] His treatment of it was brief, perhaps because it seemed so conclusive:

Mitochondrial damage has also been studied . . . Mitochondria, however, are replaceable structures. In order to 'explain' aging on the analogy of radiation-induced molecular attack we seem to require damage either to irreplaceable molecules . . . or to the copying mechanism of clonally dividing cells

When I first read this passage I already knew the data that refuted it (discussed below), but I was instantly struck by the feeling that, in the absence of that newer data, I would have abandoned on the spot the idea of mtDNA damage being a primary determinant of the rate of ageing. Mitochondria are recycled by the destruction of some and the division of others. As such, there is the opportunity for the cell to destroy those mitochondria that have sustained damage and replicate those that have not. This then places the mitochondrial population of a cell in the same boat as the cellular population of a mitotically competent organ, such as the liver: all individuals are replaceable and the global decline of the entire population can be completely prevented. One relatively recent finding serves to underscore the power of this type of preservation mechanism. Ageing is normally considered a universal characteristic of animals, except that it is hard to define ageing in unicellular creatures. But Martinez showed in a painstaking study published in 1998 that hydra, organisms with no post-mitotic cells at all, apparently do not age: they die solely from extrinsic causes, not due to increasing frailty.[21] He showed this in the most compelling way possible, by identifying conditions so benign that extrinsic mortality was almost totally absent: just one individual of his population died in the 4 years in which these conditions were maintained. Unless one is prepared to propose that a microscopic organism with a life cycle of a few days can have a mortality rate doubling time (the most standard measure of the rate of ageing) on the order of decades, this shows that elimination of some cells and their replacement by division of others is a preservation mechanism which can work indefinitely. And so, Comfort was saying, it should be for mitochondria—even mitochondria in post-mitotic cells.

Perhaps it was because Comfort's objection was buried on page 8 of a 31-page treatise; perhaps it was because others saw the weak link in his argument but never wrote it down. I suspect, however, that it was in fact because nobody could bear to give up the idea of mitochondrial mediation of ageing when nothing nearly so attractive was available as an alternative. 'It' is, of course, the fact that Comfort's objection was absolutely ignored for the next 20 years or so, during which the accumulation of mutations in the mtDNA was universally ascribed to a mechanism that was precisely of the type that Comfort had said could not be right.

The 'vicious cycle' theory

The release of superoxide ($O_2^{\bullet-}$) at the respiratory chain was the subject of intensive study during the 1970s, motivated not least by the discovery in 1969 that we have an enzyme to destroy it, superoxide dismutase (SOD).[22] It was found that two sites within the electron transport chain, near to CoQ-binding sites of Complexes I and III, were prone to release superoxide, and that the rate of this release was dependent on the degree of reduction of the relevant point in the chain. Thus, agents that block electron flow late in the chain increase $O_2^{\bullet-}$ production because of a 'logjam' of electrons at the relevant locations; ones that block electron flow early in the chain diminish $O_2^{\bullet-}$ production due to the depletion of electrons at those locations.[23,24] Later, it was shown that another factor modulates superoxide release: other things being equal it is faster when the transmembrane proton gradient is higher.[25]

All 13 proteins encoded by the mtDNA of animals are components of one or another enzyme in the respiratory chain. Thus, deleterious mutations in any of them have the capacity to alter the host mitochondrion's rate of release of superoxide (Table 13.1). A knockout of adenosine triphosphate (ATP) synthase (such as by a nonsense mutation in either of its mtDNA-encoded subunits) would raise the proton gradient and thereby increase the release of superoxide. A knockout of cytochrome *c* oxidase (COX) would lower the proton gradient, but it would also block electron flow through the complexes that are prone to release superoxide. A knockout of the one mtDNA-encoded subunit of Complex III, cytochrome *b*, might or might not increase $O_2^{\bullet-}$ production there (depending on whether the parts of the enzyme that form $O_2^{\bullet-}$ can assemble) but should increase it at Complex I, unless the diminution of proton gradient outweighs the logjam of electrons there. A mutation in a Complex I subunit

Table 13.1 Predicted effects on superoxide production rate of different types of loss-of-function mtDNA mutation. For details, see text

	Complex I degree of reduction	Complex III degree of reduction	Electrochemical proton gradient	Superoxide production rate
Complex I point mutation	?	↓	↓	↓
Complex III point mutation	↑	?	↓	?
Complex IV point mutation	↑	↑	↓	?
Complex V point mutation	↑	↑	↑	↑
Deletion or RNA point mutation	↓	↓	↓	↓↓

gene should generally reduce $O_2^{\cdot-}$ production, since it will both lower the proton gradient and deplete electrons at one or both $O_2^{\cdot-}$ -releasing sites.

This led to the following line of thought: Suppose that a cell initially has no mutant mtDNA whatever. Then a spontaneous mutation occurs. It may, if it is in the 'right' gene, cause its host mitochondrion to make more than the usual amount of $O_2^{\cdot-}$. If so, there is consequently an increased risk that nearby mitochondria (or, for that matter, the other few mtDNA molecules in the same mitochondrion) may themselves sustain mutations. Some of those mutations may also be in the right genes to make the host mitochondrion produce even more superoxide. Thus, the rate of occurrence of new mutations could in principle rise exponentially as a positive feedback loop—a vicious cycle—until all mtDNA molecules in the cell are dysfunctional and the cell is unable to respire (Fig. 13.1).[26]

As can readily be seen, however, the vicious cycle theory falls very foul of Comfort's objection. If a cell detects a mitochondrion that is not only failing to make ATP but also releasing a toxin at an elevated rate, what better stimulus can there be to destroy that mitochondrion without delay? That destruction cleanly breaks the vicious cycle and predicts a steady-state level of mtDNA damage. Thus, though one would have been unduly impulsive to reject the vicious cycle theory outright, it was in dire need of elaboration to evade this objection—elaboration which it did not receive.

It should also be mentioned that a precursor of the vicious cycle theory was published in 1980 by Miquel.[27] He proposed that mitochondria in post-mitotic cell types were progressively damaged to a point where they could not divide, leading to fewer mitochondria per cell and reduced ATP supply. This proposal has a serious problem: if a cell contains a population of mitochondria with a range of abilities to be replicated, the ones that *can* be replicated will be and the ones that cannot will not, so those that cannot be replicated will be eliminated from the cell as fast as they arise. Miquel presented and cited data indicating that mitochondrial numbers decline with age in post-mitotic cells of rodents; a more plausible interpretation for this is as a consequence of reduced physical activity, rather than a cause. *Drosophila* and *Musca* flight muscles were also noted to lose mitochondria with age; here Miquel's interpretation is more plausible (though not proven), because flies age so rapidly that damage might

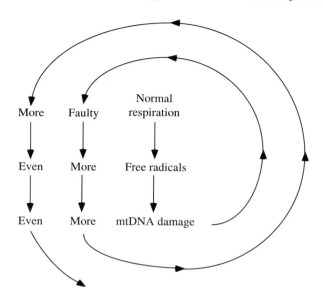

Fig. 13.1 The 'vicious cycle' theory to explain the age-related accumulation of mutant mtDNA. If mutant mitochondria produced more free radicals than wild-type ones, and if these free radicals were mutagenic to other mitochondria in the cell, there would be a positive feedback loop which would rapidly mutate all the mtDNA in the cell. However, neither prerequisite seems in fact to be true, and nor is there the intracellular spectrum of mutations that this model predicts.

be affecting all mitochondria at an appreciable rate simultaneously, so that selection could not compensate. This review will focus solely on vertebrates, however.

Mosaic loss of respiratory ability

In 1983, two papers were published initiating a series of studies that were to underpin subsequent progress in understanding how mutations in mtDNA might accumulate with age.[28,29] Both analysed the activity of the terminal enzyme of the electron transport chain, COX, in muscle biopsies from sufferers of progressive external ophthalmoplegia (PEO), a myopathy only later determined to result (in most cases) from gross deletions of the mtDNA. In all patients, there was an unambiguous loss of all COX activity in some muscle fibre segments (the muscle was cut perpendicular to the fibres, so that a thin slice of each fibre was present as a disc) while neighbouring fibres were not affected at all. In 1989 Müller-Höcker reported the same 'mosaic' COX inactivity (in a dramatically smaller proportion of fibre segments) in normal ageing.[30]

   It seems to me that the simplest interpretation of this finding is, paradoxically, that the vicious cycle theory was right after all but that Comfort was essentially right too. If the cell's reaction to a superoxide-raising mtDNA mutation is to destroy the host mitochondrion, then the amount of such destruction that it needs to be doing at any one time is a function of the number of such mutations that have occurred in the time it takes to destroy a mitochondrion.

Now, there is a chance—albeit maybe very small—that a large number of independent mutations could occur, in mitochondria of the same cell, within an interval shorter than the time it
takes for a mitochondrion to be degraded. Conceivably, if enough mutations occur in this
time, the rise in $O_2^{\cdot-}$ release might be sufficient to overwhelm the recycling machinery: the
rate at which new mutations would be occurring might exceed the rate at which they could be
eliminated by autophagy. It seems appropriate to term this the 'error catastrophe' elaboration
of the vicious cycle theory, as its dynamics are similar to those of the original error catastrophe theory of Orgel[31] concerning protein synthesis. This model would give rise to exactly
the situation that Müller-Höcker found: most cells would maintain a low and constant level
of mutant mtDNA indefinitely, whereas occasional cells that once exceeded the critical level
had plummeted to respiratory oblivion. (A concern that was immediately apparent, and will
be discussed in the concluding section of this review, was that so few fibres are affected in
normal ageing.)

This was not, however, the correct interpretation.

Clonal expansion asserted and then discovered

In the same year that Müller-Höcker published the discovery of mosaic respiratory deficiency
in normal ageing, Wallace suggested[32] that the accumulation of mutant mtDNA in mitochondriopathies was due to its having a proliferative advantage over wild-type mtDNA (wt-mtDNA).
This arose from the finding that sufferers of sporadic mitochondriopathies (ones in which the
proband's maternal lineage, including siblings, did not show symptoms) had exactly the same
mutation in every affected cell. This clonal expansion could have occurred at any time during
development, but the progressive nature of such diseases (and, indeed, the steady increase in
tissue levels of the mutant molecule) suggested that even within a single post-mitotic cell
there was a proliferation of the mutant at the expense of the wild-type molecule.[33]

The following year, Kadenbach and Müller-Höcker went a step further by considering this
phenomenon in the context of ageing.[34] They noted that the age-related increase in the number of fibres lacking COX activity was a strong indication of independent mutational events
in each affected fibre. They further observed that mitochondrial turnover in non-dividing cells
could give the opportunity for such mutant mtDNA to replicate more rapidly, eventually
depleting the cell of all its wt-mtDNA. This proposal, incorporating as it did the prediction
that different respiration-deficient muscle fibres would harbour different mtDNA mutations,
constituted a clear distinction between ageing and mitochondriopathies.

But how could clonal expansion be demonstrated? A truly conclusive demonstration could
have been very difficult, were it not for a convenient feature of loss-of-function mtDNA mutations in post-mitotic cell types: that a high proportion of them (very probably a large majority[35]) are gross deletions similar to those found in progressive external ophthalmoplegia and
other sporadic mitochondriopathies. This allows the following prediction: if one designs several DNA probes consisting of different small stretches of the mtDNA, and performs *in situ*
hybridization to a muscle sample with each such probe, one will see a mosaic distribution just
like that obtained with histochemical assays for COX. In some fibres, one of the probes will
fail to hybridize but others will give a normal signal; in other fibres a different probe will fail;
in some fibres all probes will hybridize (because the lesion is elsewhere or is a point mutation).
And in 1993, Müller-Höcker published the finding that this was exactly the situation *in vivo*[36]

(he had published essentially the same finding in a patient with a mitochondriopathy the previous year;[37] in that case all affected cells contain the same mutation, so the only distinction is between affected and unaffected cells).

The mechanistic fallout of the clonal expansion phenomenon

This discovery[36] was, in my view, the single most important experimental result in the whole history of the mitochondrial free radical theory of ageing. I give it this status for Popperian reasons:[38] because it falsified so many hitherto attractive theories, and indeed continues to be a critical observation with which any interpretation of newer results must be reconciled. It has since been confirmed in other tissues, by other labs, and using other techniques;[35,39–41] it is not in doubt.

Firstly it falsified Comfort's theory. It did not cast doubt on the idea that mitochondrial turnover preserves the *non*-DNA components of mitochondria—and indeed there is still no reason to doubt that, because mitochondrial division involves the incorporation of pristine new lipid and nuclear-coded protein components, which have not been exposed to superoxide production nearby and which therefore dilute out any oxidative damage that may be present. A steady-state level of oxidative damage to that material is thereby maintained. But the clonal expansion of a mtDNA mutation tells us that the mtDNA, which is of course synthesized by replication and so for which the above logic does not work, escapes this process. For whatever reason, the cellular process that selects some mitochondria for degradation and others for replication gets the choice wrong, and preferentially expands the mutant population rather than the wild-type one. This is as counter-intuitive to the teleologically-minded biologist as any result in biology, and it is no indictment of Comfort that he dismissed this possibility.

But secondly, it falsified the vicious cycle theory. Recall that the essence of the vicious cycle theory is a cascade of independent mutational events *in the same cell*, caused by excessive superoxide production by very nearby mitochondria that have already sustained such mutations. This is totally incompatible with the observation of only one mutant mtDNA variant in a given cell. If the vicious cycle theory were correct—whether or not the 'error catastrophe' extension of it discussed above was correct—hybridization of mtDNA probes to tissue should show a substantial signal in every cell, due to the mtDNA molecules that have suffered lesions in other regions of the mtDNA. Conceivably, the damage to mtDNA in affected cells would be so aggressive that it would be eliminated entirely, but then no signal would be present in any affected cell—that is, the distribution of signal would be the same for all probes, again contrary to what is observed. Later studies using Southern analysis[35,39] also eliminated this option.

The vicious cycle theory has been dispiritingly slow to die. It is still common to find it being referred to as the mechanism of mutant mtDNA accumulation during ageing, sometimes even in articles that also discuss clonal expansion. Bearing in mind that it was only published in concrete form[26] in the same year that Kadenbach and Müller-Höcker published their competing hypothesis,[34] I find it very hard to see why the alternative that was so rapidly shown to be incorrect received (and still receives) so much more airtime. This is especially so given that that original exposition[26] was very careful to note situations in which a vicious cycle would not occur, and the finding that the type of mutation most commonly seen *in vivo* is one that predicts just such a situation. Large deletions always remove at least one tRNA gene and thus abolish synthesis of all 13 mtDNA-encoded proteins, including those in

Complexes I and III. This will unequivocally diminish $O_2^{\cdot-}$ production: at Complex I because of the effects on electron transport and proton gradient discussed previously, and at Complex III because the absence of cytochrome *b* prevents the assembly of the Rieske protein into the complex[42] and thereby abolishes the one-electron oxidation of ubiquinol that is necessary for $O_2^{\cdot-}$ release at that complex. (Complex I also fails to assemble properly when the mtDNA-encoded subunits are missing,[43,44] but the implications of this for superoxide production are less certain than for Complex III since the precise mechanism of superoxide production at Complex I is not yet determined.)

A proposed extension of mitochondrial genetic terminology

The field of mitochondriology has hitherto made do with only one pair of words to distinguish qualitatively different mitochondrial genetic states of a cell: a cell is stated to be 'homoplasmic' for a particular mtDNA characteristic (allele, base pair, etc.) if all its mitochondrial genomes are identical in the respect in question, and 'heteroplasmic' otherwise. In what follows, however, it will sometimes be necessary to make two other distinctions, for which no terms are yet in use and for which, therefore, I introduce terms here. When all the mtDNA genomes within an *individual mitochondrion* are identical in the respect under consideration, that mitochondrion will be termed 'homochondrous' for that characteristic; mitochondria containing genomes that differ in the respect in question are 'heterochondrous'. Thus, a cell may be heteroplasmic for a given characteristic while all of its individual mitochondria are homochondrous for it, some carrying one variant and some the other. The other distinction which it will be useful to make is whether the mitochondria in a cell are identical to each other in terms of their mtDNA complement (again, with respect to some particular characteristic such as a mutation); if so, such a cell will be termed 'homokairotic', and if not, 'heterokairotic'. Thus, a cell may be (at least approximately) homokairotic even when it is highly heteroplasmic, if all its mitochondria are similarly heterochondrous. (These terms derive from the Greek *kairos*, meaning 'heddle frame', the part of a loom that controls a subset of warp threads; the motivation is that 'mito-' derives from the Greek *mitos*, meaning 'warp thread'. I am indebted to Dr James Clackson for his help in arriving at this terminology.) For clarity, the various terms (both established and new) are tabulated in Table 13.2.

Table 13.2 Extension of genetic terminology

Thing that is homogeneous or heterogeneous	Adjective for when it is homogeneous	Adjective for when it is heterogeneous	Noun for its degree of heterogeneity
The set of nuclear genomes in a cell	homozygous	heterozygous	[n/a in diploids]
The set of mtDNA genomes in a cell	homoplasmic	heteroplasmic	heteroplasmy
The set of mtDNA genomes in a mitochondrion	homochondrous	heterochondrous	heterochondry
The set of mitochondria in a cell	homokairotic	heterokairotic	heterokairoty

The alternatives that remain: 'structural' versus 'phenotype-based'

In the remainder of this review I shall leave the past behind and address what options remain for the mechanism of age-related clonal expansion of mutant mtDNA. Relevant new data and hypotheses have been appearing thick and fast in recent years and the topic has yet to reach resolution.

Before examining any of the specific proposals that have been made, it is instructive to introduce a characteristic possessed by some of them and not by others, which can itself be subjected to scrutiny of its consistency with available data. It is this: does the mechanism depend on the mtDNA-encoded proteins (or lack of them) in the mitochondria in which the mutant mtDNA resides? The vicious cycle theory certainly does depend on those proteins—partly on their lack of respiratory function, partly on their (presumed) faster release of super-oxide. Some attractive hypotheses exist, however, which do not possess this property. Hereafter, I term the latter models 'structural' and the others, such as the vicious cycle theory, 'phenotype-based'; this terminology has recently been independently proposed by Birky.[45]

The simplest and first[32] structural model was based on the observation that large deletions are common mutations both in normal ageing and in several of the best-studied mitochondriopathies. The commonest deletion in both cases is a removal of 4977 bp—that is, 30 per cent of the mitochondrial genome. Wallace pointed out that this might allow the replication of that molecule to be completed faster, and thus allow mitochondrial biogenesis to be faster. This would confer the observed selective advantage. A potential difficulty with this idea is that the mtDNA is so small (even without the deletion) that its replication—despite being much slower per base pair than nuclear or bacterial DNA replication—takes only an hour or two,[46] much faster than cell division in any human tissue *in vivo*, and enormously faster than the rate of mitochondrial turnover measured in the tissues in which mtDNA mutations mainly accumulate.[14–17] In other words, it seems that replication of mtDNA cannot be a rate-limiting step in mitochondrial biogenesis.

Birky recently proposed a highly elegant mechanism for the amplification of large deletions that escapes the above problem; unfortunately, however, it predicts amplification to levels, and at a rate, that do not match observations. He noted[45] that shortness can confer a selective advantage even without mtDNA replication being rate-limiting, because mtDNA copy number control seems to regulate total cellular mass of mtDNA, not the number of mtDNA molecules.[47] Consider, for simplicity, a cell with just two mtDNA molecules, one wild-type and one half-length, and suppose that its target mtDNA content is three times the wild-type length. Then, if genomes are chosen randomly one at a time for replication, the target may be reached with a total wild-type : deletion content of 3 : 1, 2 : 2, 2 : 3 or 1 : 4, with respective probabilities 1/3, 1/3, 1/12, and 1/4, giving on average a 25 : 27 ratio of wild-type : deletion. However, once the ratio of deleted molecules to wild-type reaches the reciprocal of the ratio of their lengths, an equilibrium situation will exist, since that ratio would only be maintained by selecting deleted molecules for replication that much more often than wild-type. For example, a cell with one wild-type and three half-length molecules and a target of five times the wild-type length will have an average wild-type : deletion ratio of 1 : 2.18 when the target is reached. This would mean that the common deletion would never rise above 60 per cent, which is incompatible with COX-negativity. Furthermore, even while such a mechanism *is* amplifying a deletion, the rate of amplification is inversely related to the number of genomes on which copy control is acting. Thus it will be exceedingly slow (which in ageing it is definitely not) in a cell with thousands of mtDNA molecules, unless (i) copy control is at the level of the individual mitochondrion, which intuitively requires mitochondrial fusion to be rare, and (ii) plenty of mitochondria are heterochondrous (since such selection could not occur in homochondrous ones), which requires that fusion be frequent. Thus, this mechanism is probably not important in ageing; it may, however, help to explain the stable heteroplasmy for deleted mtDNA in cells cultured in nonselective medium, recently reported by Schon's group.[48]

Various direct observations also challenge the idea of deleted mtDNA having an inherent replicative advantage. The earliest relevant study[49] was in yeast. Yeast cultures spontaneously generate mtDNA mutations, many of which are found to be 'suppressive'—to enjoy a selective advantage over wt-mtDNA when mutant and wild-type gametes fuse. It was found that the mutant mtDNA is generally replicated somewhat *less* frequently than the wild-type in such crosses (the important exception of hypersuppressive strains will be discussed below). More recently, Moraes *et al.*[50] performed an analogous study in cultured human cells, from which they concluded that grossly deleted mtDNA is replicated preferentially. When host mtDNA was depleted (but not eliminated) with ethidium bromide and then allowed to recover, deleted mtDNA recovered its mass several times faster than full-length mtDNA. However, this is an assay of the maximal replication rate, not the rate in the presence of a spontaneous mutation competing with a normal number of wild-type genomes in an OXPHOS-replete cell, so its physiological relevance is uncertain. Also, the ratio of recovery rates was greater than the ratio of wild-type to deleted mtDNA lengths (3 versus 1.83), but the classical strand-asynchronous model of mtDNA replication[51] suggests that maximal replication rate may be determined by the length of the major arc, which the deletion analysed reduces by a factor of 3.28, so this does not constitute evidence for faster replicability per base pair (let alone faster replication in physiological conditions) of deleted mtDNA. (The ratio of repopulation rates during the first week was calculated[50] as 7 based on linear repopulation kinetics, but the more plausible assumption of exponential kinetics gives a ratio around 3.) Finally, the same study[50] found that the presence of deleted mtDNA in host cells reduced by 68 per cent the clonability of cybrids with donor cytoplasts containing wt-mtDNA (relative to when the host cell was ρ^0), suggesting that the deleted mtDNA outcompeted the incoming wild-type; but host mtDNA carrying a loss-of-function point mutation also reduced clonability by a similar proportion, 50 per cent, again implying that mtDNA length plays at best a peripheral role.

The last-mentioned result supports a further objection to Wallace's model, noted as long ago as 1990 by Shoubridge *et al.*:[33] though large deletions are common in both ageing and mitochondriopathies, they are by no means the only mutations seen. Even if it is considered reasonable that deletions might proliferate due to having less DNA to replicate, this is not a plausible reason why point mutations should enjoy the same advantage. It is uneconomical to propose different mechanisms for the two classes of mutation, at least not in the same cell type, unless there is no alternative that could explain the phenomenon both for point mutations and for deletions. Shoubridge *et al.* suggested that the speed of mtDNA replication might not be governed solely by the quantity of DNA that must be replicated, but also by site-specific regulatory mechanisms. Specifically, there might exist *cis*-inhibitory sequences, whose disruption by point mutations or by deletions could allow unrestrained (or less restrained) mtDNA replication—possibly even runaway 'rolling-circle' replication.[52] However, this model also has a serious shortcoming: dozens of point mutations are now known that underlie mitochondrial pathologies (reviewed in, e.g. Ref. 53), as well as many that are reported to accumulate during normal ageing,[54] and these are sprinkled liberally across the whole genome. It is reasonable that some of the binding sites of proteins that regulate mtDNA replication and/or transcription might have the role proposed by Shoubridge *et al.*—and, indeed, there is now good evidence[55,56] that some such sites do confer a replicative advantage in certain circumstances—but this idea becomes hard to sustain when many regions not obviously involved in mtDNA maintenance must be postulated. (A multiplicity of such sites could perhaps be expected if coupled leading-and-lagging-strand synthesis is in fact common *in vivo*, but current evidence[57] suggests that it is restricted to situations where mitochondrial biogenesis is very rapid, which is not the case in the post-mitotic cells that accumulate loss-of-function mtDNA mutations *in vivo*.)

General challenges to structural mechanisms

In addition to the data analysed above, various observations exist that challenge the models discussed so far purely because they are 'structural', having nothing to do with the functioning of mtDNA-encoded proteins. Since these findings would thus also challenge any other structural model, it is valuable to examine them in detail.

One observation that is hard to reconcile with a structural model is the relatively high frequency of cells with just a trace (a few percent) of deleted mtDNA.[58,59] If the expansion of such mutants is independent of their phenotypic consequence, such cells should be only a short time away from becoming COX-negative, due to being taken over by that mutant mtDNA. This does not happen—the actual abundance of COX-negative cells or fibre segments rises only slowly. A phenotype-based mechanism, by contrast, is consistent with (indeed, predicts) the presence of a lot of cells with traces of mutant mtDNA, because initially that mutant mtDNA will be distributed across many mitochondria and none will be homochondrous for it. Only after homochondrous mutant mitochondria arise will their OXPHOS capacity begin to decline, and even then only gradually (by progressive dilution each time those mitochondria divide).

An even more telling inconsistency of structural models with the data is the phenomenon of 'functional dominance'. When the mosaic distribution of mitochondrial dysfunction was first discovered, it was by histochemical means (usually COX inactivity). It is straightforward to show that the same muscle fibre segments that are COX-negative are also, by and large, the ones with mtDNA deletions detectable by *in situ* hybridization: indeed, this is the most direct evidence that deletions are more common than point mutations in normal ageing.[35] But on closer examination it emerges that, even when COX activity in affected cells is absolutely eliminated, a few percent of apparently undeleted (and presumably non-mutant) mtDNA remains.[36,39] In other words, the selective pressure that caused the deleted molecule to take over the cell has not run to completion. This pressure must be very strong when it is working, because turnover rates of mitochondria are such as to allow only about 100 mitochondrial generations in the rat during its lifetime,[14,16,17] and there must be an absolute minimum of about $\log_2 1,000,000 = 20$ doublings of the mutant mtDNA population to get it from one copy to the million or so which a 1-mm-long muscle fibre segment (a typical length seen[60]) contains. Thus, the failure to complete that last scrap of expansion tells us that this strong selection is switched off at the last minute.

How is it switched off? We have only one hint: the COX inactivity. It is completely unknown why a cell that has been involuntarily deprived of nearly all its respiratory function by the proliferation of dysfunctional mtDNA should *choose* to deprive itself of the remainder, but that is the observation. [The hypothesis that I favour is that this is a side effect of the interplay between nuclear and mitochondrial gene expression: that some (though not all, we know[61]) nuclear-coded subunits of the respiratory chain cease to be transcribed when the cell detects that they are not being sufficiently incorporated into enzyme complexes. But that is beyond the scope of this review.] But then, if the mechanism of clonal expansion depends on the activity or otherwise of the oxidative phosphorylation machinery in host mitochondria, expansion would be predicted to cease when COX activity ceases. By contrast, a structural mechanism would be oblivious to the changed respiratory milieu and would proceed unabated to complete the elimination of wt-mtDNA.

A third class of observations is perhaps the most direct and forceful challenge to structural mechanisms. Mitochondrial dysfunction in skeletal muscle, both in normal ageing and in mitochondriopathies, is often associated with substantial mitochondrial hyperproliferation. Critically, structural models clearly predict that hyperproliferation should precede loss of COX activity, whereas phenotype-based models predict the opposite. The data on this point are remarkably clear: COX-negative cells are often seen that exhibit little or no mitochondrial hyperproliferation,[62,63] whereas COX-positive cells with unusually many mitochondria are almost never seen (except in the case of the MELAS mutation[64] at position 3243, which may be amplified by an unusual mechanism[56]). The cell's mtDNA copy control mechanism might delay structurally driven proliferation until OXPHOS insufficiency appears, but even then hyperproliferation should slightly precede all-out COX-negativity.

Taken together, the above observations constitute a strong argument that leads me to conclude that the mechanism underlying clonal expansion cannot be structural, so must be phenotype-based.

Mitochondrial fusion: a challenge to phenotype-based mechanisms?

Before attempting to discriminate between the various hypotheses that are unchallenged by the above arguments—the 'phenotype-based' proposals—it is necessary to consider a very general objection to the idea that clonal expansion could be phenotype-based.

Mitochondria are, of course, degenerate bacteria. Consequently, it is natural to think of the mitochondria of a cell as a population of individuals, which maintain roughly constant numbers through a balance of biogenesis by division and death by autophagy. What is not at all natural is to think of them doing the opposite of biogenesis—fusing. However, there is now very solid evidence that they sometimes do exactly that. Progress has been greatest in a very specialized aspect of mitochondrial biology, spermatogenesis, in which a gene responsible for mediating fusion was cloned in 1997;[65] this gene has homologues in all phyla yet examined and the yeast homologue also mediates fusion. In human cells, the evidence is also by now very compelling; the foremost series of studies, including recently the first *in vivo* work, is that of Hayashi's group.[66–70]

The relevance of mitochondrial fusion to the present discussion is that it makes the cell broadly homokairotic, whatever its degree of heteroplasmy. This potentially eliminates the link between genotype and phenotype among the mitochondrial population of a cell, and thereby renders any phenotype-based mechanism of selection for one genotype over another (specifically, for a mutant genotype over wild-type) out of the question. If fusion is (i) complete, so that mtDNA molecules and/or their protein or RNA products are distributed among both daughter mitochondria when the fusion product eventually redivides, and (ii) frequent, occurring at least as often as mitochondrial turnover, then at any given instant in a heteroplasmic cell there will be no significant difference between the abundance of functioning respiratory chain enzyme complexes in mitochondria that contain more mutant mtDNA and that in ones that contain less.

At present, however, there is no need to abandon the idea of a phenotype-based mechanism of clonal expansion, because no evidence exists to suggest that mitochondrial fusion *in vivo* is as frequent (or as full) as would be necessary for the above scenario, except when tissue mutant load is much higher than is ever seen in normal ageing. In fact, several types of direct evidence exist that suggest the contrary. A series of painstaking electron-microscopic studies of mito-chondria in muscle (reviewed in Ref. 71) indicates that the filamentous morphology often seen at the light microscope level may actually be a series of closely abutting but distinct units. Secondly, early work[72] using the dye JC-1, which indicates the mitochondrial membrane poten-tial by changing from red to green at a threshold level, clearly showed mitochondrial filaments with some red segments and some green segments, which is bioenergetically impossible if the filament is a continuous aqueous compartment (though one alternative, that the mitochondria *are* fully fused but JC-1 does not sufficiently precisely measure membrane potential, has not been firmly excluded). Thirdly, *in vitro* analysis of the ability of two mtDNA species harbour-ing different mutations to complement each other suggests that fusion is rare[73] (though not vanishingly so[69]). Finally, doubt has been cast on the relevance of *in vitro* observations of mito-chondrial fusion by the discovery that it is stimulated by oxidative[74] and other[75] stress: the oxy-gen tension *in vivo* is much less than when cells are cultured in air, so fusion may be greatly promoted by standard culture conditions. By analogy, it could also be promoted *in vivo* when mutant mtDNA is pathophysiologically abundant, as in mitochondriopathies (the consequent suppression of selection perhaps explaining why patients' mutant mtDNA levels typically rise rather slowly) or the recently developed mouse model of mitochondrial disease.[70]

Hypotheses for phenotype-based faster replication of mutant mtDNA

In addition to the vicious cycle theory, two other detailed, phenotype-based suggestions have been made for how mutant mitochondria might replicate more frequently than wild-type and thereby take over cells in which they arise. The first was actually set out as long ago as 1990, in the same article[33] that suggested the idea of runaway replication due to mutation of *cis*-inhibitory sequences. However, it was suggested negatively—as an unfavoured alternative to loss of *cis*-inhibition—and was thus overlooked by many, though it was later championed by Attardi's group, who named it the 'crippled mitochondrion' hypothesis.[76] The proposal was that mitochondrial biogenesis is at least partly under the control of the individual mitochon-drion, so that mitochondria initiate division (importing the relevant proteins and lipids, as well as replicating their DNA) when their microenvironment signals that this is appropriate. If so, the changes caused by a mutation-induced loss of respiratory function could perhaps be just the type of alteration to trigger biogenesis. Specifically, the depletion of intramitochondrial ATP is a plausible trigger to build more ATP-synthesizing machinery (i.e. more mitochondria) and would indeed result from a mtDNA mutation.

This hypothesis is not conclusively disproven, but it makes two quite firm predictions that appear not to be borne out by the data. One is at present only provisionally falsified: that mtDNA mutations which affect only the ATP synthase should be clonally expanded just as effectively as those which affect the electron transport chain. This is contrary to a report that examined a 5-bp region of the ATPase 6 gene.[77] The other prediction has been more decisively contradicted, however: that mitochondrial proliferation, such as can be observed with the Gomori trichrome stain or by quantifying the concentration of mtDNA, should precede loss of COX activity. In fact, the order of events appears to be the reverse,[62,63] except in the case of the MELAS mutation[64] at position 3243 which may be amplified by a different mechanism than that which amplifies typical spontaneous loss-of-function mutations such as deletions.[56] As mentioned earlier, this is also a strong general argument against structural mechanisms of amplification of deletions.

The second proposed mechanism for phenotype-based faster replication of mutant mtDNA was first put forward in 1994 in an inconspicuous forum, a conference proceedings chapter;[78] this was compensated in 1997 by its brief description in *Scientific American*.[79] It is also based on consideration of a mitochondrion's microenvironment, but does not involve any mitochondrial autonomy. If we consider a cell which contains some mutant and some wild-type mitochondria, and we assume that mitochondria travel essentially at random about the cell, we can infer that at certain times there will be unusually many mutant mitochondria near the nucleus and at other times unusually few. (We can ignore the polyploidy of mitochondria for this purpose: in any event, if mitochondrial fusion is as rare as was argued above, elementary arguments based on genetic drift show that few mitochondria will ever be heterochondrous.) Let us then make two further assumptions, both reasonable: (i) that the nucleus initiates a bout of mitochondrial biogenesis when the ATP level in the nucleus drops, and (ii) that this pulse of biogenesis is 'sub-saturating'— it involves the division of only a subset of the cell's mitochondria. Then, the beneficiaries of this pulse will preferentially be those mitochondria nearest to the nucleus, since that is where the relevant transcripts and protein products will be at greatest density—and, indeed, that is where some[46,80,81] (but not others[82]) have reported that mitochondrial biogenesis occurs. But if we consider how the pulse came about, we can see that more often than not it will occur when there are unusually many mutant mitochondria near to the nucleus, failing to supply nuclear ATP.

It is a shame when such an elegant hypothesis is very easily refuted, but such is the case here. The proposed process can be broken down into three stages, and straightforward statistical arguments show that it fails at all three. Firstly consider the situation shortly after the mutation has arisen: we can fairly presume that it segregates randomly at first, so that most mutations are destroyed before selection can affect them but a few are amplified by random chance to perhaps a few dozen copies, allowing them to reach homochondry in one or two mitochondria. But the proposed mechanism cannot start with one or two dysfunctional mitochondria: enough must accumulate that, if they all happen to be near the nucleus at the same time, they will constitute a substantial proportion of the perinuclear mitochondrial population. This is vanishingly unlikely. Secondly, even if such a situation were to arise and the mechanism thus to be allowed to begin, there is a problem of variance: the more mutant mitochondria there are, the more exactly their movements will cancel each other out, so that it is again vanishingly unlikely that the proportion of mutant mitochondria near the nucleus will ever deviate appreciably from that in the cell as a whole. And finally, if a cell did accumulate enough mutant mtDNA to be bioenergetically compromised, it would never have enough wild-type mitochondria near the nucleus to shut biogenesis down even when unusually *few* mutants were near the nucleus, so again there would be no selection for the mutant genome.

Beginner's luck: 'survival of the slowest' (SOS)

A radically different mechanism[83] was proposed by the present author in 1997. It seeks to explain not only the bald phenomenon of clonal expansion, but also two other paradoxical but long-standing observations: that expansion occurs only in non-dividing (or very slowly dividing) cell types, and that mitochondrial autophagy happens at all.

The restriction of clonal expansion to non-dividing cells is in fact a very general challenge to all the hypotheses described so far. A mechanism for preferential replication of a given mutation should, a priori, exert its influence wherever replication is occurring: it is of course possible that different mechanisms would exist in different tissues, but that is not where Occam's razor tells us to begin. It is reasonable to suppose that continuously dividing cells would not actually accumulate high enough levels of mutant mtDNA to render them bio-energetically impaired, since at that point the continued replication of the cell itself would be retarded and the contribution of those highly loaded cells to the overall mutant load in the tissue thereby capped. But we know that the excess of bioenergetic capacity in cells is substantial—in cultures heteroplasmic for mutations associated with mitochondriopathies, it is typical for cells to show no slowdown of growth until the mutant genotype exceeds about 60 per cent of the total,[84] and some cell lines grow at undiminished rates despite lacking any mtDNA whatever. By contrast, cells with a high load of clearly loss-of-function mutations are never found in rapidly cycling tissues (except cancers, discussed below).

This leads one to search for a factor in the mitochondrial life cycle which may be absent in mitotically active cells, or at least much less prevalent than in post-mitotic ones. Autophagy of mitochondria is just such a factor. It necessarily occurs at a substantial rate in post-mitotic cells, sufficient to allow the weekly to monthly half-life observed for inner membrane and matrix components;[14–17] in rapidly dividing cells, on the other hand, there is no need to make room for mitochondrial division. Critically, moreover, autophagy is a process which, if biased in favour of wild-type mitochondria, would cause the clonal expansion of mutant mitochondria even in the complete absence of any bias in the biogenesis machinery. (Autophagy has been claimed to be entirely nonselective, degrading aliquots of cytoplasm entirely at random,[85] but this teleologically implausible scenario has now been disproven in one context, the fertilized egg,[86] so may also be incorrect in post-mitotic cells.)

It was of course necessary to flesh out this abstract concept with a moderately concrete mechanism. The one that was set out[83] began from the unpopular, but (as discussed earlier) firmly predicted, notion that typical spontaneous mtDNA mutations reduce, rather than increase, the release of superoxide by their host mitochondria. This would lead to a slower rate of self-inflicted damage to the membranes of those mitochondria than to wild-type ones.

At this point it was necessary to postulate something plausible but, to my knowledge at that time, untested: that superoxide-mediated oxidation would increase a mitochondrial inner membrane's permeability to protons, thereby uncoupling its electron transport chain from its ATP synthase. (I later discovered work from the 1970s showing that, indeed, peroxidation does markedly increase a membrane's proton permeability.[87,88]) Mitochondria in such a state would be a severe liability to the cell, since their electron transport chain would continue consuming nutrients and oxygen unabated but the only release of energy would be as heat. This seemed like a highly plausible trigger for rapid lysosomal degradation of the affected mitochondrion.

These components meshed readily into a full-fledged mechanistic hypothesis (Fig. 13.2). In the absence of mutations, mitochondria succumb one by one to autophagosomes (structures

Damage Dysfunction Destruction Depletion Division

(a)

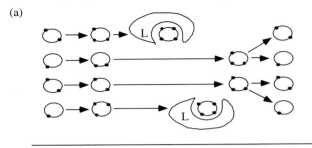

(b)

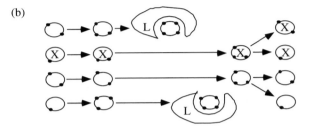

○ Mitochondrion

• Membrane damage

X mtDNA damage

L Lysosome

Damage Depletion Division Damage Depletion Division

(c)

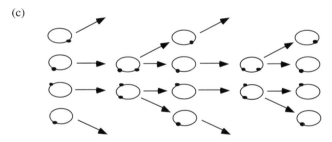

Fig. 13.2 The SOS theory to explain the age-related accumulation of mutant mtDNA, as well as its restriction to non-dividing cells and the existence of mitochondrial turnover. For details, see text.

related to lysosomes) attracted by their self-inflicted membrane damage and consequent uncoupled respiration. This depletes the cell of mitochondria until ATP supply becomes inadequate and a round of mitochondrial biogenesis is initiated (Fig. 13.2(a)). Once a mutation occurs, the same process continues, but it only rarely involves the phagocytosis of a mutant mitochondrion because the wild-type ones are eliminated more rapidly (Fig. 13.2(b)). In a population of rapidly dividing cells, cellular ATP shortage and consequent mitochondrial biogenesis is triggered by the halving of mitochondrial numbers per cell that results from each cell division, so the cycle is short-circuited and autophagy of mitochondria essentially never occurs (Fig. 13.2(c)).

This hypothesis is thus consistent with all known aspects of the clonal expansion of dysfunctional mtDNA, and it remains the only proposed mechanism that is (though another, discussed below, may amplify a class of phenotypically silent mutations). However, it has certainly not been proven correct. It makes a number of concrete predictions that are yet to be tested. One is that autophagy of mitochondria is much rarer in mitotically active tissues than elsewhere. Another is that mutations which *do* increase the rate of superoxide release are not amplified: this is one interpretation of the finding that mutations in a short region of an ATPase subunit gene do not accumulate with age,[77] but it needs more systematic examination. As noted earlier, one very direct prediction has been confirmed in yeast[49]—that mutant mtDNA is not replicated any more frequently than wild-type in most suppressive petite strains—but corresponding work on mammalian cells remains limited.

Mitotically active cells: recent developments

Arguably the weakest aspect of the SOS model in its original form was that it predicted only no selection for, not selection against, loss-of-function mtDNA mutations in mitotically active cells. Selection against such mutations would appear once they became prevalent enough to be bioenergetically meaningful, but (as was noted earlier) they do not remotely approach such levels in practice. Kowald and Kirkwood therefore proposed an embellishment of the SOS mechanism, in which there is indeed selection against mutant mitochondria even when they are in a small minority in a given cell.[89,90] Their idea was that mitochondrial biogenesis, especially the import of nuclear-coded proteins, will be slower in a mutant mitochondrion due to a relative shortage of intramitochondrial ATP and a reduced transmembrane proton gradient. This will mean that a mutant mitochondrion cannot complete division (and thus become able to initiate another round of division) as rapidly as a wild-type one. If cell division is rapid, mitochondrial biogenesis may be continuous and this difference may lead to preferential expansion of wt-mtDNA rather than mutant, purely by faster mitochondrial biogenesis. (Unlike mtDNA replication, it is unknown how long a mitochondrion takes to import all the proteins necessary to divide.)

The idea that deleterious mutations are eliminated from mitotically competent tissues has received support from several recent studies that investigated the age-related distribution of point mutations. What is found, importantly, is that this is a property not only of highly mitotic tissues but also of some rather slowly dividing ones. Both in dermal fibroblasts[91] and in tumours,[92] large deletions were absent and nearly all point mutations detected were in the non-coding D-loop region of the genome where it may be that they have no phenotypic consequence (the common deletion is found at much higher levels in tumours than in neighbouring tissue,[93] but still at under 1 per cent of total mtDNA, far less than in the above studies).[91,92] The same result was reported in an analysis of brain[94] and presumably reflects glia, which comprise over 90 per cent of the cells in most brain regions.[95] Glia and fibroblasts divide so rarely that Kowald and Kirkwood's model seems unlikely to apply. An explanation may be that cells which suffer deleterious mtDNA mutations do indeed fall into the SOS vortex but that, unlike post-mitotic cells, when they become bioenergetically incompetent they enter apoptosis at once: being more easily replaced than post-mitotic cells, they may be tuned to succumb more readily.

Interestingly, other studies of tumour mtDNA[96–101] have found numerous clear loss-of-function mutations. This may suggest that tumours vary in the stage at which their requirement for aerobic respiration becomes negligible, but a subtler explanation is indicated by the almost complete limitation of such mutations, in all these studies, to genes encoding Complex I subunits. One possibility is that tumour cells require OXPHOS not for ATP supply but only to maintain redox stability; this can be achieved in the absence of Complex I by reversing the malate/aspartate shuttle and upregulating plasma membrane electron export, but if Complexes III and/or IV are also lacking then more extreme biochemical acrobatics are needed.[102] The risk of artifactual detection in tumours of 'mutations' that are in fact nuclear pseudogenes is real—it cannot be absolutely excluded by a failure to identify the sequence in control tissue[103]—but the recent systematic identification of all such pseudogenes in the public human genome sequence[104] may diminish this risk henceforth.

Finally, a recent paper[105] points out that cells can theoretically be taken over by spontaneously mutant mtDNA even in the absence of any selection mechanism. If it is a question of pure and unbiased luck whether a given mtDNA molecule is destroyed or replicated, there is clearly a nonzero (albeit very slight) probability that a spontaneous mutation, initially present only in one copy, will defy the usual effects of genetic drift and increase to become the majority species in the cell, after which genetic drift will preferentially amplify it to homoplasmy. The mutation rate necessary for this to give rise to the frequency of COX-negative cells observed in ageing was shown to be realistic. However, this model predicts (i) that the amplification process will run to completion, contrary to the 'functional dominance' observation noted earlier, and (ii) that, when parameters are chosen that produce the observed frequency of COX-negative cells, for every cell that is entirely mutant there will be many cells that are severely heteroplasmic (say, a ratio of mutant to wild-type of between 1 : 3 and 3 : 1), which is likewise not seen.[39] If the number of mitochondrial generations is much greater, however, this selection-free model does indeed predict mostly homoplasmic cells; thus, there is no need to ascribe tumorigenic significance to the presence of such mutations,[106] as some of the aforementioned studies have tentatively done.[96,98]

The abundance of dysfunctional mtDNA in aged tissues: recent developments

There is no doubt that mtDNA mutations cause severe diseases. I have only minimally addressed such diseases in this review, partly because it seems that the population dynamics of the mutant genotype in those diseases differs in various ways from that in normal ageing. The most palpable difference is that even very elderly individuals seem to possess extremely little dysfunctional mtDNA—by most estimates, under 1 per cent of the total (but see below). The only tissue in which generally accepted techniques have found a much higher level of COX inactivity than this is the substantia nigra, where the value is about 10 per cent.[107,108] Moreover, the phenomenon of clonal expansion makes it difficult to sustain the long-standing idea that we actually have a lot of dysfunctional mtDNA but our existing detection techniques grossly underestimate it. This theory, usually termed the 'tip of the iceberg' hypothesis,[109] requires the presence of high levels of mutant mtDNA in cells that also possess enough wild-type mtDNA to exhibit good COX activity histochemically. Crucially, moreover, it requires that cells remain in this highly heteroplasmic state for long periods, since if it were unstable, rapidly moving to homoplasmy for the mutant molecule, COX activity at the tissue level would decline precipitously. But instability of a very heteroplasmic state (or rather, the consequence of that instability) is exactly what we observe in the few cells that do become wholly respiration-deficient. The only way out of this, it seems, is to propose a very strict disjunction of sister mtDNA molecules at each mitochondrial division, whereby genetic drift at the level of the mitochondrion is all but eliminated. Such a 'faithful nucleoid' system has been argued to exist on the basis of population dynamics studies in culture[52] but this interpretation of those observations has recently been suggested to be flawed[110,56] and no biochemical evidence for such a system has emerged. (It must be stressed that the evidence for nucleoids *per se*, that is, for aggregation of multiple mtDNA molecules in particulate structures, is clear—the above concerns only their 'faithfulness'.)

Direct support for the 'tip of the iceberg' hypothesis has emerged in recent years, however, with the application of novel PCR variants such as long extension PCR.[111] Several groups[112–114] have reported much higher levels of both point mutations and deletions than were found in earlier work. These reports have been severely criticized, however,[115,116] because the quantitative reliability of the techniques is unclear. A second severe difficulty, especially with the data of Ozawa's group,[113] is that most of the deletions identified leave the mutant molecule lacking one or both of the origins of replication. It has been suggested that the light-strand origin is not absolutely required for mtDNA replication,[57] but its absence is nonetheless likely to inhibit replication significantly, and the heavy strand origin is absolutely indispensable. Finally, there is the problem that the levels of mtDNA mutations reported by these groups[111–113] are so high as to seem to be at odds with the essentially undiminished bioenergetic capacity of tissue from older individuals.[117] An intriguing possibility, not yet investigated, is that much of this deleted mtDNA is in fact fragmented and in the process of being degraded. Wholesale mtDNA degradation coupled with replication of other mtDNA molecules might be an important repair mechanism; this is suggested by the finding[118] that fragmented mtDNA is abundant *in vivo* and is highly enriched in oxidatively damaged bases.

A pair of recent studies may reconcile the above observations. It was shown[59,119] that, in cardiomyocytes, at least some of the molecules identified by long extension PCR as mtDNA deletions are in fact *duplications*, which when amplified using divergent primers in the duplicated region are indistinguishable from heteroplasmic deletions (Fig. 13.3). The presence of duplications, as well as their preferential amplification in individual cells, was shown especially convincingly by Khrapko's group[59] because the sensitivity of their PCR technique was sufficient to allow use of only part of a single cell's mtDNA; thus, the breakpoints of the mutant molecule having been identified, a second sample from the same cell could be analysed using primers which lay within the putatively deleted region, and which thus would amplify nothing if the molecule really were a deletion but would amplify a characteristic, unique fragment if it were a duplication (Fig. 13.3). Jacobs's group[119] used the same technique to show the presence of duplications, but did so on DNA derived from whole tissue and thus less directly addressed the clonal expansion question. These findings allow the coexistence of large quantities of ostensibly deleted mtDNA with a very low abundance of COX-negative cells.

It is intriguing to consider the mechanism of clonal expansion of such rearrangements. It was noted earlier that in 1986, Chambers and Gingold showed[49] that suppressive petite yeast strains generally replicate their mutant mtDNA less frequently (if anything) than their wild-type, presaging the 'SOS' model of clonal expansion in mammals. But they also found that in hypersuppressive strains, whose mtDNA possesses duplicated origins of heavy-strand replication, the mutant mtDNA was indeed replicated more often than the wild-type. It seems highly likely that this would be so for the mtDNA duplications discovered in the aforementioned studies,[59,119] as has indeed been proposed previously;[120] it was recently shown[121] that both heavy-strand origins are active in such molecules.

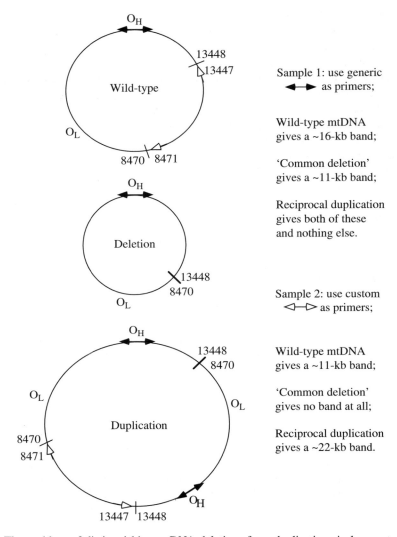

Sample 1: use generic
as primers;

Wild-type mtDNA
gives a ~16-kb band;

'Common deletion'
gives a ~11-kb band;

Reciprocal duplication
gives both of these
and nothing else.

Sample 2: use custom
as primers;

Wild-type mtDNA
gives a ~11-kb band;

'Common deletion'
gives no band at all;

Reciprocal duplication
gives a ~22-kb band.

Fig. 13.3 The problem of distinguishing mtDNA deletions from duplications in long extension PCR assays, and its solution. A duplication, when amplified with divergent primers located in the duplicated region, gives the same products as would arise from a 1 : 1 mixture of a deletion and a wild-type molecule. When a second sample from the same cell (hence containing the same mutant molecule) is analysed, primers in the unduplicated region can be used, which amplify a unique sequence from the duplication but nothing from the deficiency.

A further revelation from these studies[59,119] is that the common deletion may be mis-named—that other rearrangements may be much more common. A large proportion of the rearrangements found in both studies had one breakpoint near position 16,070 and the other in the minor arc, often near position 3260. If they are deletions, they lack the light strand origin; but if they are duplications they have it and also have two heavy strand origins. An intriguing idea, provisionally supported by both *in vivo*[122] and *in vitro* observations,[120,48] is that duplications of this sort never become homoplasmic in cells despite their replicative advantage, because they are constantly being resolved by homologous recombination into a wild-type molecule and a poorly (if at all) replicable deletion. (Machinery to do this is probably needed in order to avoid the accumulation of wild-type dimers, which may occasionally be created by mtDNA replication.[122]) If so, there will be an equilibrium level of heteroplasmy determined by the extent of the duplication's replicative advantage over wild-type. Since no bioenergetic insufficiency would be predicted to result from most such mutations, it may be that evolution has allowed their incidence to remain high relative to mutations that produce replication-competent but dysfunctional species such as the common deletion. (Clearly it is possible for a duplication to confer a loss of function, for example, if the junction sequence encodes a toxic fusion protein, and indeed mild respiratory dysfunction results from the duplications found in rare sufferers of inherited rearrangement-based mitochondriopathies,[120,123] but this can be expected to be the exception rather than the rule—see Ref. 47, for example.)

A concluding digression: the vexed question of whether mutant mtDNA matters in vertebrate ageing

If there is indeed only a negligible diminution with age in the bioenergetic capacity of almost any tissue, the question clearly arises of how it can have any pathological significance.[115] The long-standing popularity of the mitochondrial free radical theory of ageing is no accident: it arises principally from the extraordinarily consistent cross-species correlations discussed in the Introduction. However, genetically tractable mammalian models of mtDNA mutations are vital for its more detailed elucidation. Larsson's group developed a mouse model of mitochondrial disease, by flanking the gene for a mtDNA replication regulator with *loxP* sites to allow conditional deletion of this gene and consequent loss of mtDNA in a pattern defined by *cre* recombinase expression.[124] This is of great utility in the study of mitochondriopathies, but it generates respiration-deficient cells at too great a frequency to be directly relevant to studies of ageing. The same applies to the mtDNA-deletion-bearing mouse recently developed by Hayashi's group.[70] Recent work of Zassenhaus's group,[7] by contrast, provides unprecedented direct evidence that damage to mtDNA can be severely deleterious to the organism even when present at the very low levels typical of aged tissue. The synthesis of mtDNA was rendered error-prone by the transgenic introduction of a proofreading-deficient version of the mtDNA polymerase (POLG) catalytic subunit into mice. The transgene was expressed only in cardiac tissue and only after birth, and the result in young adult mice was a frequency of cardiac mtDNA point mutations of roughly one per mtDNA molecule. This sounds like a high mutation load, but one must bear in mind that only a few mitochondrial generations would have been supported by the transgenic polymerase, so homochondrous mutant mitochondria (let alone homoplasmic mutant cells) would still be rare: different mutations in different mtDNA molecules, if deleterious at all, would usually complement each other. Supporting this, respiratory function of isolated mitochondria was not detectably impaired. However, these mice exhibited severe cardiomyopathy by the age of 6 months. The significance of this finding was potentially undermined by the report[125] that transgenic overexpression of the presumed inert molecule GFP, under the same promoter used by Zassenhaus's group, also produced cardiomyopathy in a dose-dependent manner; but this loophole seems to have been closed by the subsequent report that wild-type POLG does not produce this (nor, indeed, any detectable) phenotype when expressed at similar levels under the same promoter.[134] Detailed understanding of the relevance of this finding to ageing must await careful analysis of the incidence of COX-negative cardiomyocytes and of mtDNA mutations in other tissues of these mice, but it has the potential to show definitively that mtDNA mutations really are causative in ageing.

There is thus strong motivation to seek a mechanism whereby dysfunctional mtDNA could make a major contribution to mammalian ageing even when present at extremely low levels. Two such models are presently available. One[126] revolves around the finding by Aiken's group[35,41,60] that the COX-negative segments of monkey and rat muscle fibres tend to be thinner than average, possibly indicating progress towards atrophy of the segment and eventual breakage, which could cause loss of the whole fibre. If this is correct, mtDNA mutation accumulation could be a major cause of sarcopenia (loss of muscle mass with age), a phenomenon with very pleiotropic effects in ageing due to the multifaceted role of muscle in whole-body homeostasis. However, other mechanisms (such as loss of motor neurons[127]) are presently more supported as being the primary cause of sarcopenia.

The other model, termed the 'reductive hotspot hypothesis',[128–130] is based on the production of extracellular superoxide by respiration-deficient cells. It is lacking in firm supporting evidence, though preliminary support for some of its predictions is now available.[131–133] Interestingly, the mechanism underlying the atrophy identified by Aiken's group may also be oxidative in nature, since high levels of oxidized nucleic acids were found in these regions by immunohistochemistry.[41]

The extensive and increasingly direct evidence that mtDNA damage has a significant role in ageing, coupled with the availability of multiple promising hypotheses to explain how this effect is mediated, makes this one of the most exciting areas of contemporary biogerontology. Plainly, there is an urgent imperative to test and refine these and any future elaborations of the mitochondrial free radical theory of ageing, if we are to make progress in understanding how oxygen, that small molecule without which we cannot survive for more than a few minutes, is also one *with* which we cannot survive for more than a few decades.

Acknowledgement

I am much indebted to Ian Holt and Konstantin Khrapko for numerous valuable comments on an earlier draft.

References

1. Harman D (1956). Aging: a theory based on free radical and radiation chemistry. *J. Gerontol.* **11**: 298–300.
2. Cutler RG (1991). Antioxidants and aging. *Am. J. Clin. Nutr.* **53**: 373S–379S.
3. Sohal RS, Svensson I, and Brunk UT (1990). Hydrogen peroxide production by liver mitochondria in different species. *Mech. Ageing Dev.* **53**: 209–215.
4. Sohal RS, Ku HH, Agarwal S, Forster MJ, and Lal H (1994). Oxidative damage, mitochondrial oxidant generation and antioxidant defenses during aging and in response to food restriction in the mouse. *Mech. Ageing Dev.* **74**: 121–133.

5. Pérez-Campo R, López-Torres M, Cadenas S, Rojas C, and Barja G (1998). The rate of free radical production as a determinant of the rate of aging: evidence from the comparative approach. *J. Comp. Physiol. B* **168**: 149–158.

6. Beckman KB and Ames BN (1998). The free radical theory of aging matures. *Physiol. Rev.* **78**: 547–581.

7. Zhang D, Mott JL, Chang SW, Denniger G, Feng Z, and Zassenhaus HP (2000). Construction of transgenic mice with tissue-specific acceleration of mitochondrial DNA mutagenesis. *Genomics* **69**: 151–161.

8. von Zglinicki T, Saretzki G, Docke W, and Lotze C (1995). Mild hyperoxia shortens telomeres and inhibits proliferation of fibroblasts: a model for senescence? *Exp. Cell Res.* **220**: 186–193.

9. Kristal BS and Yu BP (1992). An emerging hypothesis: synergistic induction of aging by free radicals and Maillard reactions. *J. Gerontol.* **47**: B107–B114.

10. Chèvremont M, Chèvremont-Comhaire S, and Baeckeland E (1959). Action de désoxyribo-nucléases neutre et acide sur des cellules somatiques vivantes cultivées in vitro. *Archi. Biolog. (Liege)* **70**: 811–831.

11. Nass MMK (1966). The circularity of mitochondrial DNA. *Proc. Natl Acad. Sci. USA* **56**: 1215–1222.

12. Harman D (1972). The biologic clock: the mitochondria? *J. Am. Geriatr. Soc.* **20**: 145–147.

13. Linnane AW, Marzuki S, Ozawa T, and Tanaka M (1989). Mitochondrial DNA mutations as an important contributor to ageing and degenerative diseases. *Lancet* **1**: 642–645.

14. Fletcher MJ and Sanadi DR (1961). Turnover of rat-liver mitochondria. *Biochim. Biophys. Acta* **51**: 356–360.

15. Gross NJ, Getz GS, and Rabinowitz M (1969). Apparent turnover of mitochondrial deoxyribo-nucleic acid and mitochondrial phospholipids in the tissues of the rat. *J. Biol. Chem.* **244**: 1552–1562.

16. Menzies RA and Gold PH (1971). The turnover of mitochondria in a variety of tissues of young adult and aged rats. *J. Biol. Chem.* **246**: 2425–2429.

17. Swift H and Hruban Z (1964). Focal degradation as a biological process. *Fed. Proc.* **23**: 1026–1037.

18. Rooyackers OE, Adey DB, Ades PA, and Nair KS (1996). Effect of age on in vivo rates of mito-chondrial protein synthesis in human skeletal muscle. *Proc. Natl Acad. Sci. USA* **93**: 15364–15369.

19. Comfort A (1972). *The Joy of Sex*. New York: Crown Publishers, Inc.

20. Comfort A (1974). The position of aging studies. *Mech. Ageing Dev.* **3**: 1–31.

21. Martinez D (1998). Mortality patterns suggest lack of senescence in hydra. *Exp. Gerontol.* **33**: 217–225.

22. McCord JM and Fridovich I (1969). Superoxide dismutase. An enzymic function for erythrocuprein (hemocuprein). *J. Biol. Chem.* **244**: 6049–6055.

23. Loschen G, Flohé L, and Chance B (1971). Respiratory chain-linked H_2O_2 production in pigeon heart mitochondria. *FEBS Lett.* **18**: 261–226.

24. Boveris A, Oshino N, and Chance B (1972). The cellular production of hydrogen peroxide. *Biochem. J.* **128**: 617–630.

25. Hansford RG, Hogue BA, and Mildaziene V (1997). Dependence of H_2O_2 formation by rat heart mitochondria on substrate availability and donor age. *J. Bioenerg. Biomembr.* **29**: 89–95.

26. Bandy B and Davison AJ (1990). Mitochondrial mutations may increase oxidative stress: implica-tions for carcinogenesis and aging? *Free Radic. Biol. Med.* **8**: 523–539.

27. Miquel J, Economos AC, Fleming J, and Johnson JE (1980). Mitochondrial role in cell aging. *Exp. Gerontol.* **15**: 575–591.

28. Johnson MA, Turnbull DM, Dick DJ, and Sherratt HS (1983). A partial deficiency of cytochrome c oxidase in chronic progressive external ophthalmoplegia. *J. Neurol. Sci.* **60**: 31–53.

29. Müller-Höcker J, Pongratz D, and Hubner G (1983). Focal deficiency of cytochrome-c-oxidase in skeletal muscle of patients with progressive external ophthalmoplegia. Cytochemical-fine-structural study. *Virchows Arch. A* **402**: 61–71.

30. Müller-Höcker J (1989). Cytochrome c oxidase deficient cardiomyocytes in the human heart—an age-related phenomenon. A histochemical ultracytochemical study. *A. J. Pathol.* **134**: 1167–1173.

31. Orgel LE (1963). The maintenance of the accuracy of protein synthesis and its relevance to ageing. *Proc. Natl Acad. Sci. USA* **49**: 517–521.

32. Wallace DC (1989). Mitochondrial DNA mutations and neuromuscular disease. *Trends Genet.* **5**: 9–13.

33. Shoubridge EA, Karpati G, and Hastings KE (1990). Deletion mutants are functionally dominant over wild-type mitochondrial genomes in skeletal muscle fiber segments in mitochondrial disease. *Cell* **62**: 43–49.

34. Kadenbach B and Müller-Höcker J (1990). Mutations of mitochondrial DNA and human death. *Naturwissenschaften* **77**: 221–225.

35. Lee CM, Lopez ME, Weindruch R, and Aiken JM (1998). Association of age-related mitochondrial abnormalities with skeletal muscle fiber atrophy. *Free Radic. Biol. Med.* **25**: 964–972.

36. Müller-Höcker J, Seibel P, Schneiderbanger K, and Kadenbach B (1993). Different in situ hybridization patterns of mitochondrial DNA in cytochrome c oxidase-deficient extraocular muscle fibres in the elderly. *Virchows Arch. A* **422**: 7–15.

37. Müller-Höcker J, Seibel P, Schneiderbanger K, Zietz C, Obermaier-Kusser B, Gerbitz KD, and Kadenbach B (1992). In situ hybridization of mitochondrial DNA in the heart of a patient with Kearns-Sayre syndrome and dilatative cardiomyopathy. *Hum. Pathol.* **23**: 1431–1437.

38. Popper K (1934). *Logik der Forschung. (The Logic of Scientific Discovery.)* Vienna: Springer Verlag.

39. Brierley EJ, Johnson MA, Lightowlers RN, James OF, and Turnbull DM (1998). Role of mitochondrial DNA mutations in human aging: implications for the central nervous system and muscle. *Ann. Neurol.* **43**: 217–223.

40. Khrapko K, Bodyak N, Thilly WG, van Orsouw NJ, Zhang X, Coller HA, Perls TT, Upton M, Vijg J, and Wei JY (1999). Cell-by-cell scanning of whole mitochondrial genomes in aged human heart reveals a significant fraction of myocytes with clonally expanded deletions. *Nucleic Acids Res.* **27**: 2434–2441.

41. Wanagat J, Cao Z, Pathare P, and Aiken JM (2001). Mitochondrial DNA deletion mutations colocalize with segmental electron transport system abnormalities, muscle fiber atrophy, fiber splitting, and oxidative damage in sarcopenia. *FASEB J.* **15**: 322–332.

42. Sen K and Beattie DS (1986). Cytochrome b is necessary for the effective processing of core protein I and the iron-sulfur protein of complex III in the mitochondria. *Arch. Biochem. Biophys.* **251**: 239–249.

43. Hofhaus G and Attardi G (1993). Lack of assembly of mitochondrial DNA-encoded subunits of respiratory NADH dehydrogenase and loss of enzyme activity in a human cell mutant lacking the mitochondrial ND4 gene product. *EMBO J.* **12**: 3043–3048.

44. Bai Y and Attardi G (1998). The mtDNA-encoded ND6 subunit of mitochondrial NADH dehydrogenase is essential for the assembly of the membrane arm and the respiratory function of the enzyme. *EMBO J.* **17**: 4848–4858.

45. Birky CW (2001). The inheritance of genes in mitochondria and chloroplasts: laws, mechanisms and models. *Ann. Rev. Genet.* **35**: 125–148.

46. Davis AF and Clayton DA (1996). In situ localization of mitochondrial DNA replication in intact mammalian cells. *J. Cell Biol.* **135**: 883–893.

47. Tang Y, Schon EA, Wilichowski E, Vasquez-Memije ME, Davidson E, and King MP (2000). Rearrangements of human mitochondrial DNA (mtDNA): new insights into the regulation of mtDNA copy number and gene expression. *Mol. Biol. Cell* **11**: 1471–1485.

48. Tang Y, Manfredi G, Hirano M, and Schon EA (2000). Maintenance of human rearranged mitochondrial DNAs in long-term cultured transmitochondrial cell lines. *Mol. Biol. Cell* **11**: 2349–2358.

49. Chambers P and Gingold E (1986). A direct study of the relative synthesis of petite and grande mitochondrial DNA in zygotes from crosses involving suppressive petite mutants of *Saccharomyces cerevisiae. Curr. Genet.* **10**: 565–571.

50. Moraes CT, Kenyon L, and Hao H (1999). Mechanisms of human mitochondrial DNA maintenance: the determining role of primary sequence and length over function. *Mol. Biol. Cell* **10**: 3345–3356.

51. Clayton DA (1982). Replication of animal mitochondrial DNA. *Cell* **28**: 693–705.

52. Lehtinen SK, Hance N, El Meziane A, Juhola MK, Juhola KM, Karhu R, Spelbrink JN, Holt IJ, and Jacobs HT (2000). Genotypic stability, segregation and selection in heteroplasmic human cell lines containing np 3243 mutant mtDNA. *Genetics* **154**: 363–380.

53. Howell N (1999). Human mitochondrial diseases: answering questions and questioning answers. *Int. Rev. Cytol.* **186**: 49–116.

54. Münscher C, Müller-Höcker J, and Kadenbach B (1993). Human aging is associated with various point mutations in tRNA genes of mitochondrial DNA. *Biol. Chem. Hoppe Seyler* **374**: 1099–1104.

55. Wang Y, Michikawa Y, Mallidis C, Bai Y, Woodhouse L, Yarasheski KE, Miller CA, Askanas V, Engel WK, Bhasin S, and Attardi G (2001). Muscle-specific mutations accumulate with aging in critical human mtDNA control sites for replication. *Proc. Natl Acad. Sci. USA* **98**: 4022–4027.

56. de Grey ADNJ. Stable heteroplasmy in vitro can be explained by a fusion-dependent balance between replicative advantage and respiratory disadvantage of certain mtDNA mutants. Manuscript in preparation.

57. Holt IJ, Lorimer HE, and Jacobs HT (2000). Coupled leading- and lagging-strand synthesis of mammalian mitochondrial DNA. *Cell* **100**: 515–524.

58. Schwarze SR, Lee CM, Chung SS, Roecker EB, Weindruch R, and Aiken JM (1995). High levels of mitochondrial DNA deletions in skeletal muscle of old rhesus monkeys. *Mech. Ageing Dev.* **83**: 91–101.

59. Bodyak ND, Nekhaeva E, Wei JY, and Khrapko K (2001). Quantification and sequencing of somatic deleted mtDNA in single cells: evidence for partially duplicated mtDNA in aged human tissues. *Hum. Mol. Genet.* **10**: 17–24.

60. Lopez ME, Van Zeeland NL, Dahl DB, Weindruch R, and Aiken JM (2000). Cellular phenotypes of age-associated skeletal muscle mitochondrial abnormalities in rhesus monkeys. *Mutat. Res.* **452**: 123–138.

61. Rahman S, Lake BD, Taanman JW, Hanna MG, Cooper JM, Schapira AHV, and Leonard JV (2000). Cytochrome oxidase immunohistochemistry: clues for genetic mechanisms. *Brain* **123**: 591–600.

62. Moraes CT, Ricci E, Petruzzella V, Shanske S, DiMauro S, Schon EA, and Bonilla E (1992). Molecular analysis of the muscle pathology associated with mitochondrial DNA deletions. *Nat. Genet.* **1**: 359–367

63. Johnston W, Karpati G, Carpenter S, Arnold D, and Shoubridge EA (1995). Late-onset mitochondrial myopathy. *Ann. Neurol.* **37**: 16–23.

64. Tokunaga M, Mita S, Murakami T, Kumamoto T, Uchino M, Nonaka I, and Ando M (1994). Single muscle fiber analysis of mitochondrial myopathy, encephalopathy, lactic acidosis and stroke-like episodes (MELAS) *Ann. Neurol.* **35**: 413–419.

65. Hales KG and Fuller MT (1997). Developmentally regulated mitochondrial fusion mediated by a conserved, novel, predicted GTPase. *Cell* **90**: 121–129.

66. Hayashi JI, Takemitsu M, Goto Y, and Nonaka I (1994). Human mitochondria and mitochondrial genome function as a single dynamic cellular unit. *J. Cell Biol.* **125**: 43–50.

67. Takai D, Inoue K, Goto Y, Nonaka I, and Hayashi JI (1997). The interorganellar interaction between distinct human mitochondria with deletion mutant mtDNA from a patient with mitochondrial disease and with HeLa mtDNA. *J. Biol. Chem.* **272**: 6028–6033.

68. Takai D, Isobe K, and Hayashi JI (1999). Transcomplementation between different types of respiration-deficient mitochondria with different pathogenic mutant mitochondrial DNAs. *J. Biol. Chem.* **274**: 11199–11202.

69. Ono T, Isobe K, Nakada K, and Hayashi JI (2001). Human cells are protected from mitochondrial dysfunction by complementation of DNA products in fused mitochondria. *Nat. Genet.* **28**: 272–275.

70. Nakada K, Inoue K, Ono T, Isobe K, Ogura A, Goto YI, Nonaka I, and Hayashi JI (2001). Intermitochondrial complementation: Mitochondria-specific system preventing mice from expression of disease phenotypes by mutant mtDNA. *Nat. Med.* **7**: 934–940.

71. Skulachev VP (1990). Power transmission along biological membranes. *J. Membr. Biol.* **114**: 97–112.

72. Smiley ST, Reers M, Mottola-Hartshorn C, Lin M, Chen A, Smith TW, Steele GD, and Chen LB (1991). Intracellular heterogeneity in mitochondrial membrane potentials revealed by a J-aggregate-forming lipophilic cation JC-1. *Proc. Natl. Acad. Sci. USA* **88**: 3671–3675.

73. Enriquez JA, Cabezas-Herrera J, Bayona-Bafaluy MP, and Attardi G (2000). Very rare complementation between mitochondria carrying different mitochondrial DNA mutations points to intrinsic genetic autonomy of the organelles in cultured human cells. *J. Biol. Chem.* **275**: 11207–11215.

74. Wakabayashi T, Adachi K, Matsuhashi T, Wozniak M, Antosiewicz J, and Karbowsky M (1997). Suppression of the formation of megamitochondria by scavengers for free radicals. *Mol. Aspects Med.* **18** (Suppl). S51–S61.

75. Soltys BJ and Gupta RS (1994). Changes in mitochondrial shape and distribution induced by ethacrynic acid and the transient formation of a mitochondrial reticulum. *J. Cell Physiol.* **159**: 281–294.

76. Yoneda M, Chomyn A, Martinuzzi A, Hurko O, and Attardi G (1992). Marked replicative advantage of human mtDNA carrying a point mutation that causes the MELAS encephalomyopathy. *Proc. Natl Acad. Sci. USA* **89**: 11164–11168.

77. Pallotti F, Chen X, Bonilla E, and Schon EA (1996). Evidence that specific mtDNA point mutations may not accumulate in skeletal muscle during normal human aging. *Am. J. Hum. Genet.* **59**: 591–602.

78. Wallace DC, Bohr VA, Cortopassi G, Kadenbach B, Linn S, Linnane AW, Richter C, and Shay JW (1995). Group report: the role of bioenergetics and mitochondrial DNA mutations in aging and age-related diseases. In: *Molecular Aspects of Aging* (eds K Esser and GM Martin), Chichester: John Wiley & Sons, pp. 199–225.

79. Wallace DC (1997). Mitochondrial DNA in aging and disease. *Sci. Am.* **277**: 40–47.

80. Roussev R, Christov I, Stokrova J, Sovova V, and Ivanov I (1992). A stable line of turkey bone marrow cells transformed by the myelocytomatosis virus strain MC31. Ultrastructural characteristics and localization of the DNA replication sites. *Folia Biolog.* **38**: 78–83.

81. Schultz RA, Swoap SJ, McDaniel LD, Zhang B, Koon EC, Garry DJ, Li K, and Williams RS (1998). Differential expression of mitochondrial DNA replication factors in mammalian tissues. *J. Biol. Chem.* **273**: 3447–3451.

82. Gioio AE, Eyman M, Zhang H, Lavina ZS, Giuditta A, and Kaplan BB (2001). Local synthesis of nuclear-encoded mitochondrial proteins in the presynaptic nerve terminal. *J. Neurosci. Res.* **64**: 447–453.

83. de Grey ADNJ (1997). A proposed refinement of the mitochondrial free radical theory of aging. *Bioessays* **19**: 161–166.

84. Hayashi JI, Ohta S, Kikuchi A, Takemitsu M, Goto Y, and Nonaka I (1991). Introduction of disease-related mitochondrial DNA deletions into HeLa cells lacking mitochondrial DNA results in mitochondrial dysfunction. *Proc. Natl Acad. Sci. USA* **88**: 10614–10618.

85. Seglen PO, Gordon PB, and Holen I (1990). Non-selective autophagy. *Semin. Cell Biol.* **1**: 441–448.

86. Sutovsky P, Moreno RD, Ramalho-Santos J, Dominko T, Simerly C, and Schatten G (1999). Ubiquitin tag for sperm mitochondria. *Nature* **402**: 371–372.

87. van Zutphen H and Cornwell DG (1973). Some studies on lipid peroxidation in monomolecular and bimolecular lipid films. *J. Membr. Biol.* **13**: 79–88.

88. Ivanov AS, Putvinskii AV, Antonov VF, and Vladimirov YA (1977). Magnitude of the proton permeability of liposomes following photoperoxidation of lipids. *Biophysics* **22**: 644–648.

89. Kowald A and Kirkwood TBL (1999). Modelling the role of mitochondrial mutations in cellular aging. *J. Anti-aging Med.* **2**: 243–253.

90. Kowald A and Kirkwood TBL (2000). Accumulation of defective mitochondria through delayed degradation of damaged organelles and its possible role in the ageing of post-mitotic and dividing cells. *J. Theor. Biol.* **202**: 145–160.

91. Michikawa Y, Mazzucchelli F, Bresolin N, Scarlato G, and Attardi G (1999). Aging-dependent large accumulation of point mutations in the human mtDNA control region for replication. *Science* **286**: 774–779.

92. Fliss MS, Usadel H, Caballero OL, Wu L, Buta MR, Eleff SM, Jen J, and Sidransky D (2000). Facile detection of mitochondrial DNA mutations in tumors and bodily fluids. *Science* **287**: 2017–2019.

93. Lee HC, Yin PH, Yu TN, Chang YD, Hsu WC, Kao SY, Chi CW, Liu TY, and Wei YH (2001). Accumulation of mitochondrial DNA deletions in human oral tissues—effects of betel quid chewing and oral cancer. *Mutat. Res.* **493**: 67–74.

94. Jazin EE, Cavelier L, Eriksson I, Oreland L, and Gyllensten U (1996). Human brain contains high levels of heteroplasmy in the noncoding regions of mitochondrial DNA. *Proc. Natl Acad. Sci. USA* **93**: 12382–12387.

95. Cimadevilla JM, Garcia Moreno LM, Gonzalez Pardo H, Zahonero MC, and Arias JL (1997). Glial and neuronal cell numbers and cytochrome oxidase activity in CA1 and CA3 during postnatal development and aging of the rat. *Mech. Ageing Dev.* **99**:49–60.

96. Polyak K, Li Y, Zhu H, Lengauer C, Willson JK, Markowitz SD, Trush MA, Kinzler KW, and Vogelstein B (1998). Somatic mutations of the mitochondrial genome in human colorectal tumours. *Nat. Genet.* **20**: 291–293.

97. Habano W, Nakamura S, and Sugai T (1998). Microsatellite instability in the mitochondrial DNA of colorectal carcinomas: evidence for mismatch repair systems in mitochondrial genome. *Oncogene* **17**: 1931–1937.

98. Habano W, Sugai T, Nakamura SI, Uesugi N, Yoshida T, and Sasou S (2000). Microsatellite instability and mutation of mitochondrial and nuclear DNA in gastric carcinoma. *Gastroenterology* **118**: 835–841.

99. Habano W, Sugai T, Yoshida T, and Nakamura S (1999). Mitochondrial gene mutation, but not large-scale deletion, is a feature of colorectal carcinomas with mitochondrial microsatellite instability. *Int. J. Cancer* **83**: 625–629.

100. Maximo V, Soares P, Seruca R, Rocha AS, Castro P, and Sobrinho-Simões M (2001). Microsatellite instability, mitochondrial DNA large deletions, and mitochondrial DNA mutations in gastric carcinoma. *Genes, Chromosomes Cancer* **32**: 136–143.

101. Parrella P, Xiao Y, Fliss M, Sanchez-Cespedes M, Mazzarelli P, Rinaldi M, Nicol T, Gabrielson E, Cuomo C, Cohen D, Pandit S, Spencer M, Rabitti C, Fazio VM, and Sidransky D (2001). Detection of mitochondrial DNA mutations in primary breast cancer and fine-needle aspirates. *Cancer Res.* **61**: 7623–7626.

102. de Grey ADNJ (2001). A proposed mechanism for the lowering of mitochondrial electron leak by caloric restriction. *Mitochondrion* **1**: 129–139.

103. Greenwood AD and Pääbo S (1999). Nuclear insertion sequences of mitochondrial DNA predominate in hair but not in blood of elephants. *Mol. Ecol.* **8**: 133–137.

104. Mourier T, Hansen AJ, Willerslev T, and Arctander A (2001). The human genome project reveals a continuous transfer of large mitochondrial fragments to the nucleus. *Mol. Biol. Evol.* **18**: 1833–1837.

105. Elson JL, Samuels DC, Turnbull DM, and Chinnery PF (2001). Random intracellular drift explains the clonal expansion of mitochondrial DNA mutations with age. *Am. J. Hum. Genet.* **68**: 802–806.

106. Coller HA, Khrapko K, Bodyak ND, Nekhaeva E, Herrero-Jimenez P, and Thilly WG (2001). High frequency of homoplasmic mitochondrial DNA mutations in human tumors can be explained without selection. *Nat. Genet.* **28**: 147–150.

107. Corral-Debrinski M, Horton T, Lott MT, Shoffner JM, Beal MF, and Wallace DC (1992). Mitochondrial DNA deletions in human brain: regional variability and increase with advanced age. *Nat. Genet.* **2**: 324–329.

108. Itoh K, Weis S, Mehraein P, and Müller-Höcker J (1996). Cytochrome c oxidase defects of the human substantia nigra in normal aging. *Neurobiol. Aging* **17**: 843–848.

109. Cortopassi GA and Arnheim N (1990). Detection of a specific mitochondrial DNA deletion in tissues of older humans. *Nucleic Acids Res.* **18**: 6927–6933.

110. de Grey ADNJ (2001). MitoLife: Towards a multi-purpose virtual testbed for mechanistic hypotheses regarding mitochondrial DNA population dynamics. *Mitochondrion* **1**(Suppl.): S43.

111. Barnes WM (1994). PCR amplification of up to 35-kb DNA with high fidelity and high yield from lambda bacteriophage templates. *Proc. Natl Acad. Sci. USA* **91**: 2216–2220.

112. Kovalenko SA, Kopsidas G, Kelso JM, and Linnane AW (1997). Deltoid human muscle mtDNA is extensively rearranged in old age subjects. *Biochem. Biophys. Res. Commun.* **232**: 147–152.

113. Hayakawa M, Katsumata K, Yoneda M, Tanaka M, Sugiyama S, and Ozawa T (1996). Age-related extensive fragmentation of mitochondrial DNA into minicircles. *Biochem. Biophys. Res. Commun.* **226**: 369–377.

114. Nagley P and Wei YH (1998). Ageing and mammalian mitochondrial genetics. *Trends Genet.* **14**: 513–517.

115. Lightowlers RN, Jacobs HT, and Kajander OA (1999). Mitochondrial DNA—all things bad? *Trends Genet.* **15**: 91–93.

116. Kajander OA, Kunnas TA, Perola M, Lehtinen SK, Karhunen PJ, and Jacobs HT (1999). Long-extension PCR to detect deleted mitochondrial DNA molecules is compromized by technical artefacts. *Biochem. Biophys. Res. Commun.* **254**: 507–514.

117. Barrientos A, Casademont J, Rötig A, Miró O, Urbano-Márquez A, Rustin P, and Cardellach F (1996). Absence of relationship between the level of electron transport chain activities and aging in human skeletal muscle. *Biochem. Biophys. Res. Commun.* **229**: 536–539.

118. Suter M and Richter C (1999). Fragmented mitochondrial DNA is the predominant carrier of oxidized DNA bases. *Biochem.* **38**: 459–464.

119. Kajander OA, Rovio AT, Majamaa K, Poulton J, Spelbrink JN, Holt IJ, Karhunen PJ, and Jacobs HT (2000). Human mtDNA sublimons resemble rearranged mitochondrial genoms found in pathological states. *Hum. Mol. Genet.* **9**: 2821–2835.

120. Holt IJ, Dunbar DR, and Jacobs HT (1997). Behaviour of a population of partially duplicated mitochondrial DNA molecules in cell culture: segregation, maintenance and recombination dependent upon nuclear background. *Hum. Mol. Genet.* **6**: 1251–1260.

121. Umeda S, Tang Y, Okamoto M, Hamasaki N, Schon EA, and Kang D (2001). Both heavy strand replication origins are active in partially duplicated human mitochondrial DNAs. *Biochem. Biophys. Res. Commun.* **286**: 681–687.

122. Poulton J, Deadman ME, Bindoff L, Morten K, Land J, and Brown G (1993). Families of mtDNA rearrangements can be detected in patients with mtDNA deletions: dupolications may be a transient intermediate form. *Hum. Mol. Genet.* **2**: 23–30.

123. Ballinger SW, Shoffner JM, Hedaya EV, Trounce I, Polak MA, Koontz DA, and Wallace DC (1992). Maternally transmitted diabetes and deafness associated with a 10.4 kb mitochondrial DNA deletion. *Nat. Genet.* **1**: 15.

124. Wang J, Wilhelmsson H, Graff C, Li H, Oldfors A, Rustin P, Brüning JC, Kahn CR, Clayton DA, Barsh GS, Thorén P, and Larsson NG (1999). Dilated cardiomyopathy and atrioventricular conduction blocks induced by heart-specific inactivation of mitochondrial DNA gene expression. *Nat. Genet.* **21**: 133–137.

125. Huang WY, Aramburu J, Douglas PS, and Izumo S (2000). Transgenic expression of green fluorescence protein can cause dilated cardiomyopathy. *Nat. Med.* **6**: 482.

126. McKenzie D, Bua E, McKiernan S, Cao Z, Wanagat J, and Aiken JM (2002). Mitochondrial DNA deletion mutations: a causal role in sarcopenia. *Eur. J. Biochem.* **269**: 2010–2015.
127. Faulkner JA, Brooks SV, and Zerba E (1995). Muscle atrophy and weakness with aging: contraction-induced injury as an underlying mechanism. *J. Gerontol. A* **50A**: 124–129 (Special Issue).
128. de Grey ADNJ (1998). A mechanism proposed to explain the rise in oxidative stress during aging. *J. Anti-aging Med.* **1**: 53–66.
129. de Grey ADNJ (2000). The reductive hotspot hypothesis: an update. *Arch. Biochem. Biophys.* **373**: 295–301.
130. de Grey ADNJ (2002). The reductive hotspot hypothesis of vertebrate aging: membrane metabolism magnifies mutant mitochondrial mischief. *Eur. J. Biochem.* **269**: 2003–2009.
131. Morré DM, Lenaz G, and Morré DJ (2000). Surface oxidase and oxidative stress propagation in aging. *J. Exp. Biol.* **203**: 1513–1521.
132. McArdle A, Pattwell D, Vasilaki A, Griffiths RD, and Jackson MJ (2001). Contractile activity-induced oxidative stress: cellular origin and adaptive responses. *Am. J. Physiol. Cell Physiol.* **280**: C621–C627.
133. Bassenge E, Sommer O, Schwemmer M, and Bünger R (2000). Antioxidant pyruvate inhibits cardiac formation of reactive oxygen species through changes in redox state. *Am. J. Physiol., Heart Circul. Physiol.* **279**: H2431–H2438.
134. Zhang D, Mott JL, Farrar P, Ryerse JS, Chang SW, Stevens M, Denniger G, and Zassenhaus HP (2003). Mitochondrial DNA mutations activate the mitochondrial apoptotic pathway and cause dilated cardiomyopathy. *Cardiovasc. Res.* **57**: 147–157.

Section 5 Model systems, genetic counselling, and prospectus for therapy

14   Segregation and dynamics of mitochondrial DNA in mammalian cells

Jose-Antonio Enriquez

A key aim of mitochondrial genetics is to understand the rules that govern mtDNA segregation. To this end, cells carrying more than one mtDNA genotype have been generated and the partitioning of mtDNA to daughter cells monitored. Typically, these experiments investigated the segregation of mtDNAs carrying a pathological mutation versus apparently normal mtDNA. Another approach was to create animals with two mtDNA genotypes that were non-pathological and analyse the segregation pattern of the two types of mtDNA in different tissues at various ages. Collectively, these studies demonstrate that mtDNA segregation can be non-random, yet the molecular mechanisms underlying the complex patterns of mtDNA segregation remain to be elucidated. Two levels of mitochondrial segregation can be envisioned. One is mtDNA segregation in germ cells, affecting transmission of mtDNA to the next generation. The other is segregation of mtDNA during mitosis that is somatic cells in whole animals or cells cultured in the laboratory. The Chapter reviews the current models of mitotic mtDNA segregation in mammalian cells and their experimental support. Germ line transmission of mtDNA in mammals is discussed elsewhere (Chapter 16).

Introduction

The transmission of mitochondrial DNA (mtDNA) is a complex phenomenon that is far from understood. Mitochondrial DNA's high copy number (polyploidy), typically 10^3–10^4 molecules per cell, its compartmentalization in organelles, and the fact that not all mtDNA molecules replicate in each cell cycle contribute to the complexity.[1] Moreover, mitochondria are mobile and their distribution changes within the cell during growth and division. In addition, in mammalian cells mtDNA may be organized in multicopy complexes (nucleoids) inside mitochondria,[2] as in lower eukaryotes.[3] Many of these factors are likely to play a role in determining mtDNA segregation.

Segregation and interaction of mtDNAs in cell culture models

Mitochondria have been considered to behave as an intracellular population of microorganisms. As a result, the investigation of the dynamics of mtDNA segregation was seen as a population genetics problem.[4] It was soon evident that the number of individual organelles in a cell was significantly lower than the number of mtDNA molecules. Thus, mtDNA polyploidy happens not only within a cell but also within each organelle (a typical mitochondrion in mammalian cells should host an average of five mtDNA molecules).

The norm in mammalian cells is that the sequence of all, or almost all, copies of mtDNA is identical at any given nucleotide position (homoplasmy). Thus, to be able to investigate the segregation of mtDNA in cell culture it was necessary to develop cellular models containing more than one mtDNA genotype (heteroplasmy). A number of early studies exploited drug resistance markers carried on mtDNA, most notably chloramphenicol resistance (CAP[r]).[5–10]

A major breakthrough for the analysis of mtDNA dynamics followed from the isolation of the first mammalian cell line lacking mtDNA, so-called ρ^0 cells, and the demonstration that they could be repopulated with exogenous mitochondria that carry mtDNA.[11] As heteroplasmy is common in the cells of patients with mitochondrial disease it allowed a number of human heteroplasmic cell lines to be established, either by culturing patient-derived cells directly or by transferring mitochondria from patient's cells to human ρ^0 cells, creating so-called cybrids. The cybrid approach has the advantage that mtDNA of patients with mitochondrial disease can be studied in a control nuclear background, enabling the researcher to exclude possible confounding nuclear effects on mitochondrial function. Moreover, although no one predicted it at the time, mitochondrial repopulation of ρ^0 cells gave rise to a wealth of data on mtDNA segregation that is still being assimilated.

Segregation of wild type and rearranged mtDNAs

Hayashi *et al.* performed a very interesting experiment in which mitochondria from skin fibroblasts of a CPEO patient harbouring a 5196-bp deletion (Δ-mtDNA[5,196]) were introduced into HeLa cells lacking mtDNA.[12] Three of six trans-mitochondrial clones (cybrids) isolated contained a mixture of wild-type mtDNA (wt-mtDNA) and partially deleted mtDNA (ΔmtDNA) in proportions ranging from 35 to 50 per cent. Interestingly, when grown in glucose-rich medium, the proportion of Δ-mtDNA invariably increased and then stabilized at 75–85 per cent, without any significant change in the total amount of mtDNA. This was interpreted as a replicative advantage of the Δ-mtDNA over wt-mtDNA. The positive selection of deleterious mutant mtDNA has also been observed for several different pathological variants in a number of studies[12–15] (further details discussed later in this Chapter), it appears paradoxical yet propagation of DNA by selfish mechanisms is widespread in nature.

The proportion of Δ-mtDNA remained below 50 per cent when the cells were grown in a medium where glucose was substituted by galactose (conditions that require a functional OXPHOS system). Thus, for this mutation, 50 per cent mtDNA appears to be the threshold at which OXPHOS function is compromised in cultured cells.[12] The term 'functional dominance' was coined to describe the loss of OXPHOS function in cells that retained some wt-mtDNA.[16] To explain this effect it was suggested that Δ-mtDNA and wt-mtDNA co-existed in organelles.[16] Hayashi *et al.* obtained indirect evidence for this in their cybrids when measuring cytochrome *c* oxidase (COX) function of individual mitochondria by electron microscopy.[12] All the mitochondria of a clonal cybrid line harbouring 75 per cent of Δ-mtDNA were COX-negative, suggesting that no organelle contained purely wt-mtDNA. They extended this analysis to clones with 42–72 per cent Δ-mtDNA, proportions above and below the threshold level that determines the OXPHOS competence.[17] Below 60 per cent Δ-mtDNA the majority of the organelle appeared to be COX-positive, whereas clones over

60 per cent Δ-mtDNA were uniformly COX-negative. Thus, the result suggests that in each organelle wild type and Δ-mtDNA co-exist (organelle heteroplasmy).

The observations of Hayashi *et al.*[12] in human cultured cells carrying Δ-mtDNA raised a number of important questions. What was the mechanism that maintains heteroplasmy in organelles? Why did all heteroplasmic clones accumulate Δ-mtDNA at the expense of wt-mtDNA, in the absence of selection for OXPHOS function? Was the phenomenon specific for Δ-mtDNA or a particular cell type? In 1993 Bourgeron *et al.*[18] investigated the fate of a similar Δ-mtDNA in skin fibroblasts and lymphocytes. Both immortalized cultured skin fibroblasts harbouring 60 per cent Δ-mtDNA and B lymphoblastoid cells with 80 per cent Δ-mtDNA were severely COX-deficient. The segregation behaviour of Δ-mtDNA was, however, strikingly different between the two cell types when grown in culture. Although progressive loss of Δ-mtDNA accompanied by a recovery of COX activity was seen in both, the lost was almost complete in fibroblasts, whereas it stabilized at 60 per cent Δ-mtDNA in lymphoblastoid cells.[18] Since COX-deficient cells are uridine-dependent, the effect of uridine supplementation on fibroblasts was tested. Strikingly, they accumulated Δ-mtDNA up to a level of 90 per cent after 10 passages.[18] These results indicated that heteroplasmy could be influenced by cell type (genetic effect), or growth regime (environment).

Partially duplicated mitochondrial DNA, though associated with milder pathology[19] and a milder biochemical phenotype[14] than Δ-mtDNA, displayed equally dramatic segregation bias in particular cell lines. One phenomenon was *de novo* generation of a partial triplication in one cell background, which led to the proposal that additional origins of replication can confer a selective advantage to mtDNA.[14] The other noteworthy phenomenon was the consistent loss of all rearranged mtDNA molecules in a different cell background, although it could not be determined whether this was via intramolecular recombination or via re-amplification of a very low dose of wild-type molecules. Nevertheless, it is clear from this and the other studies that genetic background can profoundly affect the fate of particular mtDNA variants.

Segregation of wild type and mutant mtDNAs harbouring point mutations

The segregation behaviour of pathological point mutations of mtDNA has been investigated widely in cell models. One of the more extensively investigated point mutation has been the mtDNA^{A3243G} transition in the human mitochondrial tRNA$^{Leu(UUR)}$ gene, associated with the MELAS syndrome.[20] In 1992, Yoneda *et al.*[15] generated 48 cybrids by transferring organelles from myoblasts obtained from four unrelated patients with MELAS to cells lacking mtDNA. When mtDNA segregation in 13 heteroplasmic clones was analysed two patterns emerged, long-term maintenance of a constant ratio of mutant to wt-mtDNA (stable heteroplasmy), or, in 5 of them, a rapid and dramatic shift to the mutant genotype. The proportion of mutant and wt-mtDNA was highly variable between subclones taken from the 'shifting' cultures whereas it lay in a narrow range in subclones taken from the stable clones. Based upon (i) the similar growth rates of cells containing wild type and those with predominantly mutant mtDNA, (ii) the constant doubling time of the shifting clones, and (iii) the speed of the shift in genotype, the authors conclude that the accumulation of mutant mtDNA was the result of intracellular selection. Since a shift to wt-mtDNA was never observed, random segregation could be excluded, and a replicative advantage of mutant mtDNA was inferred. It was proposed that the replicative advantage could only operate in cells that displayed homoplasmy for the mutant and wt-mtDNAs at the level of the organelle. The corollary was that in cells with heteroplasmic organelles the proportion of each mtDNA genotype would remain constant.[15]

Dunbar et al.[21] repeated the experiment of Yoneda et al. and obtained similar results with the same recipient (osteosarcoma) ρ^0 cell line. However, in a different (lung carcinoma) recipient ρ^0 cell line they observed the opposite behaviour namely, where a shift was observed it was towards wt-mtDNA.[21] Again, unidirectional shifting argued against a random segregation mechanism. Therefore, a replicative advantage for one or other mtDNA, determined by the nuclear background, was suggested to be the most likely explanation for the phenomena.[21]

In contrast the results of Shoubridge for the same mutation in the osteosarcoma nuclear background, were consistent with stochastic (random) segregation. Some clones increased mutant mtDNA, while others increased the amount of wild type, very few, if any, were stable.[22] Shoubridge also catalogued the distribution of the mtDNA^{A3243G} mutation in the mitochondrial-donor myoblasts, showing that all were heteroplasmic for the mutation, yet in spite of this, over half of the cybrid clones had only wt-mtDNA. Therefore, Shoubridge suggested that a preferential replication of wt-mtDNA occur during mtDNA repopulation and early clonal growth of the cybrid population. Alternatively, random segregation may have occurred in both directions in many lines, proving lethal where this led to fixation of the mutant allele.

Matthews et al.,[23] using a pure fibroblast culture as mitochondrial donor, found neither homoplasmic wt-mtDNA clones nor any significant difference in the variance of mtDNA^{A3243G} mutant load between fibroblast subclones and transformant cybrids. In a second study using pure fibroblasts, the mean proportion of mtDNA^{A3243G} in cybrids correlated well with the proportion of mutant mtDNA in the donor fibroblast cell lines.[24] Moreover, the incidence of pure wild type clones again correlated with the original amount of wt-mtDNA in donor cells. In addition, a shift towards mtDNA^{A3243G} was observed in all heteroplasmic lines,[24] albeit that the speed of segregation was up to seven-fold slower than the earlier reports.[15,21] The same mutation has also been studied in immortalized skin fibroblasts, avoiding the possible complications of cell fusion.[23] All subclones derived from patient fibroblasts that were heteroplasmic for the MELAS mutation were heteroplasmic. The interclonal variance did not increase after 15 generations indicating that the heteroplasmy was stable and arguing against any biased segregation between the two types of mtDNA in these cells.[23] In summary, after mitochondrial transfer several possible outcomes for heteroplasmic clones have been documented: stable maintenance of heteroplasmy, rapid unidirectional segregation to either wt-mtDNA or mutant mtDNA, slow unidirectional segregation to mutant mtDNA, or stochastic segregation. Presumably, specific factors (genetic and environmental) determine each outcome though none is yet known.

The majority of the published work was focussed on the behaviour of the shifting clones and scant attention was paid to the phenomenon of stable heteroplasmy. The mechanism that maintains a constant proportion of mutant and wt-mtDNA, even after years' of continuous culture, is equally perplexing to non-random segregation. Matthews et al.[23] proposed that the maintenance of stable heteroplasmy in their mtDNA^{A3243G} fibroblasts argued in favour of linked replication and segregation of the wild type and mutant mtDNAs. More recently, Lehtinen and collaborators[25] using the mtDNA^{A3243G} mutation addressed the issue of maintenance of heteroplasmy in an exhaustive work. They describe a series of experiments that demonstrate persistent stable heteroplasmy. In addition, they compared their observation with the predictions of a random partition model and deduced a very high segregation number, similar to or even greater than the mtDNA copy number of a cell. They also found that the stable genotype could be forced to shift to a limited extent by applying external selection, that is, OXPHOS-dependent growth. One of the cell lines they used carried a second mutation in some mtDNA molecules, which showed an abrupt genotype shift, analysis of a number of subclones from this cell line indicated that the shift was followed by re-stabilization at a new level of heteroplasmy.[25]

Competition between mtDNAs

A crucial issue in the understanding of mtDNA dynamics is to settle the controversy about mtDNA competition within cells, which could facilitate intracellular selection of particular mtDNAs. This is relevant not only to understanding the mitotic segregation of mtDNA but also the evolution of heteroplasmy in post-mitotic cells. Mathematical models have been developed to support the contention that relaxed replication and random drift alone can account for the accumulation and, eventual, fixation of initially heteroplasmic mtDNAs.[26,27] However, other studies indicate that mtDNA competition and intracellular selection of one or another mtDNA genotype may also play a role.[12,15,21] An excellent example of this is the apparent replicative advantage of Δ-mtDNAs. The simplest explanation for the preferential accumulation of Δ-mtDNA is that it replicates faster because of its smaller size, although this hypothesis was not supported by direct measurements of the rate of completion of Δ-mtDNA (7.5 kb deletion) and full-length mtDNA circles in a heteroplasmic cell line.[28] Nevertheless, a recent report shows how the repopulation rates of self-mtDNA, in cells that were severely depleted of mtDNA, were significantly faster for Δ-mtDNAs than for normal size mtDNA.[29] This seems to be true even if they are normalized for mass rather than copy number. It was then suggested that a competition for limiting amounts of *trans*-acting factors involved in mtDNA replication or stability could be responsible for the maintenance of mtDNA and for the regulation of its copy number.[29] This model was supported by the inability of ape mtDNA to repopulate human cells harbouring 100 per cent deleted mtDNA, even under strong cell selection for OXPHOS function.[29] This was an unexpected result, since ape mtDNA is able to repopulate human $\rho°$ cells and restore OXPHOS function.[30,31] The presumption is that a human nuclear background maintains even nonfunctional human mtDNA over functional ape mtDNA because factors limiting for replication are preferentially sequestered by human mtDNA.

Further support in favour of a model of mtDNA copy number regulation by limiting factors was recently obtained. It was reported that the mtDNA copy number in cell models harbouring full-length, partially duplicated and different forms of deleted mtDNA was inversely proportional to the size of the mtDNA. Therefore, the cell maintains a constant mass of mtDNA rather than a constant number of mtDNA genomes. Tang et al.[32] proposed that this is a multifactorial process involving trans-acting factors that initiate replication, regulation of the mitochondrial dNTP pools, and external stimuli such as hormones and intracellular ATP demands.[32]

If confirmed, the regulation of mtDNA copy number by limitation for specific factors offers a solid conceptual frame to explain intracellular competition between different mtDNA genotypes.[22,33]

Cooperation between mtDNAs

Most of the models that have been investigated up to now involved mtDNA genotypes that caused OXPHOS deficiency or that confer a growth advantage. The question of what mutant load is necessary for the expression of OXPHOS deficiency or antibiotic resistance leads us to a more general problem. Can different mtDNAs in the same cytoplasm cooperate? It was earlier observed that different types of mutation were phenotypically silent up to a threshold. Thus, Δ-mtDNA showed an abrupt threshold in cybrids, with no phenotype when the proportion of mutant mtDNA was below 50 per cent.[12] On the other hand, wt-mtDNA levels as low as 6 or 9 per cent are sufficient to protect against the phenotypic expression of the mtDNA^{A3243G} and the mtDNA^{A8344G} tRNA mutations.[34,10] In the case of Δ-mtDNA, negative cooperation by means of a partial dominant effect of the deleted molecules over the wt-mtDNAs has been proposed.[12,16] In the case of point mutations, cooperation was also suggested.

The mtDNA^{A8344G} mutation provides a useful molecular marker since this mutation induces premature terminated proteins.[35] In particular, one of these truncated proteins, which is derived from the premature termination of COI (cytochrome *c* oxidase subunit 1), appears and accumulates in parallel to declining OXPHOS phenotype.[10] In cells with 90 per cent mutant mtDNA, just below the functional threshold, the minority of wild-type molecules (10 per cent) must complement the mutant molecules. Therefore, it was suggested that intermixing and cooperation of the wild type and mutant gene products occurred in these cells.[10,36] Although no similar molecular marker is available for the mtDNA^{A3243G} mutation the similar threshold for both tRNA mutations strongly suggests that complementation follows the same pattern.[36]

The complementation patterns described above were obtained with a wt-mtDNA that coexisted with the mutation since its inception.[36] To investigate if complementation between different mtDNAs could be achieved when two genotypes were located initially in different cells, cybrid experiments were performed. Oliver and Wallace investigated the interaction between chloramphenicol (CAP) resistance, using CAP^r and CAP^s mtDNAs. They followed the synthesis of two isoforms of the subunit 3 of Complex I[37] an mtDNA-encoded polypeptide that showed different migration in SDS-electrophoresis when encoded by CAP^r or CAP^s mtDNAs. Their results indicated that CAP^r is a dominant or co-dominant character and that the presence of CAP^r mitochondrial ribosomes allows the synthesis of polypeptides encoded by CAP^s mtDNA.[38] This observation suggested that complementation between mtDNAs originally located in physically distinct organelles can occur.[38] However, others observed no evidence of interaction between CAP^r and CAP^s mtDNAs sequentially introduced in the same cell.[10]

A more robust experimental approach to evaluate the possibility of mtDNA cooperation would be to mix homoplasmic mitochondria harbouring two pathological 'recessive' mtDNA mutations derived from different cells. Since each mutation has a well-defined phenotype, restoration of function due to complementation between the two types of mtDNA could be easily evaluated. This type of experiment was performed by Yoneda *et al.*[10] They reported no evidence of mtDNA interaction between two mtDNAs harbouring recessive OXPHOS defective mutations (one the mtDNA^{A8344G} mutation in the tRNA^{Lys} and the other the mtDNA^{A3243G} mutation in the tRNA$^{Leu(UUR)}$).

Takai *et al.*[39] introduced a predominantly (>95 per cent) Δ-mtDNA^{5196}, unable to support mitochondrial protein synthesis due to the lack of five tRNAs, together with CAP^r mtDNA. Then, they studied the ability of the double cybrids to perform protein synthesis in the presence and absence of CAP. The synthesis of Δ-mtDNA^{5196} and HeLa mtDNA encoded protein markers was detected in a cybrid cell line containing 53 per cent Δ-mtDNA^{5196}. However, protein synthesis was largely although not completely inhibited by CAP. These results were interpreted as an indication of a general interaction between the two types of mtDNA. Thus, the CAP^r HeLa mtDNA provided the five tRNAs (lacking from Δ-mtDNA) and the residual resistance to chloramphenicol needed to allow expression of the genes encoded by Δ-mtDNA.[39]

The heightened sensitivity to CAP displayed by the double cybrids with respect to the parental CAP^r line is difficult to understand. It was explained by considering the resistance to CAP as a recessive trait. It should be noted however, that this is the opposite of the conclusion inferred from the earlier experiments described above, where CAP^r was apparently dominant or co-dominant[38] (see also Ref [10] and references therein). In addition, no direct test of the purity of the HeLa mtDNA in the cybrid cells was performed. It was reported that cells apparently homoplasmic for a mutant mtDNA may contain a trace of wt-mtDNA which can be selected in certain culture conditions.[40] Therefore, the possibility of coexistence of HeLa CAP^r and HeLa CAP^s mtDNA is a very common phenomenon[10,41] and therefore cannot be excluded. In addition they described a double cybrid cell line carrying 76 per cent Δ-mtDNA^{5196} able to grow under strong selective conditions that could very well be explained if Δ-mtDNA^{5196} and HeLa CAP^s mtDNA coexisted in it but remain fully segregated. In that way, the dominant effect of Δ-mtDNA^{5196} might be avoided.

These results appeared to contradict those of the earlier study that showed no restoration of OXPHOS function when two different mutant mtDNAs were introduced in the same cytoplasm.[10] Takai *et al.* reasoned that this contradiction could be because both types of organelles used previously were OXPHOS incompetent. Therefore, the mitochondria would be unable to reach the energy threshold needed to fuse. To test this possibility, Takai *et al.*[42] introduced into cells two mutant mtDNAs that caused loss of OXPHOS function when homoplasmic. Again one was the Δ-mtDNA^{5196} and the other was a mtDNA^{4269} mutant in tRNA^{Ile}.[43] Then, they tried to select cells showing partial recovery of OXPHOS activity by growing them in the absence of uridine and pyruvate. In this selection medium, a partial recovery of OXPOS would be enough to allow the survival of cells. However, no colony was obtained.[42] The experiment was repeated but without selection, two out of 98 clones analysed harboured both types of mtDNA (18 and 60 per cent of ΔmtDNA^{5196}, respectively). The clone carrying 60 per cent Δ-mtDNA^{5196} was able to show partial restoration of mitochondrial protein synthesis; despite reaching the threshold level at which Δ-mtDNA^{5196} was previously found to cause failure of protein synthesis.[12] Interestingly, five sub-clones taken from the 18 per cent Δ-mtDNA^{5196} cybrid all showed an increase in the amount of Δ-mtDNA^{5196} (40–55 per cent), and partial restoration of protein synthesis. Seemingly then, complementation between deficient mtDNAs that were originally located in separated organelles can occur.

Why then the discrepancy between the different reports designed to detect mtDNA complementation? In the HeLa cell, mtDNA interaction seems to be observed repeatedly, whereas this was not the case in osteosarcoma cells. To gain some insight into the apparent prohibition of mtDNA interaction in osteosarcoma cells, we analysed the interaction of two sets of mitochondria harbouring non-allelic recessive single point mtDNA mutations.[40] One was the mtDNA^{8344} mutation in the tRNA^{Lys} and the other was an *in vitro* isolated frame shift mutation within the gene coding for the ND4 subunit of the NADH dehydrogenase.[44] Strong selective pressure for OXPHOS competence was applied by growing cybrids in galactose containing medium to promote clones exhibiting complementation between the two mutant mtDNAs. In parallel, cell fusion frequency was determined in equivalent cybrids grown on glucose-containing medium that was nonselective for respiratory capacity. Twelve of 53 clones that were able to grow in the galactose-containing medium were studied; all had re-established normal mitochondrial protein synthesis and respiratory activity.[40] All of them showed a high proportion of tRNA[Lys] mutant mtDNA (61–86 per cent) that however never reached the previously observed threshold (91 per cent). Therefore, strong selection demonstrated that mtDNA cooperation is possible in the osteosarcoma nuclear background. Nevertheless this is a rare phenomenon at least in this cell type; it was estimated that only 0.3–1.6 per cent of the cells that received both types of mitochondria in their cytoplasm, exhibited complementation.[40]

Another advance was made by a very clever experiment carried out by Hayashi *et al.*[45] They reasoned that under nutritional selection most of the cybrids containing two types of mutant mtDNAs are excluded before respiratory function could be restored. To prevent this, hybrid instead cybrid cells were generated and selected in HAT medium by nuclear complementation between the HeLa HPRT⁻ and the Osteosarcoma TK⁻. Each cell line was also homoplasmic for a different tRNA point mutation (HeLa HPRT⁻, mtDNA[A4269G] in the tRNA[Ile], and Osteosarcoma 143B: TK⁻, mtDNA[A3243G] in the tRNA[Leu(UUR)]) this allowed to select only cells with two nuclei as well as two types of mutant mtDNA. Since OXPHOS competence was not required for growth in HAT medium, they were able to estimate the proportion of HAT[R] cells generated (cells that received two types of mtDNA). In parallel, they estimated the proportion HAT[R] cells able to grow in the absence of uridine. Fascinatingly, they found that a minimum of 10 days in uridine-supplemented medium was necessary to be able to isolate HAT[R] cells (24 per cent) that were subsequently capable of growing in the absence of uridine. More interesting still, after 14 days under no nutritional constrains the majority of their HAT[R] clones (88 per cent) were also able to survive in the absence of uridine. Predictably, the HAT[R], uridine independent cells had restored mitochondrial protein synthesis and COX activity.[45] Because the experiment combined HeLa and 143B nuclei, potential differences between the two cell types could not be addressed; nor was the influence of hybrid status on complementation behaviour or OXPHOS restoration evaluated.

These unresolved issues could be of major interest since, as discussed above, osteosarcoma derived cybrids containing two different tRNA mutations, maintained in culture more than 12 weeks under nonselective conditions were unable to recover OXPHOS competence.[10] Other work supports the idea that the osteosarcoma background tends to segregate two populations of mtDNA. Cell death was prevalent in slow-growing complemented 143B cybrid and hybrid clones.[40] Their ability to complement was lost rapidly when cells were switched from galactose to nonselective medium, and these cells died when switched back to selective medium (R Acín and JA Enriquez unpublished observations). These findings suggest that in the osteosarcoma background equilibrium exists between two counteracting forces; an inherent tendency to segregate the two mutant mtDNAs into distinct mitochondrial populations and selection for those cells with a mixture of mtDNAs appropriate for survival in galactose medium. In conclusion, the discrepancy between results outlined above is due probably to the use of different nuclear backgrounds.[46]

Segregation and complementation of mtDNAs in animal models

The extrapolation of any model developed from cell culture studies to the situation *in vivo* should be made with care. Nevertheless, it would be unwise to dismiss the segregation and complementation behaviour of mtDNA genotypes in culture as irrelevant to the progression of maternally transmitted mtDNA diseases, or fixation of pathological mutations during development. Some theoretical models propose that random intracellular drift and relaxed replication alone could account for the clonal expansion of mtDNA mutations during ageing. Therefore replicative advantage of some mtDNAs need not be invoked to explain age-related accumulation of mutant mtDNAs or increased load of mutant mtDNA in post-mitotic cells.[26,27] Nevertheless, experimental evidence strongly suggests that mtDNA segregation may not merely be random.

Since natural heteroplasmy is rare in mammals, the investigation of this issue has been addressed by the generation of artificial heteroplasmic embryos. This was achieved in mice by fusion of zygotes carrying one mtDNA haplotype with enucleated embryos carrying a different mtDNA haplotype.[47] Most reports using engineered heteroplasmic mice were devised to investigate the transmission of two mtDNA haplotypes through the germ line.[48,49] Fortunately, some groups also followed the fate of host and transferred mtDNAs in different cell types during development. Intriguingly, a variety of behaviours almost as broad as those observed in cultured cells were found. Some cell types such as colonic crypts showed a segregation behaviour compatible with a random drift model. In these cells, heteroplasmy was unstable and the general tendency over time was to reach homoplasmy. However, four tissues (liver, kidney, spleen, and blood) showed a preferential and consistent accumulation of one or other mtDNA haplotype in a tissue-specific and age-related manner.[50] Moreover, the rate of segregation was specific for each tissue. Therefore, the random-drift segregation model is not sufficient to explain the behaviour of mtDNA in somatic cells culture in the laboratory or *in vivo*.

Similar experiments also suggested that some mouse mtDNA haplotypes have a replicative advantage over others during embryonic development and differentiation, and also showed tissue-specific segregation patterns.[51] To explain the directional bias in the selection of the accumulated mtDNA haplotype, it was proposed that polymorphic mtDNAs do not behave as neutral variants. Rather, it was suggested that haplotype-dependent differences in respiratory chain function, detected at a sub cellular level, could favour the expansion of one or other mtDNA haplotype.[50] The notion of phenotypic effects associated with frequent and non-pathological mtDNA haplotypes in humans and mice has recently received strong support.[52,53] Alternatively, since no differences in respiratory chain function associated to mouse mtDNA haplotypes was observed in cell culture, factor(s) involved with mtDNA maintenance were recently proposed to play a crucial role in the direction of segregation.[54]

Maintenance of heteroplasmy over five generations was reported in one artificially generated heteroplasmic mouse.[55] Interestingly, tissue variability falls after the second generation. The stability of heteroplasmy through a number of generations and the ongoing decrease in tissue variability was interpreted as a consequence of *de novo* generation of intramitochondrial heteroplasmy. This would be achieved by fusion between the two original types of organelles.[55] Thus, a similar cause for maintenance of stable heteroplasmy was proposed for cultured cells[15] and of whole animals.[55]

Few data are yet available on the segregation patterns of heteroplasmic mtDNAs in human tissues, but they suggest that their behaviour may also be variable. Thus, a longitudinal analysis on the segregation of polymorphic or pathogenic mtDNA mutations in white blood cells and platelets showed no change in the proportion of a silent polymorphism. On the contrary, the mutation load of a mtDNA point mutation at nucleotide 3460 showed a progressive reduction with age at an overall rate of 1 per cent per year.[56] A decline in the proportion of MELAS mutant mtDNA over a period of several years in blood cells of six patients has also been reported,[57] as has tissue specific distribution of human heteroplasmic mtDNAs.[58] Therefore, it appears that different modes of mtDNA segregation occur in different cell types of whole animals, including humans, and that these represent all the variety of behaviours observed in cultured cells.

Mitochondria and mtDNA seen as a single dynamic cellular unit

Two opposite models have been proposed. One considers that mtDNA is itself mobile and able to pass between organelles in a way that is efficient and leads to a random distribution within the cell cytoplasm.[17] The model of mitochondria as a single dynamic unit arose out of a study of mitochondria pre-treated briefly with ethidium bromide (EB) to label mtDNA prior to fusion with ρ^0 recipient cells. The resultant cybrids were stained additionally with a fluorescent compound (Rhodamine 123) to label all the cybrid mitochondria regardless of whether or not they contained mtDNA.[17] Since the two fluorescent profiles (mtDNA labelled with EB and organelles labelled with Rhodamine 123) substantially overlapped, it was inferred that the donor cytoplast mitochondria had fused with organelles lacking mtDNA, spreading mtDNA throughout all the organelles, within 6 h.[17] There are a number of points that were not evaluated in this report that could compromise the interpretation of the results: (i) It is not clear whether uptake of R123 is similar for OXPHOS-competent organelles and OXPHOS incompetent organelles located in the same cytoplasm. In fact, the labelling intensity of the OXPHOS competent mitochondria was shown to be substantially higher than that of the OXPHOS incompetent organelles when they were located in different cells;[17] (ii) There is an important asymmetry in the distribution of R123 labelled organelles in OXPHOS competent and incompetent cells. Thus, ρ^0 mitochondria are poorly labelled with R123 and seem to be located chiefly around the nucleus. On the contrary, the label in ρ^+ mitochondria spreads throughout the cytoplasm. Therefore, if the two patterns are merged, ρ^+ mitochondrial fluorescence might completely hide that of ρ^0 organelles.

A second argument was raised in the same report to support the notion of mtDNA as a free and quickly moving entity between all the cell's mitochondria. This is based on electron microscopy observations of the COX activity of mitochondrial profiles in cells containing variable amount of Δ-mtDNA. Since Δ-mtDNA does not segregate in different organelles, it was inferred that individual mtDNA molecules, full-size or partially deleted, freely and continuously move between mitochondria and mix homogeneously. Again, there is alternative explanation of the data, but most importantly, the experiments are not equivalent. At the outset of the second experiment Δ-mtDNA and wt-mtDNA molecules were located in the same physical entity (i.e. the mitochondria of the patient) when transferred to a ρ^0 cell. Whereas in the EB/R123 staining experiment two physically independent types of mitochondria (ρ^0 and ρ^+) were introduced into the same cytoplasm. Therefore, to be fully comparable, it would be necessary to introduce mitochondria pure for Δ-mtDNA into a cytoplasm containing only full-size mtDNA.

Nevertheless, the single dynamic unit model is attractive, as it can accommodate the behaviour of highly stable heteroplasmic clones, that is cell lines which maintain a constant proportion of mutant and wt-mtDNA, as well as those clones that show very slow segregation of mtDNA genotypes. Inherent in the model is the assumption that each and every mtDNA molecule moves quickly and freely in the cytoplasm and that the unit of mtDNA segregation is a single molecule.[25,59] The model cannot explain rapid segregation of mtDNA that has been observed in a number of situations (see above) whatever the type of mtDNA that is preferentially accumulated. Nor can it explain the complementation behaviour of mtDNA in cultured cells even in the most favourable case. Thus in the mixed HeLa/osteosarcoma hybrids, mitochondrial profiles that had not recovered COX activity were readily apparent by electron microscopy 10 days after fusion.[45] Moreover, no hybrid was OXPHOS competent 7 days after fusion, and 20 per cent of them remained OXPHOS incompetent at day 14.[45] The concept of quick and continuous fusion of mitochondria within cells allowing rapid migration of mtDNA molecules suffers from other problems. Fusion and fission of mitochondrial membranes is known to be an exquisitely regulated process.[60] Specific proteins have the ability to promote fusion[61,62] or fission.[62] When the balance is disturbed, mitochondrial function and inheritance are compromised in yeast[62] and male sterility induced in *Drosophila*.[61] Therefore, the proposal that mtDNA behaves in all situations and every cell type as a single dynamic unit in mammalian cells seems implausible.

Making sense out of all this . . .

To gain any coherent picture from the myriad findings described above it is necessary to assume that all the apparent contradictions are in fact partial views of a complex picture. However, some extreme positions have to be jettisoned, in particular the concept of mtDNA segregation as solely passive and amenable to modelling by a population genetics approach at the cellular level.[4] By the same token, the idea that mitochondria and their DNA behave exclusively as independent entities (organelles) is fatally flawed. A recent view that is gaining ground suggests that mitochondria are capable of fusion and fission, and that they are organized in a dynamic architecture with transitions between a network-like structure and a more disperse one.[63–68] The fact that these organelles are dynamic and able to interchange material is likely to have important consequences for the interaction, and thereby segregation, of mtDNA molecules. Very recently it was demonstrated beautifully that, despite their ability for interaction, mitochondria within individual cells are morphologically heterogeneous and unconnected, allowing them to have distinct functional properties.[69] Thus, we should not presuppose that mtDNA are able to move freely between mitochondria. This would require a sophisticated molecular mechanism able to randomize the distribution of the mtDNAs throughout the mitochondrial network. On the contrary, yeast mtDNA seems to be much less mobile than other mitochondrial components.[70] Evidence is accumulating that mammalian mtDNA is also organized in stable superstructures (nucleoids). Then, how does the segregation and complementation behaviour described above fit with the organelle dynamic?

The polyploid mtDNA nucleoid as the unit of inheritance of mammalian mtDNA

Recently a model was proposed that assumes that mtDNA nucleoids each containing several copies of mtDNA are copied as a unit. A sort of mitochondrial mitosis would then be responsible for mtDNA replication and transmission, that is, after replication, the nucleoid divides, yielding two daughter nucleoids each a replica of its parent.[59]

Nucleoids could themselves be heteroplasmic or, more than one type of homoplasmic nucleoid could be present in a given cytoplasm. The first situation could arise by mutation events during replication and the second situation would correspond to engineered hetero-plasmic cells and embryos, or could evolve from nucleoids that were initially heteroplasmic.

The different segregation behaviours observed to date could be easily accommodated in this model. Thus, if the nucleoid is heteroplasmic, its faithful division would result in stable heteroplasmy or in a very slow rate of mitotic segregation, and there would be no selection of mtDNA variants. The model requires that the mtDNA copy number per nucleoid is within a narrow range, but different cell types could have different sized nucleoids. Heteroplasmy will be maintained even if some nucleoids are not replicated each cell cycle, as heteroplasmy can be shared by all nucleoids. This would accommodate the observation that mtDNA replication is relaxed. If heteroplasmy were due to the presence of two types of homoplasmic nucleoids, segregation would be very rapid and can follow a random pattern, or an intracellular selection for one or other type of nucleoid under certain circumstances:[59]

With respect to the different complementation behaviours of recessive mtDNA mutations, it is easy to imagine that the different molecules in a nucleoid can complement each other when any of its mtDNA molecules harbours a mutation. Even more, it would be possible to complement several mtDNA mutations affecting more than one gene, or to support a high proportion of one mutation, if at least one functional copy of each gene per nucleoid remains. Interestingly, for mutations that show a partial dominant phenotype, as is the case with large partial deletions, this model provides a good explanation for the fact that, even if the propor-tion of wt-mtDNA is as high as 30 per cent, no COX^+ mitochondria are observed in cells.[12] Thus if this level of heteroplasmy is due to heteroplasmic nucleoids that have an insufficient load of wt-mtDNA no random grouping of wt-mtDNA molecules would generate functional mitochondria. On the other hand, complementation between two different homoplasmic mutant nucleoids, would be much more difficult if we assume that, despite the ability of the organelles to undergo fusion or fission, the area of influence of each nucleoid remains restricted to a small portion of the mitochondrial network.

It should be remarked that the nucleoid model is not just an ad-hoc adaptation of the model that considered single organelles as the unit of inheritance of mtDNA. There is a substantial difference between them. In the former model mitotic segregation can occur by organelle division, while the nucleoid model does not allow it.

Then, what . . .?

The fact that fusion and fission of mitochondria appear to be complex and regulated processes[60] adds to the barriers that the polyploid mtDNA genome has to face in the cell. Thus, several levels of structure have to be taken into account to understand the behaviour of this genome. Those are: the mtDNA molecule itself, the organization of mtDNA molecules in nucleoids, the compartmentalization of nucleoid within the organelles, the dynamics of and structure of mitochondria in the cell. We have to keep in mind that the organization of mito-chondria at each of these levels could vary between different cell types and different physio-logical or pathological situations. These differences are likely to influence segregation and the degree of interaction among heteroplasmic mtDNAs.

Therefore, segregation behaviour depends on a number of parameters that exert their influ-ence to quite different extents in particular cell types or at particular stages of development. These are mitochondrial partition, fusion and fission, replication mechanism, recombinase expression, mtDNA copy number per nucleoid, and last but by no means least the ability to satisfy OXPHOS demand (a function of the inherent capacity to generate ATP aerobically, which depends on the mtDNA genotype, combined with ATP demand).

Acknowledgements

I would like to thank Ian Holt, Erika Fernandez-Vizarra, Carlos Moraes, Patricio Fernandez-Silva, Manuel J. Lopez-Perez and Julio Montoya for their help in discussing and correcting this review. My research is supported by the Spanish Ministry of Education grant PM-99-0082.

References

1. Bogenhagen D and Clayton DA (1997). Mouse L cell mitochondrial DNA molecules are selected randomly for replication throughout the cell cycle. *Cell* **11**: 719–727.
2. Spelbrink JN, *et al.* (2001). Human mitochondrial DNA deletions associated with mutations in the gene encoding Twinkle, a phage T7 gene 4-like protein localized in mitochondria. *Nat. Genet.* **28**: 223–231.
3. Miyakawa I, Sando N, Kawano S, Nakamura S, and Kuroiwa T (1987). Isolation of morphologically intact mitochondrial nucleoids from the yeast, Saccharomyces cerevisiae. *J. Cell. Sci.* **88**: 431–439.
4. Howell N (1999). Human mitochondrial diseases: answering questions and questioning answers. *Int. Rev. Cytol.* **186**: 49–116.
5. Bunn CL, Wallace DC, and Eisenstadt JM (1974). Cytoplasmic inheritance of chloramphenicol resistance in mouse tissue culture cells. *Proc. Natl Acad. Sci. USA* **71**: 1681–1685.
6. Bunn CL, Wallace DC, and Eisenstadt JM (1977). Mitotic segregation of cytoplasmic determinants for chloramphenicol resistance in mammalian cells. I: fusion with mouse cell lines. *Soma. Cell Genet.* **3**: 71–92.
7. Wallace DC, Bunn CL, and Eisenstadt JM (1975). Cytoplasmic transfer of chloramphenicol resistance in human tissue culture cells. *J. Cell Biol.* **67**: 174–188.
8. Mitchell CH and Attardi G (1978). Cytoplasmic transfer of chloramphenicol resistance in a human cell line. *Soma. Cell Genet.* **4**: 737–744.
9. Kearsey SE, Munro E, and Craig IW (1985). Studies of heterogeneous mitochondrial populations in a mouse cell line: the effects of selection for or against mitochondrial genomes that confer chloramphenicol resistance. *Proc. R. Soc. Lond. B Biol. Sci.* **224**: 315–323.
10. Yoneda M, Miyatake T, and Attardi G (1994). Complementation of mutant and wild-type human mitochondrial DNAs coexisting since the mutation event and lack of complementation of DNAs introduced separately into a cell within distinct organelles. *Mol. Cell. Biol.* **14**: 2699–2712.
11. King MP and Attardi G (1989). Human cells lacking mtDNA: repopulation with exogenous mitochondria by complementation. *Science* **246**: 500–503.
12. Hayashi J, *et al.* (1991). Introduction of disease-related mitochondrial DNA deletions into HeLa cells lacking mitochondrial DNA results in mitochondrial dysfunction. *Proc. Natl Acad. Sci. USA* **88**: 10614–10618.
13. Vergani L, Rossi R, Brierley CH, Hanna M, and Holt IJ (1999). Introduction of heteroplasmic mitochondrial DNA (mtDNA) from a patient with NARP into two human rho degrees cell lines is associated either with selection and maintenance of NARP mutant mtDNA or failure to maintain mtDNA. *Hum. Mol. Genet.* **8**: 1751–1755.
14. Holt IJ, Dunbar DR, and Jacobs HT (1997). Behaviour of a population of partially duplicated mitochondrial DNA molecules in cell culture: segregation, maintenance and recombination dependent upon nuclear background. *Hum. Mol. Genet.* **6**: 1251–1260.

15. Yoneda M, Chomyn A, Martinuzzi A, Hurko O, and Attardi G (1992). Marked replicative advantage of human mtDNA carrying a point mutation that causes the MELAS encephalomyopathy. *Proc. Natl Acad. Sci. USA* **89**: 11164–11168.

16. Shoubridge EA, Karpati G, and Hastings KE (1990). Deletion mutants are functionally dominant over wild-type mitochondrial genomes in skeletal muscle fiber segments in mitochondrial disease. *Cell* **62**: 43–49.

17. Hayashi J, Takemitsu M, Goto Y, and Nonaka I (1994). Human mitochondria and mitochondrial genome function as a single dynamic cellular unit. *J. Cell. Biol.* **125**: 43–50.

18. Bourgeron T, Chretien D, Rotig A, Munnich A, and Rustin P (1993). Fate and expression of the deleted mitochondrial DNA differ between human heteroplasmic skin fibroblast and Epstein-Barr virus-transformed lymphocyte cultures. *J. Biol. Chem.* **268**: 19369–19376.

19. Dunbar DR, *et al.* (1993). Maternally transmitted partial direct tandem duplication of mitochondrial DNA associated with diabetes mellitus. *Hum. Mol. Genet.* **2**: 1619–1624.

20. Goto Y, Nonaka I, and Horai S (1990). A mutation in the tRNA(Leu)(UUR) gene associated with the MELAS subgroup of mitochondrial encephalomyopathies. *Nature* **348**: 651–653.

21. Dunbar DR, Moonie PA, Jacobs HT, and Holt IJ (1995). Different cellular backgrounds confer a marked advantage to either mutant or wild-type mitochondrial genomes. *Proc. Natl Acad. Sci. USA* **92**: 6562–6566.

22. Shoubridge EA (1995). Segregation of mitochondrial DNAs carrying a pathogenic point mutation (tRNA(leu3243)) in cybrid cells. *Biochem. Biophys. Res. Commun.* **213**: 189–195.

23. Matthews PM, *et al.* (1995). Intracellular heteroplasmy for disease-associated point mutations in mtDNA: implications for disease expression and evidence for mitotic segregation of heteroplasmic units of mtDNA. *Hum. Genet.* **96**: 261–268.

24. Bentlage HA and Attardi G (1996). Relationship of genotype to phenotype in fibroblast-derived trans-mitochondrial cell lines carrying the 3243 mutation associated with the MELAS encephalomyopathy: shift towards mutant genotype and role of mtDNA copy number. *Hum. Mol. Genet.* **5**: 197–205.

25. Lehtinen SK, *et al.* (2000). Genotypic stability, segregation and selection in heteroplasmic human cell lines containing np 3243 mutant mtDNA. *Genetics* **154**: 363–380.

26. Chinnery PF and Samuels DC (1999). Relaxed replication of mtDNA: A model with implications for the expression of disease. *Am. J. Hum. Genet.* **64**: 1158–1165.

27. Elson JL, Samuels DC, Turnbull DM, and Chinnery PF (2001). Random Intracellular Drift Explains the Clonal Expansion of Mitochondrial DNA Mutations with Age. *Am. J. Hum. Genet.* **68**: 802–806.

28. Moraes CT and Schon EA (1995). In: *Progress in Cell Research* (ed. F Palmieri), pp. 209–215.

29. Moraes CT, Kenyon L, and Hao H (1999). Mechanisms of human mitochondrial DNA maintenance: the determining role of primary sequence and length over function. *Mol. Biol. Cell* **10**: 3345–3356.

30. Kenyon L and Moraes CT (1997). Expanding the functional human mitochondrial DNA database by the establishment of primate xenomitochondrial cybrids. *Proc. Natl Acad. Sci. USA* **94**: 9131–9135.

31. Barrientos A, Kenyon L, and Moraes CT (1998). Human xenomitochondrial cybrids. Cellular models of mitochondrial complex I deficiency. *J. Biol. Chem.* **273**: 14210–14217.

32. Tang Y, *et al.* (2000). Rearrangements of human mitochondrial DNA (mtDNA): new insights into the regulation of mtDNA copy number and gene expression. *Mol. Biol. Cell* **11**: 1471–1485.

33. Moraes CT (2001). What regulates mitochondrial DNA copy number in animal cells? *Trends in Genet.* **17**: 199–205.

34. Chomyn A, *et al.* (1992). MELAS mutation in mtDNA binding site for transcription termination factor causes defects in protein synthesis and in respiration but no change in levels of upstream and downstream mature transcripts. *Proc. Natl Acad. Sci. USA* **89**: 4221–4225.

35. Enriquez JA, Chomyn A, and Attardi G (1995). MtDNA mutation in MERRF syndrome causes defective aminoacylation of tRNA(Lys) and premature translation termination. *Nat. Genet.* **10**: 47–55.

36. Attardi G, Yoneda M, and Chomyn A (1995). Complementation and segregation behavior of disease-causing mitochondrial DNA mutations in cellular model systems. *Biochim. Biophys. Acta* **1271**: 241–248.

37. Oliver NA, Greenberg BD, and Wallace DC (1983). Assignment of a polymorphic polypeptide to the human mitochondrial DNA unidentified reading frame 3 gene by a new peptide mapping strategy. *J. Biol. Chem.* **258**: 5834–5839.

38. Oliver NA and Wallace DC (1982). Assignment of two mitochondrially synthesized polypeptides to human mitochondrial DNA and their use in the study of intracellular mitochondrial interaction. *Mol. Cell Biol.* **2**: 30–41.

39. Takai D, Inoue K, Goto Y, Nonaka I, and Hayashi JI (1997). The interorganellar interaction between distinct human mitochondria with deletion mutant mtDNA from a patient with mitochondrial disease and with HeLa mtDNA. *J. Biol. Chem.* **272**: 6028–6033.

40. Enriquez JA, Cabezas-Herrera J, Bayona-Bafaluy MP, and Attardi G (2000). Very rare complementation between mitochondria carrying different mitochondrial DNA mutations points to intrinsic genetic autonomy of the organelles in cultured human cells. *J. Biol. Chem.* **275**: 11207–11215.

41. Wallace DC (1986). Mitotic segregation of mitochondrial DNAs in human cell hybrids and expression of chloramphenicol resistance. *Somat. Cell Mol. Genet.* **12**: 41–49.

42. Takai D, Isobe K, and Hayashi J (1999). Transcomplementation between different types of respiration-deficient mitochondria with different pathogenic mutant mitochondrial DNAs. *J. Biol. Chem.* **274**: 11199–11202.

43. Taniike M, *et al.* (1992). Mitochondrial tRNA(Ile) mutation in fatal cardiomyopathy. *Biochem. Biophys. Res. Commun.* **186**: 47–53.

44. Hofhaus G and Attardi G (1993). Lack of assembly of mitochondrial DNA-encoded subunits of respiratory NADH dehydrogenase and loss of enzyme activity in a human cell mutant lacking the mitochondrial ND4 gene product. *EMBO J.* **12**: 3043–3048.

45. Ono T, Isobe K, Nakada K, and Hayashi JI (2001). Human cells are protected from mitochondrial dysfunction by complementation of DNA products in fused mitochondria. *Nat. Genet.* **28**: 272–275.

46. Attardi G, Enriquez JA, and Cabezas-Herrera J (2002). Inter-mitochondrial complementation of mtDNA mutations and nuclear context. *Nat. Genet.* **30**: 360; discussion 361.

47. Laipis PJ (1996). Construction of heteroplasmic mice containing two mitochondrial DNA genotypes by micromanipulation of single-cell embryos. *Methods Enzymol.* **264**: 345–357.

48. Smith LC, Bordignon V, Garcia JM, and Meirelles FV (2000). Mitochondrial genotype segregation and effects during mammalian development: applications to biotechnology. *Theriogenology* **53**: 35–46.

49. Jenuth JP, Peterson AC, Fu K, and Shoubridge EA (1996). Random genetic drift in the female germline explains the rapid segregation of mammalian mitochondrial DNA. *Nat. Genet.* **14**: 146–151.

50. Jenuth JP, Peterson AC, and Shoubridge EA (1997). Tissue-specific selection for different mtDNA genotypes in heteroplasmic mice. *Nat. Genet.* **16**: 93–95.

51. Takeda K, Takahashi S, Onishi A, Hanada H, and Imai H (2000). Replicative advantage and tissue-specific segregation of RR mitochondrial DNA between C57BL/6 and RR heteroplasmic mice. *Genetics* **155**: 777–783.

52. Ruiz-Pesini E, *et al.* (2000). Human mtDNA haplogroups associated with high or reduced spermatozoa motility. *Am. J. Hum. Genet.* **67**: 682–696.

53. Johnson KR, QYZ, Bykhovskaya Y, Spirina O, and Fischel-Ghodsian N (2001). A nuclear-mitochondrial DNA interaction affecting hearing impairment in mice. *Nat. Genet.* **27**: 191–194.

54. Battersby BJ and Shoubridge EA (2001). Selection of a mtDNA sequence variant in hepatocytes of heteroplasmic mice is not due to differences in respiratory chain function or efficiency of replication. *Hum. Mol. Genet.* **10**: 2469–2479.

55. Meirelles FV and Smith LC (1997). Mitochondrial genotype segregation in a mouse heteroplasmic lineage produced by embryonic karyoplast transplantation. *Genetics* **145**: 445–451.

56. Howell N, Ghosh SS, Fahy E, and Bindoff LA (2000). Longitudinal analysis of the segregation of mtDNA mutations in heteroplasmic individuals. *J. Neurol. Sci.* **172**: 1–6.

57. Rahman S, Poulton J, Marchington D, and Suomalainen A (2001). Decrease of 3243 A → G mtDNA mutation from blood in MELAS syndrome: a longitudinal study. *Am. J. Hum. Genet.* **68**: 238–240.

58. Chinnery PF, *et al.* (1999). Nonrandom tissue distribution of mutant mtDNA. *Am. J. Med. Genet.* **85**: 498–501.

59. Jacobs HT, Lehtinen SK, and Spelbrink JN (2000). No sex please, we're mitochondria: a hypothesis on the somatic unit of inheritance of mammalian mtDNA. *Bioessays* **22**: 564–572.

60. Jensen RE, Aiken Hobbs AE, Cerveny KL, and Sesaki H (2000). Yeast mitochondrial dynamics: Fusion, division, segregation, and shape. *Microsc. Res. Tech.* **51**: 573–583.

61. Hales KG and Fuller MT (1997). Developmentally regulated mitochondrial fusion mediated by a conserved, novel, predicted GTPase. *Cell* **90**: 121–129.

62. Sesaki H and Jensen RE (1999). Division versus fusion: Dnm1p and Fzo1p antagonistically regulate mitochondrial shape. *J. Cell Biol.* **147**: 699–706.

63. Bleazard W, *et al.* (1999). The dynamin-related GTPase Dnm1 regulates mitochondrial fission in yeast. *Nat. Cell Biol.* **1**: 298–304.

64. Wong ED, *et al.* (2000). The dynamin-related GTPase, mgm1p, is an intermembrane space protein required for maintenance of fusion competent mitochondria. *J. Cell Biol.* **151**: 341–352.

65. Bereiter-Hahn J and Voth M (1994). Dynamics of mitochondria in living cells: shape changes, dislocations, fusion, and fission of mitochondria. *Microsc. Res. Tech.* **27**: 198–219.

66. Rutter GA and Rizzuto R (2000). Regulation of mitochondrial metabolism by ER Ca^{2+} release: an intimate connection. *Trends Biochem. Sci.* **25**: 215–221.

67. Rizzuto R, *et al.* (1998). Close contacts with the endoplasmic reticulum as determinants of mitochondrial Ca^{2+} responses. *Science* **280**: 1763–1766.

68. Smirnova E, Shurland DL, Ryazantsev SN, and van der Bliek AM (1998). A human dynamin-related protein controls the distribution of mitochondria. *J. Cell Biol.* **143**: 351–358.

69. Collins TJ, Berridge MJ, Lipp P, and Bootman MD (2002). Mitochondria are morphologically and functionally heterogeneous within cells. *EMBO J.* **21**: 1616–1627.

70. Nunnari J, *et al.* (1997). Mitochondrial transmission during mating in Saccharomyces cerevisiae is determined by mitochondrial fusion and fission and the intramitochondrial segregation of mitochondrial DNA. *Mol. Biol. Cell* **8**: 1233–1242.

15 Mouse models of mitochondrial disease

Caroline Graff and Nils-Göran Larsson

Mitochondrial DNA has proved refractive to genetic engineering providing a major obstacle to creating animal models of mitochondrial DNA disease. Mitochondrial DNA (mtDNA) is located in the matrix enclosed by double membranes and there is as yet no method for introducing and stably maintaining foreign DNA in mitochondria. Most mouse models have therefore been generated by nuclear gene targeting (Table 15.1). However, it has recently been shown that it is possible to introduce isolated mitochondria into mouse embryos (Table 15.1). This strategy allows mtDNA mutations to be introduced into the germ line, provided that mitochondria carrying the desired mutation can be isolated from cell lines or tissues. Gene targeting of mtDNA remains an important goal for the future.

Mice with ANT-1 gene deficiency develop mitochondrial myopathy and cardiomyopathy

The first mouse knockout that mimicked mitochondrial disease in humans was of the adenine nucleotide translocator (*ANT*) gene. The primary function of ANT is ATP/ADP exchange between the mitochondrial matrix and the cytosol. ANT belongs to a large family of nuclear-encoded inner mitochondrial membrane carriers, which contain six membrane-spanning domains. In contrast to most proteins imported into mitochondria, ANT and other carrier proteins do not contain a mitochondrial targeting peptide. ANT has also been proposed to make up part of the mitochondrial permeability transition pore that has a role in apoptosis. There are three human ANT isoforms, all of which have tissue specific patterns of expression. *ANT1* is predominantly expressed in heart, skeletal muscle and brain. *ANT2* is predominantly expressed in kidney, spleen, liver, fibroblasts, and lymphocytes, whereas *ANT3* is ubiquitously expressed at low levels.

There are only two *Ant* genes in mice; *Ant1* is expressed in heart, skeletal muscle and brain and *Ant2* is expressed in all tissues except skeletal muscle.[1] *Ant1*-deficient mice were generated by deleting exons 1–3 of *Ant1* (*Ant1*−/−) and as predicted this allele does not show any *Ant1* expression.[2] Homozygous knockouts survived and were fertile at least until the age of 8 months.[2] Since *Ant2* is expressed in all tissues except muscle, the homozygous *Ant1*(−/−) mice were deficient of Ant in muscle and partially deficient in heart and brain.[1] The knockouts displayed ragged red fibers (RRF) and increased mitochondrial volume in skeletal muscle, classical features of mitochondrial myopathy (MM) in humans. Enzyme histochemistry demonstrated an increased activity of both succinate dehydrogenase (SDH, Complex II) and cytochrome *c* oxidase (COX, Complex IV) in skeletal muscle of the *Ant1* knockout. Patients with MM typically have RRF with increased SDH and *reduced* COX activity. The

Table 15.1 Mouse models of mitochondrial disease

Mouse model/ targeted gene	Technique	Biochemical findings and phenotype	References
$Ant-/-$	Germ line knockout	Heart: $H_2O_2\uparrow$ Gpx$\uparrow$, Aconitase$=$, HCM Muscle: CII$\uparrow$, CIV$\uparrow$, $H_2O_2\uparrow$ Gpx$\uparrow$, Sod2$\uparrow$, Aconitase$=$, Exercise intolerance, RRF, S-lactate$\uparrow$	1,2
$SOD2^{m1BCM}/$ $SOD2^{m1BCM}$	Germ line knockout	Heart: Sod1$\uparrow$, 10% DCM, Exercise intolerance CNS: Degenerative injury, Motor abnormalities Growth retardation, Anaemia	9
$Sod2tm1^{Cje}-/-$	Germ line knockout	Heart: CI$\downarrow$, CII$\downarrow$, CIII$=$, CIV$=$, Aconitase$\downarrow$, CS$\downarrow$, DCM Muscle: CI$=$, CII$\downarrow$, CIII$=$, CIV$=$, CNS: Aconitase$\downarrow$, Liver: HMG-CoA lyase$\downarrow$, Steatosis Organic aciduria, S-ketones$\uparrow$	8,10,11
$Sod2tm1^{Cje}+/-$	Germ line knockout	Liver: CIII$\downarrow$, Increased oxidative damage to mitochondrial proteins and mtDNA	12
$Tfam-/-$	Conditional knockout	Embryo: CII$=$, CIV$\downarrow$, mtDNA$\downarrow$, Apoptosis$\uparrow$ Absence of heart, Delayed neural development, Embryonic lethal	25
$Tfam+/-$	Conditional knockout	Heart: CI$\downarrow$, CII$=$, CIII$\downarrow$, CIV$\downarrow$, CV$\downarrow$, CS$=$ All tissues: mtDNA$\downarrow$ Phenotypically apparently normal	25
$Ckmm$-cre, $Tfam-$	Conditional knockout	Heart: CI$\downarrow$, CII$=$, CIV$\downarrow$, CS$=$, mtDNA$\downarrow$, Apoptosis$\uparrow$, DCM with mosaic CIV deficiency, AV heart conduction blocks Muscle CI$=$, CII$=$, CIV$=$, mtDNA$\downarrow$	26
$Myhca$-cre, $Tfam-$	Conditional knockout	Heart: CI$\downarrow$, CII$=$, CIII$\downarrow$, CIV$\downarrow$, Aconitase$=$ DCM with mosaic CIV deficiency, AV heart conduction blocks	28
RIP-cre, $Tfam-$	Conditional knockout	Pancreatic β cells: CII$=$, CIV$\downarrow$, Diabetes Mellitus, Impaired insulin stimulus-secretion coupling, β-cell loss	29
CAP^r (mt501-1)	ES cell cybrids	Germ line mice: DCM, myopathy Chimeric mice develop bilateral cataracts	23
ΔmtDNA	Cybrid fusion to embryos	Heart, muscle, and kidney: mosaic CIV deficiency Renal failure, S-lactate$\uparrow$	13
$Frda^{del4}(-/-)$	Germ line knockout	Apoptosis$\uparrow$, No iron deposits Embryonic lethal	38
MCK-cre, $Frda-$	Conditional knockout	Heart. CI$\downarrow$, CII$\downarrow$, CIII$\downarrow$, Aconitase$\downarrow$, Iron accumulation, HCM, DCM	39
NSE-cre, $Frda-$	Conditional knockout	Heart. CI$\downarrow$, CII$\downarrow$, CIII$\downarrow$, Aconitase$\downarrow$, No iron deposits, CM Brain: Aconitase$\downarrow$, Movement disorder, Defective proprioception	39
A/J mtDNA	Natural mtDNA variations	tRNA arginine gene polymorphism modifies severity of hearing impairment in mice homozygous for the A/J allele at the Ahl locus	37

CI–V, activity of respiratory chain enzyme Complex I-V; CM, cardiomyopathy; CS, citrate synthase activity; DCM, dilated cardiomyopathy; ES, embryonic stem cells; HCM, hypertrophic cardiomyopathy; Gpx, glutathion peroxidase activity/expression; RRF, ragged red fibre; Sod1, cytoplasmic superoxide dismutase activity/expression; Sod2, mitochondrial superoxide dismutase activity/expression; $=$ unchanged; $\downarrow$ reduced; $\uparrow$ increased.

hearts of the homozygous knockout $Ant1(-/-)$ mice developed a concentric hypertrophy by the age of 4–6 months with an increased heart weight and an increased number of normally appearing mitochondria. Respiration rates of mitochondria isolated from tissue homogenates of skeletal muscle showed a reduction in ADP-stimulated respiration for Complexes I (NADH dehydrogenase) and II of the respiratory chain.

The $Ant1(-/-)$ mice have also been used to study the levels and toxicity of reactive oxygen species (ROS).[1] Skeletal muscle, brain and heart mitochondria from the Ant1 deficient mice produced two- to eight-fold higher amounts of hydrogen peroxide (H_2O_2) than control mice, while liver mitochondria from the same animals had normal ROS production. Increased levels of the detoxifying enzymes mitochondrial superoxide dismutase (MnSOD or SOD2), and gluthathione peroxidase-1 (Gpx1) were found in both heart and skeletal muscle. The activity of aconitase was normal in heart and skeletal muscle indicating that the increased ROS levels did not interfere with the activity of iron–sulphur cluster enzymes. Long-extension polymerase chain reaction (LX-PCR) analyses revealed increased levels of mtDNA rearrangements in the mutant hearts comparable to the levels found in very old mouse hearts. However, it should be noted that LX-PCR analyses are prone to artefacts that make this method unreliable for quantification of mtDNA rearrangements.[3] That said, it is interesting to note that mutations in $ANT1$ is one cause of multiple deletions of mtDNA in humans (Chapter 9).

Mouse models with impaired ROS defence

The ROS are a normal byproducts of a number of cellular processes, most notably respiration. Defence mechanisms to neutralize ROS include SOD of which there are three isoforms with different locations. Cu/ZnSOD (SOD1) is located in the cytosol, extracellular SOD (SOD3) is secreted and MnSOD (SOD2) is located in the mitochondrial matrix. Gain of function mutations in $SOD1$ have been identified in cases of familial amyotrophic lateral sclerosis[4] and studies of animal models suggest that mutated $SOD1$ causes activation of caspase 1 and caspase 3 leading to neuronal cell death by apoptosis.[5] Knockout of $Sod1$ or $Sod3$ in mice did not generate any major phenotype.[6,7]

In contrast, $Sod2$ knockout mice displayed a dramatic phenotype. Two independent mouse lines with Sod2 deficiency have been generated, $Sod2^{tm1Cje}(-/-)$[8] and $SOD2^{m1BCM}(-/-)$.[9] The $SOD2^{m1BCM}$ mice were created by deleting exons 1 and 2 of $Sod2$. These knockout mice exhibited a diminished growth rate from postnatal day 2 (P2) progressing until death at P18. The mutants developed neurodegenerative changes with motor abnormalities, limb weakness, early onset fatigue, and circling behaviour. In addition, the mutants had hypocellular bone marrow resulting in anaemia, abnormal distribution of glycogen, and intracellular lipid vacuoles in hepatocytes. Approximately 10 per cent of the $SOD2^{m1BCM}(-/-)$ mutants developed dilated cardiomyopathy with widespread myocardial cell injury and abnormal mitochondria. The $Sod1$ activity was increased by ~25 per cent in mutant heart tissue probably reflecting a compensatory response to the $Sod2$ deficiency.

The $Sod2^{tm1Cje}(-/-)$ mice[8] were obtained by deletion of exon 3 and these knockouts were hypotonic, hypothermic, and paler at birth than their littermates. At P4–P5, the mutants started to die off and all showed severe growth retardation with death before P15.[8,10] The hearts were enlarged and showed signs of dilated cardiomyopathy (DCM) with dilated left ventricles and reduced left ventricle wall thickness. Histology of the myocardium showed hypertrophic and degenerative changes as well as an increased number of apparently normal mitochondria. Histochemistry showed that mutant heart and skeletal muscle had decreased SDH activity and normal COX activity. In addition, the knockout mice displayed liver steatosis and skeletal muscle lipid deposits suggesting abnormal fatty acid metabolism. There were no neurological signs, the brain appeared normal upon microscopy and there was no evidence of increased lipid peroxidation. SDH activity was reduced in skeletal muscle and heart mitochondria at P4–P6.[11] There was also a deficiency of Complex I, citrate synthase, and aconitase activities in knockout heart mitochondria, possibly caused by oxidative damage to these enzymes. There was no evidence of increased mtDNA rearrangements in heart, brain, kidney, skeletal muscle, or liver as determined by LX–PCR analyses.

The heterozygous $Sod2^{tm1Cje}(+/-)$ knockout mice did not exhibit an abnormal phenotype up to age 9 months despite a 50 per cent reduction in $Sod2$ activity in heart, brain, liver, and kidney.[12] Analysis of liver mitochondria from the heterozygous knockouts aged 2–4 months revealed increased oxidative damage to mitochondrial proteins as measured by the levels of added carbonyl groups. There was no evidence of increased protein oxidation in the cytosol. Further, $Sod2^{tm1Cje}(+/-)$ liver mitochondria demonstrated a 30 per cent increase of the oxidative adduct 8-OH-guanine in mtDNA but not in nuclear DNA. The levels of Gpx and Cu/Zn SOD were normal in liver mitochondria, which suggests that there was no compensatory increase in these ROS scavengers. The mitochondrial aconitase activity in liver was reduced ~30 per cent whereas cytosolic aconitase activity was unchanged in the heterozygotes compared with the wild type animals. Measurements of oxygen consumption in isolated liver mitochondria indicated an impairment of Complex III activity.

The $Sod2^{tm1Cje}(-/-)$ mice were rescued from DCM, neonatal death, and lipid accumulation in liver by treatment with the SOD mimetic, manganese 5, 10, 15, 20-tetrakis (4-benzoic acid) porphyrin (MnTBAP) intraperitoneally from P3.[10] The mean life span of MnTBAP treated $Sod2^{tm1Cje}(-/-)$ mice was extended from ~P8 to ~P16. Interestingly, the MnTBAP-treated mutants developed a progressive movement disorder characterized by limb ataxia accompanied by head tremor. At P21, the mice were moribund, immobile, and exhibited weight loss. Histology showed spongiform encephalopathy and neuronal vacuolization. The brain phenoype is likely explained by the inability of MnTBAP to cross the blood–brain barrier; thus, the beneficial effects of the compound are not realized in brain.

In summary, $Sod2$-deficient mice show that mitochondrial SOD activity is necessary for maintenance of respiratory chain function. The oxidative stress caused by lack of $Sod2$ is limited to mitochondria and is detrimental to the function of terminally differentiated tissues with a high-energy demand, such as brain and heart. The differences in phenotype between the two $Sod2$ knockout mouse strains may well be explained by differences in genetic background.

The hypothesized link between increased ROS production and rearrangements of mtDNA is somewhat tenuous, given the pitfalls of LX-PCR. The $Ant1$ knockouts were suggestive of such a link as these mice displayed increased hydrogen peroxide production and increased mtDNA rearrangements. In contrast, LX-PCR of the $Sod2$ knockout tissues did not identify increased levels of mtDNA rearrangements despite the fact that ROS levels are predicted to be high in these mice. The $Ant1$ knockout might promote mtDNA rearrangement via altered nucleotide balance, whereas the $Sod2$ knockout would not be expected to have this effect. Alternatively, mtDNA rearrangements may have accumulated over 16–20 months in the $Ant1$-deficient mice due to chronic exposure to high levels of ROS whereas the $Sod2$-deficient mice may simply not have lived long enough to display this phenotype. It should be noted that neither the *Ant*1 nor the *Sod*2 knockouts primarily affect respiratory chain function, but rather ADP/ATP translocation and ROS defence, respectively. There is thus a need for further studies to establish or refute the proposed link between respiratory chain deficiency, ROS production, and mtDNA rearrangements.

Heteroplasmic mice

Two approaches applied recently have succeeded in the long-held goal of establishing mixtures of mutant and wild-type mtDNA (wt-DNA) in mice and shown that the mutant mtDNA can be transmitted through the germ line.

Mice with mtDNA deletion

In a ground-breaking study, Hayashi and colleagues introduced exogenous mouse mitochondria with partially deleted mtDNA (Δ-mtDNA) into mouse zygotes by electrofusion and demonstrated that the Δ-mtDNA was transmitted through the germ line for three generations.[13] This was achieved by isolating a naturally occurring Δ-mtDNA from enucleated somatic cells or brain synaptosomes (synaptic nerve cell endings) obtained from aged mice and fusing these with ρ^0 mouse cells that lack mtDNA. One resulting cybrid clone contained 30 per cent Δ-mtDNA, which lacked a 4696-bp region encompassing six tRNA genes and seven structural genes. The mtDNA mutant load of the clonal cell line increased to 83 per cent after many cell divisions. Cybrids with high levels of Δ-mtDNA demonstrated decreased COX activity confirming that the Δ-mtDNA deletion was deleterious. In order to generate trans-mitochondrial mice, the Δ-mtDNA was introduced into pronuclear stage embryos by electrofusion of enucleated cytoplasts, containing Δ-mtDNA, and mouse embryos. The chimeric embryos were cultured for 1–2 days and subsequently introduced to the oviduct of pseudo-pregnant foster mothers. A total of 111 pups were born and 98 of these survived to adulthood. Further characterization identified 24 mice with between 6 and 42 per cent Δ-mtDNA in skeletal muscle. Five F_0 founder females with 6–13 per cent Δ-mtDNA were selected for further breeding and germ line transmission of Δ-mtDNA to their progeny was accomplished. Transmission of Δ-mtDNA was confirmed by analysis of muscle biopsy specimens from three consecutive generations, $(F_1–F_3)$. The variance in the proportion of Δ-mtDNA in progeny of mothers with a low proportion of the mutant mtDNA was greater than the variance in progeny to mothers with high levels of Δ-mtDNA. This could be explained by a replicative advantage to the Δ-mtDNA molecule over wt-mtDNA molecule. All pups had less than 90 per cent Δ-mtDNA suggesting that very high levels of Δ-mtDNA are lethal to ova or embryos.

Surprisingly, a partially duplicated mtDNA molecule was identified in all generations $(F_0–F_3)$ despite being undetectable in the cell lines used to create the mice. The partially duplicated mtDNA comprises a copy of partially deleted and a copy of wt-mtDNA. Analysis of the proportion of partially duplicated mtDNA in tissues from F_1 and F_2 mice revealed 0–17 per cent Δ-mtDNA in skeletal muscle, heart and blood whereas Δ-mtDNA was absent in other tissues such as testis, kidney, and brain. It should be noted, however, that it is possible that low levels of the partially duplicated mtDNA molecule escaped detection since the samples were analysed by Southern blotting. Therefore, it remains unclear if the Δ-mtDNA molecule was transmitted through the germ line, or whether transmission occurred via partially duplicated mtDNA molecules. After transmission the partially duplicated molecules could have been resolved via intramolecular recombination to yield wt-mtDNA and

Δ-mtDNA molecules. Alternatively, the Δ-mtDNA molecule was transmitted intact and subsequently recombined with the wt-mtDNA generating a partially duplicated molecule. In any event, partially duplicated mtDNA is known to co-exist with Δ-mtDNA in humans.

Histochemical studies in the Δ-mtDNA mice revealed that muscle fibres containing more than 85 per cent rearranged mtDNA (Δ-mtDNA and partially duplicated mtDNA) were COX-negative but these fibres did not have typical RRF appearance upon Gomori trichome staining. A mosaic pattern of COX-negative fibres was also found in the heart of mice with high levels of rearranged mtDNA. Mice with high levels of mutant mtDNA died by P200 from kidney failure. Analysis of kidneys containing 85 per cent mutant mtDNA demonstrated reduced COX activity (70 per cent reduction). The mice also presented with lactic acidosis and anaemia, which are well-recognized features in paediatric patients.

Thus, the Δ-mtDNA deletion mouse model reproduces several important features of human mitochondrial disorders such as mosaic distribution of COX-deficient muscle fibres in skeletal and heart muscle and different mutational load in different tissues of the same individual. Nevertheless, RRF that are often associated with COX-negative fibres in patients with Kearns–Sayre syndrome were absent in the Δ-mtDNA mice. Further, the levels of rearranged mtDNA were similar in most analysed mouse tissues, whereas the levels of Δ-mtDNA in human mitochondrial disorders often vary considerably between tissues. In adult humans, there are typically high levels of Δ-mtDNA in post-mitotic tissues such as heart, muscle, and brain and low or undetectable levels in blood. The findings in Δ-mtDNA mice are most similar to children with early onset multisystem mitochondrial disease who typically have a widespread distribution of high levels of Δ-mtDNA.[14]

It is important to clarify further the interrelationship between Δ-mtDNA and partially duplicated mtDNA, and the availability of mice with rearranged mtDNA should aid greatly this process. Maternal transmission of partially duplicated mtDNA has been described in several human pedigrees. In these pedigrees, the affected children suffered from multisystem disorders and had widespread tissue distribution of high levels of rearranged mtDNA.[15–17] There has been only one case-report of maternal transmission of Δ-mtDNA[18] and several reports of non-transmission of Δ-mtDNA in humans.[19,20] These observations in humans and mouse suggest that partially duplicated mtDNA molecules may predispose to the formation of Δ-mtDNA during early embryonic development. The Δ-mtDNA mouse will be a valuable tool for studying the maintenance and dynamics of rearranged mtDNA molecules in the germ line.

Chloramphenicol-resistant mice

The drug chloramphenicol specifically inhibits mitochondrial translation yet chloramphenicol resistance (CAP^r) can result from point mutations in the *16S rRNA* gene of mtDNA.[21] These mutations not only confer chloramphenicol resistance they also impair mitochondrial ribosome function. The inhibition of mitochondrial protein synthesis causes a reduction of Complex I and IV activities.[22]

Mitochondria can be introduced to embryonic stem (ES) cells by cybrid techniques, however, this requires the use of female ES cells in order to create trans-mitochondrial mice, since mtDNA is exclusively maternally inherited. In contrast, manipulation of nuclear genes usually utilizes male ES cells. Recently, it was demonstrated that the CAP^r mutation caused by a T → C transition at nucleotide 2433 (T2433C) of the *16SrRNA* gene could be transmitted through the female germ line.[23] The chimeric CAPr mice were generated in two steps. First, mouse cells carrying the T2433C mutation were enucleated and the cytoplasts were fused to female ES cells that had been deprived of their endogenous mitochondria by rho-damine-6-G treatment. All chimeric mice with significant ES-cell contribution, as determined by coat colour, developed bilateral cataracts. Electroretinograms demonstrated a reduction of both rod and cone function. Morphology in 6-month-old chimeric males did not reveal any signs of photoreceptor degeneration but there was vacuolization of the retinal pigment epithelium and the optic nerve head contained a hamartomatous-like protuberance. The mice born after germ line transmission displayed growth retardation, myopathy, cardiomyopathy (CM), and embryonic or perinatal lethality. Skeletal and heart muscle mitochondria were abnormal with inclusions. The neonatal lethality after germ line transmission of the CAP^r mtDNA prevents stable maintenance of the mutant mtDNA in the mouse.

Tfam *knockout mice*

The unsolved technical problems associated with transfection of mitochondria encouraged us to use an alternate approach whereby mtDNA expression is manipulated by targeting of a nuclear gene. Mitochondrial transcription factor A (Tfam) is a nucleus-encoded protein that is imported to mitochondria where it acts as a transcription factor.[24] It is not only necessary for transcription, but also for mtDNA replication since an RNA primer is necessary for replication initiation. We utilized the *cre-loxP* recombination system to disrupt *Tfam* since this system would allow manipulation of respiratory chain function in selected mouse tissues. The *cre-loxP* recombination technique involves two steps. First, we generated mice with *loxP* sequences flanking exons 6 and 7 of the *Tfam* gene (*Tfam^loxP^*). This was achieved by homologous recombination in ES cells, creation of mouse chimeras and subsequent transmission through the germ line.[25] The second step encompasses excision of exons 6 and 7 of *Tfam* and was accomplished by reciprocal DNA recombination between the two *loxP* sites when *Tfam^loxP^* mice were mated with transgenic mice expressing *cre*-recombinase. Insertion of *loxP* sites into the *Tfam* locus does not impair the expression of Tfam protein, mtDNA expression, or the respiratory chain function.[26]

We initially created germ line knockouts by mating heterozygous *Tfam^loxP^* mice (+/*Tfam^loxP^*) with animals homozygous for a β-*actin cre*-transgene, which ubiquitously expressed *cre*-recombinase in the preimplantation embryo.[25] This mating generated heterozygous *Tfam* knockouts (+/*Tfam⁻*) which were viable and had no observable phenotype. However, the +/*Tfam⁻* mice exhibited reduced mtDNA copy number (~30–40 per cent reduction) in all analysed tissues and reduced activities in the heart of respiratory chain complexes I, III, IV, and V, all of which contain mtDNA-encoded subunits. Still, the levels of mitochondrial transcripts and mtDNA-encoded respiratory chain subunits were unchanged in most other tissues despite the general reduction of mtDNA copy number. This may be due to a compensatory increased stability of mitochondrial transcripts and proteins.[14,27]

An intercross of +/*Tfam⁻* mice produced no homozygous mutant pups and we could determine that loss of *Tfam* was embryonic lethal between embryonic day (E)8.5 and E10.5. Analysis of homozygous knockout (*Tfam⁻/Tfam⁻*) embryos revealed absence of cardiac structures, complete absence of Tfam protein and an absence of mtDNA. Thus Tfam is essential for mtDNA maintenance *in vivo* and loss of mtDNA is not compatible with normal embryonic development.

In a series of studies, we have mated *Tfam^loxP^/Tfam^loxP^* mice to transgenic mice carrying the *cre*-recombinase gene regulated by different tissue specific promoters.[26,28,29] In the first study, we generated a mouse model for mitochondrial dilated cardiomyopathy and atrio-ventricular heart conduction blocks by heart-specific inactivation of the *Tfam* gene.[26] To selectively disrupt *Tfam* in heart and skeletal muscle, *Tfam^loxP^/Tfam^loxP^* mice were mated with muscle creatinine kinase (*Ckmm*)-*cre* transgenic mice; double heterozygous offspring were mated with *Tfam^loxP^/Tfam^loxP^* mice thus generating heart and muscle specific *Tfam* knockout animals (*Tfam^loxP^/Tfam^loxP^*, +/*Ckmm-cre*). The *Ckmm* promoter is active from E13. The mutant animals exhibited decreased spontaneous activity and growth retardation or weight loss from P10. Mean survival was 20 days and most knockouts were dead by the ages of 3–4 weeks. At autopsy, at ages 2–4 weeks, the mutant hearts were enlarged with increased weight and dilation of the left ventricular chamber, similar to human dilated cardiomyopathy. Further analysis of 2–4-week-old mutants showed a highly tissue-specific pattern with knock-out of *Tfam* and a corresponding reduction of Tfam protein levels in heart and skeletal muscle. The levels of mtDNA and mitochondrial transcripts were reduced in heart (70–80 per cent reduction) and in skeletal muscle (30–40 per cent). There was also a reduction of the mtDNA-encoded respiratory chain subunit ATP8 protein and of respiratory chain function in mutant hearts but not in muscle. None of these changes were observed in kidney or liver. Enzyme histochemistry showed a mosaic pattern with several cardiomyocytes lacking COX activity while maintaining normal SDH activity. Mutant hearts had an increased number of mito-chondria with abnormal shape and size. Electrocardiography (ECG) of mutants revealed a progressive atrioventricular (AV) heart conduction block, decreased peak aortic blood flow velocity and all mutants died within 30 min of onset of isoflurane anaesthesia. Telemetry showed intermittent periods of AV heart conduction blocks in wake mutant animals. Thus, the heart- and muscle-specific *Tfam* knockout animals reproduce important physiological fea-tures of human mtDNA disorders caused by deletions or point mutations of mitochondrial tRNA genes. It is well established that the mutation load in patients, that is, the proportion of mutated mtDNA to wt-mtDNA, can determine the severity of symptoms. For instance, a threshold level of ~60 per cent deleted mtDNA is required to cause respiratory chain defi-ciency[30] which is consistent with the data observed in the *Ckmm-cre* mutant mice. Patients with progressive external ophthalmoplegia and Kearns–Sayre syndrome caused by mtDNA deletions have an uneven distribution of COX-deficient muscle fibres directly correlated to the distribution of deleted mtDNA.[31] An analogous mechanism may account for the histo-chemical mosaicism observed in the mutant mouse hearts, such that uneven expression and/or uneven action of the *cre*-recombinase gives rise to genomic mosaicism for the *Tfam*⁻ allele. Cardiac manifestations are frequent in mitochondrial disorders. Kearns–Sayre syndrome patients often develop AV heart conduction blocks requiring prophylactic treatment with pacemaker. Similar to the cardiomyopathy mice, affected patients may develop dilated mitochondrial cardiomyopathy leading to heart failure.[32]

In the second study, we mated the *Tfam^loxP^/Tfam^loxP^* mice to animals carrying the *cre*-recombinase transgene regulated by the α-*myosin heavy chain* (*Myhca*)-promoter active from E8.[28] Double heterozygous offspring were mated to *Tfam^loxP^/Tfam^loxP^* to obtain heart-specific *Tfam* knockouts with the *Tfam^loxP^/Tfam^loxP^*, +/*Myhca-cre* genotype. This mating, referred to as 'standard mating' generated reduced litter sizes with a lower than expected number of mutant animals. Further analyses showed that 75 per cent of the mutant animals died during the first week of life and that the remaining 25 per cent of the heart-specific *Tfam* knockout mice survived for several months. Analysis of E18.5 knockouts showed that the *cre-loxP* recombination was restricted to heart, leading to a reduction of mtDNA (70 per cent reduction). The heart weights were not increased and there were no obvious malformations in the mutant hearts at E18.5. Hearts obtained from adult knockout mice at ages 2–4 months presented with markedly increased weights, significant enlargement of the heart accompanied by dilation of ventricles and atria. There was also a reduction in Tfam protein levels and mtDNA copy number (70 per cent reduction). Tissue homogenates of adult knockout hearts demonstrated a reduced activity of Complexes I, III, and IV whereas Complex II, aconitase and isocitrate dehydrogenase displayed normal activities. The COX and SDH staining of mutant hearts revealed an extensive mosaic deficiency of COX activity in cardiomyocytes. The ECG recordings revealed AV heart conduction blocks in anaesthetized and wake mutant mice.

In order to investigate whether the long-living knockouts carried some genetic resistance to developing dilated cardiomyopathy, the adult knockout animals were intercrossed. This mating, referred to as 'mutant mating', generated approximate Mendelian proportions of knockouts. More than 95 per cent of the knockouts obtained from the mutant mating survived for more than 3 months, suggesting that the life span of the knockouts was modified by some genetic determinant, possibly a recessive gene. There were clear differences in the biochemical, and histological profiles of standard and mutant mating knockouts at E18.5. The E18.5 standard mating knockout embryos had reduced Tfam protein levels, reduced ATP8 protein levels, reduced mtDNA copy number (70 per cent reduction), reduced Complex IV activity, and a profound mosaic COX deficiency in the heart. The E18.5 mutant mating knockouts displayed normal levels for most variables except for Tfam protein levels, which were reduced in two out of four analysed hearts, and COX activity, which was deficient in cardiomyocytes. In spite of these differences, there appeared to be an equal frequency of *cre-loxP* recombined *Tfam* alleles in standard and mutant mating E18.5 hearts. Adult mutant mating knockout hearts displayed markedly increased heart weights with dilation of ventricles and atria and a mosaic pattern of COX-negative cardiomyocytes.

The results from the *Tfam/Ckmm-cre* and *Tfam/Myhca-cre* studies show that the age of onset of respiratory chain dysfunction in mutant mice can be successfully manipulated by temporal regulation of *cre* expression in the heart. The data also show that the long-living mutants generated by the standard mating must carry some genetic determinant which protects their hearts from the consequences of the knockout since it is transmitted to their offspring. These genes may act to stabilize mtDNA, mitochondrial transcripts, or mitochondrial proteins. In any event, further studies of other tissue-specific *Tfam* knockouts on several different genetic backgrounds will allow researchers to systematically search for genes that modify the phenotype. Such genes may shed light on the pathogenic mechanisms of mitochondrial disorders in general and on mitochondrial biogenesis in particular.

In a third study, we disrupted the *Tfam* gene in pancreatic β-cells by mating the *Tfam^loxP^/Tfam^loxP^* mice with transgenic mice carrying the *cre*-recombinase gene regulated by the rat insulin-2 promoter (*RIP-cre*).[29] The offspring carrying the *RIP-cre* transgene were subsequently mated to *Tfam^loxP^/Tfam^loxP^* mice generating mutant mice with tissue specific knockout of *Tfam* in pancreatic β-cells (*Tfam^loxP^/Tfam^loxP^*, +/*RIP-cre*). Analysis of 7-week-old mutant mice showed the presence of the *Tfam^−^* allele in brain and pancreas. Furthermore, the knockouts had severe mtDNA depletion and severe COX deficiency in pancreatic islets. The mitochondria of β-cells were more abundant and had an abnormal appearance with tubular cristae indicative of severe respiratory chain dysfunction. Histochemical analysis of islets from 7-week-old mice demonstrated a normal distribution of endocrine cells, normal total mean surface islet area and normal mean ratio of endocrine to exocrine pancreatic tissue. The mutant animals developed diabetes as reflected in increased non-fasting and fasting blood glucose levels from the age of 5 weeks. The non-fasting blood insulin levels were reduced at 7–9 weeks, suggesting that the primary cause of diabetes in these young mice was deficient insulin secretion caused by deficient β-cell function.

The hypothesis of impaired stimulus–secretion coupling in the knockout β-cells was further investigated by physiological *in vitro* studies of isolated islets. The β-cell stimulus–secretion coupling is initiated by glucose uptake and metabolism resulting in increased cytosolic ATP/ADP ratios, closure of ATP-dependent K^+-channels, depolarization of the plasma membrane, opening of voltage dependent L-type Ca^{2+}-channels, increase in cytoplasmic free Ca^{2+} concentration $[Ca^{2+}]_i$ and exocytosis of insulin-containing secretory granules. We found decreased polarization of the mitochondrial membrane potential after glucose stimulation, impaired $[Ca^{2+}]_i$ signalling, reduced insulin secretion after glucose stimulation, and normal total insulin content in knockout islets at the ages of 7–8 weeks. However, in 27–39-week-old mutant mice the phenotype was quite different. The *Tfam*$^-$ allele could no longer be detected in pancreas, the islets had normal COX activity, β-cell mitochondria appeared normal upon electron microscopy and there was an aberrant distribution of endocrine cells with loss of β-cells and a relative increase of other islet cell types. These findings suggest that the mutant β-cells were lost with time by an unknown mechanism.

It has been estimated that approximately 0.5–1 per cent of diabetes is caused by mutations in mtDNA and these patients have a phenotype similar to that in the β-cell *Tfam* knockout mice with decreased glucose-stimulated insulin secretion and reduced β-cell mass without any evidence of inflammation or apoptosis.[33] The mitochondrial diabetes mice thus provide genetic evidence for a critical role of the respiratory chain in normal glucose-induced insulin secretion and may prove useful for future investigations of the pathogenesis and treatment of mitochondrial diabetes.

Mitochondria have a central role in programmed cell death, apoptosis, and may induce apoptosis by releasing apoptosis inducing factors from the intermembrane space to the cytosol. This initiates a cascade of events which activates caspase 3 and results in DNA fragmentation. We noticed cell loss in pancreatic islets in the mitochondrial diabetes mouse model with β-cell-specific *Tfam* knockout, and cell loss has been reported in the brainstem and pancreatic islets in humans with respiratory chain dysfunction. In a recent report, it was demonstrated that COX-negative muscle fibres from patients with high levels of single mtDNA deletions or tRNA point mutations show signs compatible with apoptosis.[34] We analysed mouse embryos completely lacking Tfam and heart tissue with tissue-specific Tfam depletion, in order to further investigate the relationship between respiratory chain deficiency and apoptosis.[35] There was a significant increase in TUNEL-positive cells in mouse hearts and embryos with respiratory chain deficiency consistent with an active apoptotic process. Apoptosis could be confirmed in *Tfam* knockout hearts by visualizing DNA fragmentation on electrophoretic gels and by demonstrating the presence of activated caspase 3 and activated caspase 7. We also found that *Tfam* knockout embryos, which lack mtDNA and respiratory chain function, displayed no apoptosis at E8.5 and massive apoptosis at E9.5 followed by resorption of the embryo at E10.5. Thus, both embryonic and terminally differentiated cells with mtDNA depletion and respiratory chain deficiency are more apoptosis prone *in vivo* than normal cells. We also found increased levels of *Gpx* and *Sod2* transcripts and increased Gpx enzyme activity in *Tfam* knockout hearts suggesting an increased ROS defence. However, we could not detect any reduction in the activity of the ROS sensitive iron–sulphur cluster containing enzymes aconitase and SDH.

We also found increased transcript levels of the glycolytic enzyme glyceraldehyde-3-phosphate dehydrogenase in *Tfam* knockout hearts suggesting that glycolytic ATP production may be sufficient to maintain the ability to undergo apoptosis in respiratory-deficient cells. The exact mechanism by which respiratory-chain-deficient cells undergo apoptosis is not clear but it is likely that the reduced oxidative phosphorylation capacity affects the mitochondrial membrane potential, perhaps making the cells more likely to undergo mitochondrial membrane permeability transition whereby apoptosis-inducing factors are released to the cytosol. However, it still remains open if cytochrome *c*-mediated apoptosis is the main *in vivo* pathway in cells lacking mtDNA or whether other cytochrome *c*-independent pathways contribute to the process.

Interactions between the nuclear and mitochondrial genomes

Mutations of mtDNA can predispose to antibiotic-induced hearing loss in humans and nuclear genes modify the mtDNA-determined phenotype.[36] A systematic scheme of backcrosses in mice with age-associated hearing impairment due to nuclear gene defects has demonstrated that the extent of hearing loss can be modified by the mtDNA genotype.[37] The three different inbred mouse strains (A/J, NOD/LtJ and SKH2/J) with age related hearing loss were crossed to (CAST/Ei) mice with normal hearing. The F1 hybrids from these crosses all had normal hearing and they were systematically backcrossed to the different hearing-impaired strains. Surprisingly, in one of the strains (A/J) the hearing impairment was worse if the trait had been transmitted through the A/J mothers than if it had been transmitted through the CAST/Ei mothers indicative of a maternally inherited component. This phenomenon was only seen in mice homozygous for the A/J allele at the *Ahl* locus on chromosome 10 (D10Mit138 *Ahl*). Sequence comparison of mtDNA in the three hearing-deficient mice strains demonstrated a single nucleotide difference in the tRNA-arginine gene. The A/J mice contained mtDNA with 10 adenine repeats, whereas NOD/Ltj and SKH2/J carried nine adenines and the wild type CAST/Ei strain carried eight adenines at this position. Further studies are necessary to demonstrate direct interaction between the nuclear *Ahl* gene product and the mutated mitochondrial tRNA gene.

References

1. Esposito LA, Melov S, Panov A, Cottrell BA, and Wallace DC (1999). Mitochondrial disease in mouse results in increased oxidative stress. *Proc. Natl Acad. Sci. USA* **96**: 4820–4825.
2. Graham BH, Waymire KG, Cottrell B, Trounce IA, MacGregor GR, and Wallace DC (1997). A mouse model for mitochondrial myopathy and cardiomyopathy resulting from a deficiency in the heart/muscle isoform of the adenine nucleotide translocator. *Nat. Genet.* **16**: 226–234.
3. Kajander OA, Kunnas TA, Perola M, Lehtinen SK, Karhunen P J and Jacobs HT (1999). Long-extension PCR to detect deleted mitochondrial DNA molecules is compromized by technical a rtefacts. *Biochem. Biophys. Res. Commun.* **254**: 507–514.
4. Rosen DR (1993). Mutations in Cu/Zn superoxide dismutase gene are associated with familial amyotrophic lateral sclerosis. *Nature* **364**: 362.

5. Pasinelli P, Houseweart MK, Brown RH, and Cleveland DW (2000). Caspase-1 and -3 are sequentially activated in motor neuron death in Cu, Zn superoxide dismutase-mediated familial amyotrophic lateral sclerosis. *Proc. Natl Acad. Sci. USA* **97**: 13901–13906.

6. Carlsson LM, Jonsson J, Edlund T, and Marklund SL (1995). Mice lacking extracellular superoxide dismutase are more sensitive to hyperoxia. *Proc. Natl Acad. Sci. USA* **92**: 6264–6268.

7. Reaume AG, Elliott JL, Hoffman EK, Kowall NW, Ferrante RJ, Siwek DF, Wilcox HM, Flood DG, Beal MF, Brown RH, Scott RW, and Snider WD (1996). Motor neurons in Cu/Zn superoxide dismutase-deficient mice develop normally but exhibit enhanced cell death after axonal injury. *Nat. Genet.* **13**: 43–47.

8. Li Y, Huang TT, Carlson EJ, Melov S, Ursell PC, Olson JL, Noble LJ, Yoshimura MP, Berger C, Chan PH, *et al.* (1995). Dilated cardiomyopathy and neonatal lethality in mutant mice lacking manganese superoxide dismutase. *Nat. Genet.* **11**: 376–381.

9. Lebovitz RM, Zhang H, Vogel H, Cartwright J, Dionne L, Lu N, Huang S, and Matzuk MM (1996). Neurodegeneration, myocardial injury, and perinatal death in mitochondrial superoxide dismutase-deficient mice. *Proc. Natl Acad. Sci. USA* **93**: 9782–9787.

10. Melov S, Schneider JA, Day BJ, Hinerfeld D, Coskun P, Mirra SS, Crapo JD, and Wallace DC (1998). A novel neurological phenotype in mice lacking mitochondrial manganese superoxide dismutase. *Nat. Genet.* **18**: 159–163.

11. Melov S, Coskun P, Patel M, Tuinstra R, Cottrell B, Jun AS, Zastawny TH, Dizdaroglu M, Goodman SI, Huang TT, Miziorko H, Epstein CJ, and Wallace DC (1999). Mitochondrial disease in superoxide dismutase 2 mutant mice. *Proc. Natl Acad. Sci. USA* **96**: 846–851.

12. Williams MD, Van Remmen H, Conrad CC, Huang TT, Epstein CJ, and Richardson A (1998). Increased oxidative damage is correlated to altered mitochondrial function in heterozygous manganese superoxide dismutase knockout mice. *J. Biol. Chem.* **273**: 28510–28515.

13. Inoue K, Nakada K, Ogura A, Isobe K, Goto Y, Nonaka I, and Hayashi JI (2000). Generation of mice with mitochondrial dysfunction by introducing mouse mtDNA carrying a deletion into zygotes. *Nat. Genet.* **26**: 176–181.

14. Larsson NG and Clayton DA (1995). Molecular genetic aspects of human mitochondrial disorders. *Annu. Rev. Genet.* **29**: 151–178.

15. Dunbar DR, Moonie PA, Swingler RJ, Davidson D, Roberts R, and Holt IJ (1993). Maternally transmitted partial direct tandem duplication of mitochondrial DNA associated with diabetes mellitus. *Hum. Mol. Genet.* **2**: 1619–1624.

16. Poulton J, Deadman ME, and Gardiner RM (1989). Duplications of mitochondrial DNA in mitochondrial myopathy *Lancet* **1(8632)**: 236–240.

17. Rotig A, Bessis JL, Romero N, Cormier V, Saudubray JM, Narcy P, Lenoir G, Rustin P, and Munnich A (1992). Maternally inherited duplication of the mitochondrial genome in a syndrome of proximal tubulopathy, diabetes mellitus, and cerebellar ataxia. *Am. J. Hum. Genet.* **50**: 364–370.

18. Bernes SM, Bacino C, Prezant TR, Pearson MA, Wood TS, Fournier P, and Fischel-Ghodsian N (1993). Identical mitochondrial DNA deletion in mother with progressive external ophthalmoplegia and son with Pearson marrow-pancreas syndrome. *J. Pediatr.* **123**: 598–602.

19. Graff C, Wredenberg A, Silva JP, Bui TH, Borg K, and Larsson NG (2000). Complex genetic counselling and prenatal analysis in a woman with external ophthalmoplegia and deleted mtDNA. *Prenat. Diagn.* **20**: 426–431.

20. Larsson NG, Eiken HG, Boman H, Holme E, Oldfors A, and Tulinius MH (1992). Lack of transmission of deleted mtDNA from a woman with Kearns-Sayre syndrome to her child. *Am. J. Hum. Genet.* **50**: 360–363.

21. Kearsey SE and Craig IW (1981). Altered ribosomal RNA genes in mitochondria from mammalian cells with chloramphenicol resistance. *Nature* **290**: 607–608.

22. Levy SE, Waymire KG, Kim YL, MacGregor GR, and Wallace DC (1999). Transfer of chloramphenicol-resistant mitochondrial DNA into the chimeric mouse. *Transgen. Res.* **8**: 137–145.

23. Sligh JE, Levy SE, Waymire KG, Allard P, Dillehay DL, Nusinowitz S, Heckenlively JR, MacGregor GR, and Wallace DC (2000). Maternal germ-line transmission of mutant mtDNAs from embryonic stem cell-derived chimeric mice. *Proc. Natl Acad. Sci. USA* **97**: 14461–14466.

24. Parisi MA and Clayton DA (1991). Similarity of human mitochondrial transcription factor 1 to high mobility group proteins. *Science* **252**: 965–969.

25. Larsson NG, Wang J, Wilhelmsson H, Oldfors A, Rustin P, Lewandoski M, Barsh GS, and Clayton DA (1998). Mitochondrial transcription factor A is necessary for mtDNA maintenance and embryogenesis in mice. *Nat. Genet.* **18**: 231–236.

26. Wang J, Wilhelmsson H, Graff C, Li H, Oldfors A, Rustin P, Bruning JC, Kahn CR, Clayton DA, Barsh GS, Thoren P, and Larsson NG (1999). Dilated cardiomyopathy and atrioventricular conduction blocks induced by heart-specific inactivation of mitochondrial DNA gene expression. *Nat. Genet.* **21**: 133–137.

27. England JM, Costantino P, and Attardi G (1978). Mitochondrial RNA and protein synthesis in enucleated African green monkey cells. *J. Mol. Biol.* **119**: 455–462.

28. Li H, Wang J, Wilhelmsson H, Hansson A, Thoren P, Duffy J, Rustin P, and Larsson NG (2000). Genetic modification of survival in tissue-specific knockout mice with mitochondrial cardiomyopathy. *Proc. Natl Acad. Sci. USA* **97**: 3467–3472.

29. Silva JP, Kohler M, Graff C, Oldfors A, Magnuson MA, Berggren PO, and Larsson NG (2000). Impaired insulin secretion and beta-cell loss in tissue-specific knockout mice with mitochondrial diabetes. *Nat. Genet.* **26**: 336–340.

30. Hayashi J, Ohta S, Kikuchi A, Takemitsu M, Goto Y, and Nonaka I (1991). Introduction of disease-related mitochondrial DNA deletions into HeLa cells lacking mitochondrial DNA results in mitochondrial dysfunction. *Proc. Natl Acad. Sci. USA* **88**: 10614–10618.

31. Lansman RA and Clayton DA (1975). Selective nicking of mammalian mitochondrial DNA in vivo: photosensitization by incorporation of 5-bromodeoxyuridine. *J. Mol. Biol.* **99**: 761–776.

32. Moslemi AR, Selimovic N, Bergh CH, and Oldfors A (2000). Fatal dilated cardiomyopathy associated with a mitochondrial DNA deletion. *Cardiology* **94**: 68–71.

33. Otabe S, Yasuda K, Mori Y, Shimokawa K, Kadowaki H, Jimi A, Nonaka K, Akanuma Y, Yazaki Y, and Kadowaki T (1999). Molecular and histological evaluation of pancreata from patients with a mitochondrial gene mutation associated with impaired insulin secretion. *Biochem. Biophys. Res. Commun.* **259**: 149–156.

34. Mirabella M, Di Giovanni S, Silvestri G, Tonali P, and Servidei S (2000). Apoptosis in mitochondrial encephalomyopathies with mitochondrial DNA mutations: a potential pathogenic mechanism. *Brain* **123**: 93–104.

35. Wang J, Silva JP, Gustafsson CM, Rustin P, and Larsson NG (2001). Increased *in vivo* apoptosis in cells lacking mitochondiral DNA gene expression. *Proc. Natl Acad. Sci. USA* **7**: 4038–4043.

36. Bykhovskaya Y, Estivill X, Taylor K, Hang T, Hamon M, Casano RA, Yang H, Rotter JI, Shohat M, and Fischel-Ghodsian N (2000). Candidate locus for a nuclear modifier gene for maternally inherited deafness. *Am. J. Hum. Genet.* **66**: 1905–1910.

37. Johnson KR, Zheng QY, Bykhovskaya Y, Spirina O, and Fischel-Ghodsian N (2001). A nuclear-mitochondrial DNA interaction affecting hearing impairment in mice. *Nat. Genet.* **27**: 191–194.

38. Cossee M, Puccio H, Gansmuller A, Koutnikova H, Dierich A, LeMeur M, Fischbeck K, Dolle P, and Koenig M (2000). Inactivation of the Friedreich ataxia mouse gene leads to early embryonic lethality without iron accumulation. *Hum. Mol. Genet.* **9**: 1219–1226.

39. Puccio H, Simon D, Cossee M, Criqui-Filipe P, Tiziano F, Melki J, Hindelang C, Matyas R, Rustin P and Koenig M (2001). Mouse models for Friedreich ataxia exhibit cardiomyopathy, sensory nerve defect and Fe-S enzyme deficiency followed by intramitochondrial iron deposits. *Nat. Genet.* **27**: 181–186.

40. Babcock M, de Silva D, Oaks R, Davis-Kaplan S, Jiralerspong S, Montermini L, Pandolfo M, and Kaplan, J (1997). Regulation of mitochondrial iron accumulation by Yfh1p, a putative homolog of frataxin. *Science* **276**: 1709–1712.

16 Transmission, genetic counselling, and prenatal diagnosis of mitochondrial DNA disease

Joanna Poulton, Vincent Macaulay, and
David R Marchington

Mitochondrial DNA is maternally inherited in humans. Thousands of copies of mitochondrial DNA are present in every cell and in most normal individuals these are virtually identical. Mitochondrial diseases may be caused by mutations in either mitochondrial or nuclear genes and hence give rise to maternal or autosomal patterns of inheritance. Antenatal diagnosis of mitochondrial diseases based on chorionic villus sampling (CVS) is available for Mendelian disorders and the syndromes caused by a limited number of human mitochondrial DNA mutations. However, prenatal diagnosis of many other maternally inherited mitochondrial diseases is less reliable because it is currently not possible to predict accurately how the level of pathological and normal mitochondrial DNA will change later in gestation or throughout life. This review focuses on the substantial progress that has been made recently in understanding transmission, genetic counselling, and prenatal diagnosis of mitochondrial diseases.

Modes of inheritance of mitochondrial diseases

Unlike nuclear DNA, where there are usually only two copies of each gene per cell, thousands of copies of mitochondrial DNA (mtDNA) are present in every nucleated cell. Normal individuals are homoplasmic (i.e. virtually all copies of their mtDNA are identical). Heteroplasmy (the presence of both normal and mutant mtDNA in a single individual, tissue, or cell) is common to many mtDNA diseases, so that the proportion of mutant mtDNA in any cell or tissue may vary from 0 to 100 per cent. Change in the level of mtDNA variants over time is termed segregation. Segregation of mtDNA mutants in the germ line is the thrust of this chapter. Segregation of mtDNA mutants in somatic tissues and cell lines is discussed in Chapter 14.

The polypeptides encoded by mtDNA are all subunits of the oxidative phosphorylation system (OPS), a highly complex array of multimeric enzymes which produce ATP (see Chapter 4). The majority of these are encoded in the nucleus, as are all the proteins involved in mtDNA maintenance and expression, and other mitochondrial functions. Hence, there are potentially a large number of diseases with a Mendelian pattern of inheritance.

Maternally inherited mtDNA diseases

Mitochondrial DNA mutants cause diverse phenotypes in different organisms due to impaired respiratory chain function: the *petit* colony morphology with loss of aerobic respiration in yeast, cytoplasmic male sterility and non-chromosomal stripe in higher plants, and neurological or multisystem disease in man. The latter include mtDNA rearrangements[1] which cause sporadic Kearns–Sayre syndrome, Pearson's syndrome[2] or maternally inherited diabetes and deafness;[3] point mutations which cause mitochondrial encephalopathy with lactic acidosis and stroke-like episodes (MELAS),[4] myoclonic epilepsy with ragged red fibres (MERRF)[5] and Leber's Hereditary Optic Neuropathy (LHON).[6] Heteroplasmy (the presence of both normal and mutant mtDNA in a single individual) is present in many such mtDNA diseases, so that the proportion of mutant mtDNA in any cell or tissue may vary from 0 to 100 per cent. In some tissues the level of mutant changes successively with time, for instance, falling in blood[7] and accumulating in non-dividing cells such as muscle.[8] In most disorders, there appears to be a threshold effect such that tissues function normally unless the proportion of mutant rises above a particular level. Heteroplasmy may underlie some of the variability in penetrance and severity of mtDNA disorders. Preferential accumulation of mutant mtDNAs in affected tissues appears to explain their progressive nature.[9,10] Such a mechanism cannot be the explanation in LHON due to the G11778A[6] mutation which is commonly homoplasmic. The MtDNA haplotype analysis in this disorder demonstrates a high degree of homogeneity, consistent with a small number of founder mutations. Hence mitochondrial genetic variation is less likely to underlie the differences than other genetic or environmental factors (see the Section on 'Involvement of mtDNA in multifactorial disorders').

The main part of this chapter will focus on mechanisms of transmission and genetic advice to individuals with maternally inherited mtDNA disease.

Mendelian mitochondrial diseases

Over the past few years there have been a number of publications on the cloning of nuclear genes for mitochondrial diseases. Mutations in genes encoding subunits of the respiratory chain or involved in its assembly have been identified in children with severe diseases presenting early in life (Table 16.1).[11] Almost all of these are autosomal recessive and hence have

Table 16.1 Summary of bottleneck estimations in humans using a single selection model

Study number	mtDNA mutant	Severity of mtDNA mutant	Proportion of mutant mtDNA in mother	Median final proportion of mutant mtDNA (%)	Estimated bottleneck size (median)	Reference
1	Polymorphism	No effect	98%	2	1–2	31
2	G8993T	Mild	Blood 50%*	99	1	32
3	A3243G	Severe	Blood 7% Muscle 18%	8		29
4	mtDNA deletions mtDNA duplications	Very severe Mild	Ovary 22%	19	9	30

a 1 in 4 recurrence risk in siblings of affected individuals. *Surf* 1 is numerically the most important. Mutations in this gene underlie 75 per cent of cytochrome oxidase deficient Leighs syndrome, that is about 10–20 per cent of all Leigh's syndrome.[12] In addition mutations have been identified in various subunits of Complex 1, in proteins involved in assembly[13] or transport of macromolecules into mitochondria.[14]

Mutations have also been identified in genes involved in mtDNA replication, repair or maintenance in association with mtDNA depletion or multiple deletions.[15] Four of these disorders present in adult life with proximal external ophthalmoplegia, neurigenic weakness and multiple mtDNA rearrangements. Mutations in thymidine phosphorylase (TP) underlie recessive MNGIE (myoneurogastrointestinal encephalomyopathy) in which mtDNA depletion and multiple mtDNA deletions co-exist. TP is a trifunctional protein involved in turnover of nucleotides.[16] Mutations in at least three different genes underlying dominantly inherited proximal external ophthalmoplegia (AdPEO) have been identified in recent years: mitochondrial DNA polymerase (POLG), the mitochondrial adenine nucleotide transporter (ANT) and a DNA helicase named Twinkle.

Mitochondrial DNA depletion is a heterogeneous group of disorders usually presenting in infancy or childhood. The mtDNA in these patients was previously held to be qualitatively normal but quantitatively reduced in affected tissues. Much as patients with TP deficiency may have mtDNA depletion in addition to mtDNA deletions, it is likely that there are low levels of heteroplasmic mtDNA mutations.[17] Most of the familial cases have been identified in a single generation in sibships and are hence likely to be autosomally recessive. However, dominant inheritance has been identified in one family. Mutations have been identified in deoxyguanosine kinase (DGUOK) in consanguinous Druze kindreds presenting with liver disease[18] and in mitochondrial thymidine kinase (TK2)[19] in patients with a pure myopathic presentation. The precise role of these proteins in the pathogenesis of the various disorders is unknown.

Involvement of mtDNA in multifactorial disorders

It is now clear that mitochondria are involved in some multifactorial and polygenic diseases. In most of the cases that have been studied, a homoplasmic mtDNA mutant is maternally transmitted and interacts with environmental or other genetic factors. Hence these are maternally inherited disorders whose penetrance is variable. For instance, maternally inherited deafness results from interaction of the 1555 mtDNA mutation with an environmental factor. Exposure to aminoglycoside antibiotics increases the penetrance and lowers the age of onset of deafness associated with this mutation. In another well-characterized example, nuclear and mitochondrial genes interact to cause deafness associated with senescence in mice. In addition to linkage to a nuclear marker, Johnson *et al.*[20] demonstrated a clear maternally inherited component, linked to a specific mitochondrial haplotype with a candidate mtDNA mutation in an ERNA gene.

We have recently demonstrated an association between a common mtDNA variant in man (henceforth the 16189 variant), and four multifactorial phenotypes: type 2 diabetes, thinness at birth, dilated cardiomyopathy and penetrance in homozygotes for the haemochromatosis C282Y allele. The increased risks are conferred by the 16189 variant arising on multiple different mtDNA haplotypes and in several different ethnic groups. This excludes a founder effect and strongly suggests that the effect is caused by the 16189 variant *per se*. The T → C transition at 16189 bp is almost always homoplasmic. It gives rise to a homopolymeric C tract that frequently results in heteroplasmic length variation near to control sequences in the large non-coding region but as yet the effect on function is unknown. The data suggest that the risk of diabetes conferred by this mitochondrial variant interacts with both genetic and environmental factors. Because the majority of mitochondrial proteins are encoded by autosomal genes such interactions are intuitively likely. They probably underlie the variability in penetrance in many mtDNA diseases where mutant load does not explain variable penetrance or tissue specificity, of which LHON is a good example (see Chapter 8).

Inheritance of mtDNA

Maternal and paternal transmission of mtDNA

Like all extra-chromosomal DNA, including chloroplast and plastid DNA, mtDNA is generally maternally inherited. In humans the term *mitochondrial inheritance* is synonymous with *maternal inheritance*. At fertilization, the sperm contributes about 500 mtDNAs, or 0.5 per cent of the total DNA to the zygote. Studies of paternal transmission in intraspecific mouse crosses, show that paternal mtDNA is lost very early in embryogenesis. Paternal mitochondria labelled with vital dyes prior to *in vitro* fertilization (IVF) are degraded by the early pre-nucleus stage apparently via ubiquitinylation. However, in mouse interspecific crosses, paternal mtDNA is detectable right from single cell embryos through to neonates albeit at low levels (<1 per cent).[21] However, the paternal mtDNA is restricted to certain tissues and is not transmitted to offspring, hence it does not enter the germ line. Transmission of paternal mtDNA in mouse thus appears to be unlikely.[22] In man the possibility of paternal transmission has become an issue because of advances in treatment of male infertility due to a deficiency in numbers of sperm (oligospermia). It is now possible to generate viable human embryos by microinjection of single sperm from oligospermic men into unfertilized human oocytes (so called ICSI for intracytoplasmic sperm injection). As the sperm tail mitochondria may be specifically excluded from the embryo during natural fertilization, this procedure might introduce more paternal mtDNA than normal. This is a real issue, because evidence is accumulating that mitochondrial dysfunction may contribute to male infertility.[23,24] The procedure may therefore increase the likelihood of injecting mtDNA carrying pathogenic mutants. However, current studies suggest that no detectable paternal contribution results from this procedure. There is however, a unique case report of a patient with mitochondrial disease where a mutation arose on paternal mtDNA.[25] No wild type paternal mtDNA was detectable in any tissue, and the mutant paternal mtDNA was detectable only in muscle where it comprised 90 per cent of mtDNA. It would thus appear that the mtDNA mutation conferred an exceptional advantage to the mutant mtDNA, but only in the myogenic lineage. Hence, it is likely that paternal transmission of mtDNA is rare. This can readily be inferred from the apparent absence of mtDNA recombination in human lineages,[26] although this is controversial.[26,27] From here onwards, we will ignore the potential paternal contribution because it is clear that the vast majority of mtDNA is maternally inherited.

Presumed benefit of uniparental inheritance of mtDNA

All mitochondrial genomes encode only a small number of polypeptides. The nucleus encodes the vast majority of respiratory chain subunits and all of the proteins needed for mitochondrial biogenesis. There are therefore potentially a large number of important interactions between mitochondrial and nuclear genomes. The constraints of these requirements may explain the high level of uniformity (homoplasmy) among mtDNAs *within* an individual, contrasting with the great diversity of mtDNA *between* individuals. The mutation rate of mtDNA is substantially higher than that of nuclear DNA. It is generally held that the vast majority of non-neutral mutations are likely to be detrimental. An organism's population of mtDNA will accumulate an increasing number of deleterious mutations by a process known as Muller's ratchet.[28] This is an irreversible 'ratchet' because once a detrimental point mutation has occurred, the chance of a compensatory or back mutation is low. Hence, if transmission is random and unrestricted, the offspring should become successively less fit. Therefore, any organism transmitting DNA uniparentally or by asexual reproduction needs a means of preventing the accumulation of detrimental mutants. Uniparental inheritance excludes accumulation of mtDNA mutations from one parent. In addition, the genetic bottleneck (restriction in the number of founder mtDNA molecules) eliminates or reduces the variation between mtDNAs in the offspring. In humans and mice, this bottleneck apparently occurs during oocyte development (see Section on 'The mitochondrial bottleneck' below).

Furthermore, the importance of homoplasmy is implied by (i) the instability of mtDNA heteroplasmy in unicellular organisms and (ii) the existence of a genetic bottleneck in multicellular organisms as diverse as maize and man.

The mitochondrial bottleneck

There are examples where all the copies of mtDNA in a mother differ from those of her offspring by a single nucleotide. Hence, complete switching of mtDNA type has occurred in a single generation. Because oocytes contain approximately 100,000 mtDNAs and yet the mutation probably only occurs once, there must be a restriction in mtDNA numbers followed by amplification, whereby the mutant mtDNA becomes the mitochondrial founder for the child. We refer to this as a genetic 'bottleneck'. After birth, there may also be segregation of mtDNAs so that affected individuals have different levels of mutant mtDNA in different tissues, different cells within a tissue and perhaps even different mitochondria. In practice, however, the mean level of mutant in the offspring and oocytes is typically close to that of the mother.[29,30] While this is probably the truest for the level in the mother's ovaries, it will also be reflected by her other tissues (see the Section on 'Is there selection of mtDNAs in the germ line?', for the limitations in the case of A3243G mutation).

The mitochondrial bottleneck in human oocytes and pre-implantation embryos
We investigated the bottleneck in normal oocytes from couples in our IVF clinic referred for male infertility. We used naturally occurring length variation in the large non-coding region of mtDNA. This region of mtDNA deviates from the rule that homoplasmy is the norm, as some individuals are heteroplasmic for different length variants. We showed that there is little or no difference in the frequency distribution of length variants between several different tissues from any normal individual. We studied a heteroplasmic length variant in oocytes from controls and from a patient with a pathogenic mtDNA mutation and showed that segregation of founder mtDNA molecules has probably occurred by the time the oocytes are mature.[31] A similar result was obtained from oocytes of a woman with the A3243G mutation.[29] We demonstrated that no such segregation occurred in multiple samples of placenta (unpublished). Further studies are essential as the apparent bottleneck size may depend on the

mtDNA mutation. For instance, segregation was very marked in a family carrying the mtDNA mutation at position T8993G[32] compared with a patient with the mtDNA rearrangement.[30] Hence the confidence limits for recurrence risks are extremely wide in the former.

If mutant mtDNA remains uniformly distributed among individual cells of the embryo it should be possible to assess the level of mutant mtDNA prenatally, by CVS or pre-implantation embryos. In a recent study, blastomeres in pre-implantation embryos derived from a woman with the A3243G mutation were analysed (RP Jansen *et al.*, personal communication), every blastomere contained very similar levels of mutant mtDNA.

Few carrier/affected foetuses have been analysed for load of mutant mtDNA in different tissues. However, the limited existing data from studies on human foetuses or neonates with pathogenic mtDNA mutations also suggest that the proportion of mutant mtDNA in different tissues is more uniform than in adults. Hence, mtDNA do not appear to segregate much during embryogenesis.[33-35]

Animal models of the bottleneck 1: polymorphic variants
Four groups have recently constructed heteroplasmic mouse models of mtDNA segregation by introducing donor cytoplasm into a fertilized recipient mouse egg.[36-39] Analysis of developing female germ cells demonstrated that the major component of the bottleneck occurs between the primordial germ cell and primary oocyte stage. As in humans, these data imply that the major component of the bottleneck has occured by the time oocytes are mature.

Blastomeres from pre-implantation embryos derived from heteroplasmic oocytes in mouse contained very similar levels of mutant mtDNA.[37,40]

In two of the animal models of heteroplasmic mtDNA segregation the proportion of each mtDNA variant was uniform in all tissues of the foetus's analysed. Taken together, these studies suggest that a major bottleneck occurs during oogenesis and that mtDNA segregates little during embryogenesis.

However, in two of these experiments there was tissue-specific, directional selection for different mtDNA genotypes in the same animal after birth.[39,41] While this type of segregation occurs in human diseases, these animal studies used non-pathogenic mtDNA: no clear defect of mitochondrial function was detectable.[42] Furthermore, when liver cells were harvested from liver that was nearly homoplasmic for one of the mtDNA types were cultured, selection went in the opposite direction. This suggests that there are tissue-specific factors conferring an advantage to one type of mtDNA *in vivo* that are different in cell culture. In summary, little segregation has been observed before birth in mice. If confirmed in humans this will simplify prenatal diagnosis. The factors governing segregation in somatic cells are discussed in more detail in Chapter 14.

Animal models of the bottleneck 2: detrimental variants
There are now mouse models of two different groups of deleterious mtDNA mutations but in neither has there been extensive analysis of mtDNA segregation or constellations of phenotypes that are classical for mtDNA disease. Mitochondria harbouring a mtDNA mutation in a ribosomal gene which confers chloramphenicol resistance (CAP[r]) and a respiratory defect in cultured cells were introduced into mouse embryonic stem (ES) cells and used to create chimeric mice. CAP[r] mtDNA was detectable in all of 10 types of tissue in 7 chimeric mice, but not in all tissues in all of the mice that we analysed. This demonstrated that transmitochondrial ES cells are still pluripotent and suggested that this method can be used to generate mice that

are chimeric and potentially transgenic for mtDNA mutants.[43] Other investigators obtained germ line transmission using a different CAP[r] mutation but found that the phenotype was severe and resulted in foetal death.[44] Survivors had myopathy and dilated cardiomyopathy and the oldest pup died at 11 days.

Another group succeeded in generating mice with rearranged mtDNA[45] (see Chapter 15). Unlike human phenotypes where mtDNA deletions are usually sporadic, transmission of this rearranged mtDNA followed a maternal inheritance pattern. There was histological but not clinical evidence of muscle involvement and the main cause of death was renal failure, a rare occurrence in human mtDNA diseases. Therefore these studies are not exact parallels of human mtDNA disease. Hayashi and colleagues also used their model to assert that complementation occurs between donor and recipient mtDNAs arguing that similar cytochrome oxidase activity in all mitochondria within a cell implies that each mitochondrion contains a similar proportion of wt-DNA and mutant mtDNA. This in turn suggests that there must be complete mixing of donor and recipient mtDNAs. While this may well turn out to be correct, the published data set is incomplete as the origin of wt-mtDNA (whether donor or recipient) was not determined, nor the precise types of rearrangement present. The presence of duplicated mtDNA may influence the segregation of rearranged mtDNAs, particularly if higher forms such as triplications are present. Such factors are very likely to influence apparent bottleneck sizes in the case of mtDNA rearrangements.[46]

Bottleneck size

Two types of mathematical model have been used to describe the mitochondrial bottleneck, differing in whether they consider a single or multiple selections (see Box 16.1). The most widely used assumes that the bottleneck occurs as a result of mtDNA segregation over 30 identical cell divisions, during which the mtDNA content of the cell partitions stochastically. The model is a poor fit in biological terms because reality does not fit these assumptions: the mtDNA content of the oocyte varies fifty to hundred-fold, indeed there appears to be no mtDNA synthesis early in embryogenesis, from zygote to blastocyst. Furthermore, there may be selection of mtDNAs based on phenotypic or selfish mechanisms. There appears to be a high degree of cytoplasmic organization in the late stages of oogenesis precluding total mtDNA mixing and stochastic partitioning. Furthermore polarity of the embryo is evident even in the zygote, suggesting that mitochondria are unlikely to segregate as single independent units even early in embryogenesis. Hence, the packaging of mtDNAs into daughter cells may reflect their location within the zygote at the time of fertilization. If the cytoplasmic organization of the oocyte is maintained during the first cell divisions, the segregation of a heteroplasmic mtDNA population would depend mostly on the mtDNAs that were founders for each cytoplasmic region. After the last mitotic division of oogenesis, oocytes undergo a massive increase in size (~twenty-fold) during which there is presumably multiclonal proliferation of mtDNAs.[47] In this case, a single selection model may be the more physiological. The best description of mtDNA segregation during oogenesis may ultimately be an iterative process drawing upon both single and multiple selection models.

In practice, both single and multiple selection models generate frequency distributions for heteroplasmic oocytes/offspring of a similar shape, even though the bottleneck size (or number of segregating unites, n) is radically different. The advantage of the single selection model is that it can be used to model recurrence risks 'on the back of an envelope' in the clinic for counselling patients.

Box 16.1

The inheritance of mtDNA lends itself to population genetic modelling in miniature. The same mathematical machinery that has been developed to describe the sampling of genes from generation to generation in a population can be invoked to treat the sampling of mtDNA genomes during oogenesis. This sampling process—the cause of the fluctuation of allele frequencies in populations ('genetic drift')—leads to changes in the proportions of heteroplasmy between a mother and her children. The Wright–Fisher model presents an idealization of the situation. Suppose a mother is heteroplasmic at some position in her mtDNA with a level of mutant equal to p_0. In the course of development of the germ line, the level of mutant can fluctuate just because of the stochastic nature of the sampling process. The intensity of fluctuation depends on the number of molecules that are sampled at each stage: small numbers lead to large fluctuations, larger numbers to less.

After one round of sampling, where N molecules are taken, the number of mutant molecules is described by a binomial distribution. After g rounds of sampling, the distribution does not take a simple mathematical form. However, some of its properties can be obtained easily. In particular, the expected value does not change from the starting value p_0, and the variance satisfies:

$$V = p_0(1 - p_0)(1 - (1 - N^{-1})^g)$$

To a good approximation, this variance only depends on g/N. That is, a tight bottleneck (N small) for a few rounds of sampling (g small) is equivalent to a mild bottleneck (N large) for many rounds (g large), at least as far as the variance is concerned.

This result has been used as a way to estimate N, by the method of moments.[48] That is, by assuming a group of siblings represent separate realizations of the sampling process, the variance can be estimated from data and the above expression inverted to obtain N (to assign g, each sampling event is assumed to correspond to a cell division in the germ line).

Since we do not really know much about the number of molecules being sampled throughout the process of oogenesis, Bendall *et al.*[49] took the view that you might as well take $g = 1$. They used a Bayesian approach to infer N in this case, within pedigrees. Even if the model is not an accurate representation of the biological processes, you can think of this number as the effective size of the bottleneck. More explicit models of oogenesis are clearly needed. Chinnery and Samuels[50] have made a start.

The above describes the picture when all mtDNAs are considered equal. The role that selection might play in the segregation process is still unclear, and more theoretical work is needed.

Is there selection of mtDNAs in the germ line?

Given the appealing view that the mtDNA bottleneck improves the biological fitness of offspring, one might assume that there would be a high rate of foetal attrition for germ cells or embryos with a high level of a detrimental mtDNA mutant. This can be investigated by looking at (i) the fertility of women carrying mtDNA mutants, which might be reduced and the difference in the mean percentage mutant mtDNA in (ii) mother and offspring or (iii) ovary and oocytes.

Two parameters must be considered before embarking upon this discussion, bottleneck size and stability of the mean level of mutant mtDNA. Firstly, if mtDNAs segregate stochastically, the progeny of cells that are heteroplasmic for two neutral mtDNA polymorphisms should tend to segregate to 100 per cent one type or the other after enough cell divisions. Hence, other factors such as phenotypic selection must be operating in cell cultures where this does not occur. For example, in cells containing mtDNA mutants that confer a severe phenotype,

100 per cent mutant mtDNA may never be reached. Secondly, segregation to 100 per cent (mutant or wild-type) will be slow where number of segregating units is large (for instance, in a cell with many thousands of mtDNAs where the number of mtDNAs per mitochondrion is 1 and mitochondria segregate independently). Hence, bottleneck sizes can appear to be large either because the number of segregating units is genuinely large, or because selective pressures are operating. Conversely, small bottleneck sizes may indicate that the number of segregating units is small, perhaps because of a mtDNA segregation defect, or because of stochastic mtDNA segregation.

Secondly, the mean level of mutant mtDNA in a population may alter either because of selection, or drift due to a small number of segregating units. A consistent tendency for the mean to shift in a specific direction suggests selection rather than drift, but stability does not indicate the absence of selection. Indeed we suggest that opposing selection pressures are the norm in cultures of cells with severe mtDNA phenotypes.

In Drosophila, it is clear that impaired mitochondrial function may reduce both male and female fertility. The fertility of women carrying the A3243G mutant appears no different from controls,[51] so if foetal attrition occurs then its effect on the whole population is small. Chinnery and colleagues collated published data on the difference in level of mutant mtDNA in blood from mothers and their offspring in some of the commonest maternally transmitted mtDNA diseases.[52] Unfortunately the interpretation of such data is hampered by several problems. Firstly, the data are subject to reporting bias, even if the proband is omitted from the analysis. Secondly, longitudinal studies suggest that the level of mutant mtDNA in blood may decline with time in the two commonest severe mutations, namely mtDNA deletions[53] and A3243G.[7] It is likely that such a decline occurs for all heteroplasmic mutations in which the level of mutant mtDNA in blood is lower than muscle.[54] For A3243G, the rate of decline is proportional to the initial load of mutant mtDNA.[7] Hence the initial maternal load will be underestimated by more than that of the offspring, particularly in mothers with a high level of mutant mtDNA in muscle. Hence neither the mean nor the distribution of the difference in level of mutant mtDNA between mothers and offspring can be used to make inferences about this process, as Chinnery *et al.* attempted to do. The only studies that are truly informative about this process are those on animals and on human oocytes. There are only four relevant studies on humans, summarized in Table 16.1. The mean level of mutant mtDNA was lower in oocytes than in ovary (study 4) or in muscle (which is likely to be closer to the level in ovary than the level in blood study 3). Both involved severe mtDNA mutations that undergo selection in cell culture (see Chapter 14) so it is likely that selection against these mutants occurred. This is consistent with the tabulated estimates of bottleneck size, which should be magnified by such processes. In contrast, the bottleneck size for a neutral polymorphism and the phenotypically mild T8993C mutation are small, suggesting that little if any selection occurs in these cases. This may be reflected by large swings in per cent mutant either up or down (studies 1 and 2). In the published mouse studies, the proportion of mtDNA types in ovary was not recorded. In a subsequent study it is clear that the proportion of the BALB mtDNA always increased in spleen (surrogate for level in blood as this comprises mainly lymphocytes) and, by analogy with pathogenic mutations in humans, is likely to be the 'fittest' of the 2 genotypes in these mice, although this must be subtle as it was not measurable.[42] The overall trend is that the level of BALB for the mother (not specifically in ovary) is lower than the level for the offspring or developing oocytes, consistent with selection against the disadvantageous type.

In conclusion, we have suggested that selection against detrimental mtDNA mutants operates during oocyte maturation, as this is the simplest explanation of the data on the human and mouse germ line. In severe pathogenic mutants this results in a trend towards a lower proportion of mutant mtDNA in the offspring/oocytes and a larger apparent bottleneck. In milder/polymorphic mtDNA variants the apparent bottleneck size is smaller and consequently swings between generations can be much larger. This contrasts with the assumptions made by previous investigators who are not able to explain the apparent differences in bottleneck sizes.[32,29,52]

Genetic management of mitochondrial disease

Estimating recurrence risks

Diseases in which the molecular basis is known
Autosomal.   Current data suggests that the recurrence risks for autosomal recessive disorders, such as MNGIE and recessively inherited mtDNA depletion are likely to be up to 25 per cent . However, as both these disorders have autosomal dominant phenocopies, molecular confirmation is important.

MtDNA rearrangements.   The recurrence risk for pure mtDNA deletions is likely to be very low (<1–5 per cent). If mtDNA duplications are present the recurrence risk is higher. We therefore suggest that excluding mtDNA duplications is an important component to genetic counselling.

8993.   Recurrence risks for the 8993 mutation depend on the base change, the T8993G being more severe than T8993A. The situation has been ably summarized by White *et al.*,[55] see Figs 16.1 and 16.2. The confidence intervals are very wide.

3243.   Recurrence risks in families carrying the A3243G mutation are particularly difficult, because the level of mutant mtDNA in different tissues is more variable than for mutations at 8993 bp. In particular, the level of mutant mtDNA falls with time in blood. This makes it difficult to assess the mother's mutant load. Published data[52] is likely to have reporting bias. We therefore favour a policy of honesty about the uncertainties. In patients with levels of <30 per cent A4354G mutant mtDNA in muscle and/or <10 per cent in blood the recurrence risk is low (maybe 15–25 per cent). In patients with symptoms (other than just diabetes and/or deafness) and/or a mutant load >50 per cent in muscle We advise a high recurrence risk >60 per cent.

8344.   Chinnery *et al.*[52] have collated useful information about levels of mutant which are around 80, 20, and 15 per cent for women with levels of 80–100, 60–80, and 40–60 per cent mutant, respectively (Fig. 16.3). Offspring of women with lower levels of mutant are at low risk.

LHON.   There is little reliable data on recurrence risks for individual LHON mutations. Most authors state the recurrence risks for the 11778 mutation and state that the levels for 3460 and 14484 are similar. In fact, the relative risk to women is higher in 3460 families as the sex ratio is less skewed to males.[56] The most comprehensive report by Harding probably overestimates risks as ascertainment is less complete than in the Australian studies. Risks to female and male offspring of affected mothers are higher than to unaffected (50, 77, 9, and 50 per cent,

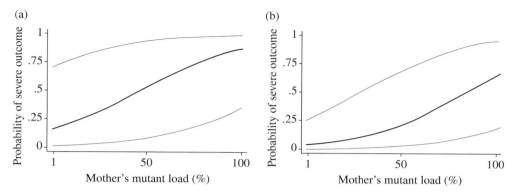

Fig. 16.1 Phenotype and mother's mutant load in blood in, 8993 mtDNA mutations; risk of severe outcome with respect to (a) T8993 G mutation and (b) T8993C mutation in the mother.

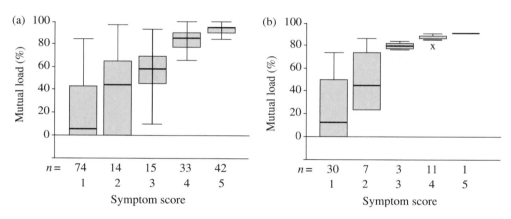

Fig. 16.2 Phenotype and mutant load in 8993 mtDNA mutations. Risk of severe outcome with respect to (a) T8993G and (b) T8993C mutation in the child. Symptom scores: 1, asymptomatic adult; 2, asymptomatic child; 3, mild symptoms like night vision or proximal weakness; 4, moderali CNS involvement; like developmental delay or movement disorder; 5, Leigh's syndrome. (Data from SA White, *et al.* (1999). *Am. J. Hum. Genet.* **65**: 474–482.)

respectively from the UK data or 30, 50, 15, and 25 per cent for the Australian ones). Furthermore, the risk decreases with age (Fig. 16.4), so that males who have reached aged 20 without problems have halved their lifetime risk. For females, this occurs at aged 27 years.[57]

Diseases in which there is a respiratory chain defect but
the precise molecular basis is unknown
Genetic counselling of this group is extremely difficult as they embrace such a wide group of disorders. In the largest study of Leigh's disease recurrence risks were between 1 in 8 and 1 in 4. If, however, a mother carries a (n unrecognized) mtDNA mutation then the recurrence risk can be much higher, for instance we advise >60 per cent in patients with MELAS.

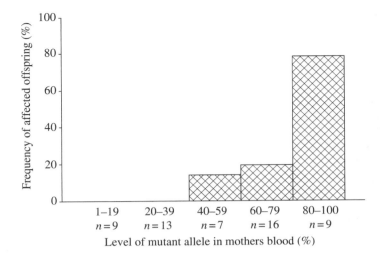

Fig. 16.3 Recurrence risks in offspring of women carrying the A8344G mutation. (Data from PF Chinnery (1998). *Brain* **121**: 1889–1894.)[52]

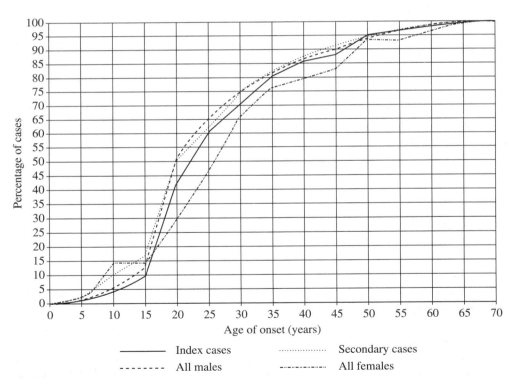

Fig. 16.4 Age onset in LHON. (——) index cases. (·········) secondary cases. (-----) all males. (-··-··-··) all females.

Prenatal diagnosis

*Prenatal diagnosis in autosomal mitochondrial diseases in which
the molecular basis is known*
Prenatal diagnosis is now available in families where a nuclear mutation has been identified, particularly in the case of severe recessive disorders. As with many other Mendelian disorders when the mutation can be identified, CVS and termination of affected foetuses can be offered. This is now routine in families with Leigh's disease caused by mutations in the *SURF*1 gene.[58,59] Other recessive disorders in which the causal mutation has been identified are collectively rare, and prenatal diagnosis has only been carried out in a handful of cases.[59,60]

Prenatal diagnosis is also theoretically available in dominantly inherited AdPEO. However, as the severity of the phenotype is variable, it is not yet clear whether families will choose this option.

*Prenatal diagnosis in diseases in which there is a respiratory chain defect but
the precise molecular basis is unknown*
Prenatal diagnosis based on respiratory chain function in amniocytes is possible in families with autosomal inheritance where the defect is present in all tissues. The main disorder where this has been feasible is systemic cytochrome *c* oxidase deficiency, which is sufficiently distinctive when clinical and biochemical features are combined. In practice this approach has largely been replaced by DNA-based diagnosis. Tissue-specific cytochrome oxidase deficiency could be caused by a heteroplasmic mtDNA mutation and may not cause a detectable respiratory chain defect in cultured CVS even from an affected foetus. Similarly, deficiencies in other complexes appear to be more heterogeneous and hence uncertainties have precluded attempts to use this method widely.

Management options and prenatal diagnosis of mtDNA disease
Precise recommendations regarding prenatal diagnosis for maternally inherited mtDNA diseases have been formulated at a recent European Neuromuscular Centre (ENMC) workshop.[61] These recommendations depend on the particular mutation and hence the recommendation of the workshop was that specialist advice be sought in counselling these patients.

Currently the options open to women with mtDNA disease are

1. *Oocyte donation.* In practice, there is a limited supply of donors, and maternal relatives such as sisters are high risk.

2. *Pre-implantation diagnosis.* Current data suggest that the varied tissue distribution of mtDNA mutants which is found postnatally has not developed in the pre-implantation embryo in which heteroplasmic mtDNA is uniformly distributed between blastomers.[37,40]

3. *Chorionic villus sampling.* Little is known regarding the tissue distribution of mtDNA mutants in the developing foetus. Such evidence as exists suggests that the mutant load in extra-embryonic tissues probably reflects that of the foetus.[55,62]

4. There may be many asymptomatic maternal relatives who feel unable to risk having children because of these uncertainties. Estimations of recurrence risks based on blood levels of mutant mtDNA are reasonable in some types of mutation but may be inaccurate for others.[63] We are using oocyte sampling to estimate recurrence risks more accurately. This has been particularly useful in families with a single affected child where the absence of mutant mtDNA in the mother's blood may be falsely reassuring. While the level of mutant

mtDNA in oocytes sampled following superovulation may give the best estimate for the likely levels in the child, it is not certain that they are truly representative of those which might develop into live babies. We have used this approach particularly in 'private mutations' where there are minimal historical data on which to base estimates of recurrence risks.

Requirements for mtDNA prenatal diagnosis

A major problem for genetic counselling is that the correlation between phenotypic severity and level of mutant is poor in many mtDNA diseases. Prenatal diagnosis would be easy if and only if there were (i) a close correlation between load of mutant mtDNA and disease severity, (ii) uniform distribution of mutant in all tissues, and (iii) no change in mutant load with time. These are fulfilled in a families with mutations at 8993 bp but not in the majority of mtDNA disorders.[54,55,63,64]

Recurrence risks for a severe phenotype based on maternal level of mutant have been estimated in a handful of disorders, most accurately for mutations at 8993 bp.[55] Predictions are limited by the accuracy with which the level of mutant mtDNA in oocytes can be predicted from the tissues available for analysis. In the case of mitochondrial encephalomyopathy, lactic acidosis, and stroke-like episodes (MELAS) due to mutations at 3243 bp, blood levels of mutant mtDNA may be very misleading. We suggest that there are situations where preconceptual genetic counselling based on oocyte sampling could be useful. It is probable that this should be restricted to women where prenatal diagnosis can subsequently be carried out.

Pre-implantation diagnosis has some theoretical advantages but is not widely available in many centres for example, the UK. As with all IVF procedures, the rate of achieving pregnancy is substantially lower than natural conception. It is therefore most applicable to women with a very high recurrence risk.

CVS has been successfully carried out in several women carrying the NARP mutation. In all cases the mutant load was either high or low, enabling accurate predictions. However, caution is needed for other mtDNA disorders in which the correlation between severity and mutant load is less precise. As with all of the options, there is a risk that CVS may be unhelpful where the mutant load has an intermediate level.

We anticipate that our understanding of the transmission genetics and segregation of mtDNA mutants will be revolutionized by new findings based on the animal models of mtDNA disease currently being developed and that prenatal diagnosis will become routine thereafter.

Precise recommendations for some common mtDNA disorders

MtDNA rearrangements.   For women with KSS due to mtDNA rearrangements, particularly those in whom rearrangements are detectable in blood (>5 per cent), we recommend CVS and Southern blotting (PCR analysis may be misleading). For women with chronic progressive external ophthalmoplegia (CPEO) and healthy women (in whom no deleted mtDNA is detectable in blood) with a single child with mtDNA rearrangements, the risk of another affected child is probably very low: CVS analysis is an option.

The NARP or Leigh's syndrome—T8993G and T8993C.   There is a relationship between mutant load in the mother and the risk of an affected offspring. Both mutations fulfil the criteria above for prenatal diagnosis and therefore CVS is likely to be informative. For symptomatic women and those with levels of mutant above 50 per cent, oocyte donation or pre-implantation genetic diagnosis should be seriously considered.

The MERRF A8344G. There is a relationship between mtDNA mutant load in the mother and the risk of an affected offspring. Severe disease is rare in offspring of mothers with a load of <40 per cent mutant mtDNA in blood. CVS should be offered to mothers with levels of >40 per cent. Oocyte donation or pre-implantation genetic diagnosis should also be considered in mothers with high mutant load.

MELAS A3243G. This is the most common and most problematic heteroplasmic mtDNA disorder because severity is not clearly related to mutant load.

1555, 11778, 3460, and 14484 mutations. As there is currently no way of predicting the clinical phenotype of patients with these mutations, prenatal diagnosis is not appropriate.

Private point mutations. In this group of patients there is no good data available from which risk can be calculated. Sampling of several tissues in the mother, including oocyte sampling, may help.

References

1. Holt IJ, Harding AE, and Morgan-Hughes JA (1988). Deletions in muscle mitochondrial DNA in patients with mitochondrial myopathies. *Nature* **331**: 717–719.
2. Rotig A, Colonna M, Blanche S, Fisher A, Deist FL, Frezai J, *et al.* (1988). Deletions of blood mitochondrial DNA in pancytopenia. *Lancet* **i**: 567–568.
3. Dunbar D, Moonie P, Swingler R, Davidson D, Roberts R, and Holt I (1993). Maternally transmitted partial direct tandem duplication of mitochondrial DNA associated with diabetes mellitus. *Hum. Mol. Gen.* **2**(10): 1619–1624.
4. Goto Y-I, Nonaka I, and Horai S (1990). A mutation in the tRNA leu(UUR) gene associated with the MELAS subgroup of mitochondrial encephalomyopathies. *Nature* **348**: 651–653.
5. Shoffner JM, Lott MT, Lezza AM, Seibel P, Ballinger SW, and Wallace DC (1990). Myoclonic epilepsy and ragged red fiber disease (MERRF) is associated with a mitochondrial DNA tRNA(Lys) mutation. *Cell* **61**(6): 931–937.
6. Wallace DC, Singh G, Lott MT, Hodge JA, Schurr TG, Lezza AM, *et al.* (1988). Mitochondrial DNA mutation associated with Leber's hereditary optic neuropathy. *Science* **242**(4884): 1427–1430.
7. Rahman S, Poulton J, Marchington D, and Suomalainen A (2001). Decrease of 3243 A–>G mtDNA mutation from blood in MELAS syndrome: a longitudinal study. *Am. J. Hum. Genet.* **68**(1): 238–240.
8. Poulton J and Morten K (1993). Noninvasive diagnosis of the MELAS syndrome from blood DNA [letter]. *Ann. Neurol.* **34**(1): 116.
9. Poulton J, O'Rahilly S, Morten K, and Clark A (1995). Mitochondrial DNA, diabetes and pancreatic pathology in Kearns–Sayre syndrome. *Diabetologia* **38**: 868–871.
10. Weber K, Wilson J, Taylor L, Brierley E, Johnson M, and Turnbull D (1997). A New mtDNA mutation showing accumulation with time and restriction to skeletal muscle. *Am. J. Hum. Genet.* **60**: 373–380.
11. Smeitink J vdHL (1999). Human mitochondrial complex I in health and disease. *Am. J. Hum. Genet.* **64**: 1505–1510.
12. Tiranti V, Jaksch M, Hofmann S, Galimberti C, Hoertnagel K, Lulli L, *et al.* (1999). Loss-of-function mutations of SURF-1 are specifically associated with Leigh syndrome with cytochrome c oxidase deficiency. *Ann. Neurol.* **46**(2): 161–166.
13. Papadopoulou LC SC, Davidson MM, Tanji K, Nishino I, Sadlock JE, Krishna S, Walker W, Selby J, Glerum DM, Coster RV, Lyon G, Scalais E, Lebel R, Kaplan P, Shanske S, De Vivo DC,

Bonilla E, Hirano M, DiMauro S, and Schon EA (1999). Fatal infantile cardioencephalomyopathy with COX deficiency and mutations in SCO2, a COX assembly gene. *Nat. Genet.* **23**: 333–337.

14. Koehler CM LD, Merchant S, Renold A, Junne T, and Schatz G (1999). Human deafness dystonia syndrome is a mitochondrial disease. *Proc. Natl Acad. Sci. USA* **96**: 2141–2146.

15. Zeviani M, Servidei S, Gellera C, Bertini E, DiMauro S, and DiDonato S (1989). An autosomal dominant disorder with multiple deletions of mitochondrial DNA starting at the D-loop region. *Nature* **339**(6222): 309–311.

16. Nishino I, Spinazzola A, and Hirano M (1999). Thymidine phosphorylase gene mutations in MNGIE, a human mitochondrial disorder. *Science* **283**: 689–692.

17. Barthelemy C, De Baulny O, and Lombes A (2002). D-loop mutations in mitochondrial DNA: link with mitochondrial DNA depletion? *Hum. Genet.* **110**(5): 479–487.

18. Mandel H, Szargel R, Labay V, Elpeleg O, Saada A, Shalata A, *et al.* (2001). The deoxyguanosine kinase gene is mutated in individuals with depleted hepatocerebral mitochondrial DNA. *Nat. Genet.* **29**(3): 337–341.

19. Saada A, Shaag A, Mandel H, Nevo Y, Eriksson S, and Elpeleg O (2001). Mutant mitochondrial thymidine kinase in mitochondrial DNA depletion myopathy. *Nat. Genet.* **29**(3): 342–344.

20. Johnson KR, Zheng QY, Bykhovskaya Y, Spirina O, and Fischel-Ghodsian N (2001). A nuclear-mitochondrial DNA interaction affecting hearing impairment in mice. *Nat. Genet.* **27**(2): 191–194.

21. Kaneda H, Hayashi J, Takahama S, Taya C, Lindahl KF, and Yonekawa H (1995). Elimination of paternal mitochondrial DNA in intraspecific crosses during early mouse embryogenesis. *Proc. Natl Acad. Sci. USA* **92**(10): 4542–4546.

22. Shitara H, Hayashi JI, Takahama S, Kaneda H, and Yonekawa H (1998). Maternal inheritance of mouse mtDNA in interspecific hybrids: segregation of the leaked paternal mtDNA followed by the prevention of subsequent paternal leakage. *Genetics* **148**(2): 851–857.

23. Ruiz-Pesini E, Lapena AC, Diez-Sanchez C, Perez-Martos A, Montoya J, Alvarez E, *et al.* (2000). Human mtDNA haplogroups associated with high or reduced spermatozoa motility. *Am. J. Hum. Genet.* **67**(3): 682–696.

24. Rovio AT, Marchington DR, Donat S, Schuppe HC, Abel J, Fritsche E, *et al.* (2001). Mutations at the mitochondrial DNA polymerase (POLG) locus associated with male infertility. *Nat. Genet.* **29**(3): 261–262.

25. Schwartz M and Vissing J (2002). Paternal inheritance of mitochondrial DNA. *N. Engl. J. Med.* **347**(8): 576–580.

26. Macaulay V, Richards M, and Sykes B (1999). Mitochondrial DNA recombination-no need to panic. *Proc. R. Soc. Lond. B Biol. Sci.* **266**(1433): 2037–2039; discussion 2041–2042.

27. Hagelberg E GN, Lio P, Whelan S, Schiefenhovel W, Clegg JB, and Bowden DK (1999). Evidence for mitochondrial DNA recombination in a human population of island Melanesia. *Proc. R. Soc. Lond. B Biol. Sci.* **266**(1418): 485–492.

28. Colato A and Fontanari JF (2001). Soluble model for the accumulation of mutations in asexual populations. *Phys. Rev. Lett.* **87**(23): 238102.

29. Brown D, Samuels D, Michael E, Turnbull D, and Chinnery P (2001). Random genetic drift determines the level of mutant mtDNA in human primary oocytes. *Am. J. Hum. Genet.* **68**(2): 533–536.

30. Marchington D, Hartshorne G, Barlow D, and Poulton J (1998). Evidence from human oocytes for a genetic bottleneck in a mitochondrial DNA disease. *Am. J. Hum. Genet.* **63**: 769–775.

31. Marchington D, Hartshorne G, Barlow D, and Poulton J (1997). Homopolymeric tract heteroplasmy in mtDNA from tissues and single oocytes: support for a genetic bottleneck. *Am. J. Hu. Genet.* **60**: 408–416.

32. Blok R, Cook D, Thorburn D, and Dahl H (1997). Skewed segregation of the mtDNA nt 8993 (T → G) mutation in human ocytes. *Am. J. Hum. Genet.* **60**(6): 1495–1501.

33. Suomalainen A, Majander A, Pihko H, Peltonen L, and Syvanen AC (1993). Quantification of tRNA3243(Leu) point mutation of mitochondrial DNA in MELAS patients and its effects on mitochondrial transcription. *Hum. Mol. Genet.* **2**(5): 525–534.

34. Harding AE, Holt IJ, Sweeney MG, Brockington M, and Davis MB (1992). Prenatal diagnosis of mitochondrial DNA8993 T—G disease. *Am. J. Hum. Genet.* **50**(3): 629–633.

35. Matthews PM, Hopkin J, Brown RM, Stephenson JB, Hilton-Jones D, and Brown GK (1994). Comparison of the relative levels of the 3243 (A → G) mtDNA mutation in heteroplasmic adult and fetal tissues. *J. Med. Genet.* **31**(1): 41–44.

36. Laipis P (1996). Construction of heteroplasmic mice containing two mitochondrial DNA genotypes by micromanipulation of single-cell embryos. *Methods Enzymol.* **264**: 345–357.

37. Jenuth J, Peterson A, Fu K, and Shoubridge E (1996). Random genetic drift in the female germline explains the rapid segregation of mammalian mitochondrial DNA. *Nat. Genet.* **14**(2): 146–151.

38. Meirelles F and Smith L (1997). Mitochondrial genotype in a mouse heteroplasmic lineage produced by embryonic karyoplast transplantation. *Genetics* **145**: 445–451.

39. White S (1999). Molecular Mechanisms of Mitochondrial Disorders [PhD]. Melbourne: University of Melbourne.

40. Molnar M and Shoubridge E (1999). Preimplantation diagnosis for mitochondrial disorders. *Neuromusc. Disord.* **9**(6–7): 521.

41. Jenuth J, Peterson A, and Shoubridge E (1997). Tissue-specific selection for different mtDNA genotypes in heteroplasmic mice. *Nat. Genet.* **16**: 93–95.

42. Battersby BJ and Shoubridge EA (2001). Selection of a mtDNA sequence variant in hepatocytes of heteroplasmic mice is not due to differences in respiratory chain function or efficiency of replication. *Hum. Mol. Genet.* **10**(22): 2469–2479.

43. Marchington D, Barlow D, and Poulton J (1999). Transmitochondrial mice carrying resistance to chloramphenicol on mitochondrial DNA: developing the first mouse model of mitochondrial DNA disease. *Nat. Med.* **5**: 957–960.

44. Sligh JE LS, Waymire KG, Allard P, Dillehay DL, Nusinowitz S, Heckenlively JR, MacGregor GR, and Wallace DC (2000). Maternal germ-line transmission of mutant mtDNAs from embryonic stem cell-derived chimeric mice. *Proc. Natl Acad. Sci. USA* **97**: 14461–14466.

45. Inoue K, Nakada K, Ogura A, Isobe K, Goto Y, Nonaka I, *et al.* (2000). Generation of mice with mitochondrial dysfunction by introducing mouse mtDNA carrying a deletion into zygotes. *Nat. Genet.* **26**(2): 176–181.

46. Poulton J and Holt I (1994). Mitochondrial DNA: does more lead to less? *Nat. Genet.* **8**: 313–315.

47. Jansen R (2000). Germline passage of mitochondria: quantitative considerations and possible embryological sequelae. *Hum. Reprod.* **15**(Suppl 2): 112–128.

48. Solignac M, Genermont J, Monnerot M, and Mounolou J (1987). Drosophila mitochondrial genetics: evolution of heteroplasmy through germ line cell divisions. *Genetics* **117**: 687–696.

49. Bendall K, Macaulay V, Baker J, and Sykes B (1996). Heteroplasmy in the human mitochondrial DNA control region in twin pairs. *Am. J. Hum. Genet.* **59**: 1276–1287.

50. Chinnery PF and Samuels DC (1999). Relaxed replication of mtDNA: a model with implications for the expression of disease. *Am. J. Hum. Genet.* **64**(4): 1158–1165.

51. Moilanen J and Majamaa K (2001). Relative fitness of carriers of the mitochondrial DNA mutation 3243A > G. *Eur. J. Hum. Genet.* **9**(1): 59–62.

52. Chinnery P, Howell N, Lightowlers R, and Turnbull D (1998) MELAS and MERRF. The relationship between maternal mutation load and the frequency of clinically affected offspring. *Brain* **121** (Pt 10): 1889–1894.

53. Larsson NG, Holme E, Kristiansson B, Oldfors A, and Tulinius M (1990). Progressive increase of the mutated mitochondrial DNA fraction in Kearns–Sayre syndrome. *Pediatr. Res.* **28**(2): 131–136.

54. White S, Collins V, Dahl H, and Thorburn D (1999). The level of mutant mtDNA in patients with mutations at NT8993 remains stable. *J. Inherit. Metab. Dis.* **22**: 899–914.

55. White S, Collins V, R RW, Cleary M, Shanske S, DiMauro S, *et al.* (1999). Genetic counseling and prenatal diagnosis for the mitochondrial DNA mutations at nucleotide 8993. *Am. J. Hum. Genet.* **65**: 474–482.

56. Black G, Craig I, Oostra R, Norby S, Rosenberg T, Morten K, *et al.* (1995). Leber's Hereditary Optic Neuropathy: Implications of the sex ratio for linkage studies in families with the 3460 ND1 mutation. *Eye* **9**: 513–516.

57. Harding A, Sweeney M, Govan G, and Riordan-Eva P (1995). Pedigree analysis in Leber hereditary optic neuropathy families with a pathogenic mtDNA mutation. *Am. J. Hum. Genet.* **57**(1): 77–86.

58. Poulton J, McShane A, Pike M, Seller A, Marchington D, Kennedy S, *et al.* (2001). Advances in Genetic Management of Patients with Mitochondrial Disease. *J. Neurol. Sci.* **187**: S 435.

59. Amiel J, Gigarel N, Benacki A, Benit P, Valnot I, Parfait B, *et al.* (2001). Prenatal diagnosis of respiratory chain deficiency by direct mutation screening. *Prenat. Diagn.* **21**(7): 602–604.

60. Niers L, Smeitink J, Trijbels J, Sengers R, Janssen A, and van DHL (2001). Prenatal diagnosis of NADH : ubiquinone oxidoreductase deficiency [In Process Citation]. *Prenat. Diagn.* **21**(10): 871–880.

61. Poulton J and Turnbull DM (2000). 74th ENMC international workshop: mitochondrial diseases 19–20 november 1999, Naarden, the netherlands. *Neuromuscul. Disord.* **10**(6): 460–462.

62. Wardell T, Morris A, Wright C, and Turnbull D (1999). Studies in oocytes from a female infant with Pearson's syndrome. In: *EUROMIT; 1999*; Cambridge (UK), p. 232.

63. Chinnery PF, Howell N, Lightowlers R, and DMT (1998). The inheritance of MELAS and MERRF: the relationship between maternal mutation load and the frequency of affected offspring. *Brain* **121**: 1889–1894.

64. Chinnery PF HN, Lightowlers R, and Turnbull DM (1997). Molecular pathology of MELAS and MERRF: the relationship between mutation load and clinical phenotype. *Brain* **120**: 1713–1721.

17 Gene therapy for mitochondrial DNA disorders

B Bigger, RW Taylor, DM Turnbull, and RN Lightowlers

Mutations of the mitochondrial genome (mtDNA) cause a variety of progressive clinical disorders for which there is no effective treatment. Consequently, novel therapeutic approaches are being considered. Mitochondrial genetics is complex, with single cells containing many hundreds or thousands of mtDNA molecules and in the disease state there are often populations of mutated and wild type mtDNA coexisting in the same cell or tissue. As the defective genome is expressed within the mitochondrial matrix surrounded by two membranes, any therapeutic molecule must reach this compartment. Concepts for treatment include transfection and expression of wild type mitochondrial genes from the nucleus (allotopic expression) and reducing the load of mutated mtDNAs in heteroplasmic cells by a variety of means. Although there has been some success in manipulating levels of heteroplasmy by cell replacement or concentric exercise techniques, no one method will be effective for treating all patients with mtDNA disease.

Introduction

In the past few years, there have been numerous reports of nuclear gene defects that cause mitochondrial disease (see Chapters 9 and 10). Whilst this group of disorders is highly significant, strategies for potential gene therapy are similar to those proposed for other nuclear gene defects and will not be reviewed in this chapter. The aim here is to focus on disease due to primary mutations of the mitochondrial genome and how the genetic aspect of these disorders presents unique difficulties for gene based therapy. Although several chapters in this book deal admirably with mtDNA genetics, it is important to revisit some of the peculiarities of mitochondrial genetics and their relevance to disease.

Disorders of the mitochondrial genome

As has already been discussed, there is great interest in mtDNA disease and the possible involvement of mitochondrial dysfunction in common neurodegenerative disorders and the ageing process (see Chapters 12 and 13). Mutations of the mitochondrial genome (point mutations or rearrangements) lead to the production of aberrant mitochondrial translation products, incorrect processing and maturation of mitochondrial transcripts, or general defects in intramitochondrial protein synthesis. As all mitochondrially encoded polypeptides are required for efficient oxidative phosphorylation, such defects manifest as deficiencies in cellular respiration.

Despite the fact that the first patient with symptoms resulting from defects in the mitochondrial genome was only identified in 1988[1,2] the involvement of mtDNA mutations in disease has rapidly been recognized as considerable. Given its size, mutations in the mitochondrial genome are responsible for a disproportionately large amount of mitochondrial disease, for which over 100 pathogenic mutations and rearrangements have been identified.[3] In the North East of England, the incidence of mtDNA disease is 1 : 17,000 and 1 in 8000 individuals carry a potentially pathological mutation.[4] This is particularly striking when compared to the incidence of myotonic or Duchenne dystrophy (approx. 1 : 20,000 and 1 : 31,000, respectively) and similar to Huntington's disease.

Mitochondrial cytopathies resulting from mtDNA mutations can present as a multitude of clinical phenotypes affecting mainly heart, skeletal muscle, or central nervous system (CNS). Interestingly, the same mutation may cause varied clinical phenotypes in different individuals or pedigrees. This is often due to variation in the proportions of defective and wild type mtDNA. With 10^3–10^4 copies of mtDNA in a typical mononuclear cell, the threshold of disease manifestation is believed to be dependent upon the percentage of mutated versus wild type mtDNA molecules in individual cells and tissues. Pathological mtDNA mutations are mostly recessive that is the *threshold* for disease manifestation is usually greater than 50 per cent. In some patients who have had serial biopsies taken over a period of several years, the ratio of mutated to wild type mtDNA (wt-DNA) increased, that is, segregation to mutated mtDNA occurred. It is therefore essential that any gene therapy strategy designed to target mitochondrial DNA disease must take into account both mutant load and segregation bias.

Gene therapy for mtDNA disorders

As all mtDNA-encoded polypeptides are essential components of oxidative phosphorylation enzymes, defects associated with pathogenic mtDNA mutations may be difficult to overcome by pharmacological intervention. Consequently, radical concepts for treating these chronic progressive disorders need to be developed. Recently, several novel hypotheses have been contemplated:

- Redesigning mitochondrial genes for expression from the nucleus
- Methods for manipulating mtDNA heteroplasmy
- Introduction of mitochondrial mini-vectors

Each approach has its advantages and disadvantages and is considered below.

Redesigning mitochondrial genes for expression from the nucleus

Pathogenic point mutations are most commonly found in mt-tRNA or mt-mRNA genes. There is a great deal of interest in being able to exploit the endogenous protein and nucleic acid import pathways to treat these disorders. The basic concept is simple—identify the mutated gene product, introduce a wild type version of the gene into the nucleus and import normal copies of the gene product into mitochondria from the cytosol. Expression of a gene in a foreign location in this manner is termed allotopic expression.

Allotopic expression of mitochondrially encoded proteins

Most nuclear encoded gene products targeted and imported into mitochondria possess a short N-terminal amphipathic protein sequence that is removed after import (reviewed in Chapter 3). The products of mtDNA, however, do not require a targeting signal as they are synthesized in the mitochondrial matrix. It had been known for many years that various non-mitochondrial polypeptides could be relocated to the mitochondrial matrix simply by adding a targeting sequence to their N-terminus. Nevertheless, important questions remained. Could endogenous mitochondrial gene products be translocated to the matrix when translated in the cytosol and fused to an N-terminal targeting signal? If so, was the imported protein integrated successfully into a multi-subunit complex involved in oxidative phosphorylation? In addition to engineering the gene to encode a presequence, there was a further problem—the gene must also be modified to take account of differences in the mitochondrial and standard genetic codes. Codon recognition in human mitochondria differs slightly from the standard genetic code—the triplet AUA specifies methionine in mitochondria (in contrast to isoleucine in the cytosol). Critically, AGA and AGG do not specify arginine rather they are recognized as translation *termination* codons in mitochondria. Conversely the stop codon TGA in the standard code specifies tryptophan in the mitochondrial genetic code. In 1988, Nagley et al.[5] overcame the real and imagined difficulties of allotopic expression in yeast. They recoded the mitochondrial *ATP8* gene from *Saccharomyces cerevisiae* and fused it with the N-terminal targeting signal of ATPase 9 of the fungus *Neurospora crassa*. When the engineered gene was inserted into the nucleus of *S. cerevisiae*, the allotopically expressed ATPase 8 protein was successfully targeted and imported into mitochondria, restoring respiratory function to a strain lacking the normal mitochondrial gene product.

This impressive piece of work demonstrated that allotopic expression was a viable method of restoring respiratory function, at least in yeast. But could this approach be used to restore oxidative phosphorylation in human cells? After many years of trying to repeat this feat in higher eukaryotes by several research groups, Manfredi et al.[6] have now reported some success. In a subset of patients with the mtDNA disease termed NARP (*Neurogenic Ataxia and Retinitis Pigmentosa*), a point mutation in the *MTATP6* gene at np 8993 causes a defect in ATP synthase.[7] Manfredi et al. recoded a wild type copy of the *MTATP6* gene and added a presequence from human COXVIII. Working with cell lines carrying the NARP mutation, the chimeric gene was introduced by viral transfection into the nucleus and the wild type fusion protein was reported to partially rescue the biochemical phenotype (Fig. 17.1).

A second exciting approach is to transfect human cells with a respiratory gene from a different species and to rectify a respiratory defect by mitochondrial import of the gene product. This has been attempted with the relatively simple rotenone-insensitive NADH : quinone oxido-reductase (roughly equivalent to mammalian Complex 1) which is expressed from a single nuclear gene (*NDI1*) in *S. cerevisiae*.[8] Using the adeno-associated virus, Yagi and colleagues were able to transfect human cell lines with the yeast *NDI1* gene. The transfected cell lines imported the yeast respiratory Complex 1 into the mitochondrial matrix and were able to show the enzyme was fully functional.[9] This work has recently been extended using human cell lines lacking the essential mtDNA-encoded ND4 gene product. Transfectants expressing the targeted NDI1 gene product demonstrated NADH-dependent and rotenone-insensitive respiration, which was antimycin sensitive, showing the NDI1 protein to be incorporated into an active respiratory chain.[10] Although technically impressive, NDI1 does not pump protons

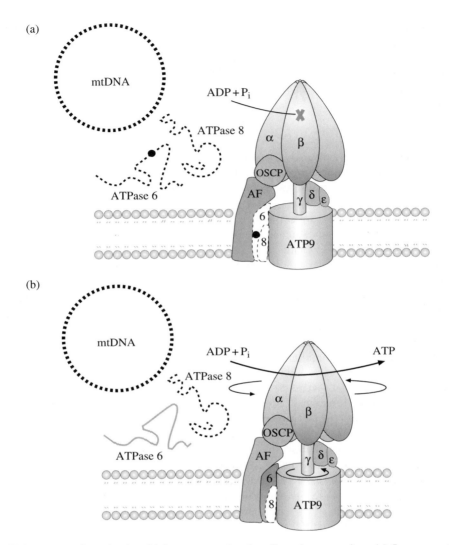

Fig. 17.1 Rescue of a mitochondrial gene mutation by allotopic expression. (a) In man, mtDNA encodes two polypeptides (ATPase 6 and ATPase 8) that are components of the F_0F_1 ATP synthase (shown as dashed lines in the figure). All other members of the complex are encoded by the nucleus, translated in the cytosol and translocated to mitochondria. In this example, expression from a mutated *MTATP6* gene produces a defective ATPase 6 gene product (mutation shown as a black dot). When the subunit is integrated into the complex, the enzyme is unable to synthesize ATP normally. (b) By recoding MTATP6 to allow correct cytosolic translation and adding an N-terminal preprotein to target the gene product to mitochondria, the chimeric gene product can now be expressed from the nucleus (allotopic expression). The fully functional MTATP6 encoded in the nucleus is shown as a continuous line. The various subunits of the complex are designated according to the standard nomenclature for yeast. AF, associated factors.

across the inner membrane, and this was reflected in a lowered P : O ratio for NADH-dependent coupled respiration. Therefore, it is unlikely that allotopoically expressed NDI1 would be an effective gene therapy for Complex I deficiency, as oxidative phosphorylation would remain far less efficient than normal. Furthermore, although mutations in Complex 1 genes are commonly associated with Leber's hereditary optic neuropathy (LHON), it is not clear that the pathology is a direct result of Complex I deficiency.

Allotopic expression of mt-tRNA genes

In many patients with mtDNA disease the defective gene encodes a mt-tRNA. How could such patients be treated by allotopic expression? It has been known for many years that most plant and protist species import from the cytosol some or all tRNAs involved in mitochondrial translation.[11,12] This is not the case in humans, where all mt-tRNAs are encoded by the mito-chondrial genome and there is no requirement for tRNA import. Nevertheless, Tarassov, Martin and colleagues embarked upon a series of experiments to examine the validity of tRNA import as a gene therapy strategy for mitochondrial diseases. First they investigated tRNA^{Lys} of *S. cerevisiae* (tRK1), as this is the only tRNA in yeast transcribed from nuclear DNA and imported into mitochondria. Then they went on to demonstrate that tRK1 and derivatives can be imported into isolated human mitochondria.[13] Import requires the tRNA^{Lys} to be aminoacyl-ated and for the import mixture to contain the mitochondrial precursor of the yeast lysyl tRNA synthetase and other undefined factors.[14] The same group have recently found that certain nuclear-expressed tRNAs can be targeted and imported into mitochondria of cultured human cells (I Tarassov, personal communication). In addition to import of tRNAs, there is evidence to suggest that the RNA components of MRP RNase and RNase P are translocated into mam-malian mitochondria. Finally, some 5S rRNA co-localizes with mitochondria.[15] By identifying the important *cis*-acting elements required for successful RNA import, it is envisaged that novel vectors will be designed to import tRNAs, antisense RNAs or even ribozymes that may be able to modulate levels or expression of mitochondrial transcripts.

The allotopic expression of both mitochondrial proteins and mt-tRNAs is a potentially exciting method for treating patients with defects of the mitochondrial genome. However, the correctly engineered genes must be delivered, recombined into the nucleus and faithfully expressed in a large number of human cells for this approach to be viable.

Manipulation of mtDNA heteroplasmy

Many patients suffering from mtDNA disorders harbour two populations of mtDNA, (hetero-plasmy). In addition to the molecule carrying the pathogenic mutation, the patient carries wild type copies. As mutations are often recessive, it is striking that these patients contain a cure within their own body. A cure would result if wt-mtDNA were propagated at the expense of mutated mtDNA. But how can mutant molecules be eliminated? Three approaches have been taken. First, cell replacement therapies have been considered. Second, the mutated mtDNA has been targeted either by engineering and targeting restriction endonucleases to the mitochondrial matrix or by using sequence-selective peptide nucleic acids to inhibit the replica-tion of the pathogenic molecule. Third, the mutated mtDNA could be repaired using a mis-match repair system. Another potential, and in principle straightforward, mechanism would be to employ factors that influence segregation bias, that is, induce or overexpress a nuclear gene whose product promotes propagation of wt-DNA over mutated mtDNA. Although the existence of such factors is implied by the outcome of segregation studies in cultured human cells (see Chapter 14), as yet no such factor has been identified.

Cell replacement therapy

Patients suspected of having a mitochondrial disorder are often subjected to a muscle biopsy. Sections of this material can be retained for histochemical and biochemical analysis, molecular genetic diagnostics, and used to establish primary myoblast cultures. Several groups in the 1990s reported that some pathological mutations were absent from primary cell lines cultured in the laboratory.[16,17] The mutations were heteroplasmic in patients' muscle and associated with the classic mosaic pattern of cytochrome *c* oxidase (COX) activity of mitochondrial disease. The mutations were sporadic and somatic and there was no instance of disease transmission. Cells from the muscle biopsy that proliferate in culture are myogenic progenitors known as satellite cells, which make up a relatively small mass of the mature myofibre. Exactly why the mutation is not present in primary cultures established from muscle with greater that 95 per cent mutant load remains unresolved. However, this phenomenon has been exploited to remove the mutated mtDNA from at least a small section of tissue.[18,19] Muscle degenerants such as the anaesthetic bupivicaine have been used on a limited amount of vastus lateralis muscle from a patient with a myopathy due to a mutation in mt-tRNA[Leu(CUN)]. Muscle regenerated due to activation of satellite cells, and the newly formed fibres displayed normal COX activity and a remarkably low level of mutated mtDNA. The success of such cell replacement therapy is tempered by the knowledge that the pathogenic molecule is likely to be present in the majority of cells within the body of a patient. Even in cases where the mutant population of mtDNA is restricted to muscle, the mutation is likely to be present at high levels in all muscle blocks and it is currently not known what quantity of muscle degeneration can be repaired by endogenous satellite cell regeneration. Nor is it known if the mutated mtDNA will reaccumulate in the regenerated muscle.

An interesting variation on this concept has been explored by Taivassalo *et al.*[20] again studying heteroplasmic patients with low levels of pathogenic mtDNA in satellite cells. Instead of using chemical muscle degenerants, these authors were able to show that by inducing muscle hypertrophy with short bursts of concentric exercise, satellite cells apparently devoid of mutated mtDNA were incorporated into myofibres, increasing the proportion of fibres with normal respiratory activity. Although the number of patients assessed is still low, the effect of a simple treatment such as concentric muscle exercise is highly encouraging.

Targeting mutated mtDNA

Sequence selective cleavage with restriction endonucleases

By standard cybrid fusion techniques, Srivastava and Moraes generated a heteroplasmic rodent cell line containing mtDNA from both rat and mouse. Crucially, the mouse mtDNA contained two cleavage sites for the restriction endonuclease *Pst*1, whilst the rat genome was devoid of any *Pst*1 site. By fusing the presequence of human COXVIII to the endonuclease and transfecting cells with the engineered gene, it was successfully targeted to mitochondria and the cell lines revealed a significant shift of heteroplasmy towards the rat genome, consistent with the endonuclease cleaving the mouse mtDNA.[21] This is encouraging, but what is the relevance to mtDNA disease? In rare situations, pathogenic mutations introduce unique restriction sites into the mitochondrial genome. For example, a T → G transversion at np 8993 which causes a maternally inherited Leigh Disease or NARP (see also above) results in a unique *Sma*1 site. Tanaka and colleagues were also able to produce an endonuclease (*Sma*1) fused to a mitochondrial preprotein. When expressed in a human cell line heteroplasmic for mtDNA carrying the T → G transversion, the endonuclease is imported correctly and has been shown to selectively degrade the pathogenic molecule, allowing the wild type to propagate.[22] Therefore transfection of the chimeric endonuclease into patients harbouring the 8993 transversion could rectify the disorder.

Inhibiting replication of the mutated genome with peptide nucleic acids
Even assuming that it is possible to express the targeted endonuclease in sufficient numbers of cells to treat a patient, one major drawback is that only a very small subset of patients harbours pathogenic molecules that contain unique restriction sites. Ideally, any treatment for heteroplasmic disorders should be amenable to all mutations. One possible panacea for all heteroplasmic mutations would be to use an agent that could bind selectively to any pathogenic molecule and inhibit its replication. As mtDNA is believed to turnover throughout life, inhibiting replication of the pathogenic mtDNA would allow the wild type to propagate, similar to the situation where the mutated molecule is selectively digested. This hypothesis is simple and compelling (Fig. 17.2). Mitochondrial DNA replication is believed to be initiated by synthesizing one strand of the duplex historically referred to as the heavy (H-) strand and is primed by a short RNA species originating from the light (L-) strand promoter.[23] Synthesis of the L-strand does not occur until the origin of L-strand replication (O_L) is uncovered after about two-thirds of the new H-strand has been synthesized,[24] that is, lagging-strand synthesis is delayed (although this has recently been challenged).[25] As a consequence of this delay the H-strand template is single-stranded for much of the replication process, providing an excellent target for any agent that can base-pair selectively to mutated mtDNA. There are, however, substantial barriers to be addressed before treatment of patients can even be considered. First, an agent must be identified that can show selective targeting under physiological conditions, even when a molecule is identical except for a single base pair. Second, the agent must be able to inhibit mtDNA replication. Third, the agent must be capable of entering the cell, and thence mitochondria.

For a single point mutation, an agent must be identified that will selectively target molecules differing in sequence from the normal copy by only a single base pair. Paradoxically, deleted mtDNA would seem to provide an easier target for selective inhibition, but it is complicated by the deletion mechanism involving repeat sequences. In the 'common' deletion, for example, two repeat sequences of 13 bp, separated by almost 5 kb, nucleate the deletion event, with the resolved 'deleted' molecule retaining a single copy of the 13 bp repeat.[26] To promote binding selectivity, an agent must be designed which recognises the unique nucleotide sequence around the mutation. At physiological temperatures, it is difficult to design any standard oligonucleotide that will show meaningful binding specificity, although bridging oligomers designed to span the deletion sequence do show some binding cooperativity.[27] Peptide nucleic acids (PNAs), however, are ideally suited for binding selectivity at such temperatures. These molecules carry regular nucleobases on a repeating aminoethyl glycine backbone.[28] Due to their unusual composition, PNAs are not degraded by nucleases or peptidases and are relatively stable in serum and cell extracts.[29] PNAs are able to perform standard Watson–Crick base interactions with complementary DNA or RNA oligomers.[30] Crucially, they are uncharged, promoting increased binding affinity with complementary molecules.

(a)   Mutated mtDNA

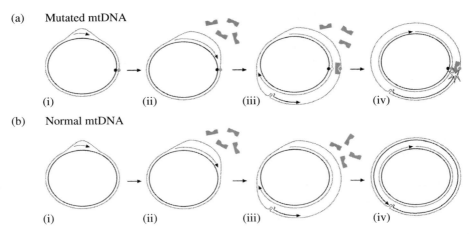

(b)   Normal mtDNA

Fig. 17.2 The antigenomic approach to mtDNA disease. Two mtDNA molecules found in a typical heteroplasmic state. (a) Mutated mtDNA; (b) the wild type copy. The L-strand strand of mtDNA is shown as a closed bold line and the H-strand as a dotted line. Arrows indicate the direction of synthesis of the new DNA strand. The two molecules are identical except for a single pathogenic mutation, represented by the filled circles (a). The antigenomic agent is shown as a grey rectangle with a semicircular inset to highlight its binding selectivity. In (i), the two molecules are ready to replicate. A short nascent H-strand is shown in the displacement loop, initiating from the origin of H-strand replication; (ii) The new H-strand is extended in a clockwise fashion, with the L-strand acting as template and the old H-strand being displaced. (iii) Further extension displaces the region of the H-strand which carries the mutation (shown as a grey circle). This single-stranded region spanning the mutation is a perfect template for the antigenomic molecule which binds to the mutated template. Due to the single base pair mismatch, it is unable to interact with the normal mtDNA. The H-strand has now been extended beyond the origin of L-strand replication, which, after displacement, forms a stem-loop structure. This structure is recognized by mtDNA primase and synthesis of a new L-strand is initiated (bold line with arrow). (iv) As the new L-strand is extended further, the replication complex on the mutated mtDNA will encounter the tightly bound antigenomic molecule straddling the mutation on the old H-strand. If the complex is unable to remove the bound molecule, replication will be truncated, as shown in the upper panel. The antigenomic agent is unable to bind to normal mtDNA and replication of both H- and L-strand are completed as shown in (b). This illustration is simplified and does not show how the two fully replicated molecules are resolved. Although the truncated replication intermediate shown in (a iv), contains a complete L-strand with a new and complete H-strand, it is possible that this duplex is never resolved from the complex. Even assuming correct resolution, replication of a mutated mtDNA can only produce one daughter molecule, unlike the uninhibited normal molecule that will produce two daughter mtDNA molecules. (Figure reproduced from Smith PM, *et al.* (2002). The use of PNAs and their derivatives in mitochondrial gene therapy. In: *Toward Gene Therapy & Functional Genomics with Synthetic Organic Polymers: Peptide Nucleic Acids, Morpholinos, and Related Antisense Biomolecules* (eds M During and CG Janson), Landes Bioscience.)

Furthermore, single base mismatches have a dramatic effect on binding affinities, making PNAs ideal agents for differential binding of templates differing by only a single base pair at physiological temperatures.[31] Previously, a short 11-mer PNA which spans the A8344G mutation known to cause MERRF (myoclonus, epilepsy with ragged red fibres) has been shown to bind selectively to a template carrying the MERRF mutation and not a template identical except for a single nucleotide. MtDNA polymerase gamma-driven run off replication of the MERRF template was shown *in vitro* to be inhibited by the PNA.[32] Inhibition was unaffected by template DNA being coated by single-stranded binding protein, confirming the PNA as an excellent candidate for an antigenomic agent.

PNAs have been shown to be imported into a variety of cells, albeit with low efficiency, however they are not localized to mitochondria. Conjugation to a 29-mer COXVIII presequence successfully targeted PNAs to mitochondria in cultured cells, but matrix import could not be demonstrated in isolated organelles.[33] It has recently been possible to overcome this problem by taking advantage of the uncharged nature of PNAs. Addition of a caged lipophilic cation, such as a triphenylphosphonium moiety, to PNAs facilitates membrane potential-driven uptake into the matrix.[34] Although very encouraging, whilst uptake can be shown in isolated organelles and into mitochondria of cultured cells, addition of high concentration TPP–PNAs to heteroplasmic cell lines has yet to result in altered levels of heteroplasmy.

There are only two possible explanations for these results—the PNA does not bind to mtDNA, or the PNA binds mtDNA but is removed from the template during or prior to replication. To circumvent the latter possibility, TPP–PNA derivatives have now been synthesized with the uv-inducible photocrosslinking moiety, benzophenone and constructs are being made around the chemotherapeutic drug chlorambucil (Fig. 17.3).

Mismatch repair of mutated mtDNA

An entirely hypothetical approach is to target the mutated molecule and repair it using a wild type oligonucleotide as template. The concept is simple. An imported 'wild type' oligonucleotide would hybridize across the mutation site as the mtDNA becomes single-stranded during replication, generating a heteroduplex. This is recognized by the mismatch repair machinery and providing there is no strand bias, repair will restore the wild type sequence or mutate the oligonucleotide. Although seductive, there are numerous problems associated with this approach. First, it has yet to be shown convincingly that human mitochondria possess mismatch repair activity. Second, even assuming there is such activity, it is not known whether this activity will show a strand bias. Third, an oligonucleotide must be imported and hybridized to mtDNA to produce a heteroduplex that can act as a substrate for the mismatch repair machinery. Recently, chimeric RNA–DNA hybrid oligonucleotides (chimeroplasts) have been used to correct single nucleotide nuclear gene defects possibly by a process involving the mismatch repair machinery[35,36] with levels of success *in vivo* ranging from as much as 40 per cent correction,[37] to a more generally achieved level of 1 per cent.[38] Steer and colleagues have also reported some success with RNA/DNA chimera-targeted gene conversion of mutated kanamycin and tetracycline resistance genes using rat liver mitochondrial lysates.[39] We now also have some data to suggest that mismatch repair activity does occur in human mitochondria and that the repair activity does not show any strand bias (PA Mason and RN Lightowlers, unpublished experiments).

It is exciting to contemplate the use of mismatch repair in treating mtDNA disorders, but it is clear that there is a great deal of experimentation is needed before this concept can progress.

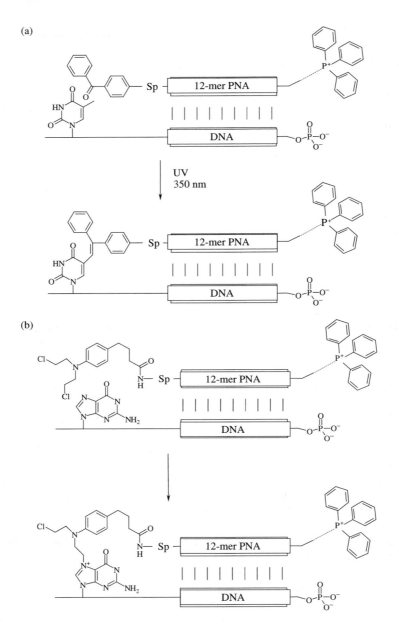

Fig. 17.3 Covalent attachment of inhibitory PNAs to DNA Peptide Nucleic Acids exhibit sequence selectivity which can be used to target pathogenic mtDNA molecules differing from their wild type counterparts by only a single nucleotide. By derivatizing the PNA with a caged lipophilic cation such as triphenylphosphonium (shown attached to the right of the PNA), the molecule can be targeted to mitochondria and translocated into the matrix. Unfortunately, experiments with heteroplasmic cells in culture, have shown no modulation of heteroplasmy levels in the presence of the triphenylphosphonium–PNA derivative. To tackle the possibility that bound PNA could be removed by the replication or transcription machinery, molecules have been designed to covalently attach to ssDNA after hybridization. (a) A benzophenone moiety has been added to the PNA–TPP derivative. After irradiation with long wave UV the molecule becomes covalently bound via the methyl group of thymine residues. (b) Chlorambucil linked to PNA–TPP. When brought into proximity with a guanine residue, chloride is lost resulting in covalent attachment of PNA–TPP to DNA.

Design and introduction of mitochondrial mini-vectors

A logical means of treating mtDNA defects is to rectify the mutation by introducing a wild type copy of the defective gene(s) into mitochondria and expressing it within the matrix. Once the gene has been successfully targeted to the mitochondrial matrix, expression must be maintained. This can be achieved in various organisms by selection for homologous recombination events. Unfortunately, the current view is that although there has been a report of recombinase activity in mammalian mitochondrial lysate,[40] it is not clear that recombination is a common occurrence, as it is with yeast mtDNA. If recombination is a very rare event, the only way of maintaining targeted genes is by engineering constructs that will be replicated autonomously. Designing such a construct is fraught with difficulty as the *cis*-acting elements important for mtDNA replication, maintenance, and resolution have yet to be fully catalogued.

Mitochondrial DNA vectors

Mitochondrial vectors for yeast mitochondria have been available for some time. Biolistic bombardment has been employed to transform yeast mitochondria lacking mtDNA (ρ^0) with a plasmid containing the *OXI*1 gene flanked by its control regions. Internalized mtDNA was shown first to be replicated in concatamers within mitochondria, and also to be able to rescue an mtDNA-encoded *OXI*1 point mutation by recombination.[41] A yeast mitochondrial expression vector termed pMIT was also devised, composed of an in frame fusion of the RNA maturase coded in introns 1 and 2 of yeast mitochondrial *COX*I.[42] In plants, electroporation of isolated wheat mitochondria with plasmids containing a *luciferase* gene or a *COX*II gene has been successfully transcribed, whilst the mRNA of the latter was also efficiently processed and edited.[43]

In addition to the concerns due to absence or low level recombination activity, there are other problems with applying this information to mammalian mitochondrial vector design. First, both *S. cerevisiae* and wheat mitochondrial DNA possess genes with individual promoters, introns, and terminators. Mammalian mitochondrial DNA is intronless and has only three transcription initiation sites, all within the D-loop region. Transcription from these sites generates large polycistronic RNA units from which individual RNA species are processed and matured (see Chapter 2). Second, *cis*-acting elements crucial for resolving mtDNA following replication and the mechanism of mtDNA resolution are not currently known. Finally, it is considerably more difficult to introduce DNA into mammalian mitochondria than into yeast or plant mitochondria by the techniques of electroporation and biolistic bombardment (see delivery section, below) making it difficult to assess functionality of vectors.

Despite this depressing prognosis, recoding of reporter or exogenous genes has been attempted with the aim of expression within mammalian mitochondria. The cDNA of the human ornithine transcarbamylase *(OTC)* gene was recoded and ligated to a bacterial vector containing the entire mouse mitochondrial genome. This construct has had progressively larger segments removed, including the bacterial backbone, to create mitochondrial minicircles.[44] Electroporation of these and other constructs into isolated mouse mitochondria results in the vector reaching a mitochondrial location that is insensitive to added DNase,[45] but no mitochondrial *OTC* transcription has been observed to date. There are several possible reasons for the lack of transcription. First, electroporation may not be a reliable method for targeting nucleic acids to the correct microenvironment for gene expression. It is interesting to note that using similar electroporation parameters to,[45] McGregor *et al.*[46] showed that following electroporation of *in vitro* transcribed *mt-luciferase* RNA, the transcript reached an RNase-insensitive environment in mitochondria, but no translation of this RNA could be demonstrated. Second, the mitochondrial mini-vector, unlike the endogenous mtDNA is completely double stranded. *In vivo*, it is believed that half of the major non-coding region is triplex in a substantial fraction of mtDNA molecules. Although this entire third strand does not act as a primer for DNA synthesis, it is possible that it is required to produce a replication competent DNA configuration. However, runoff transcription of fully duplex mitochondrial mini-plasmids such as pTER has been demonstrated *in vitro* using a post-100,000-g mitochondrial lysate.[47] Third, it may also be essential to maintain the mtDNA in a supercoiled form to promote transcription.[48] In support of this argument, electroporation of supercoiled DNA results in the internalization of predominantly open circular and linear DNA.[45] Assuming that supercoiled DNA is required for transcription, it is unclear if mitochondrial helicases can act sufficiently in the time frame of the experiments to permit successful transcription.[49]

It should also be noted that despite modern cloning methods, manipulation and cloning of entire mammalian mitochondrial genomes, and in particular, human mtDNA remains problematic.[50] This has undoubtedly hampered research efforts in this area. To our knowledge, complete human mtDNA has only been cloned in the last 2 years. Ideally, the production of a mammalian mitochondrial GFP or luciferase vector would permit direct visualization of transient expression. Further, the use of selectable markers such as the chloramphenicol resistance mutation (CAP^r) in the 16S rRNA gene[51] or oligomycin resistance due MTATP6 mutations,[52] will hopefully provide a much needed handle for longer-term mitochondrial transfection procedures.

Delivery of vectors to mitochondria

Trials to assess the efficacy of any novel mitochondrial mini-vector require the delivery of a large polyanion across a double membrane to the mitochondrial matrix. Standard approaches to gene therapy for nuclear genetic disorders rely on effective systems of DNA delivery to the nucleus. Much of the current success in this field is owed to a wide range of naturally occurring gene delivery vectors, namely viruses. Viruses have developed highly specialized strategies for entry into mammalian cells, escaping or avoiding the lysosomal pathway, nuclear localization and directing high levels of gene expression. As such they present a powerful approach to gene transfer. Mitochondria, by contrast do not appear to have any specific viral pathogens. On the basis of electron microscopy data in the late 1960s and 1970s, intramitochondrial viruses, such as Rous sarcoma virus were postulated[53,54] but the evidence for true intramitochondrial location was contested even then[55,56] and does not appear to be supported by any further data. A mitochondrial virus occurs in the fungus causing Dutch Elm disease but this appears to be the result of a freak event, as the isolated virus is non-infectious.

In the absence of viral delivery, several others methods have been attempted with limited success.

Utilizing the endogenous protein import system

By adding a short target peptide, which is recognized by components of the mitochondrial translocation machinery, it is believed to be possible to import nucleic acids. Vestweber and Schatz fused the presequence of yeast COX subunit IV to a modified mouse dihydrofolate reductase and showed it could be imported and cleaved by yeast mitochondria.[57] A short, 24-mer single or double stranded oligonucleotide was chemically coupled to the target peptide and was internalized via the protein translocation complex. Following submitochondrial fractionation and nuclease/protease treatment, the authors concluded that a subset of the DNA-protein conjugate had reached the matrix. The original work has been extended using 322 nucleotides of duplex DNA coupled to the target peptide of rat OTC. The DNA was radiolabelled and following submitochondrial fractionation, radiolabel was detected in the mitochondrial matrix.[58] A similar approach has recently been used to demonstrate that liposome-mediated cellular delivery of an oligonucleotide coupled to a target peptide reaches mitochondria.[59]

Despite this, no effective progress on the import of large DNA sequences has been reported, suggesting that the translocation system will not be useful for importing self-replicating mitochondrial mini-vectors.

Cationic liposomes

One of the most popular non-viral methods for introductng DNA into cells is mediated by cationic liposomes.[60] Most cationic lipid formulations consist of lipid soluble tails and a positively charged headgroup, which binds in a charge specific manner to the phosphate backbone of the nucleic acid. For optimal transfection, these nucleic acid–liposome complexes require a net positive charge[61] and appear to be condensed into a stable structure,[62] which is often resistant to nuclease digestion.[63] Cationic liposome/DNA complexes and derivatives have been noted to localize to a certain extent to mitochondrial sites,[64] probably due to the mitochondrial membrane potential. However, although DNA delivery through the outer mitochondrial membrane is feasible, the double membrane barrier is unlikely to permit matrix import of DNA by this route.

Amphiphiles with delocalized cationic charge centres, such as the triphenylphosphonium derivatives, have been used to pull small electroneutral molecules into the mitochondrial matrix in a membrane-potential-dependent manner, but dealing with a large polyanion like DNA is altogether another prospect. There has been some interest in coating large nucleic acids, such as potential mini-vectors, to the self-assembling cationic amphiphile, dequalinium.[65] Once formed, these DQAsome assemblies are predicted to cross the plasma membrane and localize to mitochondria where they will release their nucleic acid cargo. It has been postulated that the released DNA could then be imported into the mitochondrial matrix via the protein translocation machinery.[66]

Biolistic bombardment

Yeast mitochondria have been transformed with DNA using a method developed for plant cells. Biolistic bombardment of plant cells with 0.5–1 μm diameter tungsten coated beads results in internalization of the DNA into cells (reviewed by Klein *et al.*).[67] Adaptation of this technique for mitochondrial transformation with plasmid DNA containing the *OXI3* gene, resulted in successful complementation of the *OXI3*⁻ respiratory-deficient yeast strain after homologous recombination with the deficient mitochondrial gene.[68] However, the efficiency of this technique was only about $1 : 10^5$, highlighting the limitations of biolistic bombardment.

This technique has also been used to transfect ρ^0 yeast mitochondria with a plasmid containing the *OXI*1 gene and demonstrate complementation after forming a diploid with a strain carrying point mutations in *oxi1*.[41] More recently, this technique has also been used to introduce a pathogenic tRNA mutation in an attempt to produce a simple model for mtDNA disease.[69]

There has been no report of successful biolistic-bombardment induced transformation of mammalian mitochondria. This may be due to the relatively small size of individual mitochondria in relation to the bombarding particles.[70] Alternatively, biolistic bombardment may not have been attempted with valid self-replicating mini-vectors. Recent advances in biolistic bombardment technology, permitting successful transfection of mammalian cells *in vivo*, in particular fibroblasts,[71–73] however, suggest that it may be worth revisiting this technology, particularly once we learn more of the essential *cis*-elements for mammalian mtDNA maintenance.

Electroporation

The transformation of isolated mammalian mitochondria with plasmid DNA by electroporation is currently under development. Respiratory competent mitochondria have been subjected to electroporation with a 7.2-kb plasmid, using field strengths of between 8 and 20 kV/cm.[45] The functional integrity of electroporated mitochondria was retained at up to 12 kV/cm, at which point electron microscopy showed that approximately half of the retained plasmid appeared to be present on the inner membrane or mitochondrial matrix. Most of the apparently internalized DNA proved to be nicked or linear, with no detectable supercoiled DNA, despite having used the supercoiled form for electroporation. Addition of DNase 1 to mitochondria post-electroporation also showed a subset of the vector to have accessed a DNase-insensitive location. Electroporation of isolated mitochondria with vectors of between 8.6 and 20 kb also produced data consistent with internalization in a size-dependent manner.[44]

Despite these apparently successful experiments, transcription or translation of any vector has not been possible following electroporation of mammalian mitochondria. This is in contrast to results recently obtained for electroporation of isolated wheat mitochondria, where vectors were transcribed and the transcript was both correctly spliced and edited[43] (see Section on 'Manipultion of mtDNA heteroplasmy').

Conclusion

Disorders of the mitochondrial genome are now recognized as relatively common genetic disorders. Defects cause lesions in respiration and ATP synthesis. The absence of pharmacological therapies for patients suffering from these chronic progressive disorders has forced the research community into considering more radical proposals, many of which are highly original. Due to its location within the mitochondrion, many approaches to treatment of mtDNA disease require targeting and import of therapeutics. Advances have been made in this area, including highjacking the protein translocation system or conjugation of nucleic acid to delocalized lipophilic cations. Progress in mitochondrial transfection has, however, been limited by the absence of unequivocal evidence for the functionality of any nucleic acid that has been claimed to be imported. It is clear that to make substantial contributions towards the goal of therapy, we need first to increase our limited knowledge of the molecular mechanisms underlying mtDNA maintenance and expression.

One approach that does not require the transfection of mitochondria is that of cell replacement. It is encouraging that activation of satellite cells in myofibres decreases the level of pathogenic mtDNA in some patients with heteroplasmic disorders. However, this approach is unlikely to be of any benefit to the majority of patients who have multisystem disorders.

The challenge of treating patients with mtDNA disorders is technically and intellectually demanding. Many exciting new ideas have been considered in the past few years, but it is clear that we are still very far from being able to treat patients with these disabling, progressive disorders.

References

1. Holt IJ, Harding AE, and Morgan-Hughes JA (1988). Deletions of muscle mitochondrial DNA in patients with mitochondrial myopathies. *Nature* **331**: 717–719.
2. Wallace DC, Singh G, Lott MT, Hodge JA, Schurr TG, Lezza AMS, Elsas II LJ, and Nikoskelainen EK (1988). Mitochondrial DNA mutation associated with Leber's hereditary optic neuropathy. *Science* **242**: 1427–1430.
3. MITOMAP: a human mitochondrial genome database (2001). Center for Molecular Medicine, Emory University, Altanta, GA, USA.
4. Chinnery PF, Johnson MA, Wardell TM, Singh-Kler R, Hayes C, Brown DT, Taylor RW, Bindoff LA, and Turnbull DM (2000). The epidemiology of pathogenic mitochondrial DNA mutations. *Ann. Neurol.* **48**: 188–193.
5. Nagley P, Farrell LB, Gearing DP, Nero D, Meltzer S, and Devenish RJ (1998). Assembly of functional proton-translocating ATPase complex in yeast mitochondria with cytoplasmically synthesised subunit 8, a polypeptide normally encoded by the organelle. *Proc. Natl Acad. Sci. USA* **85**: 2091–2095.
6. Manfredi G, Fu J, Ojaimi J, Sadlock JE, Kwong JQ, Guy J, and Schon EA (2002). Rescue of ATP synthesis deficiency in mtDNA-mutant human cells by transfer of MTATP6, a mtDNA-encoded gene, to the nucleus. *Nat. Genet.*
7. Holt IJ, Harding AE, Petty RKH, and Morgan-Hughes JA (1990). A new mitochondrial disease associated with mitochondrial DNA heteroplasmy. *Am. J. Hum. Genet.* **46**: 428–433.
8. de Vries S and Grivell LA (1988). Purification and characterization of a rotenone-insensitive NADH:Q6 oxidoreductase from mitochondria of Saccharomyces cerevisiae. *Eur. J. Biochem.* **176**: 377–384.
9. Seo B, Wang J, Flotte T, Yagi T, and Matsuno-Yagi A (2000). Use of the NADH-quinone oxidoreductase (NDI1) gene of *Saccharomyces cerevisiae* as a possible cure for complex I defects in human cells. *J. Biol. Chem.* **275**: 37774–37778.
10. Bai Y, Hajele P, Chomyn E, Chan E, Seo BB, Matsuno-Yagi A, Yagi T, and Attardi G (2001). Lack of complex I activity in human cells carrying a mutation in MtDNA-encoded ND4 subunit is corrected by the *Saccharomyces cerevisiae* NADH-quinone oxidoreductase (NDI1) gene. *J. Biol. Chem.* **276**: 38808–38813.
11. Dietrich A, Weil JH, and Marechal-Drouard L (1992). Nuclear-encoded transfer RNAs in plant mitochondria. *Annu. Rev. Cell Biol.* **8**: 115–131.
12. Schneider A and Marechal-Drouard L (2000). Mitochondrial tRNA import: are there distinct mechansims? *Trends Cell Biol.* **10**: 509–513.
13. Kolesnikova O, Entelis N, Mireau H, Fox T, Martin R, and Tarassov I (2000). Suppression of mutations in mitochondrial DNA by tRNAs imported from the cytoplasm. *Science* **289**: 1931–1933.
14. Entelis N, Kolesnikova O, Dogan S, Martin R, and Tarassov I (2001). 5S rRNA and tRNA import into human mitochondria. Comparison of *in vitro* requirements. *J. Biol. Chem.* **276**: 45642–45653.

15. Magalhaes P, Andreu A, and Schon EA (1998). Evidence for the presence of 5S rRNA in mammalian mitochondria. *Mol. Biol. Cell* **9**: 2375–2382.
16. Bidooki SK, Johnson MA, Chrzanowska-Lightowlers Z, Bindoff LA, and Lightowlers RN (1997). Intracellular mitochondrial triplasmy in a patient with two, heteroplasmic base changes. *Am. J. Hum. Genet.* (in press).
17. Weber K, Wilson JN, Taylor L, Brierley E, Johnson MA, Turnbull DM, and Bindoff LA (1997). A new mtDNA mutation showing accumulation with time and restriction to skeletal muscle. *Am. J. Hum. Genet.* **60**: 373–380.
18. Clark KM, Bindoff LA, Lightowlers RN, Andrews RM, Griffiths PG, Johnson MA, Brierley EJ, and Turnbull DM (1997). Reversal of a mitochondrial DNA defect in human skeletal muscle. *Nat. Genet.* **16**: 222–224.
19. Fu K, Hartlen R, Johns T, Genge A, Karpati G, and Shoubridge EA (1996). A novel heteroplasmic tRNAleu(CUN) mtDNA point mutation in a sporadic patient with mitochondrial encephalomyopathy segregates rapidly in skeletal muscle and suggests an approach to therapy. *Hum. Mol. Genet.* **5**(11): 1835–1840.
20. Taivassalo T, Fu K, Johns T, Arnold D, Karpati G, and Shoubridge E (1999). Gene shifting: a novel therapy for mitochondrial myopathy. *Hum. Mol. Genet.* **8**: 1047–1052.
21. Srivastava S and Moraes C (2001). Manipulating mitochondrial DNA heteroplasmy by a mitochondrially-targeted endonuclease. *Hum. Mol. Genet.* **10**: 3093–3099.
22. Utsumi K and Inoue M (eds) (2001). New Mitochondriology. Tokyo: Kyoritsu Publishing, pp. 369–375.
23. Chang DD and Clayton DA (1985). Priming of human mitochondrial DNA replication occurs at the light-strand promoter. *Proc. Natl Acad. Sci. USA* **82**(2): 351–355.
24. Hixson JE, Wong TW, and Clayton DA (1986). Both the conserved stem-loop and the divergent 5'-flanking sequences are required for initiation at the human mitochondrial origin of light-strand replication. *J. Biol. Chem.* **261**(5): 2384–2390.
25. Holt IJ, Lorimer HE, and Jacobs HT (2000). Coupled leading- and lagging-strand synthesis of mammalian mtDNA. *Cell* **100**: 515–524.
26. Schon EA, Rizzuto R, Moraes CT, Nakase H, Zeviani M, and DiMauro S (1989). A Direct Repeat Is a Hotspot for Large-Scale Deletion of Human Mitochondrial DNA. *Science* **244**: 346–349.
27. Taylor RW, Wardell TM, Connolly BA, Turnbull DM, and Lightowlers RN (2001). Linked oligodeoxynucleotides show binding cooperativity and can selectively impair replication of deleted mitochondrial DNA templates. *Nucleic Acids Res.* **29**: 3404–3412.
28. Nielsen PE and Egholm M (eds) (1999). Peptide Nucleic Acids: Protocols and Applications. Horizon Scientific Press: Wymondham, England.
29. Demidov VV, Potaman VN, Frank-Kamenetskii MD, Egholm M, Buchardt O, Sonnichsen SH, and Nielsen PE (1994). Stability of peptide nucleic acids in human serum and cellular extracts. *Biochem. Pharmacol.* **48**(6): 1310–1313.
30. Egholm M, Buchart O, Christensen L, Behrens C, Freier SM, Driver DA, Berg RH, Kim SK, Norden B, and Nielsen PE (1993). PNA hybridizes to complementary oligonucleotides obeying the Watson-Crick hydrogen-bonding rules. *Nature* **365**: 566–568.
31. Orum H, Nielsen PE, Egholm M, Berg RH, Buchardt O, and Stanley C (1993). Single base pair mutation analysis by PNA directed PCR clamping. *Nucleic Acids Res.* **21**(23): 5332–5336.
32. Taylor RW, Chinnery PF, Turnbull DM, and Lightowlers RN (1997). Selective inhibition of mutant human mitochondrial DNA replication in vitro by peptide nucleic acids. *Nat. Genet.* **15**: 212–215.
33. Chinnery PF, Taylor RW, Diekert K, Lill R, Turnbull DM, and Lightowlers RN (1999). Peptide nucleic acid delivery to human mitochondria. *Gene Ther.* **6**(12): 1919–1928.
34. Muratovska A, Lightowlers RN, Taylor RW, Turnbull DM, Smith RAJ, Wilce JA, Martin SW, and Murphy MP (2001). Targeting of peptide nucleic acid (PNA) oligomers to miitochondria within cells by conjugation to lipophilic cations: implications for mitochondrial DNA replication, expression and disease. *Nucleic Acids Res.* **29**: 1852–1863.

35. Cole-Strauss A, Yoon K, Xiang Y, Byrne B, Rice M, Gryn J, Holloman W, and Kmiec E (1996). Correction of the mutation responsible for sickle cell anemia by an RNA–DNA oligonucleotide. *Science* **273**: 1386–1389.

36. Woolf T (1998). Therapeutic repair of mutated nucleic acid sequences. *Nat. Biotechnol.* **16**: 341–344.

37. Kren B, Bandyopadhyay P, and Steer C (1998). In vivo site-directed mutagenesis of the factor IX gene by chimeric RNA/DNA oligonucleotides. *Nat. Med.* **4**: 285–290.

38. Alexeev V, Igoucheva O, Domashenko A, Cotsarelis G, and Yoon K (2000). Localised in vivo genotypic and phenotypic correction of the albino mutation in skin by RNA–DNA oligonucleotide. *Nat. Biotechnol.* **18**: 43–47.

39. Chen Z, Felsheim R, Wong P, Augustin L, Metz R, Kren B, and CJ S (2001). Mitochondria isolated from rat liver contain the essential factors required for RNA/DNA oligonucleotide-targeted gene repair. *Biochem. Biophys. Res. Commun.* **285**: 188–194.

40. Thyagarajan B, Padua RA, and Campbell C (1996). Mammalian mitochondria possess homologous DNA recombination activity. *J. Biol. Chem.* **271**: 27536–27543.

41. Fox TD, Sanford JC, and McMullin TW (1988). Plasmids can stably transform yeast mitochondria lacking endogenous mt DNA. *Proc. Natl Acad. Sci. USA* **85**(19): 7288–7292.

42. Anziano P and Butow R (1991). Splicing-defective mutants of the yeast mitochondrial COXI gene can be corrected by transformation with a hybrid maturase gene. *Proc. Natl Acad. Sci. USA* **88**: 5592–5596.

43. Farre J and Araya A (2001). Gene expression in isolated plant mitochondria: high fidelity of transcription, splicing and editing of a transgene product in electroporated organelles. *Nucleic Acids Res.* **29**: 2484–2491.

44. Bigger B, Tolmachov O, Collombet J, Fragkos M, Palaszewski K, and Coutelle C (2001). An araC-controlled bacterial cre expression system to produce DNA minicircle vectors for nuclear and mitochondrial gene therapy. *J. Biol. Chem.* **276**: 23018–23027.

45. Collombet J, Wheeler V, Vogel F, and Coutelle C (1997). Introduction of plasmid DNA into isolated mitochondria by electroporation. A novel approach toward gene correction for mitochondrial disorders. *J. Biol. Chem.* **272**: 5342–5347.

46. McGregor A, Temperley R, Chrzanowska-Lightowlers Z, and Lightowlers R (2001). Absence of expression from RNA internalised into electroporated mammalian mitochondria. *Mol. Genet. Genomics* **265**: 721–729.

47. Micol V, Fernandez-Silva P, and Attardi G (1996). Isolation and assay of mitochondrial transcription termination factor form human cells. *Methods Enzymol.* **264**: 158–173.

48. Buzan J and Low R (1988). Preference of human mitochondrial RNA polymerase for superhelical templates with mitochondrial promoters. *Biochem. Biophys. Res. Commun.* **152**: 22–29.

49. Hehman GL and Hauswirth WW (1992). DNA helicase from mammalian mitochondria. *Proc. Natl Acad. Sci. USA* **89**: 8562–8566.

50. Bigger B, Tolmachov O, Collombet J, and Coutelle C (2000). Introduction of chloramphenicol resistance into the modified mouse mitochondrial genome: cloning of unstable sequences by passage through yeast. *Anal. Biochem.* **277**: 236–242.

51. Kearsey S and Craig I (1981). Altered ribosomal RNA genes in mitochondria from mammalian cells with chloramphenicol resistance. *Nature* **290**: 607–608.

52. Slott EF, Shade RO, and Lansman RA (1983). Sequence analysis of mitochondrial DNA in a mouse cell line resistant to chloramphenicol and oligomycin. *Mol. Cell. Biol.* **3**: 1694–1702.

53. Nass M (1977). Studies on the synthesis and structure of mitochondrial DNA in cells infected by Rous sarcoma viruses and on the occurrence of intramitochondrial virus-like particles in certain RSV-induced tumour cells. *Mol. Cell. Biochem.* **14**: 121–128.

54. Mach O and Kara J (1971). Replication of Rous sarcoma virus and the biosynthesis of the oncogenic subviral ribonucleoprotein particles (virosomes) in the mitochondria isolated from Rous sarcoma tissue. *Biochem. Biophys. Res. Commun.* **44**: 162–169.

55. Bader A (1973). Role of mitochondria in the production of RNA-containing tumor viruses. *J. Virol.* **11**: 314–324.
56. Ogura H and Oda T (1977). Search for virus specific DNA sequences and viral particles in mitochondria of avian leukemic myeloblasts. *Acta Med. Okayama* **31**: 121–128.
57. Vestweber D and Schatz G (1989). DNA-protein conjugates can enter mitochondria via the protein import pathway. *Nature* **338**: 170–172.
58. Seibel P, Trappe J, Villani G, Klopstock T, Papa S, and Reichmann H (1995). Transfection of mitochondria: strategy towards a gene therapy of mitochondrial DNA diseases. *Nucleic Acids Res.* **23**(1): 10–17.
59. Geromel V, Cao A, Briane D, Vassy J, Rotig A, Rustin P, Coudert R, Riguat JP, Munnich A, and Taillandier E (2001). Mitochondria transfection by oligonucleotides containing a signal peptide and vectorized by cationic liposomes. *Antisense Nucleic Acid Drug Dev.* **11**: 175–180.
60. Felgner P and Ringold G (1989). Cationic liposome-mediated transfection. *Nature* **337**: 387–388.
61. Behr J, Demeneix B, Loeffler J, and Perez-Mutul J (1989). Efficient gene transfer into mammalian primary endocrine cells with lipopolyamine-coated DNA. *Proc. Natl Acad. Sci. USA* **86**: 6982–6986.
62. Radler J, Koltover I, Salditt T, and Safinya C (1997). Structure of DNA-cationic liposome complexes: DNA intercalation in multilamellar membranes in distinct interhelical packing regimes. *Science* 275: 810–814.
63. Wheeler J, Palmer L, Ossanlou M, MacLachlan I, Graham R, Zhang Y, Hope M, Scherrer P, and Cullis P (1999). Stabilized plasmid-lipid particles: construction and characterization. *Gene Ther.* **6**: 271–281.
64. Cudd A and Nicolau C (1985). Intracellular fate of liposome-encapsulated DNA in mouse liver. Analysis using electron microscope autoradiography and subcellular fractionation. *Biochim. Biophys. Acta* **845**: 477–491.
65. Weissig V and Torchilin V (2001). Cationic bolasomes with delocalised charge centres as mitochondria-specific DNA delivery systems. *Adv. Drug Deliv. Rev.* **49**: 127–149.
66. Weissig V, Lizano C, and Torchilin V (2000). Selective DNA release from DQAsome/DNA complexes at mitochondria-like membranes. *Drug Deliv.* **7**: 1–5.
67. Klein T, Arentzen R, Lewis P, and Fitzpatrick-McElligott S (1992). Transformation of microbes, plants and animals by particle bombardment. *Biotechnology* **10**: 286–291.
68. Johnston S, Anziano P, Shark K, Sanford J, and Butow R (1988). Mitochondrial transformation in yeast by bombardment with microprojectiles. *Science* **240**: 1538–1541.
69. Rohou H, Francisci S, Rinaldi T, Frontali L, and Bolotin-Fukuhara M (2001). Reintroduction of a characterized Mt tRNA glycine mutation into yeast mitochondria provides a new tool for the study of human neurodegenerative diseases. *Yeast* **18**: 219–227.
70. Butow RA and Fox TD (1990). Organelle transformation: shoot first, ask questions later. *Trends Biol. Sci.* **15**: 465–468.
71. Johnston S and Tang D (1993). The use of microprojectile injection to introduce genes into animals cells in vitro and in vivo. *Genet. Eng (NY)* **15**: 225–236.
72. Ibrahim M, St-Ammour A, Celio M, Mauch F, and Menoud P (2000). Construction and application of a microprojectile system for the transfection of organotypic brain slices. *J. Neurosci. Methods* **101**: 171–179.
73. Steele K, Stabler K, and VanderZanden L (2001). Cutaneous DNA vaccination against Ebola virus by particle bombardment: histopathology and alteration of CD3-positive dendritic epidermal cells. *Vet. Pathol.* **38**: 203–215.

Index